FAMILY HEALTH & MEDICAL GUIDE

BY THE EDITORS OF CONSUMER GUIDE®

WITH
IRA J. CHASNOFF, M.D.,
JEFFREY W. ELLIS, M.D.,
AND ZACHARY S. FAINMAN, M.D.

CONTENTS

INTRODUCTION 4

1 STAYING HEALTHY 6

2 YOU AND YOUR DOCTOR 29

3 COPING WITH SYMPTOMS 47

4 FACTS ABOUT INFECTIOUS DISEASES 69

5 FACTS ABOUT ALLERGIES AND THE IMMUNE SYSTEM 102

6 THE BRAIN AND NERVOUS SYSTEM 119

Medical Consultants:
  Ira J. Chasnoff, M.D., Pediatrics
  Jeffrey W. Ellis, M.D., Obstetrics and Gynecology
  Zachary S. Fainman, M.D., Internal Medicine
Consultant for Prescription Drugs:
  Nicola Giacona, Doctor of Pharmacology

Cover Design: Inez Smith
Illustrations: Teri J. McDermott, M.A., Medical Illustrator

Notice:
In this book, the authors and editors have done their best to outline the indicated general treatment for various conditions, injuries, diseases, ailments, and their symptoms. Also, recommendations are made regarding certain drugs, medications, and preparations; and descriptions of certain medical tests and procedures are offered.

Different people react to the same treatment, medication, preparation, test, or procedure in different ways. This book does not attempt to answer all questions about all situations that you may encounter.

Neither the Editors of CONSUMER GUIDE® and Publications International, Ltd., nor the authors or publisher take responsibility for any possible consequences from any treatment, procedure, test, action, or application of medication or preparation by any person reading or following the information in this book. The publication of this book does not constitute the practice of medicine, and this book does not attempt to replace your physician. The authors and publisher advise the reader to check with a physician before administering any medication or undertaking any course of treatment.

7	THE SKIN	150
8	BONES AND MUSCLES	177
9	THE EYE AND VISION	201
10	EAR, NOSE, AND THROAT	218
11	THE LUNGS AND RESPIRATORY SYSTEM	236
12	THE HEART AND CIRCULATORY SYSTEM	255
13	THE DIGESTIVE SYSTEM	313
14	THE KIDNEYS AND URINARY SYSTEM	347
15	THE ENDOCRINE SYSTEM	363
16	THE MALE REPRODUCTIVE SYSTEM	387
17	THE FEMALE REPRODUCTIVE SYSTEM	395
18	PROBLEMS OF COUPLES	429
19	PREGNANCY AND CHILDBIRTH	443
20	CARING FOR YOUR CHILD	460
21	EMOTIONAL HEALTH AND MENTAL ILLNESS	498
22	HEREDITY AND INHERITED DISEASES	519
23	CANCER	537
24	FACTS ABOUT MEDICAL TESTS	552
25	FACTS ABOUT PRESCRIPTION DRUGS	572
	INDEX	581

INTRODUCTION

Family Health and Medical Guide is designed to help the one person who is responsible for your health and the health of your family—*you*. You are the only one who can observe your health and regulate your personal health habits on a daily basis. You are the one who decides what you eat, how you exercise, when you sleep, and where you go when a medical problem occurs. You are the one who wants to protect your good health and prevent illness. You are the one who wishes to avoid unnecessary trips to the doctor while at the same time becoming informed about when you should see a physician and what the field of medicine can do. How can you intelligently fulfill these goals?

This book provides the answers. Its wide coverage of health and medical topics shows you how to design and plan your health care and that of your family. As medical costs continue to rise and medical testing becomes both more sophisticated and more expensive, average people in

need of medical care often find it impossible to keep up with what needs to be known to assure good health for themselves and their families. This book provides a guide to medical care and health practices that will help you make the right decisions about what you and your family need.

Family Health and Medical Guide is not a substitute for your doctor. Rather, it gives you the information you need to make the best use of modern medical care —whether you are trying to select the right doctor for your family, decide on which specialist you need to see, or simply make sure that you and your family stay healthy.

You will find advice on how to find a doctor and how to make certain that he or she is the best doctor for you. You will also find an explanation of all of the specialties in medicine—from anesthesiology (the study of painkilling substances used in surgery) to urology (the study of disorders of the urinary tract).

You will learn the difference between clinical and laboratory tests and be able to familiarize yourself with the commonly administered tests. If you have to have tests done, you will know what to expect, how to prepare yourself for as little discomfort as possible, and what the results may indicate.

If your doctor prescribes a medication, you will learn how to read the prescription and interpret the directions. You can read about buying drugs—and saving money on your prescriptions—as well as about storing your medications.

In addition to providing information about modern medical care, *Family Health and Medical Guide* offers facts and explanations about the human body. The book is divided into sections based on systems of the body (for example, the digestive system). Each section covers diseases, disorders, conditions, syndromes, diagnostic procedures, treatments, and medical terms pertaining to that body system. Preceding these individual entries is an introduction to the body system—a description of its parts and of how the system as a whole normally functions in a healthy body. These introductions give you a reference point for becoming familiar with the way your body should work. To understand disease as a departure from the normal healthy state of an organ or system, you should understand what is normal and healthy.

In fact, the book begins with a section on how to stay healthy with nutrition and lifestyle suggestions. There are also other separate sections on recognizing and coping with common symptoms, infectious diseases, and inherited conditions.

In those entries that discuss a disease or disorder, the description of the problem, the cause (if known), the symptoms, the treatment, the prognosis, and the risk factors are discussed. In addition, preventive action is outlined, if appropriate or possible. In those entries that define a term or discuss a procedure, the explanation includes examples to illustrate the concept or idea. In short, each entry attempts to be as inclusive as possible without being technical and hard to understand.

The aim of this book is to help you take charge of your health care and that of your family. This book will help you develop a personal health plan that fits your life as well as meets your health and medical needs. Equally important, this family health guide will help you communicate with your doctor as he or she diagnoses your ailments and prescribes treatment for them. It will help you describe your problem more accurately, thus enabling the doctor to help you with greater understanding.

Maintaining good health is a team effort between you, your doctor, and the other members of your family who need medical care. Remember, however, that the final responsibility for your health is yours. The best way to help yourself and your family is to be informed about your medical needs. You can gain that knowledge by reading *Family Health and Medical Guide*.

And if you need medical care, see your doctor. This book will tell you when and why.

STAYING HEALTHY

Medicine and health care today are based on the premise that definite physical factors are responsible for diseases and disorders. The discovery in the nineteenth century that viruses and bacteria accounted for many infectious diseases led to remarkable advances in the management and treatment of disease. So for many years, the public relied on the miracles of medicine to cure and to prolong life as much as possible.

However, it has been discovered in this century that noninfectious diseases — cancer, heart disease, hypertension, congenital problems — have become the major causes of sickness and death. Modern medical research shows more and more that, despite the advances of medicine, it is what individuals do for themselves and how they take care of their bodies that make the greatest difference in the length and quality of their lives.

Most people are born healthy with bodies meant to last a lifetime. Many diseases and disorders can be prevented with a healthy lifestyle. That includes eating nutritious well-balanced meals, exercising regularly, controlling weight, getting adequate sleep and rest, avoiding hazardous substances and bad habits, and scheduling regular physical examinations.

The effects of abusing our health by such practices as smoking cigarettes, consuming a high-fat diet, or overindulging in alcohol do not usually show up until years later. At that point, however, it is often too late to reverse the ill effects.

On the other hand, following the simple guidelines to a healthy lifestyle produces immediate results — better looking bodies, more energy, and less need for expensive medical care. Even those born with genetic or inherited tendencies to certain disorders can decrease the chances of developing problems by taking good care of themselves.

Good health in the future depends upon the care taken of the body today. Practicing preventive health care does not guarantee that a person will live past 100 years of age or run marathons at age 90. But neither does it mean living a life of constant denial or deprivation. It does involve changing some habits and learning new ways. Many people, however, find that, once they try it, they prefer the taste of foods with less sugar or salt.

Be an active participant and take responsibility for your health You have taken the first step by picking up this book. Read it and learn more about how the body functions. Be aware of the seven warning signs of cancer and be attuned to the changes in your body that could be symptoms of illness. Think about the quality of your life and the improvements that could be made within your family to practice preventive medicine and stay healthy. Talk about what you learn with others.

A man who was celebrating his 100th birthday was asked what advice he could give about living a long life. The man replied, "Keep breathing!" Good advice, but as you will learn in this chapter, although living a long *healthy* life is not quite that simple, the efforts are well worthwhile.

EATING TO STAY HEALTHY: GOOD NUTRITION

Your body is made up of billions of cells—the basic building blocks of the body. To survive, each cell needs a continual supply of energy or fuel, oxygen with which to burn the fuel, water, and nutrients (certain chemical substances). These requirements are extracted from food as it passes through the digestive system.

Nutrition refers to the way the body uses food to maintain itself and grow. Planning good nutrition involves learning what nutrients the body needs and identifying and eating the foods that supply those nutrients.

There is a division of labor among the cells in the body's various systems that accomplishes the care and feeding of cells. The process of digestion breaks down all food that is swallowed until it is small enough to pass through the wall of the small intestine and be absorbed into the bloodstream. The bloodstream carries the nutrients to each cell in the body, where they are broken down and sorted. Some nutrients provide energy, others help form new tissues, and others enable the body to grow or restore itself.

Nutrients

There are six categories of nutrients, and all are present in many foods. In order of predominance they are water, carbohydrates, fats, proteins, vitamins, and minerals. The body is composed of similar materials in about the same order of predominance. So a person who weighs 125 pounds would contain about 75 pounds of water; 25 pounds of fat; and 25 pounds of protein, carbohydrates, vitamins, and minerals.

The body requires varying amounts of all six categories of nutrients to maintain body heat, to move, to build and restore bones and tissues—in short, for any function or activity.

Calories—body energy

Fuel supplied by nutrients is measured in calories. When a person consumes more nutrients or calories than the body burns up during basic body functions or exercise, the excess is stored as fat.

So good nutrition also involves consuming sufficient amounts of all the nutrients the body needs to keep growing and functioning without adding extra weight.

To eat all the essential nutrients without consuming too many calories, a person must learn to select foods wisely. Foods that provide more nutrients than calories are said to have *nutrient density*. For example, three ounces of steak and three ounces of sardines provide the same amount of iron, but the steak contains 330 calories while the sardines have only 175 calories. The sardines have more nutrient density.

On the other hand, 12 ounces of beer has almost no nutritional value but provides 150 calories of energy that, if not used, is converted to fat. Thus, beer is not the wisest food choice.

Making wise choices

There is growing evidence that excessive amounts of cholesterol, animal fats, sugar, and salt are underlying factors in major diseases such as heart attack, hypertension, diabetes, cancer of the colon, and kidney and liver diseases. Yet the average American diet is laden with these items. How do you know what nutrients you need to stay healthy?

The federal government has established Recommended Dietary Allowances (RDAs), a list of appropriate nutrients and the amounts in which they are needed, based on the latest scientific information available. It also sets average caloric needs to maintain certain weights according to an individual's height and age. The RDAs are guidelines, not requirements, for healthy people. The needs of pregnant women, older people, or those with medical problems often differ from the RDAs guidelines.

Labels on packaged goods usually list the nutritional values of the items and the percentages of the RDAs that they meet. In addition, many recipes now include nutritional and caloric data. All this information helps you keep tabs on and control your intake of calories and nutrients.

On the other hand, it's not necessary to count nutrients when making diet choices. Foods are grouped by their similarities in nutritional content. After learning to recognize the groups to which items belong, a person can maintain a well-balanced diet by eating from the four food groups each day: two servings of meat or fish protein; two servings of milk or dairy products; four servings of fruits or vegetables; and four servings of grains, breads, or cereals.

Those who prefer a vegetarian diet must select their nutrients from fewer food groups. The lacto-ovo-vegetarian—*lacto* means milk and *ovo* means egg—excludes animal flesh (meat, fish, and fowl) but can substitute other protein-rich foods such as milk, eggs, legumes, or peanut butter. The strict vegetarian, who also eliminates dairy products, must add other supplements to the diet.

Keeping up-to-date about nutrition

In recent years, research has uncovered more and more information about nutrition. Although the volume of new facts may seem to complicate the choices, the more knowledge you have access to, the better you can make decisions in your own best interest. To keep abreast of the most recent scientific data, read and listen to as many informed sources as possible and become aware of the differences in information.

For instance, some figures strongly suggest certain assumptions but do not scientifically prove them. Studies reveal that in cultures in which people consume foods containing a lot of fiber, there are virtually no colon disorders compared to countries whose people subsist on low-fiber food. These facts suggest but do not prove that a high-fiber diet has beneficial effects.

The flood of new information has also stirred much debate. A prime example is the controversy that surrounds the non-sugar sweeteners, considered food additives. The government banned cyclamates in 1969 because some tests showed they could potentially cause cancer. But when the government tried to prohibit saccharin eight years later for the same reason, consumers protested that the benefits were greater than the potential risks. The ban has been suspended so consumers are free to use the product if they want. Now a third approved sweetener, Aspartame, has come under scrutiny by the public because of reported side effects.

Despite these and other controversies, most packaged groceries contain additives — many of which are natural substances — considered safe by the government. The additives prevent spoilage; maintain or add vitamins, minerals, and proteins; enhance the flavor and appearance; or help in the preparation of the food. Additives are listed on package labels along with other ingredients — an important point for people with allergies to certain ingredients or for those who must follow strict sugar-free or salt-free diets.

More data are being reported lately that warn of the possible perils of excessive use of substances that are safe or even necessary to use in moderation. Two of these are salt (sodium) and caffeine. The body requires small daily amounts of sodium to maintain the volume and constant flow of blood in the blood vessels. But too much sodium seems to contribute to the development of high blood pressure (hypertension), a disorder that often produces no symptoms but that can lead to kidney failure, stroke, and heart disease. Caffeine, an ingredient in coffee, tea, many colas, and nonprescription medicines, is a great pick-me-up in small doses. However, it is also a habit-forming stimulant that, in larger doses, may lead to nervousness, insomnia, and irregular heartbeat.

Studies are linking caffeine to certain birth defects and to fibrocystic breast disease in women, a condition characterized by noncancerous lumps in the breast.

Be wary of the many health food quacks. They promote gimmicks, worthless products, and megadoses of vitamins with claims of preventing and curing all sorts of nutritional deficiencies or problems, building muscles without exercise, and melting away pounds without dieting.

Reliable information is available, often free of charge, from national and local health and food associations or organizations; food producers; the U.S. Department of Agriculture; or registered dietitians (R.D.s) listed in the Yellow Pages.

With so many advances being made in the area of nutrition, what applies today may change tomorrow. However, one fact will not become outdated: it is less expensive and less time-consuming to prevent the diseases that result from nutritional deficiencies than it is to cure them.

So practice these rules of good nutrition — it's never too late to change bad eating habits:
• Eat well-balanced, nutrition-rich meals, including breakfast;
• Limit calories sensibly to lose weight;
• Read labels to learn the ingredients of packaged goods;
• Drink plenty of water;
• Cut out or moderate intake of animal fats, caffeine, sugar, salt, alcohol, and any other substances that add calories without nutritional benefit or that pose possible hazards;
• Learn as much as possible about

how your body functions; and
• Stay alert to new findings.

The following section will explain in more detail some of the more important and interesting nutrition-related topics.

Amino acids

Amino acids are the main building blocks of proteins and are found in all living cells. There are 20 or more different kinds of amino acids, each of which contains carbon, hydrogen, oxygen, nitrogen, and in some cases sulfur. Each protein molecule is made up of thousands of amino acid molecules, linked to each other in chains.

Functions

In the body, food proteins in the small intestine are broken down to their amino acids, which are transported through the bloodstream to form, repair, and maintain body protein. Sometimes they are also used as fuel. In the cells, enzymes (substances, often proteins, which stimulate body processes) break down some amino acids into simpler compounds, use some for structure, and form others into chains of new proteins.

Types

Nutritionists divide amino acids into two groups:
• nonessential amino acids, which can be manufactured by the body if we don't eat enough of them, and

- essential amino acids, which must be included in our diets if we are to remain healthy.

Rich sources of amino acids include meat, fish, fowl, egg white, milk, cheese, and various peas and beans. The proteins from animal sources are much more complete — that is, they contain more essential amino acids in the right proportions—than those from plant sources. Thus the person who avoids meat and dairy products should include substantial amounts of two or more plant proteins in each day's meals.

Carbohydrates

Carbohydrates are organic substances made up of carbon and a two to one ratio of hydrogen and oxygen. Carbohydrates are a basic fuel source for the body, producing heat and energy. They come in the form of sugars, starches, and glycogen (a storage form of carbohydrates). Non-food carbohydrates are gums and cellulose (plant fiber).

Sugars such as sucrose, glucose, fructose (fruit sugar), and lactose (milk sugar) can be used very quickly by the body. Starches must be turned into sugars by digestive juices before they can be used. Sugars travel through the bloodstream and are stored in the liver and muscles (as glycogen) for later use, or are incorporated into fat for more permanent storage.

Potatoes, rice, and wheat are rich sources of starch; they are made up of 90 percent starch, after the water is removed. Fruits and vegetables generally have less starch and more fiber.

Starches and sugars are essential to life, but they have a poor reputation because many of them are refined before use and stripped of some of their vitamins, minerals, and bulk. Thus, the bran and the germ of wheat are removed, as is the husk of rice, all rich in vitamins, minerals, and fiber. Refined sugar provides calories without some other food benefits. That is why a diet that includes whole grain breads and cereals enriched with added vitamins and minerals, plus a well-balanced selection of fruits, vegetables, meats, and other basic foods, is advised for good nutrition.

Cholesterol

Cholesterol is a fatlike substance, found in all animal fats and oils. It is manufactured by the liver from saturated fats and is a basic ingredient in the formation of normal male and female hormones, Vitamin D, cell membranes, brain tissue, the sheaths that protect nerve fibers, blood, liver bile, and other body substances. After the first six months of life, the liver can make all of the cholesterol the body needs — about 1,000 milligrams a day. However, the average American consumes about 600 milligrams a day of cholesterol from such sources as eggs and meat.

High cholesterol level and disease

Eating cholesterol—and also saturated fats, which are found in dairy products, animal fat, and oils such as coconut and palm — can raise the level of cholesterol in the

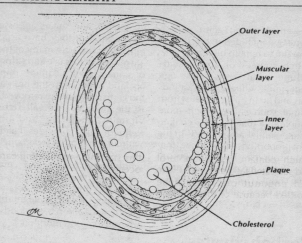

Cholesterol (fat) particles invading the inner wall of a blood vessel may eventually form hard yellowish plaque that may impede the blood flow.

blood. When the blood contains too much cholesterol, or when there is an inherited defect that interferes with the body's ability to use or process cholesterol and fats, the risk of heart attack and blood-vessel disease rises.

Hardening of the arteries (atherosclerosis), which causes most heart attacks, first begins with an injury to an artery wall. Normally a blood clot forms over the injury and heals it. But when there is too much cholesterol in the blood, cholesterol deposits itself in the wound and promotes the formation of a plaque. The plaque, made up of cholesterol, dead and dying cells, connective tissue, and a calcium cap, may grow to obstruct an artery. If the blockage is in one of the arteries nourishing heart muscle, it can cause a heart attack.

Normal levels of cholesterol in the blood are generally considered to be in the range of 100 to 250 or 280. However, many dietitians and doctors recommend keeping the cholesterol level below 200; a few researchers suggest that the healthiest range is 100 to 150, usually possible only on a vegetarian diet. Studies show that heart attack risk rises almost in direct relation to the amount of cholesterol in the blood.

Not all people with high blood cholesterol levels, however, develop heart disease or hardening of the arteries. This seems to be due to the *kind* of cholesterol most of them have. They possess high levels of a fraction of cholesterol known as high-density lipoprotein (HDL), which transports excess cholesterol to the liver where it is eliminated. Some people have high HDL levels because of heredity. Exercise raises HDL levels, as does one or two drinks of alcohol a day. Cigarette smoking lowers HDL.

Lowering the cholesterol level

You can reduce the cholesterol in your diet by avoiding fatty meats, cutting back on eggs, and eating more fish and poultry, which contain less cholesterol and saturated fat than meats. Palm and coconut oils should be avoided because of their content of cholesterol-raising saturated fat. Taking off excess weight, exercising regularly, and quitting smoking also help.

Fluoride

Fluoride is a compound of fluorine, a chemical element. Fluorine is found in soil and is necessary to plant life and to the formation of teeth and bones in animals, including humans.

In the human body, traces of fluoride are found in the bones, the teeth, the thyroid gland, and the skin. However, it has been found that larger amounts of fluoride than are naturally present in the teeth will help prevent and/or reduce tooth decay.

Preventing tooth decay

The best source of fluoride for prevention of tooth decay is fluoridated drinking water. Water with a fluoride content of one part per million is considered safe and effective, especially if given to children while their teeth are developing. The maximum benefit is obtained when the child drinks fluoridated water daily from birth until the permanent teeth are complete (between the ages of ten and 13). However, if fluoride intake is excessive before the permanent teeth erupt while the tooth enamel is forming, the enamel may become stained and mottled. If the teeth have erupted, this staining and mottling cannot occur.

Effects on other diseases

There has been some controversy over the fluoridation of drinking water. Most health scientists today believe that a fluoride level of about one part per million does not damage either teeth or other body tissues. Some dentists report that fluoridation prevents dental diseases other than cavities, such as periodontal diseases (diseases of the gum and bone supporting the teeth) and abnormal positioning of the teeth. Many physicians and researchers also find that fluorides may play a significant role in the treatment and prevention of osteoporosis, an abnormal thinness and brittleness of the bones, common in women after menopause and in both men and women over the age of 65. One recent study of over 1000 persons age 45 and older shows that osteoporosis is less frequent in those who have lived most of their lives in areas where the drinking water has a high fluoride content. There was also significantly less arteriosclerosis (hardening of the arteries often because of calcium deposits) in these persons, suggesting that fluorides help keep calcium deposited in the hard tissues of the body and not in the soft tissues. It would seem, therefore, that fluorides play an important role in preventing osteoporosis and arteriosclerosis, two of the main diseases of aging.

Other pros and cons

Opponents of fluoridation point to the long-range and unknown effects of adding fluoride to the water supply and to infringements on freedom of choice in imposing this "compulsory medication" on scores of children and adults. Supporters counter these charges by pointing out that fluorides are not medications but preventives, used in the same way that chlorine is used to kill bacteria in water supplies. Fluorides, they also assert, are normally found in teeth and bones as well as in water, and other methods of consuming fluorides are more costly and less effective in the long run than obtaining them from one's water supply.

Obesity

Obesity is a term commonly applied to body weight that is 20 percent or more above normal weight. It has been linked statistically to high blood pressure, diabetes, cardiovascular disease, and chronic back and joint pains, among other ailments, and it is a potentially serious condition that shortens life span.

The risk of disease and death among the obese is greater for men than for women, but for both it increases in direct proportion to the degree of overweight. For example, among those who are 20 percent overweight there are 25 percent more deaths for men and 21 percent more for women than among those of normal weight in a given age group; and for those 30 percent overweight, there are 42 percent more deaths for men and 30 percent more for women.

Obesity tends to occur more frequently in some families than in others. This may indicate a hereditary tendency, or it may be due to family food patterns and attitudes toward food. Women tend to gain weight after the menopause and men gain in middle age. Overweight children often grow up to be overweight adults. This is particularly true when food is used as a reward for a child or is withheld as a punishment. Food may then come to represent security and love — an attitude toward food that often continues into adult life.

Causes

The cause of obesity is virtually always the direct result of taking in more food than is "burned off" in activity. Certain glandular disturbances can affect the appetite or the distribution of fat on the body, but these conditions are uncommon. The appetite for food is influenced by habit as well as by emotional factors, and it is not always prompted by hunger. The appetite center, or feeding center, is the area in the brain that controls the appetite. It is thought to be located in the brain area called the hypothalamus. The coined term "appestat," suggested by the word "thermostat," has been used for the mechanism of appetite control.

The connection between smoking, appetite, and weight gain is unclear. Smoking has been said to inhibit, or decrease, appetite, so that giving up smoking is often thought to be followed by increased appetite and weight gain. The gain in weight that may follow when smoking is stopped has also been attributed to the dependence of some smokers on oral satisfaction; when they stop smoking, they are impelled to substitute the oral satisfaction of eating for that of smoking.

Treatment

The treatment of obesity is twofold: eat less and exercise more. A low-calorie diet that is nutritionally well-balanced and that can form the basis of permanent eating habits is the first step. Combined with a regular exercise program, such a diet can eliminate obesity. Anyone embarking on such a program, however, should consult a doctor for a checkup and for guidance.

Appetite-decreasing drugs can be harmful and should be taken only under medical supervision. Even physicians who use them in selected cases recognize that these drugs are at best only a temporary prop and not an answer to the problem of overweight over a period of time.

Crash diets and fad diets can lead to vitamin and nutritional deficiencies; if they are effective at all, it is basically only because they furnish fewer total calories. The quick weight loss that many such diets promise is often merely a loss of fluid from the body tissues, and the weight lost will quickly be regained as the fluid is replaced.

Massage is not effective in removing or redistributing local fat deposits. Hot baths and sweating serve only to remove water from the tissues, which will soon be replaced.

In extreme cases surgery is sometimes resorted to to remove excessive layers of fatty tissue, such as pendulous breasts; however, the expense of the operation and the inherent dangers of any surgery make this a treatment used only as a last resort. The same caution should be exercised with stomach-stapling surgery or intestinal bypass surgery.

Prevention

It is particularly important for parents to teach children good eating habits and to control any tendency to overweight before it has become a serious problem. The old notions that children should have food urged on them and that a fat child is a healthy child should be recognized as not only false but harmful. Older people, too, need to take special care to avoid overweight. They tend to be less active than in their younger days, yet may continue to follow their established eating patterns. Reduced activity may make it necessary for the elderly to seek out means of regular exercise — whether it be calisthenics or sports such as swimming, bicycling, bowling, or hiking—that are suited to their capacities and tastes.

One safeguard for those of all ages is to control overweight strictly, at an early stage, by weighing daily and embarking on a diet-and-exercise plan as soon as the weight is three to five pounds above the norm for the individual's height and body type. It is far easier to take off a few pounds than to wait until massive obesity requires a protracted and difficult struggle. Increased life span and improved health and vigor—not to mention improved appearance — will be a satisfying reward.

Vitamins and minerals

Vitamins and minerals are substances that are essential in small amounts to maintain good health, to promote growth, and to regulate body functions. Most vitamins and minerals are supplied by the diet, but sometimes they are formed in the body.

A balanced and varied diet usually provides all the necessary vitamins and minerals without the need for supplements. Green leafy vegetables, yellow fruits and vegetables, citrus fruits, and whole grain products along with dairy products, meats, seafood, and dried beans and peas supply adequate quantities of vitamins and minerals as well as other nutrients.

A carefully selected diet with its vitamins and minerals is essential for everyone but is especially vital for those individuals with special needs. Pregnant and nursing women, newborns and growing children, and the elderly and ill have special nutrition requirements. Most of these needs can be met by a varied diet, and it is important to remember that during periods of physical growth and change or during illness a nutritious diet is imperative.

Deficiency

Occasionally, a person may experience a vitamin or mineral deficiency—an intake insufficient to maintain good health. There may be several reasons for such a deficiency of a vitamin or mineral:

• An unbalanced diet that features too many vitamin- or mineral-deficient foods. For example, some vegetarians omit all protein sources and are either careless about or unaware of the proper balance of vegetable nutrients.

• An inadequate diet that lacks the proper amounts of nutritious foods. People on strict weight-reducing programs or those who restrict their diets for religious reasons may be susceptible to deficiencies.

• An inability of the body to absorb or utilize vitamins or minerals despite a nutritious diet.

• An unusual need for vitamins or minerals, for example, during pregnancy or illness.

• Occasionally, excessive intake of one vitamin that may adversely affect the body's use of another vitamin even though the second vitamin is present in normal amounts. For instance, some studies have shown that large amounts of Vitamin E may change the body's use of Vitamin K, even to the point of causing a deficiency of K.

All of these reasons point out the importance of careful attention to balance in the diet. In addition, it is necessary to understand that vitamins fall into one of two categories: fat-soluble (Vitamins A, D, E, K) and water-soluble (B vitamins, folic acid, niacin, Vitamin C). Fat-soluble vitamins are stored in the body, whereas water-soluble vitamins are eliminated from the body daily. It is, therefore, not difficult to see that a deficiency of water-soluble vitamins might occur more easily if these elements are not replenished daily.

Toxicity

On the other hand, vitamin toxicity is more likely to occur from fat-soluble vitamins that can accumulate to toxic levels in the body tissues where they are stored. In general, water-soluble vitamins, because they are excreted daily, are considered nontoxic, although occasionally unusually large doses may cause side effects, especially large doses of Vitamin B_6.

Vitamin and mineral toxicity can be as dangerous as a deficiency. Again, a balanced and adequate diet is the key to preventing any toxic effects of vitamins and minerals.

VITAMINS

A vitamin is any of a large group of unrelated organic substances often identified as "enzyme components," which are found in many foods in small amounts and are necessary for normal body functioning. Many vitamins help to regulate the rate at which chemical reactions take place in the body.

Vitamin A

Vitamin A is found in fish liver oils, liver, butter, egg yolks, cheese, and yellow vegetables and fruits. Deficiency of this vitamin in the diet causes inadequate production of rhodopsin, or "visual purple," a substance important in the retina's functioning, resulting in night blindness. Vitamin A deficiency can also result in epithelial (surface) tissue disorders and lessened resistance to infection.

Vitamin B

The name Vitamin B may refer to any member of the Vitamin B complex, including thiamine, riboflavin, niacin, niacinamide, the B_6 group, biotin, pantothenic acid, folic acid, para-aminobenzoic acid, inositol, cyanocobalamin (or B_{12}), and choline.

Vitamin B_1, or *thiamine*, is found in whole wheat, enriched flour, meat, and fish. A deficiency can result in beriberi, a disease characterized by abnormal heart functions, swelling, and inflammation of the nerves.

Vitamin B$_2$, *riboflavin*, is found in milk, organ meats (liver, kidneys, brains), eggs, malt, and various algae. It acts as a catalyst in bodily processes that involve oxidation (the body's use of oxygen). Dietary deficiencies may result in stomatitis (inflammation of the mucous tissue in the mouth), cheilitis (inflammation of the lips), eye-related malfunctions, and dermatitis (skin inflammation).

Vitamin B$_6$ is a group of substances (including pyridoxine, pyridoxal, and pyridoxamine) widely distributed in animal and plant tissues. These substances are involved in amino acid (a building block of protein) metabolism and in the breakdown of glycogen (a stored sugar). Vitamin B$_6$ appears in wheat, bran, yeast, seeds, and corn. A deficiency can result in functional disturbances of the nervous system.

Vitamin B$_{12}$, *cyanocobalamin*, affects the formation of red blood cells and is found in all animal products, especially liver, fish meal, and eggs. When Vitamin B$_{12}$ is absent from the diet or is not absorbed by the body, anemia (red cell deficiency in the blood) may result.

Vitamin C

Vitamin C, or *ascorbic acid*, is found in many vegetables and fruits, especially such green vegetables as green peppers and most citrus fruits. It is an essential element in the human diet. A deficiency may result in a disease called scurvy, in which the victim suffers anemia, spongy gums, bleeding, and hardening of the leg muscles. An overdose of Vitamin C is potentially dangerous and may result in diarrhea, kidney stones, decreased fertility for both men and women, spontaneous abortion in women, liver damage, bone fractures, drug interactions, a B$_{12}$ deficiency and iron poisoning.

Vitamin D

Vitamin D includes any of several related anti-rickets compounds. These compounds are present in fish liver oils, in butter, egg yolks, fortified milk, and are also produced in the body on exposure to sunlight. A Vitamin D deficiency may cause rickets in children and *osteomalacia* (softening of the bones) or *osteoporosis* (decreased bone mass) in adults.

Vitamin E

Vitamin E is necessary in human diets for normal muscular and reproductive functioning and development, normal red blood cell functions, and other necessary biochemical processes. Vitamin E is found in milk, wheat germ oils, cereals, egg yolks, beef liver, muscle meats, leafy green vegetables, and other foods.

Vitamin K

Vitamin K is a group of vitamins found in their natural state in alfalfa, spinach, cabbage, and other green, leafy vegetables; also in hog-liver fat, egg yolk, putrefied fish meal, and hemp seed. These vitamins promote clotting of the blood by increasing the production of prothrombin, the blood's clotting agent. A deficiency can result in blood coagulation abnormalities.

Vitamin supplementation

Vitamins are not themselves direct sources of energy. As enzyme components, they can act only in the presence of food-contained nutrients. Hence taking massive doses of supplements without eating food is useless and may even be dangerous.

In general, vitamin megadoses (abnormally large doses far beyond daily requirements) are not needed. Many reputable nutritional guides suggest that for restricted-calorie diets below 1,000 to 1,200 calories daily, a multivitamin preparation may be useful, but higher potency or "therapeutic" formulas are not generally necessary. The prescribed multivitamin dosage is based on amounts of individual vitamins equal to the recommended daily allowances.

Recommended dietary allowances.

A table, compiled by the Food and Drug Administration, is issued periodically as "United States Recommended Daily Allowances" (USRDA). This table suggests the following daily vitamin dosages for adults and children four years and older: Vitamin A, 5,000 international units; B_1, 1.5 milligrams; B_2, 1.7 milligrams; B_6, 2 milligrams; folacin, 0.4 milligrams; biotin, 0.3 milligrams; niacin, 20 milligrams; pantothenic acid, 10 milligrams; ascorbic acid, 60 milligrams; Vitamin D, 400 international units; and Vitamin E, 30 international units.

MINERALS

Minerals are natural, nonorganic solid substances that have a definite chemical composition and characteristic crystalline structure, color, and hardness. Like vitamins, they are essential for health and growth and perform two functions in the body: minerals build (bones and soft tissues) and regulate (the cardiovascular system, the internal pressure of body fluids, nerve responses, and oxygen conduction).

The body requires some minerals in relatively large amounts; these macrominerals are calcium, phosphorus, sodium chloride, potassium, magnesium, and sulfur. Others are called trace minerals because they are needed only in minute (tiny) quantities: iron, manganese, copper, iodine, zinc, cobalt, fluorine, and selenium. Still other minerals are harmful: lead, mercury, and cadmium.

Mineral supplementation

Although minerals are necessary, they are essential only in certain small amounts and can be harmful if taken in excess. Those who use mineral supplements should take care not to surpass the daily requirement. An overload can upset the balance of other minerals and block their performance; can result in decreased physical ability; and can contribute to such conditions as anemia, bone demineralization (mineral depletion) and brittleness, nervous system disease, and fetal abnormalities. With certain minerals, even consuming twice the daily requirement or taking one day's requirement all in one dose can lead to severe illness. Excessive minerals are especially risky for children, pregnant or nursing women, and the elderly.

Calcium

Calcium is the most prevalent mineral in the body; in fact, bones and teeth together contain an average of two to three pounds. It regulates certain body processes—normal nerve function, muscle tone, and blood clotting. Good sources of calcium include milk and milk products, green leafy vegetables, citrus fruits, and dried peas and beans.

Phosphorus

Phosphorus coexists with calcium in the bones and teeth but is also present in most body tissues. Phosphorus is present in so many foods that a deficiency is rare; it is most abundant in meat, poultry, fish, eggs, and whole-grain foods.

Sodium chloride

Sodium and chloride combine to form sodium chloride (table salt) yet each element functions separately. Sodium maintains regular water balance both inside and outside the cells and is found in blood plasma and fluids outside the cells. Foods rich in sodium include meat, fish, poultry, eggs, milk, and processed foods like ham, bread, and crackers. Chloride, part of hydrochloric acid which is basic to the digestive system, is concentrated in gastric (stomach) juices. People who perspire heavily may have to add salt to their diet, but generally most people eat too much salt because of their high consumption of processed food and added table salt. Surplus salt increases the body's water retention (edema) and is associated with high blood pressure, kidney disease, cirrhosis of the liver, and congestive heart disease.

Potassium

Potassium, mainly present in the fluid in cells, regulates the balance and volume of body fluids in tandem with sodium. Most foods, both plant and animal, are rich in potassium so a deficiency is very rare, although it may show up in conjunction with prolonged diarrhea, use of diuretics (medication that removes water from the body), or a diet that lacks protein.

Magnesium

Magnesium is contained mostly in bones although it is present in all body tissues. It is vital to the enzymes that help convert food into energy. Magnesium deficiencies usually occur only in post-surgical patients, alcoholics, and others who do not eat a well-balanced diet. Magnesium-rich foods include bananas, whole-grain cereals, dry beans, milk, nuts, peanuts, peanut butter, and most dark green vegetables.

Sulfur

Sulfur, found in all tissues, is a part of several important amino acids and of the vitamins thiamine and biotin. It is not yet understood how it works in the body.

Most trace elements rely on organic compounds for transport, storage, and function.

Iron

Iron is apparent throughout most of the body, chiefly in the blood, liver, spleen, and bone marrow. It is an integral part of the compounds that are necessary to transport oxygen to the cells and to regulate its use there. These foods provide significant amounts of iron: liver, meat products, egg yolks, fish, green leafy vegetables, peas, beans, dried fruit, whole-grain cereal, and food made from iron-rich cereal.

Manganese

Manganese is fundamental for the normal building of tendons and bones and is part of some enzymes. Food rich in this mineral include bran, coffee, tea, nuts, peas, and beans. Manganese deficiency in humans is virtually unknown.

Copper

Copper, an element involved with the storage and release of iron to form the oxygen-carrying hemoglobin for red blood cells, is most vital in the early months of life. If a pregnant woman's intake is sufficient, her baby will be born with enough copper. It is most available in processed food as well as in organ meats, shellfish, nuts, and dried peas or beans.

Iodine

Iodine is only necessary in minute amounts but is indispensable for the normal working of the thyroid gland. A shortage can result in thyroid enlargement (goiter). Before the introduction of iodized salt in the United States in 1924, iodine-deficiency goiter was common in inland areas. Food harvested from the sea is abundant in iodine.

Zinc

Zinc is a fundamental part of the enzymes that move carbon dioxide in the red blood cells from the tissues to the lungs for exhalation. A deficiency of zinc may show up as a loss of the sense of taste or delayed healing of wounds. Associated with protein, zinc is found in meat, poultry, cheese, dry beans, nuts, cocoa, fish, egg yolks, and milk. Although it is available in whole-grain cereal, it is not likely to be absorbed because of the presence of other substances.

Cobalt

Cobalt, not needed in the body by itself, is part of the nutrient Vitamin B_{12}, available in meat, eggs, and dairy products.

Chromium

Chromium acts with insulin in the use of glucose (sugar). A shortage produces a diabetic-like condition. It is present in dried brewer's yeast, whole-grain cereals, and liver.

Selenium

Selenium works in conjunction with Vitamin E. Not much is known about selenium, except that it is important in the body and that it is found in animals and plants where it is accessible in the earth.

Fluorine

Fluorine is important to the formation of teeth and resistance to dental caries (cavities), especially in children, and helps maintain calcium in the bones of the elderly. It is available in small and varying amounts in water, soil, vegetables, and meat.

AVOIDING HAZARDOUS SUBSTANCES TO STAY HEALTHY

The nation's leading recreational drugs are alcohol, cigarettes, and marijuana. All three are used by both adults and minors, although only two are legal — and only for adults. They are powerful substances to which young and old alike can become addicted and which have the capacity to injure or destroy the body.

Alcohol

Drinking alcohol is a generally socially acceptable way for adults to unwind, feel happy, and enjoy themselves. Done in moderation, drinking alcohol is a fairly harmless practice for most people. In fact, there is evidence that one or two drinks a day may help prevent heart attacks by easing tension. And statistics show that those who drink moderately live longer than those who either abstain totally or drink heavily.

However, alcohol is a central nervous system depressant. The short-term effects can disrupt mental and motor skills, resulting in bad judgment, poor coordination, and a tendency to have accidents. Consumed heavily on a regular basis, alcohol damages internal organs, especially the liver and the heart.

Alcoholism is an addiction to liquor in which the alcoholic continues to drink despite the problems it causes in any area of the person's life. Alcoholism is not a cause for shame or embarrassment, nor is it a sign of failure or degeneracy. It is a disease that, like any other, requires professional treatment. Many alcoholics are respectable employed persons whose problem has developed over time. Yet every alcoholic touches and strongly affects the lives of at least four other people, be it family, employer, or friends.

The fact that alcohol is so prevalent and acceptable in our society makes it easier to form a dependence on it—a good reason why those who drink should examine their drinking habits from time to time.

Marijuana

All of the impacts of smoking or ingesting marijuana are not yet known because long-term studies on its effects are still underway. It is known that marijuana affects the brain by interfering with the ability to think—to understand, to judge, and to solve problems. Marijuana also slows reaction time and hinders coordination and visual perception.

Because marijuana cigarettes do not have filters, their smoke irritates lung tissue much more than the smoke of regular filtered cigarettes. Marijuana cigarettes also contain more tar and more benzopyrene, a cancer-causing agent in tobacco. In addition, marijuana raises the heart rate by as much as 50 percent and lowers the sex hormone and fertility levels in both males and females.

Moderate use of marijuana does not appear to pose highly dangerous long-term effects. However, there are several reasons for concern about the use of this substance. First, much of the marijuana used is smoked by young people in their formative years; they tend to use the drug more regularly than adults. Second, improved cultivation is turning out harvests of the plant that are increasingly more potent. Third, unlike alcohol, the mind-altering chemical in marijuana can remain and accumulate in the body for a week or more. Fourth, because the substance is illegal, there are no quality controls over its content; quantities of marijuana have been found to be contaminated with pesticides or laced with other more dangerous or addictive narcotics.

Tobacco

Despite the proven medical risks of smoking tobacco in cigarette, cigar, or pipe form, many smokers who want to quit just can't seem to break the habit.

Help is available, for those who cannot do it on their own, through several sources. Quit Smoking Clinics are held locally through the American Cancer Society. The society also produces do-it-yourself "Quitters' Aides." The American Lung Association co-sponsors clinics and produces two self-help manuals, one to help in quitting and one to keep from restarting. The American Health Foundation sponsors a five-day program called the Stop Smoking System.

If you want to try quitting by yourself, it may help first to figure out why you smoke and then to substitute other activities or substances when you feel the urge to light up. Smokers' motivations tend to fall within these categories: anxiety, having something to do with the mouth and hands, stimulation, relaxation, addiction or craving, and habit.

There doesn't seem to be any one method that is right for everyone. Ex-smokers have quit in a variety of ways. If one plan fails, then try another; if you don't succeed the first time, keep trying. Remember, smoking is a learned behavior that can be changed.

The important point is there are many situations that threaten our good health that we cannot prevent or undo: the problems of aging, contact with a certain number of viruses and bacteria, inherited disorders, and unavoidable accidents. But the risks posed by the substances discussed in this section can be controlled — cigarettes and marijuana by keeping the products out of our mouths and alcohol, by using but not abusing it.

The following pages will discuss each of these substances and their effects in more detail.

Alcoholism

Alcoholism is a disorder in which a person repeatedly drinks excessive amounts of alcoholic beverages, with resulting harm to health, relations with other people, and work performance. The person becomes physically dependent upon alcohol as well as psychologically dependent. There is a genuine craving for alcohol, and unpleasant symptoms such as delirium tremens (a syndrome of fever, hallucinations, tremors, and a tremendous stress response) are seen. Withdrawal seizures or convulsions are also common. These and other withdrawal symptoms may follow an attempt to stop drinking "cold turkey."

Causes

Various causes of alcoholism have been suggested. These include a shy, lonely, immature, or dependent personality; depression; and self-hate. Some societies and groups within those societies encourage overuse of alcohol as recreation and as an escape from life's problems. It has been suggested but not proved that a tendency to alcoholism may be inherited or is the result of a chemical defect in one's makeup. Whatever the cause, alcoholism is a self-damaging disease and an ineffective way to deal with life. An estimated one American in ten suffers from alcoholism at some time in life.

Symptoms

The fact that a person is an alcoholic (one who suffers from alcoholism) is not always obvious.

Alcoholics often do not recognize their own alcoholism and commonly hide symptoms from spouses, family, friends, and employers. Signs of alcoholism include:

- Frequent drunkenness
- Tolerance to alcohol (a great deal of liquor is required before the person shows signs of intoxication; however, this is not true in all cases, especially where alcohol has damaged the liver)
- Physical dependence, resulting in withdrawal symptoms a day or more after stopping drinking; symptoms may range from tremors and physical pain to seizures and visions of bugs or strange creatures
- Continued drinking even when it is harming the person's health and personal life
- Poor job performance
- Depression.

Other signs may include an odor of liquor on the breath in the morning; "sneaked" drinks; suspicious work absences (due to sleeping off hangovers); and frequent falls, accidents, and cigarette burns on hands and body (caused by drunken carelessness). Several years of alcoholism can cause permanent damage to the liver, brain, heart, and nervous system. Heavy drinking by a pregnant woman (six drinks a day, perhaps fewer) can result in mental retardation, low birth weight, and birth defects in her baby.

In the worst cases, in which the alcoholic has been drinking as much as a gallon of beer or a pint of whiskey a day for several months, sudden withdrawal of alcohol may even result in death because of convulsions and/or delirium tremens.

Treatment

Treatment of severe alcoholism involves two stages: immediate and long-term. Both require a physician's attention.

The first step is to stop the drinking while treating the symptoms of withdrawal. Sometimes, with the patient's consent, a drug known as disulfiram is taken daily by mouth; it causes vomiting if the patient drinks anything alcoholic. It stops the person from drinking, but the patient may refuse to continue it because of its unpleasant results. In a crisis situation, withdrawal is best done in a hospital alcoholic unit. Under a doctor's care, psychological support and reassurance may be enough to comfort the patient during the withdrawal stage. But frequently other measures are needed. The patient may be undernourished from drinking so much and eating so little and may need replacement doses of vitamins, particularly thiamine (Vitamin B_1). Fluids containing glucose (a sugar) and salt water may be added to the blood, which has been robbed of water and glucose by the effects of overuse of alcohol. Tranquilizing drugs may be given to help ease withdrawal symptoms, which may continue for days.

Long-term treatment may include psychiatric help to treat the problem that caused the alcoholism in the first place, such as depression or mental illness. For many alcoholics the solution is to join an organization known as Alcoholics Anonymous (AA). Members help each other overcome their drinking problems and vow to stay away from alcohol completely. In helping each other, they develop badly needed confidence and positive feelings about themselves.

Prevention

Alcoholism is a significant social and medical problem that cannot be easily stopped. However, it may be diminished if people:

- learn the extent of its dangers;
- find more healthful ways to deal with life's problems and disappointments — by facing, rather than avoiding, them;
- learn to recognize the symptoms of alcoholism; and
- seek help for problem drinking from their physicians and/or a group like Alcoholics Anonymous.

Marijuana

Marijuana, or cannabis, is the dried flower clusters, stems, and leaves of the Indian hemp plant (also known as *Cannabis sativa*), which look like coarse tobacco. It is also known as "weed," "pot," "grass," "tea," and "Mary Jane," as well as a number of other slang equivalents.

Marijuana has been smoked, drunk, eaten, or sniffed throughout recorded history. When marijuana is rolled into a cigarette, it is called a "joint" or a "reefer." When it is smoked, it smells like burning rope.

Immediate effects

Marijuana relaxes the body and the mind. It gives a feeling of exhilaration, inner joy, and euphoria. However, it also produces mood swings. In addition, marijuana heightens perceptions. Colors are brighter, music is more intense, and time is extended. These effects can be accompanied or followed by panic, depression, hallucinations, and fear of death, particularly if marijuana is being used in combination with other drugs. Marijuana does not, however, increase intellectual functioning or creative capacity. Marijuana impairs judgment, and driving a car while under the influence of marijuana is dangerous.

Visible symptoms of marijuana use include red eyes, dilated pupils, and lack of physical coordination. Sometimes, users feel lethargic and nauseous. Reactions to use of the drug differ. The person may be happy, talkative, and silly, or may become withdrawn.

Long-term effects

Users of marijuana often become psychologically dependent upon the drug because it represents a way to avoid facing the problems and stresses in individual lives. Marijuana users do not, however, become physically addicted to it and do not suffer serious withdrawal reactions when they abstain from its use. Most users of marijuana do not progress to use of hard drugs, such as heroin or cocaine, although that risk does exist.

It is believed that use of marijuana may cause long-term physical effects, including damage to the brain, heart, lung, and reproductive system, as well as a decrease in motivation.

Smoking

Smoking usually begins as a social behavior and results in significant physical consequences to the body. Cigarette smoke is much more influential in this regard than pipe or cigar smoke. Cigarette smoking tends to be habit-forming and the accumulated effects increase the risks for development of life-threatening disease.

The chemical makeup of cigarette smoke is complicated and still under scientific investigation. One of the chemicals in tobacco is tar, a powerful cancer-causing agent that is, therefore, called a carcinogen. Another chemical in tobacco, nicotine, produces harmful effects on the nervous system. Other chemicals in tobacco interfere with biochemical changes such as gas exchange and with other functions in breathing.

Links to cancer

Smoking of cigarettes, pipes, and cigars is linked to oral cancers. The most common oral cancers include those of the mouth, lip, salivary gland, tongue, and throat. Symptoms of oral cancers include a persistent sore, which may be accompanied by bleeding; a thickened area; discoloration; difficulty chewing or swallowing; and/or persistent sore throat. Such symptoms require a physician's attention.

Cigarette smoking is also implicated in lung cancers. Initially, cigarette smoke may destroy tiny hairs which normally function in clearing away mucus in the respiratory tract. The bronchial lining may then undergo changes that result in cancerous cell production. The most common lung cancers associated with smoking are typed the squamous cell carcinoma and undifferentiated small or oat cell carcinoma. Early symptoms of lung cancer are variable but may include coughing, wheezing, and/or chest pain. Anyone with a smoking history should be alert to these symptoms. If you have not smoked cigarettes, your chances of developing lung cancer are extraordinarily reduced. If you do have a history of smoking, stopping will decrease your risk of developing lung cancer.

Links to chronic respiratory diseases

Emphysema and chronic bronchitis are most often caused by smoking. Both of these diseases are considered chronic obstructive pulmonary diseases in which there is airway blocking. Emphysema and chronic bronchitis frequently coexist. In emphysema, the air sacs of the lungs accumulate abnormal amounts of air. Expiration of air is especially impaired. In chronic bronchitis, the structure and function of the bronchi undergo changes that impede the air flow.

The initial symptom of emphysema is shortness of breath. This may or may not be accompanied by a persistent cough. Progression of the disease, usually occurring over a course of years, results in severe difficulty breathing and restriction in activity. In chronic bronchitis, a persistent cough develops initially and is usually accompanied by mucus production. If you experience shortness of breath or develop a persistent cough, consult your physician. Stopping smoking will generally provide the best means of slowing the course of these diseases.

Links to circulatory disorders

Stopping smoking can also significantly reduce the incidence of arteriosclerosis in which the walls of the arteries thicken and lose elasticity. This is associated with heart attacks and strokes.

Effects on some medications

Smoking can also produce indirect adverse reactions in the body. Chemicals in smoke can interfere with the action of some medications. These drugs may be altered in absorption rate by the body and in duration of effect. One example of such a drug is a particular type of diuretic prescribed to control fluid retention and high blood pressure. It is prudent to discuss smoking habits with a physician when drugs are prescribed. The physician will then be able to make the proper adjustments in dosage.

Effects on nonsmokers

Nonsmokers who encounter cigarette smoke of others are known as passive smokers. Research thus far reveals that even a passive smoker can suffer from the body's reaction to cigarette smoke. Passive smokers develop increased heart rates and blood pressure levels, and some people develop constriction of the bronchi in the lungs. Children are especially vulnerable potential passive smokers.

In almost every case, stopping smoking is beneficial even if there are no signs of disease. Never starting is even better.

YOU AND YOUR DOCTOR

Most people never think about how to choose a doctor until they need one in a hurry. When a person is injured or suddenly becomes ill, finding a good doctor is a necessity, and there is often no time to spare in finding one.

If a person does not have a family doctor, injury or sudden illness means a quick visit to an emergency room or outpatient section of the nearest hospital, where staff physicians who know nothing about the patient's personal medical history must treat him or her symptomatically and, more often than not, on an urgent basis. This is usually not a good way to establish a lasting physician-patient relationship.

A better way to assure yourself of medical care is to have a personal physician who is familiar with you and your family's medical history and who is available (or has associates who are available) when you need care. This way, your health needs are being met by someone who knows you and whom you know.

The best time, then, to choose a doctor is when you don't need one. You should never wait until you have no choice about the doctor you see. How do you choose a doctor? Here are some guidelines on making an informed choice.

Choosing a family doctor

Many families want a doctor who is familiar both with family members as individuals and with the family as a group. Doctors who have specialized in family medicine are called family practitioners. They have evolved from what used to be called "general practitioners," and their education and training have been expanded to enable the family practitioner not only to provide medical care, but also to recognize and handle the social, emotional, and psychological factors that affect the health and well-being of their patients and their families. Whereas in the past, general practitioners usually had only one year of internship (postgraduate clinical hospital training usually divided among several branches of medicine) before entering general practice, today's family practitioner completes the one-year rotating internship and a two-year residency in family practice, during which he or she receives more intensive training in general surgery, internal medicine, obstetrics/gynecology, and pediatrics among other fields.

Family practitioners care for all

the members of a family so that there is often no need for a different specialist for each individual. A family practitioner is well equipped to handle routine care such as Pap smears, uncomplicated pregnancies, immunizations, and routine physicals. A family practitioner can diagnose and treat all of the common ailments as well as many of the uncommon ones and can also guide you to the right specialist when you need one.

In addition to comprehensive medical care for all family members, today's family practitioner is interested in maintaining your good health and preventing illness. He or she is as interested in preventing disease as in curing or treating it. This interest is part of the family practitioner's overall goal to view and treat the patient and the family as an individual or an entity with physical, emotional, and social needs as well as medical requirements.

How can you find a family practitioner who is right for your family? You can call the county medical society or your local chapter of the American Medical Association. These organizations have uniform requirements for physicians to be admitted to their lists, for example, board certification, level of training, and so forth. They also can tell you where you can find a specialist. However, these societies do not offer an opinion on the overall quality of a physician. This is something you must assess for yourself, and the questions listed below will help you make this assessment.

You should also ask people in your neighborhood about the doctor they see. They may be able to offer suggestions based on their personal experience with local physicians. In addition, if you live in a city, you may find that there is a local organization that evaluates the medical profession on behalf of the consumer. Neighborhood consumer groups often will make medical referral information available to you at no charge and will steer you toward physicians who have a proven record of treating their patients with respect and concern.

In the process of selecting a family physician, you should draw up a list of basic questions to ask the doctor:

- Will the doctor treat all family members?
- Does the doctor provide care during pregnancy and perform deliveries?
- Does the doctor have staff privileges at a nearby accredited hospital?
- Does the doctor perform surgery and, if so, what types of surgery?
- Does the doctor encourage preventive medicine, such as routine checkups, immunizations, and follow-up tests?
- Does the doctor make emergency house calls for bedridden family members?
- Does the doctor have office hours that are convenient for your family, especially for those who work or attend school?
- What arrangement does the doctor have for a substitute when he or she is unavailable?
- What are the fees for the various services?
- Is the doctor certified by the American Board of Family Prac-

tice (or a specialty board of another area)?

The answers to these questions, along with the recommendations of friends and neighbors, will help you select the right doctor for you and your family.

How to choose a specialist

In approaching the problem of finding a specialist, you should remember that most specialists receive their patients through referrals from family doctors or from other specialists. Many have a policy of not accepting a patient who has not first been examined and referred by a family doctor. This is a method of making sure that those who really need specialists see them, and those who do not need them do not incur the expense that seeing a specialist would entail.

Whether or not you should see a specialist, then, is usually a medical decision: it is a decision made by your doctor about whether your medical complaint needs the attention of somebody who specializes in that particular area. For example, if you have a mild inflammation of the ear (perhaps as a result of a fungus infestation of the ear canal from swimming in the ocean), your family doctor is more than capable of treating it, prescribing for it, and assuring you of complete recovery in a short time. On the other hand, if you have a chronic inflammation of the ear canal, have suffered a partial loss of hearing, or your doctor has discovered a large abscess

along the mastoid bone under the ear, he or she will probably refer you to an ear specialist.

You must also remember that difficulties in one area of the body affect other areas, so it is not always a specialist who is needed to find out what is wrong. For example, visual problems may be limited to abnormalities in the eye itself, but they may also be the result of a wide variety of causes, including diabetes, arteriosclerosis (hardening of the arteries), strokes, or even a brain tumor in that part of the brain that controls vision. The human body is an organic system. Changes in one part of that system affect other parts of the system. No part of the system functions in isolation. Consequently, the first task in diagnosing an illness is to discover the real causes of the ailment. When the culprit is found, *then* you may be referred to a specialist who deals with the specific area of the body that is causing the problem.

So the first line of action in selecting a specialist is to follow your family doctor's advice. He or she will know whether or not you need a specialist. However, you can always ask for a second opinion or seek out a specialist on your own. If for no other reason than knowing that you did all that you were able to do, you should always try to get as much information as possible about your own or a family member's illness. You may even find something that one of the doctors missed.

If your family doctor refers you to a specialist, or if you seek one on your own, you should know what each specialty consists of and what to expect when you see each specialist. The following section gives you a brief description of each of over 30 medical and surgical specialties. As you read about each one, remember that an internship is the period, immediately after a doctor graduates from medical school, during which he or she receives supervised practical experience in a hospital setting. A residency, also supervised in a hospital setting, follows an internship, and it is a period of advanced training in a doctor's chosen medical specialty. The length of a residency varies, depending on the specialty. Board certification means that a doctor is certified as meeting the professional standards of a medical specialty organization called a board, which usually requires a residency in an accredited institution (hospital); a rigorous set of examinations; and, in some fields, a year or two of clinical experience.

Allergy and immunology

This branch of medicine is concerned with the study, diagnosis, and treatment of disorders related to immunity (the body's ability to resist disease or other threatening substances) and to the body's immune system. The body's immune system fights against the intrusion of outside forces, whether they be in the form of irritating substances that cause allergic reactions or of microorganisms that cause infection. This is the system that helps us fight off illness every day of our lives. Modern immunological research indicates that many infections can be as much a result of defects in a person's immune system as they are a result of exposure to viruses or bacteria.

Immunologists are also studying the role of the immune system in cancer growth. It may someday be possible to prevent cancer by modifying the immune system to reject the introduction of cancerous growth in the body.

In addition, immunologists are interested in the opposite effect of the immune system: the rejection of foreign substances at times when it would be better for the body if they were not rejected. The most obvious examples are the rejections of organ transplants. Immunologists are seeking to find ways to effect *selective* operation of the immune system: to reject cancer, but to accept a new heart, kidney, or liver.

The best-known branch of immunology deals with allergies, which are responses of the body's immune system to an irritating environmental substance. Doctors who practice as allergists are involved in identifying environmental irritants causing symptoms and formulating a plan of treatment. Allergists may treat allergies by suggesting environmental modifications to eliminate the offending substance, by the use of drugs to relieve the symptoms, or by a program of desensitization. Desensitization involves injecting minute amounts of the offending agent to make the immune system less sensitive to it. Once this program is set up, your family doctor can often give the injections. Allergists also consult in the management of diseases such as asthma.

An immunologist will complete a residency in internal medicine or pediatrics after graduating from medical school. After this residency he or she completes a two-year fellowship program of training in allergy and immunology. Specialty board examinations are also required.

Anesthesiology

Modern surgery is done without pain during the procedure. While many minor procedures may be done with a local anesthetic — a painkiller that is usually injected into or rubbed onto the affected area—other more complex procedures require that the patient be unconscious.

An anesthesiologist is a specialist in those drugs that cause a cessation of the experience of pain. The word "anesthesia" is derived from two Greek roots: *ana*, meaning the loss or lack of something; and *esthesia*, the act or process of sensing. Hence, "anaesthesia" means, literally, a lack of sensation.

Anesthesiologists, like other medical specialists, have completed medical school, an internship, and a residency in their specialty — anesthesiology — before starting their practice. They may also receive some training in a field other than anesthesiology, such as internal medicine, pediatrics, or obstetrics. Some of them also do tours of surgical residency, in order to broaden and deepen their knowledge of surgical techniques and needs.

Bariatrics

Bariatrics is a relatively new field in medicine, brought into popularity by the public's keen interest in the problems of being overweight.

Bariatricians have been making advances in what is known about being over- or underweight, by dispelling myths and substituting hard scientific evidence. Their training usually involves an internship in internal medicine, with a special residency in bariatrics. In addition, bariatricians are certified by their specialty group, the American Society of Bariatric Physicians, which issues its own standards of practice.

Cardiology

Cardiology is a branch of internal medicine that deals with the diagnosis and treatment of diseases of the heart. It covers the entire field of heart and circulatory system difficulties that may stem from birth abnormalities, childhood diseases, or advancing age.

Cardiology and heart surgery complement each other. Over the years, doctors in each of these fields have worked closely together in the treatment of heart diseases. For example, the cardiologist may determine that a child has been born with a hole between the chambers of the heart. The heart surgeon, also called a cardiovascular surgeon, is the one who will repair this hole through open heart surgery.

Cardiologists may take care of a variety of heart conditions such as rheumatic heart disease in children and congestive heart failure and heart attacks in adults.

There have been many medical advances in the last few years in both the medical treatment and surgical treatment of heart disease. All of this means that a cardiologist must be acquainted not only with anatomy and physiology, but also with modern computerized diagnostic equipment as well. As research progresses in the field of artificial or mechanical hearts, we can expect even more to be demanded of the cardiologist.

Training in cardiology involves a residency in internal medicine, followed by at least two years of specialized training in cardiology.

Cardiovascular surgery

The cardiovascular surgeon performs surgery on the heart and blood vessels of the body. Open heart surgery came into its own during the 1950s and underwent further refinement in the 1960s and 1970s. It has been nearly two decades since the first heart transplant. In 1983, a successful implantation of an artificial heart took place.

The cardiovascular surgeon performs many different types of surgery on the heart, including the replacement of heart valves and bypasses of blocked coronary arteries.

Training in cardiovascular surgery involves the completion of a general surgery residency followed by two or three years of specialized training in all aspects of heart and blood vessel surgery.

Dentistry

Dentistry is the prevention, diagnosis, and treatment of diseases, disorders, and malformations of the teeth, mouth, and jaws. Most people select a dentist with a general practice who can provide routine dental care and, if necessary, recommend a dental specialist for those needing specialized treatment. Some of the dental specialties include:

• orthodontia—straightening of teeth
• periodontia—treatment of gums
• endodontia — root canal treatment
• exodontia—extraction of teeth.

A dentist planning to establish a general practice will complete four years of dental school and perhaps an optional one-year general residency. Dental specialists will have specific training in their specialty.

Finding a family dentist is much like finding a family doctor. You should ask friends and neighbors for recommendations or contact your local dental society. Often, too, your family doctor can suggest a dentist.

Dermatology

Dermatology is the diagnosis and treatment of skin diseases. This is another relatively recent addition to the specialties of medicine. All dermatologists will have had training in allergies, since over the years many skin conditions have been recognized as allergic reactions instead of skin diseases.

Other skin disorders diagnosed and treated by dermatologists range from acne and contact dermatitis (skin inflammation caused by contact with irritating substances) to psoriasis (drying and scaly skin) and skin cancer.

As with all specialists, the dermatologist must also be completely knowledgeable about all of the diseases, disorders, and conditions involving other parts of the body that may have some bearing on the condition of the skin.

Dermatologists are required to do an internship, usually in internal medicine, followed by at least a three-year residency in dermatology.

Endocrinology

When we think of "messages" being sent throughout the body, we usually think of the nervous system. But there is another communication system in the body, called the endocrine system. It is made up of the ductless glands including the pituitary gland, the adrenal glands, the thyroid gland, the parathyroid glands, the islet cells in the pancreas, the ovaries (in women), and the testes (in men). These glands secrete hormones that travel as messengers throughout the body to direct and integrate a vast number of bodily functions.

An endocrinologist is a specialist in the diagnosis and treatment of disorders of the endocrine system. He or she must know the symptoms that such disorders exhibit and the specific treatment that such symptoms call for. This means an internal medicine internship and residency, with solid competency in bio-

chemistry, followed by two years of training in endocrinology.

Epidemiology

This medical field deals with the outbreak, frequency, distribution, and control of communicable diseases in the human community. The unofficial headquarters of this activity is the Center for Disease Control (once the Communicable Disease Center) in Atlanta, Georgia.

Epidemiology not only deals with disease communication in general, but also with the specific conditions under which certain diseases seem to flourish. For example, the relatively new field of Urban Epidemiology specifically addresses itself to those diseases and conditions peculiar to city settings. In addition, epidemiologists work to devise ways of preventing disease, such as developing vaccines against the contraction and spread of disease.

In addition to diseases, epidemiology also studies other causes of illness. For example, lead poisoning in children as a result of eating lead-base paint was a major cause of brain damage among children before epidemiologists ferreted out the cause. Epidemiologists have led the medical field in seeking environmental causes for a host of disorders once attributed to bacteria or other sources. Lead poisoning is only one of these causes. Air and water pollution, toxic substances in foods, toxic substances used in the manufacture of a variety of products — all of these subjects come under the scrutiny of the modern epidemiologist.

Epidemiology attracts physicians not only from internal medicine, but from other fields as well, such as immunology, occupational medicine, pediatrics, and others. An epidemiologist will usually have completed three years of specialized training and a year of independent research or teaching.

Gastroenterology

A gastroenterologist specializes in the diagnosis and treatment of diseases and disorders of the esophagus, the stomach, and the intestines. The word comes from two Greek words: *gastro*, meaning stomach or belly; and *entero*, meaning inner tubular structure. A gastroenterologist also specializes in related organs that help in the digestive process such as the liver or pancreas. Gastritis (inflammation of the stomach), enteritis (inflammation of the intestinal tract), ulcers, inability to digest certain foods, constipation, diarrhea, hyperacidity, "heartburn," and a host of other disorders make up the gastroenterologist's diagnostic and treatment arena.

Gastroenterologists are the specialists who do the procedure called endoscopy. Endoscopy is the technique of directly viewing hollow organs, such as the esophagus, stomach, and colon, through flexible tubes. Diagnosis and treatment of many conditions, such as ulcers and polyps, are done with this procedure. Biopsies (gathering tissue samples for testing) are also carried out with these instruments.

These specialists are trained as internists or pediatricians with an additional two-year residency in gastroenterology.

Hematology

Hematology is the study of blood and diseases and disorders of the blood and the blood-forming organs such as the bone marrow and the spleen. A hematologist is proficient in a wide range of diagnostic techniques in which blood samples are used to shed light on disorders in the rest of the body. Blood analyses can aid a diagnostician in developing treatment for a patient. The hematologist's primary concern, however, is the host of diseases and disorders of the blood itself: inability to carry oxygen, inability to help in the fight against invading microorganisms, and the inability of the body to produce normal blood levels. The first set of problems centers around the function of red blood cells, the second centers around the disease-fighting characteristics of white blood cells, and the last centers around the manufacture of blood cells by bone marrow. The hematologist is also an expert in cancers of the blood (leukemia) and in blood clotting problems (hemophilia).

The hematologist must be firmly grounded not only in internal medicine, anatomy, and physiology, but in biochemistry as well. Today this means a sound knowledge of computerized diagnostic equipment associated with biochemical analyses.

A hematologist completes an

internship and a residency in internal medicine plus two years of training in hematology. Many, if not most, hematologists today are also trained as and practice as oncologists (cancer specialists).

Internal medicine

Internal medicine is the branch of medicine that deals with the diagnosis and treatment of diseases of adults except for those conditions that require a surgeon or obstetrician. Along with the family practitioner, the internist is trained to handle a wide range of illnesses; in fact, many people select an internist as their family doctor. The internist is specifically trained to deal with chronic (long-term) illnesses, such as diabetes or high blood pressure, and acute (short-term) diseases, such as infections. In addition, an internist has both the range and depth to diagnose illnesses that might escape a specialist if they lay outside his or her special field. For this reason, internists are often called diagnosticians because they make diagnoses, treat the patient, and then may route patients to other specialists if necessary.

After graduating from medical school an internist completes one year of internship, followed by two years of residency in internal medicine. Internal medicine is also the basis for many of the specialties mentioned here (for example, cardiology, endocrinology, gastroenterology, hematology, and nephrology). This is the reason that these branches are often referred to as subspecialties and the doctors as subspecialists.

In order to become a subspecialist, the internist does at least two years of additional training, referred to as a fellowship, in his or her chosen subspecialty and is then eligible for subspecialty board certification.

Nephrology

Nephrologists treat kidney disorders. Their patients are usually referred to them by internists, as kidney problems become evident and are diagnosed as needing special care. While many nephrologists are associated with hospitals (where they perform diagnoses, treatment, research, and teaching), many are associated also with dialysis centers, located outside hospitals.

In treating kidney disorders, the nephrologist may make use of medicines or dialysis (in which machines take over the kidney's function). Referral for surgery (for example, if a transplant is indicated) is also initiated by a nephrologist. In addition, nephrologists perform kidney biopsies that are used to diagnose, treat, and follow a number of kidney diseases other than cancer.

Nephrologists are thoroughly grounded in internal medicine, with special attention to the physiological processes performed by the kidneys. These specialists must be equally well-grounded in biochemistry and the tools of modern biochemical analysis, because of the complex nature of kidney functions. An internship and residency in internal medicine is the required procedure, followed by a two-year training period in nephrology plus specialty board exams. A nephrologist will be more than familiar with all of the latest computerized testing equipment, as well as the latest in dialysis machines.

Neurology

Neurology is the field of medical science that studies the nervous system—the brain, the spinal cord, and the body's complex network of nerves. Clinical neurology concerns itself with the diagnosis and treatment of diseases of the nervous system. When a physician calls himself or herself a neurologist, that person usually means a clinical neurologist.

In order for a neurologist to do diagnostic work, he or she must be aware of the entire range of physical and psychological causes of human behavior and symptoms. Diseases and disorders of other parts of the body can affect the nervous system, and diseases of the nervous system can affect the functioning of other parts of the body. The neurologist must draw these two ends of the diagnostic spectrum together in order to get at the root of the patient's problems.

Training in neurology involves a one-year internal medicine internship, followed by a three-year residency in neurology.

Obstetrics/gynecology

The fields of obstetrics and gynecology are closely related, and physicians generally practice these specialties together. While gynecology involves the diagnosis and treatment of disorders of the female reproductive system, obstetrics specifically deals with pregnancy and childbirth and related conditions.

Many obstetricians are members of a group practice. Most obstetric groups make sure that every doctor in the group either has seen or is familiar with each patient during the pregnancy period. Thus, when it comes time for delivery, the mother will generally be taken care of by a doctor that she knows.

After medical school, an obstetrician/gynecologist completes a four-year residency. During this time, he or she will also receive some training in internal medicine, general surgery, and care of the newborn infant.

The obstetrician/gynecologist often acts as the primary care giver for women. He or she will also work closely with other medical specialists if specific problems occur that do not directly involve the reproductive system.

Occupational medicine

This is a relatively new field of medicine, not to be confused with "occupational therapy" in which patients are given tasks to help them overcome the aftereffects of disease or trauma. Occupational medicine began with industrial and business clinics, which were usually staffed with a physician (who may have only visited the clinic periodically, if the business or industry was small) and an industrial nurse (one who has specialized in the care of patients within a working environment).

As more is discovered about the effects of the working environment on employees, occupational medicine has grown to include the study, diagnosis, and treatment of a vast range of illnesses caused by the industrial environment itself. Asbestos-induced cancer, "black lung" (in which coal dust literally turns the inside of the lung black, with accompanying damage to the lung), allergic reactions to industrial fibers, eye damage from welding arcs, and injury to the feet from jobs that require standing are but a few of the hundreds of disorders treated by occupational medicine physicians.

People in the field have a strong background in internal medicine, with special training in the causes of industrially-related illnesses. In many cases, these specialists have completed a public health training program. Often, these doctors will finish medical school and an internship and then complete a public health program before going on to their specialty residency.

Oncology

Oncology is the study of tumors, particularly cancer. This is a relatively new field and is often associated with hematology (the study of the blood). The reason for this association is that, strictly speaking, oncology deals only with solid tumors and not with cancers of the blood. Today, however, many in the field are now trained as hematologist-oncologists so that they are certified to deal with both types of cancer.

Oncology embraces a large number of medical and technical disciplines, from surgery to nutrition, from immunology to biochemistry, from diagnosis of symptoms to treatment with nuclear radiation. A thorough knowledge of modern computerized diagnostic instruments is also required of the oncologist. The oncologist may also coordinate other specialists in the management of cancer, such as radiotherapists and surgeons.

There are many subdivisions of oncology. The medical oncologist is primarily responsible for prescribing and implementing chemotherapy, along with diagnosing and treating complications unique to cancer. Surgical oncologists perform cancer surgery. Pediatric oncologists diagnose and treat cancer in children. Gynecological oncologists deal with cancer in the female reproductive system.

After graduating from medical school, a medical oncologist completes an internship and residency in internal medicine, followed by an additional training program in oncology, which includes training in hematology and chemotherapy. Surgical oncologists are usually general surgeons who have completed a subspecialty fellowship in cancer surgery. Pediatric and gynecological oncologists are certified first in their respective fields and then go on to oncology fellowships in their fields.

Ophthalmology

An ophthalmologist is a medical doctor who diagnoses and treats diseases and injuries of the eyes. Most ophthalmologists are also eye surgeons. They perform a variety of operations, some of which include the reattachment of detached retinas, removal of cataracts, repairing injuries, relieving pressure caused by glaucoma, repairing blood vessel ruptures, and removing eyes that have been injured beyond repair.

An ophthalmologist may have a background in both internal medicine and surgery. This specialty requires an additional three-year residency in ophthalmology after a one-year internship, either rotating (through many specialties) or in internal medicine, and specialty board examinations. (To clarify the roles of various eye specialists: an *optometrist* tests the eyes for the purpose of properly fitting a person with glasses or contact lenses. An *optician* is a person who makes or fits glasses. Most ophthalmologists test the eyes to determine the proper lens prescription if their patients need glasses. An optometrist, however, is not a medical doctor and therefore is not permitted to treat diseases of the eye or to prescribe drugs. An optician takes the ophthalmologist's or the optometrist's recommendations and fits glasses.)

Orthopedics

Orthopedics is the branch of surgery that specializes in the diagnosis and treatment of diseases or disorders of the bones and joints. The orthopedist treats broken bones, disorders of the bones and joints that can be corrected surgically, and bone tumors, as well as other problems of the skeletal system. In addition, because of his or her knowledge of the functioning of the skeletomuscular system, the orthopedist often treats sports injuries and may serve as the physician for amateur and professional athletic teams.

The orthopedist is required to complete four years of training in orthopedic surgery along with a one-year internship in general surgery, followed by a year of independent practice before specialty board examinations.

Otorhinolaryngology

This specialty combines the study of the ear (*oto*), the nose (*rhino*), and the throat (*laryngo*) into a single discipline called *otorhinolaryngology*, often referred to as "ENT" (ear, nose, and throat) for short. Years ago, before ophthalmology became fully established as a separate discipline, eye doctors also did ENT work.

The ear and throat are connected by the eustachian tube, which leads from the inner ear to the throat. The nose leads directly into the part of the throat referred to as the nasopharynx. Inflammations of the nose may spread to the throat and vice versa. Inflammations of the throat often spread through the eustachian tube to the ears. Consequently, any infection in any of these areas could result in an infection in all of them.

Ear, nose, and throat specialists are primarily surgeons. They perform such varied procedures as rhinoplasty ("nose job"); removal of tumors from the oral, nasal, and neck areas; reconstructive ear surgery; and sinus surgery. They also function as diagnosticians of diseases of the head and neck excluding the brain and eyes.

Medical school is followed by a one-year residency in general surgery and a four-year residency in otorhinolaryngology.

Pathology

Pathology is the study of the intrinsic nature of diseases: the changes in tissue brought about by disease and the ways in which these changes in tissue provide clues not only to the causes of disease or death, but also to ways in which the spread of disease may be checked.

There are a variety of specializations within pathology, including the following:

- Cellular pathology, in which cells are the focus of study
- Clinical pathology, in which laboratory methods are used to aid clinical diagnoses
- Comparative pathology, in which human diseases are compared to those of the lower animals
- Experimental pathology, in which artificially-induced diseases or disorders are studied in order to shed light on naturally-induced diseases and disorders
- General pathology, which is the study of the processes that may occur in various diseases

- Forensic pathology, in which the results of pathologic examinations (such as autopsies, tissue samples, and chemical analyses) are used as evidence in legal proceedings.

Much of the pathologist's work is done with the microscope, preparing and interpreting biopsies (tissue samples). Pathologists are charged with deciding whether a tissue specimen is malignant or not. They also perform autopsies to determine the cause(s) of death. The pathologist is knowledgeable both in the cause and course of disease.

Pathologists ordinarily do work in both internal medicine and surgery during their training. A strong laboratory background is a necessity, with extensive training in modern instrumentation. Three- to four-year residencies in pathology are required, depending on the particular subspecialty.

Pediatrics

Pediatricians specialize in the diagnosis and treatment of diseases of children. They care for a child immediately upon birth through adolescence.

A pediatrician treats childhood illnesses and administers the appropriate immunizations to prevent disease. In addition, pediatricians perform other important tasks: they watch for any abnormalities that may appear during the growth of the child and they advise parents about the child's social and psychological needs, as well as the physical needs.

Pediatricians have at least two

years of training in general pediatrics plus an additional year of training in a pediatric subspecialty or in a field other than pediatrics. This is followed by another two-year period of further training or practice and finally an examination by the specialty board.

Peripheral vascular diseases

In addition to cardiovascular (heart and circulatory) diseases, there are many diseases of the vascular (circulatory) system alone, outside of the heart and its vessels. Physicians who specialize in these peripheral vascular diseases treat chiefly the following disorders:

- Arteriosclerosis, in which the normal artery walls become abnormally thickened or hardened (in advanced cases, the arteries may become partially or completely blocked)
- Arterial occlusion and embolism, in which undissolved material in the bloodstream (such as clumps of clotted blood, bacteria, or tissue fragments) block or occlude the flow of blood in the artery, causing a loss of blood to and possibly the death (gangrene) of the tissue beyond the blockade (when flow in a vessel is blocked, there is said to be an "occlusion"; when that block is made up of clotted blood, it is called a "thrombus"; when small bits of material break off the main clump and travel to other parts of the body, they are referred to as "emboli" or an "embolism")

- Carotid occlusive disease, in which the carotid arteries (the arteries in the neck that supply the brain with blood) become blocked (one cause of stroke)
- Aortic and femoral artery occlusive disease, in which the aorta (the main artery from the heart going through the chest and abdomen) and/or the femoral artery (a tributary artery of the aorta carrying blood to the legs) become blocked
- Venous thrombosis, in which the veins become clogged, usually with blood clots, with resulting pain and swelling of the affected extremity (when venous thrombosis occurs, it is often associated with inflammation, and this is called thrombophlebitis; if the vein becomes inflamed without thrombosis, it is referred to as phlebitis)
- Pulmonary embolism, in which clots travel to the lungs.

Specialists in this area can be internists with extensive cardiovascular training. For the most part, they are vascular surgeons.

Physical medicine and rehabilitation

The field of physical medicine and rehabilitation is concerned with the diseases and disorders of the neuromuscular (nerves/muscles) system. This specialist is skilled in using heat, cold, water, electricity, massage, and exercise to help patients regain use and function of those parts of the body damaged by injuries, stroke, severe arthritis, or spinal injury.

The physical medicine and

rehabilitation specialist is required to complete at least three years of training in the specialty, followed by two years of independent practice. Specialty board examinations are required.

Podiatry

Podiatrists concentrate on diseases in and injuries to the feet. Only recently have all the states recognized podiatry as a legitimate healing field. Doctors in this area have degrees in podiatric medicine, but not M.D. degrees; they have not attended medical school. Many podiatrists have joined the ranks of sports medicine practitioners, since many foot injuries result from popular sports activities.

Many podiatrists are qualified to perform surgery on the feet when it is indicated. They also fit a variety of orthotic devices (corrective devices inserted into shoes) to correct foot problems. The boom in jogging and running that has characterized the fitness movement has increased the demand for the services of podiatry.

Preventive medicine

The relatively new field of preventive medicine seeks to prevent illnesses from happening, in addition to diagnosing and treating them after they occur. Physicians from every field have made contributions to preventive medicine. Practitioners range from immunologists (who seek to prevent illness by inoculations) to urban epidemiologists (who search out the causes of widespread illnesses—such as childhood lead poisoning — and try to alter the environment so that the illnesses can be prevented).

Preventive medicine advocates often recommend regular or periodic physical examinations, prescribe certain regimens, and warn against toxic environments. Critics of the field claim that there are no safeguards against some types of illnesses. Advocates of the field point out that the same was said of infections before antibiotics.

Occupational medicine and public health specialists are important members of this field of medicine. In addition, preventive medicine is concerned with reviewing present health services and anticipating and planning future medical needs.

Preventive medicine specialists complete at least three years of specialized training, one year of research or teaching, and examinations by their specialty board.

Proctology

The proctologist specializes in diseases and disorders of the end of the digestive tract: the anus and rectum. The rectum is the last portion of the large intestine; the anus is the opening to the outside from the rectum. Some of the conditions a proctologist treats include hemorrhoids (enlarged blood vessels around the anus) and rectal cancer.

Proctologists complete a residency in general surgery plus a one- or two-year training period in colon and rectal surgery.

Psychiatry

A psychiatrist is a medical doctor — with the authority to write prescriptions and make medical decisions—who deals with mental disorders. Psychologists, on the other hand, do not have to have a medical degree and cannot prescribe drugs. Many psychiatrists do psychoanalysis as part of their therapeutic or diagnostic method and all psychiatrists have intensive training in psychology.

There are four chief branches of psychiatry: (1) descriptive psychiatry, which is based on the observation of external factors that may be the cause of mental illness; (2) dynamic psychiatry, which is the study of the processes, origins, and mechanisms of emotional states; (3) forensic psychiatry, which deals with the legal aspects of mental illness; and (4) orthomolecular psychiatry, which is the study of the molecular bases of mental illnesses.

Psychiatrists go through the usual medical sequence: medical school, internship, and residency. The psychiatrist may spend over five years in specialized training in psychiatry and neurology.

Pulmonary medicine

This field deals with the lungs and their related passages. Among the diseases included are:

- Lung cancer
- Tuberculosis
- Pneumonia, an inflammation of the lungs
- Bronchitis, an inflammation of the bronchi (passageways from the windpipe into the lungs)
- Tracheitis, an inflammation of the trachea (windpipe)
- Black lung, lungs clogged with coal dust
- Pleurisy, an inflammation of the lining of the lungs and the chest cavity
- Emphysema, destruction of lung tissue, causing air to become trapped within the lungs, often accompanied by severe breathing problems.

These specialists also perform bronchoscopy (viewing the trachea and bronchial passages directly through flexible tubes) and specialize in managing ventilators or respirators, artificial breathing machines.

The pulmonary specialist trains in internal medicine, followed by two years of special training in pulmonary disorders.

Radiology/radiotherapy/ nuclear medicine

A radiologist is a medical doctor who uses X rays to diagnose diseases and other disorders. A radiologist is primarily concerned with the administration and interpretation of X rays. Many perform sophisticated procedures, such as arteriography of peripheral arteries and arteries of the brain. Some choose to subspecialize in areas such as neuroradiology ("neuro" means nerves).

Radiologists have training in physics and instrumentation as well as in biochemistry and the effects of radiation on human tissue. A radiologist will have completed a three- or four-year residency in diagnostic radiology plus a one-year internship in a medical field other than radiology.

A radiation therapist is primarily concerned with the application of radiation in the treatment of cancer. A radiation therapist will have completed a one-year internship, either rotating or in internal medicine, followed by a three-year residency in the specialty.

Nuclear medicine is the field in which radioactive substances, called isotopes, are used to diagnose and treat diseases, such as an overactive thyroid. Specialists in this field are trained in the use of scans as opposed to X rays for diagnosis. A nuclear medicine specialist completes a two-year training period in either internal medicine, pathology, or radiology plus a two-year residency in nuclear medicine.

Rheumatology

Rheumatology is the field of medicine concerned with the study, diagnosis, and medical treatment of diseases and disorders of bones, joints, and muscles. These disorders are often characterized by inflammation or degeneration and include such conditions as arthritis, gout, lupus erythematosus, and other diseases of the connective tissues.

A rheumatologist has completed an internship and residency in internal medicine, followed by two or more years of training and experience in rheumatology.

Sports medicine

This is one of the newest fields in medicine and has come into its own largely as a result of two factors: the training and rehabilitation needs of both amateur and professional athletes, and the tremendous growth in fitness and sports-related activities among members of the public. Doctors from a variety of fields now list themselves as sports medicine practitioners. Exercise physiology has become an integral part of medical and sports training programs, and what was once a collection of lore on how to get the most out of your body in a game has become a field of medical research and practice.

Sports medicine has made great contributions to the general public welfare, by producing hard evidence of the benefits of healthful exercise. As a consequence, information about subjects such as nutrition, kinesiology (the study of movements), and biomechanics (study of lever systems and their effect on performance) has come to be available to the average weekend athlete. Training need no longer be haphazard; by using the information developed by sports medicine practitioners, you can train for strength, power, endurance, and speed without incurring injuries. Each goal calls for a different kind of training method. Sports medicine and exercise physiology have made a science out of athletic training.

In one sense, with the advent of sports medicine as a medical field, athletics serves the same function for ordinary people that auto racing serves for the development of new ways to make the family car better: high performance calls for research and ingenuity in converting research into practical applications. Sports medicine converts the lessons learned on the playing field into insights into the medical problems of ordinary people who want to play a little golf, tone up, and trim down.

You'll find sports medicine practitioners in the training rooms of pro ball clubs, and you'll also find them on the running track. Many of them have trained as orthopedists since that specialty field is concerned with the mechanics of muscular and skeletal function.

Surgery

Surgery is the branch of medicine that uses surgical operations to treat disease, injury, or deformity. Surgeons go into the human body by way of incisions through the skin and muscles to alter, correct, or remove and/or replace the offending organ or tissue. There seems to be a surgical specialty for almost every region of the body:

- General surgery (including the abdomen and breasts)
- Thoracic surgery (of the chest)
- Heart surgery (often included in thoracic surgery)
- Oral surgery (of the mouth), usually performed by dentists with a subspecialty in oral surgery
- Neurosurgery (of the nervous system, particularly the brain and the spinal cord)
- Plastic or cosmetic surgery (to correct damage caused by injury or for reasons of appearance)
- Orthopedic surgery (of the bones, joints, ligaments, tendons)
- Eye surgery (for repair or treatment of eye problems)
- Foot surgery (usually performed by a podiatrist or orthopedist).

Surgeons work closely with internists, pathologists, radiologists, anesthesiologists, and other related specialists. In a very real sense, everything that physicians know about diagnosing and treating illnesses is relevant in an operating room.

Surgeons have the usual four years of medical school followed by a general surgery internship and a varying time period in a general surgery residency. In addition, surgeons must also complete additional training in their specific field of surgery.

Urology

Urology deals with diseases and disorders of the urinary tract, the kidneys, the prostate gland, and the male sex organs. The urologist's skills include knowledge of diagnostic procedures and surgical techniques, as well as the ability to treat infections of the urinary tract and the male reproductive system.

After completing medical school, the urologist has two years of training in general surgery, followed by a three-year training period in urology and urologic surgery and an 18-month period of practice. Specialty board exams are then required.

COPING WITH SYMPTOMS

Most of us are aware of what we need to do to promote good health; proper diet, appropriate exercise, and adequate rest are only a few of the good health habits that contribute to fitness and vigor. However, many of us forget that understanding illness is also important to maintaining health and vitality. If we learn to recognize symptoms of illness, we can better prevent, identify, and treat problems that threaten our good health.

A symptom is evidence of a disease or disorder; it indicates a departure from the normal well-being of the body. Sometimes a symptom is a disorder in and of itself. For example, indigestion may simply be the temporary result of eating too much or too fast or of eating fatty or spicy foods. On the other hand, indigestion can be a sign of another disorder such as ulcers or even of more serious disorders such as heart attack or cancer in the intestinal tract. In these cases, indigestion is more than a temporary disorder in and of itself, and you need to be able to tell the difference.

At other times, a symptom is a defensive reaction of the body — an attempt to restore the body to normal functioning. Falling into a faint in an overheated room, for instance, is the body's method of restoring adequate blood supply

to the brain by lowering the head to the same level of the heart. However, fainting may also be a sign of a serious illness, and again you need to know when fainting should be reported to your doctor.

Observing symptoms

Your ability to recognize and understand symptoms of illness is important in helping your doctor diagnose and treat disorders. When you go to the doctor with a medical problem, you should be prepared to describe your symptoms exactly. You should note the time of their onset and the nature of your activity when they occur (such as after eating, upon awakening from sleep, after strenuous exercise like shoveling snow, or when lying down). Be prepared to describe the rapidity with which your symptoms appear. Sometimes the symptoms themselves provide fewer clues than does the manner in which they occur.

To do all of this well, you must learn to be observant about your body. The following descriptions of some of the more common symptoms will help you become alert to changes in your body. This section also offers some guidance on when to seek medical attention for symptoms. As an additional aid, you may want to read the introductions to the chapters in this book that discuss the various systems of the body. Those introductions explain the normal functioning of the body systems and may help you recognize when your body is not working the way it should.

Chest pain

Chest pain is a major symptom in many disorders, including heart disease, heartburn, and pleurisy.

Heart disease

In heart disease, chest pains may be the temporary discomfort of angina pectoris or the similar but more severe and long-lasting signs of a heart attack. In both cases the discomfort is felt as an aching or crushing sensation beneath the breastbone and may radiate into the left shoulder and arm. On some occasions it may also be felt in the back, throat, jaws, and teeth, or spread to the abdomen. In angina the discomfort typically is brought on by exertion and disappears in a few minutes with rest or with the taking of nitroglycerin. In a heart attack, the pain is usually much more intense and deep and is not relieved by nitroglycerin; in addition, the patient is restless, pale, and perspiring. When in doubt about a possible heart attack, call your doctor and go immediately to the hospital emergency room.

Often the symptoms of angina or even a heart attack, spreading to the abdomen, are mistaken for those of indigestion. Sometimes indigestion, ulcer pains, or a gallbladder attack will bring on angina, or be mistaken for a heart attack. Again, when in doubt about a heart attack, call your doctor and go to the emergency room.

Heartburn

Heartburn, felt as a burning pain beneath the breastbone, has nothing to do with the heart. It develops when some food from the stomach, mixed with digestive acids, backs up into the esophagus (the food tube from the mouth to the stomach). The acids burn the lining of the esophagus, producing pain. Heartburn may be treated by using antacids, by raising the head of the bed so that food is not as likely to back up when you are lying down, by avoiding foods like coffee and alcohol that stimulate acid production, or by taking drugs that help keep the esophagus outlet closed.

Pleurisy

The chest pains of pleurisy, which may be sharp and stabbing or vaguely uncomfortable, may occur with every breath or only when the patient breathes deeply or coughs. The pains are caused by inflammation of the pleura, the membrane that surrounds the lungs and lines the chest cavity. The pains may appear only over the site of the infection or may radiate to the lower chest and abdomen.

COPING WITH SYMPTOMS 49

Other causes

Among other causes of chest pain are rib injuries, pneumonia, blood clot in the lung, inflammation of the tissue surrounding the heart, inflammation of the nerves supplying the chest wall, and tenderness of the chest muscle after injury or exertion.

It is important that you report to your doctor any prolonged or severe chest pain, since prompt evaluation and treatment may be lifesaving.

Constipation

Constipation is a condition in which the feces (stool) are hard and their elimination from the bowels is infrequent and difficult. This condition is often more uncomfortable than harmful, although occasionally a relatively sudden change in the bowel movements, involving prolonged constipation or extreme discomfort, can be a symptom of such serious illnesses as cancer, intestinal obstructions, disease or injury of the nervous system, and endocrine gland disorders.

It is important to remember, however, that it is not absolutely necessary to have a bowel movement every day. From three bowel movements per day to three per week is considered normal.

Causes

Common causes of constipation are physical inactivity; lack of fiber or roughage in the diet; inadequate fluid intake; emotional stress, particularly depression; drug side effects; and the habit of postponing the bowel movement until some time after the urge has disappeared.

Symptoms

Conditions that often accompany constipation are difficulty and strain in producing a bowel movement, a full or bloated feeling, abdominal cramps, headache, gassiness, and hemorrhoids (swollen veins near the anus, the opening from the intestine to the outside of the body).

Treatment

The treatment of constipation usually depends on its cause. In mild cases that are not related to other disorders, simple methods of recommended treatment include adding more fiber foods (such as bran, fruits, vegetables, and other forms of roughage) to the diet; drinking eight to ten glasses of water daily; increasing exercise; and developing good bathroom habits. This last recommendation may involve an attempt to have a bowel movement at the same time every day, usually 30 to 60 minutes after breakfast. Early morning is a good time because food that enters an empty stomach activates and increases normal intestine contractions; also, residue from the previous day's meals has moved by this time to the rectal area for elimination.

Laxatives and enemas are usually not recommended for treating simple constipation. Laxatives, in particular, should be used only when absolutely necessary because overuse can lead to irritation of the lining of the rectum, and, more importantly, dependence by the intestine to the point that it cannot function properly without laxatives. Frequent enemas can also lead to dependence.

Prevention

Drinking plenty of water, getting adequate exercise, eating fibrous foods, and recognizing the urge for a bowel movement as soon as it is felt should be beneficial in promoting regular elimination and preventing constipation.

Cough

A cough is a normal reflex of the body to clear the airways. Coughing can result from inhaling dust, dirt, or irritating fumes; from breathing icy air; or from mistakenly drawing food into the airways. It can also be caused by mucus and other secretions from such respiratory disorders as the common cold, influenza, pneumonia, or tuberculosis. Persistent coughs (those that last more than two or three weeks) without other respiratory symptoms may, on occasion, suggest diseases of other organs, such as the heart. A cough may also be an early sign of congestive heart failure.

Types

The type of cough — productive or nonproductive—partially determines how it should be treated. Productive coughs—those that produce fluid or mucus—are often caused by a lung infection. When microorganisms attack the lungs, the lung tissue produces large amounts of secretions in defense. These accumulated secretions irritate the lungs, resulting in coughing that brings up fluid or mucus. A yellowish or reddish fluid in particular may indicate infection or other serious problems and requires a doctor's attention.

Nonproductive coughing does not bring up fluid. It occurs when secretions from nasal passages drip into the throat or when smoke, dust, pollen, or other irritants enter the respiratory system. Irritations such as foreign bodies or tumors may also cause a nonproductive cough, as can any inflammation of the airways and/or lung tissue, infectious or not. Another cause of nonproductive coughing is insufficient moisture in the air. The airways become dry and irritated, and coughing develops. This is particularly common in winter, when humidity is lowest. A humidifier or vaporizer that adds moisture to the air may provide more relief than any cough-suppressing drug.

Treatment

Because coughing has the vital function of clearing the airways, it should never be totally suppressed. In fact, suppressing a cough in an individual with chronic lung disease may be dangerous. Furthermore, indiscriminate use of cough suppressants may mask important symptoms. However, controlling a cough that disrupts sleep or aggravates other conditions may sometimes be necessary. This may be accomplished by using a cough suppressant and/or an expectorant. A suppressant helps to inhibit the cough by depressing the cough center in the brain. An expectorant eases the discharge of mucus from the respiratory tract, thus perhaps shortening the course of the illness.

For other than the mildest cough with obvious causes and certainly for persistent coughs, a doctor should be consulted to determine the cause and to suggest appropriate treatment.

Dehydration

Dehydration is a condition in which the body or certain body tissues suffer from lack of water.

Causes

Tissue dehydration may occur in dry climates and during the winter heating season: extremely dry air causes the rapid evaporation of water from the skin and from the mucous linings of the respiratory (breathing) system. The results are discomfort and sometimes cracking of the skin, unless it is protected by natural lubrication or lotions, and increased susceptibility of the respiratory system to infections.

Dehydration of the entire body can be life-threatening. Illnesses that produce diarrhea and vomiting are common causes of dehydration, since both of these conditions expel excessive body fluids. Cholera, which results in extreme diarrhea and vomiting, can kill through dehydration. Other causes of dehydration include diabetes; kidney disease; excess diuretics (drugs which remove excess water from the blood); liver disease resulting in an accumulation of fluid in the abdominal cavity; inflammation of the abdominal cavity, resulting in fluid accumulation; and burns. Tissue beneath a burn swells with body fluid. If the burn covers much of the body, the buildup of fluid in burn tissue draws considerable water from the blood. This can decrease its volume so much that circulation to the outer parts of the body collapses, a condition known as shock.

Symptoms

Symptoms of dehydration in addition to thirst include sudden weight loss; rough, dry skin; dry mucous membranes; rapid heartbeat and low blood pressure; lack of energy; and weakness. In an extreme case the patient is in shock, with pale skin; bluish lips and fingertips; rapid and shallow breathing; and a weak, rapid, irregular pulse. Blood tests reveal a thickening of the blood because of decreased water content.

Treatment

Treatment of mild to moderate dehydration is to have the patient drink more water with some salt added. However, if the individual suffers from vomiting or diarrhea or is unconscious, it may be necessary for medical personnel to administer saline solution (salt water) intravenously (through the vein). The intravenous method is always used in severe cases of dehydration. The goal is to replace totally the lost fluid within 48 to 72 hours, together with the valuable mineral salts that have also been lost.

Diarrhea

Diarrhea is abnormally frequent and excessively liquid bowel movements. This is often the body's defensive attempt to rid itself of irritating or toxic substances. It is a symptom that accompanies many disorders, both mild and serious.

Types

There are two basic types of diarrhea: acute (or short-term) diarrhea, the more common form, which comes on quickly and usually lasts no more than two or three days, although it can last as long as two weeks; and chronic (or long-term) diarrhea, which may also appear suddenly but lingers for many weeks or months with symptoms either constantly present or appearing and disappearing.

Both acute and, particularly, chronic diarrhea can become a serious problem because of the excessive loss of body fluids and salt (called dehydration) as well as loss of nutrients. It may also be a symptom of a disorder such as inflammatory bowel disease (Crohn's disease, ulcerative colitis).

Causes

The reasons for the consistency of the stool in diarrhea are complex. In an infection, the intestine may pour out massive quantities of fluids and salts in response to a bacterial toxin (poison) or other irritant. In inflammatory bowel disease, protein, blood, and mucus are lost through the inflamed lining of the colon, taking large quantities of water along. Other disorders speed up the normal movement of the colon, thereby not allowing time for absorption of fluids. Yet another type of diarrhea is caused by poor absorption of a type of sugar (called lactose), which draws fluid out of the colon. Finally, many diarrhea conditions are combinations of these biologic mechanisms.

Other causes of diarrhea include changes in the diet, drugs taken for other disorders (particularly antibiotics which upset the bacteria balance of the intestine), stress, and food allergies.

Symptoms

The symptoms often experienced with the characteristic loose and frequent bowel movements are nausea, cramps or pain in the abdomen, gassiness, fatigue, and fever.

Diagnosis

Diagnosis of the cause of this problem will require a report to the doctor concerning the patient's normal diet, emotional state, and recent changes in the daily habits. In addition, a sample of the bowel movement may be examined for color, consistency, odor, chemical content, and presence of blood. Stool cultures are often done to determine the offending microorganism if infection is suspected.

Treatment

Treatment for diarrhea usually involves removing or correcting the cause of the condition. If diarrhea lasts for more than three days or is a recurring problem, a doctor should be consulted, as this may be a warning sign of a more serious illness. Antidiarrhea medications can be prescribed for particularly bothersome or persistent diarrhea, but these are to be used only with caution, particularly in some infections where they may prolong the course of the illness.

The discomfort of occasional bouts of acute diarrhea, however, is usually treated with simple remedies: adequate rest; increased intake of liquids to replace lost fluids; a diet consisting of light meals, perhaps soups or broth at first, eaten more frequently; and, as solid food is added to the diet, the avoidance of irritating foods such as bran, fruits and vegetables, fried foods, coffee, and alcoholic beverages.

Dizziness and vertigo

Dizziness and vertigo are sensations of disorientation and distorted perception. Occasional episodes are not serious, but recurrent dizziness or vertigo can be symptoms of a variety of disorders, particularly those involving the eye, ear, or nervous system.

Dizziness and vertigo are sometimes confused with one another. Dizziness is an uncomfortable, distorted, or unsteady sense of the environment; the word *dizziness* is often used to describe a sensation of lightheadedness or a faint feeling. Vertigo is a false sense of movement, often the perception that one is spinning or that one's environment is whirling around. Vertigo is often accompanied by nausea.

Causes

Dizziness and, particularly, vertigo can be caused by a malfunction in one of the parts of the body that is responsible for giving the brain information on balanced posture, position, and movement. These parts include the eye, a balance-sensing mechanism in the ear, and certain areas of the brain. Thus, balance can be disturbed by any injury, impairment, or disorder involving the eyes, ears, and certain areas of the brain, as well as the nerves leading to these areas. A wide variety of problems such as injury to the head, ear infections, and migraine headaches can display dizziness or vertigo as their symptoms. Also, occasional mild upsets to the body can cause dizziness (but usually not vertigo), including such harmless factors as being overheated, overtired, tense, or nervous, as well as standing up too quickly after lying or sitting for some time.

Symptoms

Dizziness is characterized by feelings of unsteadiness, swaying, light-headedness, weakness, faintness, and, at times, nausea and vomiting. Vertigo is marked by feelings of spinning and may be associated with unsteady walking; a tendency to veer to one side while walking and, in severe attacks, falling down; paleness; sweating; and continuous rapid eye movement.

Prevention and treatment

Simple cases of dizziness can be easily avoided. Getting up slowly after lying or sitting, leaving overheated rooms to get some fresh air, eating a balanced diet, and getting adequate rest should all help to prevent common episodes of dizziness. Recurrent dizziness, however, should be investigated.

True vertigo, on the other hand, may be a sign of physical disease that can range from an inflammation of the balance mechanism in

the ear (labyrinthitis) to a brain disorder. Frequently, however, no cause will be found, and the vertigo is treated symptomatically with drugs. In all cases, any episode of true vertigo should be reported to a physician.

Edema

Edema is the accumulation of excessive amounts of fluid within the body's tissues. It is a symptom, rather than a cause, of many other conditions that can be minor or serious.

The fluid that accumulates comes from the blood. Normally, there is a constant exchange of body fluid between the blood vessels and other body tissues. The blood removes any extra fluids and carries them to the kidneys where they are excreted. Edema occurs when that exchange does not function properly, either allowing too much liquid to leave the blood vessels or too little fluid to enter the blood vessels from body tissues.

Causes

A change in pressure within the blood vessels because of heart disease, high blood pressure, blocked or damaged vessels, or kidney problems may trigger an imbalance in fluid exchange.

Mild edema is common before menstruation and during pregnancy when the blood volume increases. Excess weight, tight clothing, and hot weather may also lead to edema. Edema occurring under these circumstances is normal and should not be a cause for alarm.

Forms of edema

Edema can be confined to a small area of the body or become generalized. Some forms are more noticeable than others, depending upon their cause and location. For example, the swelling that appears around a splinter in the skin is edema. However, generalized edema results in widespread body swelling and puffiness, usually first noticed in the fingers and feet. The most serious forms of edema occur within the internal organs of the body. Heart disease, for example, may result in internal edema of the heart and lungs, causing swelling that puts tremendous strain on these organs, even to the point of becoming dangerous.

Treatment

Simple or temporary edema may be relieved by decreasing salt intake, since the sodium in salt causes the body to retain fluid. More severe or internal edema may be treated with a diuretic, a drug that stimulates the kidneys to produce more urine and thus rid the body of excess fluid. Edema that is symptomatic of an underlying disorder will often disappear with management of the condition.

Prevention

Controlling weight gain, eating a balanced diet low in salt, and wearing loose clothing may prevent milder forms of edema. Any prolonged edema not attributable to causes such as hot weather or menstruation needs investigation by a physician to determine the cause.

Fainting

Fainting is a temporary loss of consciousness and is often the supply extra needed blood to the brain. Fainting can be a symptom of a relatively mild condition (such as hunger) or a serious disorder (such as arrhythmia).

When the brain experiences a temporary reduction of its blood supply, the body reacts defensively by, in effect, causing itself to fall down, thus bringing the head to the same level as the heart thereby minimizing the effect of gravity that favors pooling of blood in the lower extremities. The net effect of this is an increase in the amount of blood coming back to the heart which allows the heart to pump blood to the brain more easily.

Causes

Fainting can be caused by an interference with any one of several internal mechanisms that protect and maintain the brain's blood supply by working against gravity and its tendency to allow blood to pool in the lower parts of the body. An example of one of these mechanisms is the "muscle pump." The muscles of the legs, when in motion, act to squeeze the veins in the legs thereby actually forcing the column of blood up toward the heart. If a person stands motionless for a long period of time without using these muscles, pooling of blood in the legs takes place, reducing the amount available to the brain. This reduction frequently causes fainting or loss of consciousness. In addition, the ability of the heart to increase its rate and force of contraction when under stress is another built-in protective mechanism.

These protective functions are impaired by a variety of causes, among them certain conditions such as an overheated or crowded environment; emotional stress; hunger; extreme fatigue; various drugs, particularly some high blood pressure medications; as well as certain diseases, including anemia, hypoglycemia (low blood sugar), heart disease, and blood loss.

Symptoms

The symptoms that usually precede actual fainting are lightheadedness; confusion; spots before the eyes; white or grayish coloring of the face; cold, moist, or clammy skin; and, at times, nausea and vomiting.

Treatment

Fainting is treated by taking several simple steps to make the person more comfortable. The patient should be lying down,
preferably with the feet higher than the head (to help blood return) and the clothing loosened. The patient should have plenty of fresh air to breathe. Recovery should occur within a few seconds of fainting, but a sense of disorientation may linger for several minutes. Spirits of ammonia and smelling salts are not usually recommended for fainting, as they may be ineffective or may cause vomiting.

Recurrent fainting should be reported to a doctor, as more testing may be needed to diagnose another disorder that is causing the fainting.

Prevention

Fainting can be prevented by lying down, preferably with legs up, or hanging the head down between the knees and breathing deeply as soon as any of the warning symptoms are noticed. These precautions help to lower the brain to the level of the heart, thus increasing the blood supply to the brain.

Fatigue

Fatigue may be physical or mental exhaustion, an overwhelming feeling of weariness, or a lack of energy and enthusiasm for even pleasant activities. It is a symptom of a vast number of diseases and disorders.

Fatigue should not be confused with weakness, which is an actual, physical loss of strength.

Causes

Fatigue and tiring rapidly with minimal activity are often the first signs or among the early signs of an approaching illness. Fatigue is a warning signal of a variety of diseases and disorders: the common cold, influenza, hepatitis, infectious mononucleosis, and other infectious diseases; heart disease; lung disorders such as emphysema; some gland diseases; anemia and nutritional deficiencies; and some diseases of the nervous system. Overwork, either physical or mental, may also cause fatigue, as can psychological disorders or emotional stress.

Symptoms

The symptoms of fatigue can include nervousness, anxiety, depression, irritability, headache, diminished sexual function, and difficulty in concentrating. When fatigue is due to psychological problems, sleep disorders are common associated symptoms, including insomnia, as well as frequent nighttime and early morning waking.

Treatment

Fatigue is best treated by treating the physical disorder or psychological problem that is causing it. Some types of fatigue, particularly that due to physical overexertion, can probably be prevented by getting adequate exercise and rest, as well as eating well-balanced meals and coping with stress and overwork.

Fever

Fever is an abnormally high body temperature.

A fever is present when the body temperature rises above the normal range of 98.6°F to 99.6°F; that is, if the body temperature is more than 101.5°F when measured with a rectal thermometer, 100.5°F when measured with an oral thermometer, or 99.5°F when measured under the arm, it is considered abnormal.

Fever is a symptom of illness and often appears to be an undesirable condition, but in fact fever acts as a defense mechanism for the body when it is being attacked by a bacterium or virus. Fever occurs when a regulatory center in the brain, whose job it is to maintain a constant body temperature regardless of the surrounding environment, responds to an illness or infection such as the common cold or influenza and sets the body temperature higher as a means of killing the invading microorganisms. It is thought that the microorganisms cannot survive these higher temperatures.

Causes and symptoms

Infections are the most common cause of fever. But a fever can also be a symptom of heart attack, some forms of cancer, and disorders in the portion of the brain that regulates temperature (such as stroke, brain tumor, or brain injury).

The early signs of fever include chills or hot flashes, flushed skin, increased pulse and breathing rates, headache, and aching muscles or joints. A slight fever may show none of these symptoms, a high fever may result in delirium or convulsions, and a prolonged fever may cause weakness and dehydration (excess loss of body fluids).

Treatment

Treatment of fever depends on its severity, duration, and cause. Immediate emergency medical treatment should be sought if fever is more than 105°F (although fever is usually higher in very young children) or if convulsions have occurred. A doctor should be consulted if a fever is high (103°F to 104°F, lasting for 12 to 24 hours); if a moderate fever (101°F to 102°F) lasts for several days; if the body temperature fluctuates widely; or if the fever disappears, then returns several days later, usually signaling a new or additional infection.

The goal of treating a fever is actually to diagnose and treat its cause. Merely lowering a mild fever may do more harm than good, as it reduces the protection that the fever may be providing in fighting off the infection; it may also mask a fever when its cause is unknown or disturb the natural course that would have been taken by the underlying illness, thus hindering diagnosis. Therefore, treating a fever should never be confused with treating its cause.

However, at times fever does need to be lowered to keep the patient comfortable and to prevent weakness and dehydration that can result from prolonged fever. Increasing fluid intake and taking aspirin or an aspirin substitute such as acetaminophen will lower a fever; tepid, not cold, baths and comfortable but not overly warm clothing and blankets will help to lower the fever but also keep the patient from feeling chilled.

It should be noted that any drug treatment for fever, especially for children, should be undertaken only after consulting with a doctor. For instance, although it has not been proven that aspirin causes or promotes a disorder called Reye's syndrome, it is recommended that aspirin not be given to children with chicken pox or influenza.

Heartburn

Heartburn is an uncomfortable, burning pain felt behind the lower part of the breastbone, sometimes extending up into the upper chest or lower neck. Despite its name, it is not caused by pain in the heart or by a heart attack. In fact, heartburn is often triggered by simple digestive upsets, although an occasional severe case may be a symptom of a more serious disorder such as peptic ulcer.

Causes

Heartburn occurs when the

acid digestive juices and partially digested food from the stomach back up into the lower esophagus and irritate its tissues.

Heartburn most often develops ten minutes to one hour after eating. It may be caused by overeating; smoking; lying down or bending over after eating, which allows the backup of stomach acids and food into the esophagus; alcoholic drinks; coffee; spicy or highly seasoned foods; acidic fruits or fruit juices; and aspirin. Heartburn is a common problem during pregnancy because the growing baby presses on the stomach and esophagus, encouraging digestive juices to move up toward the throat; this disappears after childbirth.

Symptoms

The major symptom of heartburn is the characteristic burning sensation behind the breastbone and up toward the throat; it may be accompanied by gassiness, belching, and an uncomfortable, tight feeling in the chest.

Heartburn can usually be relieved by merely standing or sitting upright or by drinking milk or something soothing to the stomach. Nonprescription antacids may also be helpful in more severe cases (but not in the presence of kidney disease, because one of the ingredients in antacids may interfere with kidney function). Any persistent, uncontrollable, or severe heartburn should be reported to a doctor, as it may be a sign of a more severe condition such as peptic ulcer.

Prevention

Heartburn can often be prevented by avoiding spicy, acidic, or other troublesome foods, as well as coffee or alcoholic beverages if they seem to trigger it. Eating smaller meals more frequently and refraining from smoking at mealtimes are also beneficial in avoiding heartburn. Sleeping with the back and head propped up on pillows may prevent stomach contents from flowing into the esophagus.

Indigestion

Indigestion, also called dyspepsia, is the discomfort caused by difficulty in digesting food. It is an uncomfortable feeling of fullness, pressure, slight pain, or gassiness and is usually related to eating. (Constipation, diarrhea, heartburn, and nausea are *not* indigestion, although they may be related to the problem.)

Causes

Indigestion is usually caused by an eating problem such as eating too fast or too much; inadequate chewing; eating in an emotionally upsetting environment; eating particularly bothersome foods, such as spicy, fatty, or oily foods, or those that may cause an allergic reaction; and smoking, especially immediately before or after a meal. Indigestion can also be caused by serious disorders such as cancer, ulcers, and diseases involving the organs associated with digestion (the esophagus, intestines, gallbladder, liver, stomach, and pancreas). In addition, heart attack, tumors, and emotional problems can be accompanied by symptoms that are similar to indigestion.

Any case of indigestion that lingers for some time or that cannot be controlled in any way should be reported to a doctor for diagnosis and appropriate treatment.

Diagnosis

The cause of indigestion is diagnosed predominantly by observing the symptoms and the conditions under which they occur. A doctor will want a description of the symptoms and of the patient's usual dietary habits; of the time, length, and location of the discomfort as well as the circumstances surrounding it and foods eaten preceding it; and of the emotional environment that usually exists during meals and snacks. X rays or stool analysis may also be used to make a diagnosis of the cause of indigestion.

Treatment

Antacids often relieve indigestion (but they should not be used by people who have kidney disease, since one of their ingredients, magnesium, may interfere with kidney function).

Prevention

However, the best treatment consists of preventing indiges-

tion in the first place. Eating balanced meals in a relaxed setting, eliminating foods that may be causing indigestion problems, and refraining from smoking during mealtime should be beneficial in the prevention of indigestion.

Insomnia

Insomnia is the inability to sleep during normal sleeping hours, when there is no apparent reason for wakefulness. The insomnia may vary from simple restlessness to wakefulness on and off throughout the night to total sleeplessness.

Causes

Although the condition is most often associated with psychological or emotional problems, it can also be related to physical disorders or even to conditions in the immediate environment.

Depression and anxiety are often the cause of insomnia. Among physical disorders that can lead to insomnia are urination problems, heart trouble, high blood pressure, infection, hardening of the arteries, spastic colon, and leg cramps. Less serious causes of insomnia can be found in the person's immediate environment — bright lights, noise, overheated or underheated bedroom, lack of ventilation. Insomnia may also be caused by too many or too few bed clothes; constipation; hunger; and too much coffee, tea, cola, or other beverage containing caffeine, which is a stimulant.

Strangely, drugs to promote sleep can cause insomnia. The careless or inappropriate use of tranquilizers and sedatives can disrupt sleep patterns. If high doses of tranquilizers or sedatives are taken, the wake-sleep rhythm or pattern can be reversed and sleep can become irregular. The person may doze throughout the day and then be unable to sleep at night.

Diagnosis and treatment

A person who has chronic or persistent insomnia should consult a physician so that the underlying cause of the insomnia—emotional or physical—can be diagnosed and treated.

Prevention

Ways of preventing or coping with simple insomnia include taking a ten or 15 minute walk before bedtime, taking a warm bath, drinking warm milk (milk contains a substance called tryptophan that naturally promotes drowsiness), reading, or watching TV. Taking sleep-promoting medications should be discussed with a doctor.

Itching

Itching is an uncomfortable or irritating sensation felt by the nerve endings located on the surface of the skin, accompanied by the urge to scratch. It has been described as a pricking, stinging, burning, or crawling feeling.

Causes

The biological reactions that lead to itching are not clearly understood, but it is known that this stimulation of the nerve endings can be caused by both physical and psychological factors.

Itching can be caused by insect bites; small cuts or scrapes; hives and other allergic reactions; a fungus infection; the rash that often accompanies infectious diseases such as chicken pox; dry skin, often stemming from bathing or showering too frequently or using harsh soaps; reactions to drugs; and psychological stress.

Symptoms

Itching is characterized by an uneasy discomfort on the skin, the urge to scratch, and possibly redness, peeling, and other irritations of the skin as a result of scratching. Itching of just the scalp and forearms with no obvious cause may be triggered by psychological stress.

Treatment

Treatment of itching depends on its cause. Itching from dry skin is usually treated by applying skin lotions or creams to small areas and using body lotions or bath oils for larger areas; reducing showers and baths to only twice weekly, as water tends to dry the skin; and trying new brands of soap or shampoo.

If itching seems to be a reaction to a drug, the doctor should be consulted before making any changes in medication. (A patient should *never* stop taking a drug without the consultation of a doctor.) The doctor will either lower the dosage to relieve the itching or give advice on treatment of the itching while maintaining the original dosage.

If no visible symptoms or outside substances seem to be triggering itching, psychological stress may be the cause, and the best treatment will involve removing the stress or learning how to deal with it.

If itching persists for more than a week after attempts at self-treatment, a doctor should be consulted because persistent itching with no visible cause may be a symptom of diabetes, thyroid disease, kidney failure, liver disease, or cancer.

Prevention

Some itching can be prevented. Limiting bathing to twice weekly and using humidifiers to keep the air moist should help prevent the itching caused by dry skin.

Loss of appetite

Loss of appetite (also known as anorexia) is a disinterest in and lack of desire for food. Loss of appetite should not be confused with the willful suppression of the urge to eat (called anorexia nervosa), which often occurs in young women. Rather, loss of appetite is a common symptom that accompanies many illnesses.

Causes

Appetite is controlled by two areas of the brain—the "feeding" center and the "fullness" center—that work to regulate feelings of hunger depending on the body's need for food. Appetite loss can, very rarely, be caused by damage to these areas of the brain, but more commonly it results from fatigue, the common cold, and psychological problems such as anxiety and depression. Serious disorders that may lead to longer periods of appetite loss include certain types of cancers as well as glandular and intestinal diseases.

Symptoms

Loss of appetite is indicated by a general disinterest in food or eating, reduced food intake, and, in severe cases, weakness and a decrease in the body's natural resistance to disease.

Treatment

A doctor's advice should be sought if appetite loss stems from emotional or psychological problems, if it lasts for long periods, or if it seems to have no obvious cause. Counseling may be beneficial for those who have emotional problems.

Nasal congestion

Nasal congestion occurs when the blood vessels in the nose enlarge, thus taking up more space in the nasal cavity and allowing less air to pass through with each breath. These enlarged blood vessels also leak fluid into the surrounding tissues, which fills the nasal cavity and further impairs breathing.

Nasal congestion is not a serious problem in itself, although it may be bothersome enough to interfere with daily activities and sleep. Persistent cases should be reported to a doctor, as nasal congestion may be a symptom of mild infections or more serious disorders.

Causes

The common cold, influenza, allergy, and bronchitis are the most frequent causes of nasal congestion. Persistent cases may be caused by structural abnormalities in the nose or by the daily use of certain drugs, particularly those often prescribed for high blood pressure, which act to enlarge all blood vessels, including those in the nose.

Treatment

Occasional nasal congestion is often treated with nonprescription decongestants such as nasal sprays, nose drops, and nasal inhalers, all of which act to shrink swollen blood vessels in the nose and stop fluid secretion. However, they also may shrink blood vessels elsewhere in the body, resulting in increased blood pressure and heart rate, as well as in nervousness and insomnia. For this reason, over-the-counter decongestants should not be used by those with high blood pressure, heart disease, diabetes, or thyroid disorders.

Also, those who do use decongestants for nasal congestion should use them only for brief periods, perhaps three days at the most; since they act to constrict the blood vessels, their overuse tends to tire the blood vessels, relaxing them completely and making the nose more congested than it was before decongestants were used. This is called rebound congestion.

In addition, specific medicine that is inserted in the nose may be prescribed by a doctor. Also, the use of vaporizers or humidifiers is often beneficial in relieving some of the discomfort of nasal congestion.

Nausea and vomiting

Nausea is an extremely uncomfortable or queasy feeling in the stomach area, often accompanied by an urge to vomit. Vomiting is the forceful ejection of the contents of the stomach through the mouth.

Both nausea and vomiting can be symptoms of relatively mild upsets in the body chemistry, such as motion sickness, or of very serious disorders, such as peptic ulcer.

Nausea and vomiting originate in an area of the brain called, interestingly, the vomiting center.

The vomiting center receives impulses from the network of nerves extending throughout the body. When nerves which supply information from both the digestive system and the inner ear (part of which controls balance) deliver the message that vomiting is necessary, the person will vomit.

Nausea and vomiting are usually temporary conditions and are sometimes beneficial, because they result in the expulsion of something potentially harmful to the body. However, persistent or recurring vomiting can lead to a dangerous loss of fluids and salts (called dehydration) and of nutrients, as well as to damage to the esophagus (the passageway from the mouth to the stomach) or upper stomach.

Causes

Several relatively mild conditions and disorders may cause nausea and vomiting, including motion sickness, the morning sickness of pregnancy, excessive alcohol intake, emotional upset, drug side effects, eating too much, eating especially bothersome foods such as oily or greasy foods, and eating spoiled food. More serious conditions that may be accompanied by nausea and vomiting are severe injury or pain, serious disorders of the digestive system (such as peptic ulcer or gastritis), heart disease, and gland disorders. Additionally, vomiting without the feeling of nausea preceding it may be a symptom of brain injury or brain tumor.

Symptoms

The symptoms that accompany nausea include a "sour" or queasy stomach, chills, perspiration, drowsiness, headache, rapid heartbeat and breathing rates, and salivation (excess saliva).

Treatment

Most nausea and vomiting will require little or no treatment, as these symptoms will subside when the factor causing them is removed or corrected. However, if vomiting occurs regularly or frequently without an obvious cause, or if blood or red or dark brown spots appear in the vomitus, medical treatment should be sought immediately and a sample of the vomitus may be examined.

Home remedies will often help to relieve the discomfort of occasional bouts of nausea and vomiting. Drinking tea, non-cola beverages, especially ginger ale, and soup or broth is often suggested because liquids need to be replaced because of the fluid loss experienced during vomiting. Solid food usually is not recommended, but when vomiting subsides, toast or crackers may be tried before returning to a normal diet.

Several medications can successfully control the urge to vomit, but they need to be prescribed by a doctor and should only be used with caution. In addition, any woman who is pregnant or thinks she may be pregnant should consult with her doctor before taking this or any type of medication.

Occult blood

Occult blood is a term referring to amounts of blood so minute (small) that they cannot be seen by the naked eye and are only detectable with a chemical test or a microscopic examination. The term is generally used in reference to blood in the stools, or feces, that indicates bleeding along the gastrointestinal tract.

Symptoms

Often, the only symptom of occult bleeding is the fatigue caused by the loss of oxygen-carrying red blood cells. Between 50 and 200 milliliters (3 to 15 tablespoons) of blood can be passed in one stool with no visible indication that it is present.

Diagnosis

Such bleeding is not always constant, so tests are typically run on three samples of stools if a problem is suspected. The patient must not eat red meat for three days before taking the samples because even cooked blood from meat can test as positive for occult blood.

Occult blood may also be present in the urine, indicating bleeding at some point in the urinary system, such as in the kidneys or bladder.

Pain

Pain is an unpleasant or uncomfortable sensation that can range from mild irritation to excruciating agony. It is probably the most commonly reported symptom and is linked to innumerable disorders and diseases. (A symptom is an abnormal physical or psychological condition that accompanies or results from a disease or disorder, and that often serves as a clue in diagnosis.)

Causes

Pain occurs when specialized nerve endings are stimulated; within a fraction of a second this pain "signal" travels through a network of nerves to the brain. Pain can be a warning sign, indicating impending damage to the body, or it can be a protective mechanism, causing the person feeling pain to remove the cause or reflexively draw away from the source. Most healthy people have occasional, brief twinges of pain that have no specific cause and are usually harmless. However, bothersome, recurring, or persistent pain can be caused by thousands of factors. Most commonly, pain is a symptom of disease, injury, or abnormal changes in the body.

Types

There are many types of pain. Pain can be dull and constant, sharp and sudden, crushing, burning, piercing, or aching. When it is felt in areas other than the location of the disorder (for example, when the pain of heart attack is felt in the arm), it is called "referred pain." Unexplainable pain should be reported promptly to a doctor for investigation and possible treatment.

Diagnosis

Diagnosing the cause of a pain may be difficult. It is best to observe any accompanying symptoms and to keep in mind the answers to two questions that a doctor may ask in trying to diagnose the pain: "What brings on the pain?" and "What brings relief?"

Treatment

The ideal treatment for pain consists of finding and correcting its source. In some cases, however, such as in widespread cancer, this would be impossible, so the pain itself needs to be treated, most commonly with analgesic drugs (painkilling medications). Aspirin and acetaminophen are probably the most common painkillers that can be obtained without a prescription. Other more potent painkillers, such as narcotics, must be prescribed by a doctor. Other drugs, both prescription and nonprescription, are designed to treat and relieve the pain of a specific disorder.

If the pain comes from the muscles such as in overexertion or from injury to soft tissues such as

a bruise, adequate rest of the affected area may bring relief.

Rash

A rash is an eruption on the surface of the skin, covering either small areas of the body or extensive areas, in the form of red spots, patches, or blisters. Often, a rash causes itching, but this is not always the case. A rash is usually a temporary condition, appearing and disappearing within a few days if not sooner. If so, there is little need for worry; however, a rash can also be a symptom of infectious diseases or other disorders.

Causes

Rashes may be caused by exposure to the sun, heat and cold, the chemicals in household cleansers or detergents, fabrics, or certain foods (these are called allergic rashes). A rash can appear as a symptom of certain diseases, including allergies, measles, rubella (German measles), chicken pox, shingles, and some sexually transmitted diseases.

Rashes that appear regularly with no other symptoms may indicate the presence of an allergy; if a rash is accompanied by other symptoms, it is more likely that the cause is an infectious disease.

Treatment

Any rash that lasts for more than a few days should be examined by a doctor. A rash will usually disappear when its underlying cause is treated. In the case of allergy, perhaps the only possible treatment will be something to relieve minor itching and irritation, but a diagnosis and allergy testing may at least indicate which irritant (allergen) to avoid in the future.

Sore throat

A sore throat is a painful irritation in the throat, often a symptom of a cold. A sore throat can range from mild scratchiness to severe pain and difficulty in swallowing.

Causes

A sore throat is most frequently seen as a symptom of the common cold, when the nasal passages are congested and the person is forced to breath through the mouth, leaving the throat dry and irritated. Coughing may also irritate the throat, as will the secretions that drain into the throat from the back of the nose during a cold.

Irritating environmental substances such as smoke, pollen, pollution, and dust can cause a sore throat when inhaled; also, a sore throat may result when hot liquids or foods are swallowed.

A severe sore throat may be caused by a bacterial (usually strep) infection of the throat, middle ear, nose, or sinuses. Left untreated, strep throat can lead to rheumatic fever, a disease that can affect the heart valves.

Symptoms

A sore throat is characterized by dryness and scratchiness in the throat and pain when swallowing. A doctor should be notified if a sore throat lasts more than a week, if it occurs without a cold, or if no obvious irritant can be found, since this type of sore throat may be a symptom of a serious disease, a blood disorder, or a severe infection. If a sore throat is accompanied by fever, achiness, and fatigue, or if the throat and mouth are very red or develop yellow or white spots, a bacterial infection is probably present.

Treatment

A simple sore throat accompanying a cold is treated by relieving the other cold symptoms. A nasal decongestant may be used if the nose is congested; a cough suppressant may be used if coughing is irritating the throat (although cough suppressants are not always recommended because they allow mucus to accumulate and thus may trigger further complications); sour, hard candy can stimulate saliva production; and gargling with warm salt water every half hour soothes the irritated tissue of the throat.

If a strep infection is the cause of the sore throat, antibiotics are prescribed to treat the infection.

Vital signs

Vital signs is a term used in diagnostic medicine to include four observable phenomena in patients: temperature, pulse, respiration rate, and blood pressure. These four items are all important indicators of disease and are easily obtainable information for the physician. Separately or together, they offer important clues to the patient's physical condition and may point toward other tests or diagnostic procedures that need to be performed.

Temperature

Temperature is a useful index to a patient's condition, since a fever, or an abnormal rise in body temperature, is usually a significant indicator of disease. Fever is generally a sign of infection, but it can be present whenever there is tissue destruction—from a severe sunburn, for example, or when large amounts of tissue deteriorate for lack of blood supply.

Pulse rate

The *pulse rate* is another easily obtainable and important piece of information about a patient's condition. The heart rate varies with a person's level of physical activity. For example, it beats faster during exercise and more slowly during rest. An inappropriate heart rate, or pulse, may indicate disease. A feverish patient will show an increased heart rate, while a weak but rapid pulse is characteristic of severe blood loss or diseases of the heart itself. Irregular pulse (arrhythmia) also suggests conditions ranging from malfunction of the heart to stress, anxiety, or overconsumption of caffeine.

Respiratory rate

Respiratory rate, or rate of breathing, is a vital sign that changes with disease. Patients with fever show an increased respiratory rate (hyperventilation) which lowers body temperature. Hyperventilation is also a common response to pain or stress. Also, any condition which leads to acidosis, or higher acid levels in the body than basic levels, similarly drives the respiratory rate upward. Diseases of the lungs, with simultaneous inability to oxygenate the blood, also increase respiratory rate.

Blood pressure

The fourth vital sign, *blood pressure,* is equally significant. It indicates to the physician the amount of blood in circulation. A decrease in circulating blood volume, as is true in cases of severe bleeding, lowers blood pressure and deprives the body tissues of adequate blood flow. Reflexes then are initiated that compensate in part for the reduced blood volume and pressure. For example, the heart rate increases and compensates partially for the sudden reduction in blood volume. Also, peripheral blood vessels in areas such as the abdomen constrict, thus diverting the remaining blood to vital areas such as the brain. And finally, unusual elevation of blood pressure constitutes a disorder in its own right: *hypertension.*

FACTS ABOUT INFECTIOUS DISEASES

The human body is both surrounded by and inhabited by many living organisms. Most are so small that they are invisible to the naked eye. For this reason, they are called *microorganisms.* Many microorganisms are harmless or even beneficial; for example, certain bacteria that normally live in the digestive system help digest food. Occasionally, however, a microorganism capable of causing a disease invades the body. Diseases caused by such microorganisms are called infectious diseases.

Infectious diseases are contagious; that is, they can be passed from one person to another. They can be transmitted by skin contact, by contaminated food or drink, or by airborne particles containing the microorganisms. Animal or insect bites are another means of transmission. (If an insect, for example, bites an infected person, the insect can carry the microorganism and pass the disease by biting another person.)

Bacterial infections

Bacteria are one-celled, microscopic organisms. They nor-mally exist in the body by the billions. Most are harmless; some, like those in the digestive tract, perform useful functions. On the other hand, some bacteria are disease-causing, or pathogenic. Disease-causing bacteria either (1) attack the body's tissues directly or (2) cause damage by secreting poisonous substances called toxins.

Fortunately, bacterial infections are frequently curable; certain bacteria can be killed by drugs called antibiotics. Other bacterial diseases can be prevented by vaccination. (Bacteria will be discussed later in this section.)

A virus is the smallest known microorganism. Viruses are responsible for diseases as prevalent and relatively harmless as the common cold and as serious as meningitis. Viruses live and reproduce only within living cells, and only certain cells are susceptible to a specific virus. You may be host to many viruses without suffering any adverse effects, but if enough cells are attacked, you may become sick.

There is no effective medical treatment for viral infections. Because a virus lives inside a cell, any treatment designed to kill the virus is also likely to harm the cell.

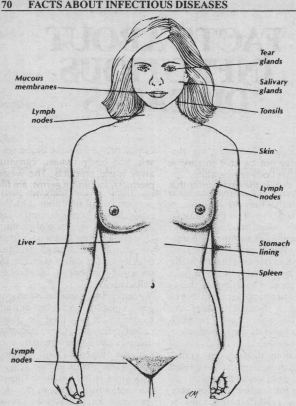

Tear glands

Salivary glands

Mucous membranes

Tonsils

Lymph nodes

Skin

Lymph nodes

Liver

Stomach lining

Spleen

Lymph nodes

The body has many natural defense mechanisms to fight infection.

In addition, there are thousands of different viruses — each with different properties — and an agent effective against one virus probably will not affect the others. Although there are vaccinations for some viral diseases, therapy for most viral diseases is limited to treating the symptoms.

The body's defenses

Despite the prevalence of disease-causing microorganisms, your body is not defenseless against these invaders. The body fights infections in three ways: by preventing these organisms from entering the body; by attacking those that do manage to enter; and by inactivating those organisms it cannot kill. Sometimes, too, the body fights disease by developing defensive symptoms. Fever is an example. During an illness, the body's temperature regulator may respond to the illness by raising the body's temperature. It is thought that the microorganism causing the disease may not be able to survive the higher body temperature.

The skin is the first barrier that guards the underlying tissues of the body. Additional protection is offered by sweat, which contains antiseptic (germ-killing) substances. Where there are natural openings in the skin, there are also defenses. For example, tear glands in the eyes secrete and bathe the eyes with fluid that contains bacteria-fighting properties. The saliva glands in the mouth and the tonsils in the throat help prevent microorganisms from attacking the mouth and throat. Many openings in the body as well as internal passages are lined with mucous membranes. These delicate layers produce mucus, a slippery secretion that moistens and protects by repelling or trapping microorganisms.

Internally, certain body organs fight infection. For instance, the liver and the spleen (a large gland-like organ located in the abdomen) filter out harmful substances from the blood flowing through them. The lining of the stomach produces acids that attack germs in food that has been eaten. And the body's lymph system manufactures white blood cells whose job it is to attack and kill invading organisms.

The lymph system

The lymph system is a network of vessels that carries lymph, a watery fluid containing white blood cells, throughout the body. Lymph drains from the blood vessels and body tissues, carrying away waste products. The waste products, including germs, are filtered out of the lymph by small glands called lymph nodes. Within the lymph nodes, unwanted microorganisms are trapped, attacked, and destroyed by white blood cells. This is one of the body's primary and most efficient lines of defense.

The lymph system also manufactures antibodies. Antibodies are protective substances that the body produces in response to an invasion of a hostile organism. Antibodies counteract invading bacteria or viruses by inactivating them so that they are powerless. Antibodies that neutralize toxins (poisons) produced by bacteria are called antitoxins.

The body's production of white blood cells and antibodies in response to an invading disease organism is called the immune reaction. Immunity is the body's ability to resist an invasion of disease-causing bacteria and viruses. Once antibodies have been made to fight a certain microorganism, that germ no longer poses a threat to the body. That is why one attack of a disease often prevents that same disease from infecting the body again. The first attack causes antibodies to be produced, and these antibodies protect the system against subsequent attacks.

Immunization

Immunity can also be provided artificially. This is the underlying basis of immunization or vaccination. A vaccine is a preparation containing the offending organism — usually in a weakened form that will not cause the actual disease. When introduced into the body, the vaccine stimulates the body to produce antibodies against the disease. These antibodies remain in the system for a long time (often for life), and the body is thus prepared to resist the actual disease.

Medications

Besides vaccination, there are other measures that can be used to help the body's natural defenses fight off infectious diseases. Bacterial infections can often be conquered by medications called antibiotics. Antibiotics, too, are products of nature. They are substances produced by living microorganisms that kill other microorganisms. Penicillin, for example, comes from a living mold called *Penicillium*. Penicillin is one of the most commonly used antibiotics, along with streptomycin, tetracycline, and erythromycin. Each of these is effective against specific diseases. Antibiotics work either by destroying bacteria or by preventing their reproduction.

Sulfonamides (or sulfa drugs) are synthetic drugs that are also effective against infections. This type of drug is often prescribed for general infections of the body or for localized infections in the urinary and intestinal tracts.

Unfortunately, these medications do not attack viruses. Viruses, therefore, account for most of the infectious illnesses today, since no effective cures have been developed. However, some viral diseases can be prevented by immunization. There are vaccines for polio, measles, rubella (German measles), mumps, and some strains of influenza — all of which are viral diseases. Researchers are working on a vaccine for chicken pox and shingles; however, this vaccine is not yet available to the public.

Researchers are continually searching for new ways to help the body combat infectious diseases. Medical advances against these diseases have already been dramatic; not too many years ago infectious diseases were uncontrollable and thus a constant danger. The understanding and control of infections has been one of medicine's greatest accomplishments.

Disease-causing microorganisms and the more common infectious diseases are discussed in greater detail in the following pages.

Bacteria

Bacteria are one-celled microscopic organisms. Some exist as chains or clumps of single cells.

Some of the many different kinds of bacteria cause disease in humans and animals, but many others are beneficial. Bacteria dispose of organic waste, enrich the soil, and ferment wine and beer. They help make vinegar, cheese, and yogurt. In human beings certain beneficial bacteria live in the intestine where they help digestion.

Bacteria are different from viruses in that they are able to multiply on their own outside a living cell whereas viruses can grow and multiply only in living cells. Bacteria are different from two other causes of infection — protozoa (one-celled animals) and fungi (plant-like organisms)— in two ways: they have a primitive nucleus (center where their genetic material is kept) rather than a well-defined one with an enclosing membrane and chromosomes; and they reproduce simply by splitting in two, as opposed to reproducing by means of a complex process (mitosis) in which their genetic material is duplicated prior to splitting.

Types

There are two main types of bacteria, classified by shape:
- Rod-shaped bacteria are known as *bacilli*. They often have one or many waving projections known as flagella, which propel them about. Some form small thick-walled cells known as "spores," which can survive for long periods even after the "parent" bacteria have been killed by freezing, disinfectants, or other harsh forces. When condi-

tions are favorable, the spores come to life and generate new bacteria. Typhoid fever is caused by a bacillus bacterium.
- Round or egg-shaped bacteria are known as *cocci*. They occur singly (micrococcus), in chains (streptococcus — the cause of strep sore throat), in pairs (diplococcus), in irregular bunches (staphylococcus — the cause of many infections), and in cube-shaped packets (sarcina).

Bacteria also exist as comma-shaped organisms called vibrios (the organism responsible for cholera) and as spirals such as the spirochete of syphilis.

Aerobic or anaerobic

Another way to classify bacteria is by whether or not they can live in the open air. Those who can are called *aerobic*. Those who cannot are called *anaerobic*. Some can live either with or without air and are called *facultative*. Tetanus (lockjaw) is an example of a disease caused by an anaerobic bacterium that is common in the soil. It poses no danger to humans unless it enters the body through a wound, particularly a puncture wound such as that made by a dirty nail. The air then cannot get to the tetanus organisms to destroy them and so they multiply within the body unless the infected person is vaccinated against tetanus.

How bacteria are transmitted

Disease bacteria enter the body in many different ways. Those that cause pneumonia and sore throat are carried in droplets that an infected person sneezes or coughs into the air; the bacteria are then inhaled and deposited on the mucous membranes of the throat or lungs by a healthy person where they multiply and eventually cause disease unless checked by the body's immune system. The bacteria of intestinal diseases like cholera and typhoid can be transmitted by foods that have been handled by an infected person or by water tainted by body wastes from an infected individual. Another important route for infection is any break in the skin, which is why it is important to clean any cut in the skin as soon as possible.

What bacteria do

Once inside the body, disease bacteria do their damage in two main ways: by direct destruction of tissue or by producing toxins, or poisons, that poison remote parts of the body. Certain white blood cells known as lymphocytes produce substances called antitoxins, which neutralize the toxins of the bacteria, and antibodies, which are tailored to cause the destruction and removal of the invading bacteria (once created, the antibodies to a specific disease can persist in the body or be reproduced when needed creating continuous immunity to the invading disease organism — sometimes for life). Still other white blood cells known as phagocytes entrap and destroy the bacteria. The phagocytes literally eat and digest the bacteria.

Bubonic plague

Known as the "Black Death" in the Middle Ages, bubonic plague is said to have killed three-fourths of the population of Europe and Asia in 20 years during the fourteenth century. In recent times, only limited numbers of people have been infected, mostly in Southeast Asia. Rare cases have been reported in the west and southwestern United States.

Causes

The disease is caused by a bacterium, *Yersinia pestis,* which is carried by wild rodents including rats, mice, prairie dogs, and squirrels. Infected fleas transmit the disease from animals to humans by their bite. Infected humans with plague sores in their lungs can pass the bacteria to other people when they cough. The result of this direct infection of the lungs is known as *primary pneumonic plague.*

Symptoms

In bubonic plague transmitted by flea bite, chills and high fever occur after an incubation period— the time between exposure to the disease and the development of symptoms—that is usually two to five days (although it can vary from a few hours to 12 days). However, the chief symptom is the development of enlarged, painful lymph glands (called buboes) that fill with pus and may later rupture. The patient is often restless, delirious, and uncoordinated.

Without treatment, 60 percent of victims die, as the plague bacteria rapidly spread to affect all organs of the body, usually in three to five days.

Primary pneumonic plague kills even more quickly. Two or three days after being infected, the victim experiences high fever, chills, rapid heartbeat, and headache. A cough develops, with blood specks in the mucus discharge that eventually turns red and foamy. Breathing is rapid and irregular as pneumonia develops. Untreated persons usually die within 48 hours.

Treatment

Immediate treatment as soon as plague is suspected can reduce the death rate to below 5 percent. Streptomycin or tetracycline antibiotic is given around the clock every six hours for seven to ten days. Patients with primary pneumonic plague need to be isolated and watched closely. Anyone who is in contact with a plague victim should also be closely watched for the development of fever, cough, and painful lymph glands. Preventive antibiotics, to prevent the onset of the infection, should generally be given to those exposed to plague victims.

Prevention

To prevent plague, travelers to the parts of Southeast Asia and India, where bubonic plague is present, should be immunized with killed plague vaccine. Insect repellants help prevent bites from infected fleas, and rodent control can reduce the source of infection.

Candida albicans

Candida albicans is a fungus that is normally present on the skin and on membranes of the mouth, throat, intestines, and vagina. It becomes an infecting agent only when there is some change in the body environment that allows it to multiply and to invade tissue.

Causes

The most common cause may be the use of antibiotics that destroy beneficial as well as harmful microscopic organisms in the body and permit *Candida* to multiply in their place. The resulting infection is known as candidiasis, candidosis, or moniliasis. In the mouth, it becomes thrush; on the skin, an inflamed rash such as diaper rash; in the vagina, vaginitis, moniliasis, or yeast infection; and in or next to the nails, candidal onychomycosis or paronychia, respectively. It can also infect the esophagus (food pipe) and the digestive tract. In rare instances, when body resistance is low, *Candida albicans* enters the bloodstream and causes serious infection of the vital organs.

Those at risk

Drug addicts, diabetics, and patients receiving chemotherapy are especially at risk. So are those whose natural defenses are weakened by certain drugs meant to suppress the immune system (such as are given to those who receive transplanted organs). Pregnant women are often susceptible to moniliasis, and babies passing through an infected birth canal may develop thrush.

Symptoms and treatment

Symptoms and treatment for the various forms of *Candida* infection follow:

- Vaginitis is characterized by a white or yellow discharge, with inflammation of the wall of the vagina and of the vulva (external genital area). A white, cheesy substance may cling to the wall of the vagina. Occasionally the infection will be passed to the woman's mate, causing irritation, redness, and soreness of the head of the penis and sometimes a slight discharge. Treatment is with an antifungal drug, such as nystatin, inserted deep in the vagina and if necessary applied to the entire region around the entrance to the vagina. Both sexual partners should use the medication when one has a recurring infection.
- Thrush appears as creamy white or bluish white patches on the tongue, which is also inflamed and sometimes beefy red; on the lining of the mouth; or in the throat. Treatment is with nystatin oral solution or drops five times a day until all patches have disappeared and then for a few days afterward.
- Diaper rash caused by *Candida* can be treated by keeping the baby dry with frequent diaper changes. In severe cases, rubber pants and disposable diapers should be avoided.
- Nail infections appear as red, painful swelling around the nail; later, pus develops (paronychia). After the area is treated with hot compresses and drainage, if necessary, and the nail cut back, an antifungal lotion is applied. The nail itself may be involved (appearing hard, yellow, and dull), making treatment more difficult and perhaps requiring long-term oral drugs.
- Systemic infection (when infection enters the bloodstream and affects the kidneys, heart, lungs, eyes, or other organs) can result in high fever, chills, anemia, and sometimes a rash or shock. Disease in the lungs can cause bloody sputum (mucus discharge); in the kidneys, blood in the urine; in the brain, seizures; in the heart, murmurs and valve damage; and in the eye, pain and blurred vision. An antifungal medicine, is usually given intravenously (into the vein).

In all cases, the underlying condition that caused the outbreak of *Candida* needs to be removed, if possible. This may mean stopping the use of antibiotics or controlling diabetes. The same approach is used to prevent future infections.

Chicken pox

Chicken pox is an extremely contagious disease that is characterized by a blistery rash. It occurs most frequently in children between the ages of five and eight with less than 20 percent of the cases in the United States affecting people over 15 years old. Chicken pox is transmitted so easily that almost everyone gets the disease at some time.

Chicken pox is caused by infection with the virus varicella zoster. The virus creates symptoms that can be mild or severe depending upon the infected person's age.

Anyone can contract chicken pox by touching either an infected person's blisters or anything that is contaminated by them. Chicken pox is also thought to be airborne since it may be caught from an infected person before the rash develops. Yet, some researchers contend that one or two spots from the disease may be present before the rash is recognized on the body. Another way to get chicken pox is by exposure to shingles, which is a nerve disorder caused by the same virus. The incubation period for chicken pox—the time between being exposed to the illness and actually showing symptoms — is 10 to 21 days. Chicken pox is contagious for about six to eight days after the rash appears.

Symptoms

The first symptom of chicken pox is usually a rash that can be very itchy. It begins as small, red spots on the trunk. Within hours, the spots become larger, fluid-filled blisters and begin spreading out from the trunk to the face, scalp, arms, and legs. Over the

The first symptom of chicken pox is an itchy rash that begins as small red spots on the trunk. Within hours the spots begin spreading out from the trunk to the face, scalp, arms, and legs.

next few days, the blisters continue to fill with pus, burst, and then form a scab or crust. New spots appear periodically during a two- to six-day period. They may occasionally spread to the soles and palms. The rash may even affect the eyes, mouth, throat, vagina, and rectum.

Another main symptom is a mild fever (101°F to 103°F) that rises and disappears as the rash comes and goes. Some children have a slight fever and feel sluggish a few days before the rash begins. However, this warning is more common in adults. Adults usually have higher fevers, a more severe rash, headaches and muscle aches, and they take longer to recuperate than children. Recovery from all symptoms takes ten days to two weeks.

Complications

Complications with chicken pox seldom develop in otherwise healthy people. The most common complication is infection of the blisters. The blister is scratched, and bacteria enter where the skin breaks. In some instances, the rash spreads to the eyes and causes pain and possible damage. Generally, the chicken pox rash heals without leaving scars unless scratched or infected. A doctor should be consulted if breathing problems, high fever, extreme drowsiness, severe headache, vomiting, or unsteadiness occur within the course of the disease or within several weeks of recovery. These symptoms may indicate further complications.

Treatment

Since there is no known cure for chicken pox, treatment constitutes reducing the effects of the symptoms. Soothing lotion, such as calamine lotion, lessens itchiness. Baths in warm (not hot) water keep the skin clean and reduce risk of infection in the rash. Baths also destroy virus in water, thereby controlling spread of the rash. If itching is severe, fingernails should be trimmed and gloves worn at night to minimize unconscious scratching. Children may

need to wear gloves all day for the duration of the rash.

Although it has not been proven that aspirin causes or promotes Reye's syndrome, a type of brain inflammation, it is recommended that aspirin not be given to a child with chicken pox. A doctor can suggest an aspirin substitute if needed.

Prevention

Researchers are trying to develop a vaccine to prevent chicken pox, but there is nothing available as yet. Although almost everyone contracts the disease once, most people do not get it again. The same organism that causes chicken pox causes the body to manufacture antibodies to combat the virus. Antibodies prevent the disease from recurring. Nevertheless, the same virus may cause shingles later in life. Why shingles occurs in some people many years after they have had chicken pox is not understood.

Coxsackie viruses

Coxsackie is the term for a group of viruses that cause a wide variety of usually brief illnesses particularly common to children. Together with two other groups of viruses that have been isolated from the gastrointestinal system, the echoviruses and the polioviruses, they are known as enteroviruses (entero means "intestine"). Coxsackie virus infections occur most often in summer and fall and can be spread by means of the mouth or infected human feces (solid waste). There are 24 group A coxsackie viruses and six group B coxsackie viruses. The following diseases are among those frequently caused by coxsackie viruses (some are also caused by other enteroviruses).

Herpangina

An epidemic disease in infants and young children, herpangina is marked by sudden high fever, headache, sore throat, vomiting, and grayish spots on the soft palate (rear roof of the mouth), tonsils, or throat that become shallow ulcers and heal in three to six days.

Hand, foot, and mouth disease

Common in young children, this is similar to herpangina except that little blisters erupt over all of the mucous membrane in the mouth and also on the hands, feet, and sometimes in the diaper area.

Epidemic pleurodynia (Bornholm disease)

Sudden, recurrent pains in the lower chest (or abdomen in 50 percent of the cases) signal the onset of this illness, often accompanied by fever, headache, nausea, abdominal tenderness, and sore throat. There may be muscle swelling of the involved area, which may be painful to the touch. Occasionally the disease spreads to cause pleuritis (inflammation of the membrane sac surrounding the lungs and lining of the chest cavity), pericarditis (inflammation of the sac around the heart), and, rarely, aseptic meningitis (see below).

Aseptic meningitis

This inflammation of the membrane covering the brain causes headache, pain and stiffness in the neck and back, fever, nausea, vomiting, drowsiness, a general sick feeling, and, rarely, muscle paralysis. Occasionally death results in newborns, but most patients recover in a week or so.

Paralytic disease

Various coxsackie viruses, echoviruses, and polioviruses produce a muscle weakness or paralysis that is similar to the paralysis of polio and is treated in the same manner. However, the paralysis is usually temporary.

Respiratory disease

Coxsackie and other enteroviruses appear to cause respiratory illnesses with head cold, fever, sore throat, and sometimes vomiting and diarrhea.

Rubella-like rash

A mild rash like that of rubella (German measles), but lasting longer, this usually occurs in epidemic form and only on the face, neck, and chest. Fever is common and meningitis can develop, but usually this is a mild disease.

Myocarditis and pericarditis

Heart failure in newborns may result from infection of the heart muscle by coxsackie or echoviruses transmitted to the baby before birth by the mother. Myocarditis (infection of the heart muscle) or pericarditis (infection of the sac around the heart) in older children and in adults may also be caused by a coxsackie virus, but patients usually make a complete recovery. (However, congestive heart failure can occur in the acute phase of these diseases.)

Although they produce a great deal of temporary discomfort, the coxsackie viruses generally do not cause lasting illness. In general the only treatment necessary is to make the patient as comfortable as possible, with plenty of liquids, bed rest, lukewarm sponge baths, and drugs such as acetaminophen to control fever until the illness has passed. Careful handwashing and proper disposal of human wastes can help prevent the spread of infection.

Diphtheria

Diphtheria is a sudden, severe, and highly contagious disease that primarily affects the tonsils, upper airways, and larynx (voice box) and is marked by formation of a membrane on the infected tissue. Complications can include inflammation of the heart (myocar-ditis), sometimes resulting in heart failure, and temporary neuritis (nerve inflammation). Diphtheria-type bacteria also infect skin wounds, but cannot invade intact skin.

Cause

Diphtheria is caused by a bacterium known as *Corynebacterium diphtheriae*, which is transmitted through the air or otherwise on droplets of moisture from the throats and noses of infected persons. It is most common during the colder months when schools are in session and people are in closer contact. Frequently, the bacteria are transmitted by carriers—people who have no symptoms and do not even know they harbor the disease. The incubation period (the time between exposure to the infection and appearance of the first symptom) is only one to seven days. Diphtheria bacteria destroy the outer layer of the mucous membrane of the throat or larynx; the slush of dead cells, bacteria, and white blood cells remaining coagulates to form the membrane that is the chief sign of the disease.

Symptoms

Symptoms include a mild sore throat, hoarseness, a rasping cough, pain on swallowing, and a mild fever. Children may be nauseous, vomit, and have chills and headache as well as fever and other symptoms. The membrane that forms is typically tough, adheres tightly, and causes bleeding if removed. It appears in patches and can vary from yellowish to grayish green or dirty gray (the most common color). Some people have little or no characteristic membrane. If the membrane extends from the throat to the trachea (windpipe), larynx, or bronchi (air tubes in the lungs), it can become detached and obstruct the passage partially or completely, choking off the air supply. Signs of this life-threatening emergency are rapid breathing, shrill breathing sounds, and blue lips and fingertips. A narrowed air passage is also caused by edema (swelling of fluid-filled tissue) in the lining of the larynx and throat.

Treatment

Treatment is with diphtheria antitoxin (a solution of refined and concentrated protective antibodies taken from the blood of horses that have been immunized against the poisons created by the diphtheria bacteria. This should be done at once, after a skin test to determine that the patient is not allergic to horse serum (blood fluid). (A patient who is found to be allergic is desensitized with great caution by a series of diluted doses of antitoxin.) After the antitoxin is given, antibiotics such as penicillin or erythromycin are given for at least a week to eliminate the diphtheria organisms. The patient remains isolated (no visitors) until two cultures (24 hours apart) of the nose, throat, or other involved area indicate that the infection is gone.

Because of the possible severe or even fatal complications of diphtheria, patients with symptoms need to be placed in a hospital intensive care unit for complete rest and careful attention. There must be constant observation for signs of airway obstruction, along with access to facilities for performing an immediate tracheostomy (creation of a hole in the neck to breathe through), to pass an air tube down into the lungs and to supply oxygen as needed. Frequent checking of the heart and nervous system is needed to identify complications. In severe cases, these can include heart irregularities, cardiac arrest (heart stoppage), and early and late nervous system disorders such as swallowing difficulty caused by paralysis of swallowing muscles due to inflammation of their nerves.

Those who have been close contacts of the patient and who have not been immunized should receive throat cultures and be immunized with vaccine. These people should be watched carefully for the development of symptoms and be given antitoxin should symptoms occur. Another approach is to give antitoxin immediately (after allergy is excluded). In people who have been immunized, a booster of vaccine will be sufficient. All contacts of patients with diphtheria should have cultures done of their nose, throat, and/or open wounds. Carriers of diphtheria should be given seven to ten days of an appropriate antibiotic (usually erythromycin) and recultured. If the organism is still present, another course of drug therapy is given. If this fails, tonsillectomy may be needed.

Prevention

Fortunately, widespread immunization has made diphtheria a rare disease. To maintain this status, children should be immunized in a series of shots (usually combined diphtheria-tetanus-pertussis—DTP) beginning in infancy.

Gonorrhea

Gonorrhea is the most frequently reported sexually transmitted disease, also known as venereal disease. It is a highly contagious infection spread primarily through direct sexual contact.

Gonorrhea predominantly affects the penis in men, the vagina in women, and the throat and anus (opening from the intestine to the outside) in both sexes. Left untreated, it can lead to a generalized blood infection, sterility (inability to conceive children), arthritis, and heart trouble. Additionally, in men it can spread throughout the prostate gland and the male duct system, causing painful inflammation.

Gonorrhea can also lead to eye infections if the eyes come in contact with the genital secretions — for instance, if the person rubs the eyes after handling the infected genital organs. Moreover, during the birth process, a baby passes through the mother's potentially infected birth canal; most states therefore require that a few drops of silver nitrate or penicillin be placed in the eyes of all newborns to prevent infection and possible blindness.

Causes

Gonorrhea is caused by a bacterial infection and is spread by direct sexual contact with an infected person.

Symptoms

In females, this disease may exist entirely without symptoms, but in many cases it is marked by a discharge from the vagina and urethra; frequent, painful urination; cloudy urine; vomiting; and diarrhea. Gonorrhea often leads to pelvic inflammatory disease (PID), which, in turn, often causes sterility. (PID results when an infection in the lower reproductive or urinary tract moves to the fallopian tubes, forming scar tissue and blocking the tubes, thereby preventing conception. Its symptoms are lower abdominal pain, fever, chills, and vaginal discharge.)

The symptoms of gonorrhea in men are a yellowish discharge from the penis within two to ten days of exposure to the disease, accompanied by painful and burning urination.

Gonorrhea of the anus is marked by an often bloody or mucus-filled discharge from the anus and pain during bowel movements. Gonorrhea of the throat may have no noticeable symptoms or may reveal itself only by a scratchy, sore throat.

Diagnosis

Diagnosis is accomplished by taking a "smear" (sample) of the discharge, examining it under a microscope to identify the gonorrhea bacterium, and confirming the diagnosis with a culture of the smear (a technique in which the sample is placed in a special substance that encourages the growth of bacteria).

Treatment

Gonorrhea is usually treated with penicillin, either injected or taken orally. A synthetic antibiotic is prescribed for those who are allergic to penicillin or who have contracted a penicillin-resistant strain of gonorrhea.

While under treatment, the patient should abstain from sexual activity until further tests have confirmed that gonorrhea is no longer present. This is usually done one week after treatment begins and sometimes again two weeks later. If signs of the disease are still present, drug therapy can be reinstated with the same antibiotic at higher dosages or perhaps with a different antibiotic.

Another sexually transmitted disease called nongonococcal urethritis (NGU) sometimes occurs simultaneously with gonorrhea, but NGU is not affected by penicillin. So if symptoms persist after regular treatment for gonorrhea, it may be that the gonorrhea is cleared up but NGU also is present and should be treated with another antibiotic, often tetracycline.

Treatment of gonorrhea, as well as of all forms of sexually transmitted disease, requires that every sexual partner of the infected person also be examined and treated if necessary. In addition, men being treated for gonorrhea should avoid alcoholic beverages, as it has been recently shown that drinking may increase the chance of developing an inflammation of the urethra.

Prevention

Gonorrhea can be prevented, obviously, by avoiding sexual contact with someone who has the disease. However, since this is not always possible, it should be remembered that the chances of contracting the disease increase with the number of different sexual partners a person has, so limiting the number of partners may be beneficial in preventing gonorrhea as well as other sexually transmitted diseases.

Herpes

Herpes is a sexually transmitted disease, perhaps even more widespread than gonorrhea. A sexually transmitted disease, also known as venereal disease, is a highly contagious illness spread primarily through direct sexual contact.

Herpes can be treated but not cured. Its symptoms appear briefly, then disappear, and the disease lies dormant in the nerve cells until it is reactivated by stress or illness. It is contagious only during these active periods. Persons taking drugs that suppress the body's immune system (for instance, cancer or organ transplant patients) are at a higher risk of developing herpes because their bodies are in a weakened state. There is also some evidence that links herpes with a higher rate of cancer of the cervix in women.

Although herpes is spread primarily by direct sexual contact, it can also be transmitted to an infant during childbirth, causing brain damage or death. Thus, if a woman shows signs of the active disease while in labor, the baby will be delivered by cesarean section (delivery through a surgical incision in the walls of the uterus and abdomen) rather than through the vagina where the herpes blisters may be present.

Cause

Herpes is caused by an infection with the herpes simplex type 2 virus, similar to, but not the same as, the virus that causes cold sores and fever blisters on the lips.

Symptoms

The predominant symptom of herpes is the outbreak of painful, itching blisters filled with fluid on and around the external sexual organs. Females may have a vaginal discharge. Symptoms vaguely similar to those of the flu may accompany these outbreaks.

The blisters will disappear without treatment in about two to ten days, but the virus will remain, lying dormant among clusters of nerve cells until another outbreak is triggered by stress, a cold, fever, or, in women, menstruation. Many patients can anticipate an outbreak by a warning sign, a tingling sensation called a "prodrome" of the approaching illness. Herpes is contagious only during actual outbreaks, so sexual activity should be avoided while symptoms are present.

Diagnosis

Diagnosis of herpes is accomplished by microscopic examination and culture of the fluid contained in the blisters.

Treatment

Herpes cannot be cured as can other sexually transmitted diseases, because any medication that will attack the virus while it lies dormant in the nerve cells will also damage the nerve cells. However, there is treatment for acute outbreaks now available that involves the use of either the antiviral drug acyclovir or laser therapy, both of which will heal blisters, reduce pain, and most importantly, kill large numbers of the herpes virus. Acyclovir has also been found to reduce the reproduction of the virus in initial outbreaks, thus possibly lessening the number of subsequent outbreaks. It should be noted, however, that to be effective, laser therapy must be started immediately after the first sores appear. In addition, herpes, as well as all forms of sexually transmitted disease, requires that every sexual partner of the infected person be examined and treated if necessary.

Prevention

Herpes can be prevented, obviously, by avoiding sexual contact with an infected person whose disease is in its active period. It should be remembered that the chances of contracting this or any other sexually transmitted disease increase with the number of different sexual partners a person has. Therefore, limiting the number of partners can be somewhat beneficial in preventing herpes.

Histoplasmosis

Histoplasmosis is an infection following the inhalation of spores from the fungus *Histoplasma capsulatum*. The parts of the body principally affected are the lungs, the liver, and the spleen.

Cause

The *Histoplasma capsulatum* spore is found in soil and in the air. There is no practical defense against breathing the spores. Development of symptoms seems to be a matter of individual immune system response.

Symptoms

In most instances, histoplasmosis does not reach a point that symptoms appear. People may have the disease, but, because of the action of their immune system, never have enough damage to make the symptoms noticeable, much less create an acute condi-

tion. However, when symptoms do appear, they can be serious, especially if left unattended. The most common symptoms are as follows:

- Acute pneumonia, which is an inflammation of the lungs, accompanied by the escape of fluid and/or debris in the lungs, and severe interruption of normal lung functions
- Influenza-like illnesses, with lethargy, cough, fever, and lung involvement
- Enlargement of the liver and the spleen, with accompanying interruptions in the normal functions of those organs
- The development of fibrous scar tissue in affected organs

Histoplasmosis can become inactive, and then be reactivated at a later date. In cases of reactivated histoplasmosis, the lungs, meninges (linings of the brain and spinal cord), heart, peritoneum (lining of the abdominal cavity), and the adrenal glands can be affected, with interruptions of the normal functioning of these organs.

Probably most affected people have histoplasmosis in a dormant form (within their bodies, but not at a stage where symptoms are evident). Fatalities occur only in cases of massive infection (which also implies massive breakdown of the body's immune system, or an immune system that is not functioning properly).

Diagnosis

Treatment for histoplasmosis begins with diagnosis. The best procedure is to cultivate growths of the *Histoplasma capsulatum* from tissue or fluid samples. Another method is by noting the rise in the body's antibody production, the protective substances produced by the body to resist the disease.

Treatment

Drug therapy is the usual treatment of chronic disease. Drugs will help control the disease, but appear to have little effect on the fibrous scarring that often accompanies advanced cases.

Prevention

There is no known preventive against histoplasmosis.

Infectious mononucleosis

Infectious mononucleosis, or mono, is a contagious viral disease that initially attacks the lymph glands in the neck and the throat. When these glands, which normally manufacture white blood cells that fight invading organisms, are weakened, sore throat, swollen glands, and fever result.

Description

Mono is caused by a virus named Epstein-Barr virus after the scientists that first identified it in the mid-1960s. The virus enters the lymph glands and attacks the lymphocytes, the white blood cells manufactured in the lymph glands. As the white blood cells come into contact with the virus, they change shape and multiply. At first there are no symptoms, because it takes several weeks before enough of the altered cells can accumulate to generate a reaction. Gradually, however, symptoms appear. First, there is a mild sore throat, sluggishness, and fever. The symptoms worsen as the body tries to fight the infection by creating more white blood cells. Finally, symptoms diminish and disappear after about six to eight weeks.

Mono spreads by contact with moisture from the mouth and throat of the infected person. Kissing, sharing drinking glasses and toothbrushes, or touching anything that has been near the mouth of an infected person transmits the disease.

Those at risk

Teenagers and young adults seem most susceptible to mono. Sometimes, children become infected, but the disease seldom affects anyone over 35.

Symptoms

In all cases, the infection develops so slowly with such mild symptoms that it may be initially indistinguishable from a cold or the flu. However, a sore throat that lasts two weeks or more; swollen glands around the neck, throat, armpit, and groin; a persistent fever (usually about 102°F); and tiredness indicate mono. Mono symptoms can be mild or so severe that throat pain can impede swallowing and fever may reach 105°F. Some people also experience a rash, eye pain, or discomfort in bright light (photophobia).

Complications

Most mono runs an uncomplicated course. Occasionally, however, the infection spreads to other parts of the body besides the throat and lymph glands. For example, mono may lead to hepatitis, an infection of the liver. Jaundice, a symptom of this complication, appears as a yellow discoloration of the skin and whites of the eyes. Another sign the infection has traveled is pain or tenderness in the abdomen. This discomfort may mean a swollen spleen (part of the lymph system) that could rupture or burst. Any of these symptoms should be reported to a physician for immediate attention.

Diagnosis

When diagnosing infectious mononucleosis, a doctor takes two blood samples, two weeks apart. The first sample determines if there is an excessive number of white blood cells, whether they are abnormally shaped because of the virus, and if the body is making antibodies (protective substances) to fight the Epstein-Barr virus. The second blood test shows whether the white blood cell count is still high, indicating disease is present. It is only completed if the first test shows signs of the disease.

Treatment

Once mono is confirmed, standard treatment for its symptoms is prescribed. Antibiotics are ineffective since the disease is caused by a virus that does not respond to antibiotics. As long as there are no complications, the best treatment is to stay in bed, drink plenty of liquids until the temperature returns to normal, and then gradually resume normal activities as strength returns.

Antibiotics may be indicated if a bacterial infection develops in addition to mono because bacteria do respond to antibiotics. In severe cases, corticosteroid drugs that reduce swelling are prescribed. If the spleen is swollen, a doctor may recommend avoiding strenuous activities, such as lifting or pushing, that may cause sudden rupture of the spleen. Hospitalization is necessary for severe complications.

Most people recover in six to eight weeks, but some cases take as long as six months for complete recovery. A tired feeling, which may include depression, is the last symptom to disappear. Mono may return in a milder form of the initial infection within a few months. Fortunately, it almost never reappears after a year.

Influenza

Influenza, more commonly called the flu, is a contagious disease that is accompanied by respiratory problems and fever. It is an uncomfortable illness that is usually not dangerous to otherwise healthy people.

Causes

Two types of viruses cause influenza: influenza A and influenza B. Each type encompasses several different strains that are named for the place where they were first identified, for example, "Hong Kong flu" and "Russian flu."

The unusual characteristic about flu virus is that once one strain spreads throughout a population, the virus strain changes in structure. Therefore, it becomes a new strain carrying a new form of influenza. The antibodies, or protective substances, produced by the body to combat the virus no longer work against recurrence of that virus because the virus has taken on different qualities. Scientists are generally able to predict what type of altered virus to expect each year, but about every ten years an entirely new strain appears.

Because influenza is thought to be transmitted by airborne particles from an infected person's respiratory system, large numbers of people in a community or even in a country can easily contract the disease in a relatively short period of time. Understandably, crowds encourage transmission of the flu. In addition, since flu spreads most easily where temperatures and humidity are low, most cases of influenza occur in fall or winter.

Symptoms

Once the body is exposed to the virus, flu symptoms develop in one to three days. Some people acquire symptoms in as short a time as 18 hours. Fever, chills, headache, muscle aches, and total exhaustion can begin suddenly. Although fevers of 100°F to 104°F are more common, body temperature may rise to 106°F.

Frequently, people experience a dry cough and runny or congested nose as their initial symptoms begin to subside. These respiratory symptoms worsen and remain for three to four days. The cough, weariness, and sometimes depression may persist for two weeks or more after the other symptoms disappear.

Complications

The most common complications result from the virus settling in parts of the respiratory system. For example, adults may get pneumonia (infection of the lungs) and children may get croup (infection of the larynx). If the patient has extreme difficulty in breathing, blood in the coughed-up phlegm, bluish skin, or a bark-like cough, a physician should be consulted immediately to prevent further complications.

One life-threatening complication that affects children between the ages of two and 16 years is Reye's syndrome. It is a type of inflammation of the brain (encephalitis) that is accompanied by deteriorating changes in the liver.

Treatment

Influenza cannot be cured, but usually only treated by relieving symptoms. However, there is an antiviral drug that is effective against influenza A virus symptoms and in some cases the disease itself. The drug can produce unpleasant side effects, so physicians prescribe it only when a patient is susceptible to additional complications.

In most cases, treatment for flu is the same as treatment for a bad cold or fever. Physicians recommend bed rest, extra fluids, and an aspirin substitute to reduce fever and muscle aches. Aspirin is not recommended for a child with flu. Although it has not been proven that aspirin causes or promotes Reye's syndrome, it is recommended that aspirin not be given to a child with influenza. Acetaminophen, however, has not been linked to Reye's syndrome and can be used. Nasal sprays or drops, when used sparingly so nasal tissues are not damaged, and cough medicines help relieve cold-like symptoms. A vaporizer in the patient's room that adds moisture to the air relieves congestion.

Prevention

Each year, researchers prepare an influenza vaccine in an attempt to prevent spread of the virus. The vaccine is composed of several different virus strains and provides protection against influenza from these strains. Regrettably, protection is not necessarily afforded against new or different strains. Vaccines are typically between 67 and 92 percent effective.

Some people have reactions from the vaccine that range from inflammation at the site of the injection to mild flu symptoms. On rare occasions, nervous system disorders result. Children receive injections in two smaller doses four to eight weeks apart to lessen chances of any reactions.

Measles

Measles is a contagious disease that mainly affects the respiratory system, skin, and eyes. It was once considered one of the more dangerous childhood diseases because the threat of serious complications was so great. Fortunately, development of a vaccine to prevent measles has drastically reduced its occurrence.

Causes

Another name for measles is rubeola. Rubeola is caused by a virus that invades the body and infects living cells. The virus comes from the respiratory system of an infected person and is spread via droplets of moisture that travel through the air. Some researchers contend that the virus enters the body through the eyes.

Incubation period for measles— the time between being exposed to the illness and actually showing symptoms — is eight to 12 days.

The measles rash—dark red spots that blend together as they spread — usually begins on the face, neck, and behind the ears and then spreads over the body as far as the knees.

During this time the infected person is contagious up to four days before symptoms begin and up to six days after the rash develops.

Symptoms

Measles usually begins much like a cold with runny nose, nasal congestion, sneezing, a dry cough, and fever between 102°F and 104°F. After three or four days, eyes may become sensitive to bright light as they grow red and swollen. Then the fever drops. At this time, red spots with tiny white centers appear in the mouth. These are called Koplik's spots.

By the fourth or fifth day, the fever increases again, and a rash appears. The rash usually starts on the face, neck, and behind the ears before spreading to the rest of the body. As the spots multiply, they grow larger, become raised, and sometimes blend together. Their color turns dark red and then brown before the skin begins to fall off in small flakes. This process takes about one week after the rash first emerges, although skin discoloration can last as long as two weeks. Other symptoms usually disappear within seven to ten days from the start of the disease.

Complications

Breathing problems, increased coughing, earache, or extreme drowsiness may indicate complications that warrant consulting a doctor immediately. The more serious complications are pneumonia (infection of the lungs) and encephalitis (inflammation of the brain). Additionally, subacute sclerosing panencephalitis (SSPE), a rare but often fatal disease of the brain, has been linked to measles. Severe ear infections can also result, particularly in young children. In addition, bronchitis, laryngitis, and swollen neck glands can complicate measles and make the course of the illness last longer or even return after apparent recovery.

Diagnosis

Generally, physicians diagnose measles by the initial symptoms.

To confirm diagnosis, nasal discharge, blood, or urine can be tested for signs of the virus.

Treatment

Measles, being caused by a virus, does not respond to antibiotics. For this reason, treatment focuses upon relieving uncomfortable symptoms. A vaporizer in the patient's room eases cold-like symptoms by adding moisture to the air. If the eyes are irritated, warm compresses may relieve the inflammation. Also, dim lights are easier on the eyes. When washing, soaps that may irritate the skin should not be used. A doctor may suggest adding baking soda to bath water or applying a soothing lotion, such as calamine lotion, to the rash to relieve itching. Most physicians recommend an aspirin substitute to reduce fever.

Prevention

Today, measles has been almost eliminated because of a vaccine given to children as an injection around 15 months of age. The vaccine, which is prepared from measles virus, stimulates antibody (protective substance in cells) action within the body to produce immunity or resistance to the disease. A low vaccine effectiveness rate in very young children is the reason that babies are not vaccinated before 15 months of age. Most babies under six months of age already have immunity that they acquired from their mothers before birth. Should a baby be exposed to measles, however, a doctor should be consulted. Measles is dangerous for anyone under three years of age or for anyone with chronic (long-term) disease.

Mumps

Mumps is a highly contagious viral disease that is usually contracted during childhood. More than 85 percent of the cases occur before age 15, especially between six and ten years of age.

Cause

Mumps is caused by a virus that attacks cells of the parotid (saliva) glands. This invasion results in painful swelling of the face beneath the ear along the jawline. Mumps virus spreads by contact with airborne moisture from the infected person's nose or throat. Sometimes, the infection comes from someone who either has the disease without symptoms or who is not yet aware of the symptoms. The disease occurs most often during spring months, though it can happen any time of year.

Symptoms

Symptoms can be so mild that they are nonexistent or they can be very severe. Fever (101°F to 103°F), headache, and loss of appetite usually develop first, followed by earache. Then the characteristic swelling of the saliva glands appears. Swelling may start on one side of the face

Parotid gland

Outline of jaw bone

Mumps is caused by a virus that infects the salivary glands, especially the parotid gland. The infection causes a painful swelling of the face in front of the ear.

and then appear on the other side within a few days. Sometimes, however, only one side swells. The inflammation may cause soreness and difficulty in eating or swallowing.

Other glands, such as the sex glands, may become swollen as well. Boys who have one or both testes inflamed may be in considerable pain. The affected testicle may shrink somewhat, but it always returns to normal size in time. Medically, this condition is known as orchitis. Contrary to popular belief, mumps uncommonly leads to sterility in males. Girls may have swelling in the ovaries (female sex organs), but there is seldom any severe discomfort. In addition, swelling may occur in other glands and organs including the breasts, other saliva glands, liver, and the brain.

Complications

Although mumps can be unpleasant, it rarely has long-term complications. If they do occur, encephalitis (inflammation of the brain) is the most dangerous complication of mumps because it carries the risk of death. Another possible result of mumps encephalitis is hearing loss or even deafness. However, hearing may return to normal after several months. A milder form of brain complication is meningoencephalitis (inflammation of the brain or its covering, the meninges). This disease causes stiff neck, headache, high fever, drowsiness, bright light sensitivity, and possible delirium — all symptoms that usually disappear without damage to the brain.

Pancreatitis, or inflammation of the pancreas, can also result from mumps. Symptoms of this complication are stomach pain, vomiting, chills, fever, and extreme weakness. Although these signs usually vanish and leave no damage, diabetes can result in rare cases. Other complications of mumps include nerve inflammation, heart problems, and nervous system disorders — all usually temporary.

Diagnosis

A doctor diagnoses mumps by examining the characteristic form and texture of the swollen parotid glands. Boys may have swelling and tenderness in the testes. Exposure to the disease is also a clue. Incubation — time between exposure to the virus and signs of symptoms — is 14 to 21 days. If mumps is suspected, secretions from the saliva glands can be tested for mumps virus.

Treatment

Treatment for mumps involves relieving discomfort of the symptoms, since there is no cure for the disease. Bed rest is usually not necessary. Soft foods and liquids may be easier to swallow. However, fruit juices with high acid content, like orange or grapefruit, may sting.

If glands are severely swollen, a physician may prescribe painkilling drugs. Steroid drugs may be recommended for men or boys with extremely swollen testes, but these drugs may prove ineffective. Warm or cold compresses including an ice pack may relieve some pain. Most mumps symptoms disappear within about ten days.

Prevention

There is a vaccine that is 95 percent effective in preventing mumps. The vaccine encourages antibodies (protective substances) to be produced by the body to resist the disease. Mumps vaccine is usually combined with measles and rubella (German measles) vaccines and given to children as a shot during their second year.

Reiter's syndrome

Reiter's syndrome is a simultaneous occurrence of *urethritis* (an inflammation of the urethra, the tube from the bladder to the outside of the body), *conjunctivitis* (an inflammation of the conjunctiva, which is the membrane that covers the front of the eyeball and the insides of the eyelids), and *arthritis* (an inflammation of the joints). It is a condition that affects males more often than females. Diarrhea occurs in some cases.

Cause

The syndrome develops from sexual transmission, but is not caused by the gonorrhea microbe. Instead, it is thought that Reiter's syndrome is caused by a virus-like organism called chlamydia.

Symptoms

Reiter's syndrome exhibits multiple symptoms, any one of which might be mistaken for another disease. The conjunctiva becomes inflamed, with corresponding discomfort around the eyes. The intestinal tract exhibits the symptoms of diarrhea, with a corresponding loss of water (which should be replaced immediately). Urethritis causes discomfort during urination. Arthritic symptoms appear, with swelling and pain in the joints. Furthermore, most victims develop fever, lesions (on the palms of the hands, the soles of the feet, the trunk, and the mouth), watery growths on the skin, and iritis (an inflammation of the iris, the part of the eye that gives it color).

Treatment

Treatment for Reiter's syndrome is similar to that for rheumatoid arthritis: aspirin or, if aspirin is ineffective, anti-inflammatory drugs such as indomethacin or phenylbutazone. The antibiotic tetracycline may help control the urethritis. Conjunctivitis may be treated with cortisone eyedrops.

Rubella

Rubella, or German measles, is a relatively mild viral infection with cold-like symptoms and a short-lived rash. The disease is contagious, but it is usually not dangerous. One exception is when rubella infects pregnant women. In this instance, the virus can also affect the unborn child, causing serious long-term problems. However, rubella outbreaks are infrequent since the development of a vaccine to prevent the illness.

Cause

Rubella results from a virus that invades the cells of the body. The virus spreads from one person to another by contact with airborne moisture from the infected person's respiratory system. An infected person can spread the virus as early as one week before the rash appears and as late as five days after the rash fades. A baby with congenital rubella syndrome can transfer the virus until the child is about 12 to 18 months old. Although instances of second infections have been reported, rubella seldom occurs twice in the same person.

Complications

Although rubella is generally a mild infection, some complications can arise. Encephalitis, or inflammation of the brain, occurs in one in 5000 cases. Thrombocytopenic purpura, a blood disease, can prove fatal when it accompanies rubella. High or prolonged fever and extreme fatigue should be reported to a physician to prevent further complications.

Another serious complication of rubella is congenital rubella syndrome, or rubella infection that is present at birth. Here the pregnant woman transmits the disease to the fetus (unborn child) during pregnancy. Rubella virus may cause one or more serious organic and growth disorders, particularly if contracted during the first three months of pregnancy when the fetus is forming. The most common problems include congenital heart defects, hearing and vision problems, blood disorders, and

The light pink rubella rash first appears on the face and the neck and then gradually spreads over most of the body.

Symptoms

The first symptoms of rubella are runny nose, swollen neck glands, and low fever (up to 101° F). About two days after these signs, a rash with very small red or pink spots appears on the face and neck. The spots are flat initially. Then they become slightly raised and fade within a day or two. As the first spots fade, more spots develop until the rash gradually spreads over most of the body. The rash lasts only two to three days, but swollen glands may persist for as long as a week. All other symptoms usually disappear by then. When there is joint pain, discomfort may last another week.

Diagnosis

Under normal circumstances, rubella is difficult to diagnose because the symptoms are so mild and variable. Sometimes a rash is absent and the disease resembles a cold. Other cases may be so severe that the infection may be confused with measles. A doctor identifies the virus by taking a blood test and tracing any history of exposure to the disease. Incubation, or time between contact with the virus and beginning of symptoms, is 14 to 21 days.

Treatment

Most patients require little or no treatment for rubella because the symptoms are so mild. Aspirin or an aspirin substitute may afford relief for any joint pain. Otherwise, drugs are not needed. Some patients may want bed rest, but most people feel well enough to be somewhat active.

Prevention

Rubella rarely occurs now because children routinely receive rubella vaccine at about 15 months of age. The vaccine is combined with measles or mumps vaccine in one injection. Rubella vaccine works in the body to stimulate antibodies (protective substances) that fight the disease.

Women who want to become pregnant should take a blood test to determine whether they are already immune (resistant) to the disease. If not, they too, can receive a vaccination. Vaccinations are not recommended for pregnant women because of a risk of infection to the fetus. For this reason also, doctors caution women to wait at least three months after vaccination before becoming pregnant.

Scarlet fever

Scarlet fever (also known as *scarlatina*) is a highly contagious childhood bacterial disease caused by Group A hemolytic streptococci.

Symptoms

The symptoms of scarlet fever include fever; sore throat; widespread scarlet rash beginning in the armpits and groin and spreading to the neck, chest, back, extremities, and even the tongue; and peeling and scaling of the skin, even on the palms and soles. The incubation period is two to four days.

Treatment

Scarlet fever in the past was an often fatal disease, but today it is easily treated with penicillin and complications are rare. In addition to the penicillin, bed rest and a nourishing diet with plenty of fluids help speed recuperation.

Septicemia

Septicemia, often called blood poisoning, is a form of bacteremia, or invasion of the blood circulation by bacteria.

Causes

The causes of septicemia usually are traceable to some surgical procedure, to the use of intravenous devices or catheters, or to childbirth injury complicated by streptococcus infection or other infections. Septicemia is also a common side effect of intravenous drug injections, particularly in drug abusers. Other diseases and disorders often associated with septicemia include endocarditis (inflammation of the lining of the heart); genito-urinary tract infections; and sometimes diseases of the skin, bones, and joints.

Symptoms

Few symptoms are unique to septicemia, so it is often confused with other illnesses. However, fever, often variable and intermittent, is generally present. Chills may occur at the outset of the disease. Skin eruptions are common and may be petechial (small, red dots or splotches), purpuric (purple and bruise-like), or may take any of several other forms. Often septicemia begins abruptly with chills, fever, nausea, vomiting, diarrhea, and general collapse.

Diagnosis

The diagnosis of septicemia is established by blood cultures, which test for various kinds of bacteria. Normally, there should be no bacteria in the blood. A single negative culture does not exclude septicemia; in some patients who have had prior antibiotic therapy, there is never a single positive blood culture. Bone marrow culture is actually the most sensitive diagnostic tool.

Treatment

Treatment of septicemia relies heavily on antibiotics. Therapy should continue until the patient has been free of symptoms for at least one week.

Shingles

Shingles, or herpes zoster, is a painful viral infection of one or more nerves. The infection produces a blistery, itchy skin rash above the affected nerve.

Causes

Shingles rash looks identical to the rash of the chicken pox virus. Shingles and chicken pox are caused by the same virus called varicella zoster. Moreover, previous infection with chicken pox is necessary in order to develop shingles. Why shingles occurs in certain people and not others at any given time is unknown. Scientists believe that after recovery from chicken pox the varicella zoster virus lies dormant in the body. One theory contends that the virus is reactivated after injury to the affected area or other emo-

tional or physical upset to the body. Sixty-five percent of the cases studied confirm this.

Another theory proposes that with shingles the number and strength of antibodies (protective substances) produced by the body to fight the varicella zoster virus may diminish after a bout of chicken pox. This reduction in force makes some individuals susceptible to another attack of the virus. Because some antibodies endure, the person gets shingles rather than chicken pox. Yet, if someone is exposed to the virus as an adult and has not had chicken pox, he or she will get chicken pox, not shingles.

Incidence of the disease increases with age. Shingles rarely occurs in people under age 15. More than 50 percent of those who get shingles are over 45 years of age.

Symptoms

Shingles begins with a prickling or tenderness in the skin over the infected nerve. Burning or shooting pain in the same area is also an early symptom. Within two to four days a rash with small, red spots appears over the affected part of the body. As the spots enlarge, they blister and sometimes blend together. Eventually they fill with pus, burst, and crust over much the same as with chicken pox rash. With shingles, however, the process takes longer and is confined to the skin area above the affected nerve.

Shingles rash is very itchy. In addition, pain increases as the

Shingles is an infection of a nerve characterized by a blistering skin rash following the path of the affected underlying nerve. The rash itself is identical to the rash of chicken pox, since both diseases are caused by the same virus.

area beneath the rash becomes more red and swollen. Shingles attacks nerves on the chest, back, neck, arm, or leg most often. However, facial nerves are involved frequently. The rash appears in a band or strip following the path of the nerve, usually on one side of the body. The rash persists two to three weeks before clearing, while the pain continues for three or four weeks. Sometimes, pain may linger for a month or more. In people over 60, pain may persist for several months after the rash disappears.

Complications

Occasionally, shingles rash becomes generalized and spreads over the entire body. This develops most often in people who have underlying disease such as Hodgkin's disease or leukemia (cancer of the blood). When these serious disorders already exist, shingles can cause death, but this is rare. A signal that such extreme illness may be present is recurrence of shingles, since the condition seldom occurs more than once.

The most common complication of shingles is a bacteria infection in the rash. This can prolong the rash and cause skin scars.

Less common complications follow a shingles attack on facial nerves. Eye disorders and Bell's palsy (a disease that temporarily paralyzes one side of the face) can result.

Treatment

Since there is no known cure for shingles, treatment focuses on reducing pain. An analgesic, or painkilling drug, may relieve burning. Some physicians prescribe steroid drugs to reduce nerve inflammation in older patients. In order to be effective, steroids must be taken soon after shingles begins. Steroid treatment is not recommended for people with underlying disease because steroids can interfere with natural resistance to infection.

Preventing infection is also important. Baths in warm (not hot) water soothe and clean the skin. For severe itching, patients should cut their fingernails and wear gloves when asleep to control unconscious scratching.

Syphilis

Syphilis is a serious, highly contagious disease spread primarily through direct sexual contact. Syphilis is caused by spiral-shaped bacteria called spirochetes.

Over time, syphilis can affect all parts of the body, the brain, bones, spinal cord, and heart as well as the reproductive organs. If left untreated, blindness, brain damage, heart disease, and even death can result. Syphilis can also be passed from a mother to her unborn baby, causing congenital syphilis in the child, which may eventually result in blindness and deafness, among other serious consequences. Syphilis in a pregnant woman must be treated prior to the eighteenth week of the pregnancy in order to prevent passage of the disease to the fetus.

Stages and symptoms

Syphilis is a progressive disorder that passes through four stages: primary, secondary, latent, and late or tertiary. Each of the four stages of syphilis is marked by a distinct set (or lack) of symptoms.

Primary syphilis is characterized by the appearance of a painless, open sore (called a chancre) ten to 90 days after exposure to the disease. As a rule, there is usually only one sore (although occasionally there are several), appearing most commonly on the genital organs, but also at times on the rectum, cervix (the opening to the uterus), lips, tongue, fingers, or anywhere that direct contact was made. The chancre first appears as a red bump, sometimes surrounded by a red ring and oozing clear fluid; it soon erodes into a painless ulcer and disappears within several weeks without treatment. Although the chancre is gone, the disease is still active in the body.

Secondary syphilis appears

within six weeks to six months of initial contact. Symptoms resembling the flu such as fever, sore throat, headache, fatigue, aching joints, and enlarged lymph nodes are common. Syphilitic meningitis (an infection of the membranes lining the brain and spinal cord) can also be seen in this

Secondary syphilis is also characterized by extremely contagious, grayish-white erosions that can be seen on the lining of the mouth, the penis, the external female sexual organs, the anus, and warm, moist areas such as the underarms; by growths resembling warts in the genital area (not to be confused with the more common nonsyphilitic genital warts); and by a rash on the palms or soles in the form of round reddish spots that occur in patches and do not itch. These sores, growths, and rashes heal within three to six weeks without treatment, and the disease enters the third stage.

In the latent stage (latent means present but not manifesting itself), all symptoms disappear, the patient appears to be healthy, and the disease is probably not contagious (except in the case of pregnant women, who can still pass it on to their offspring). The latent stage can go on indefinitely, but it is felt that one third of those with latent syphilis will progress to the final stage of the illness.

By the late or tertiary stage of syphilis, the disease is in all likelihood no longer contagious, but the entire body may come under siege. Late syphilis can damage the brain, bones, spinal cord, and heart, commonly causing blind-

ness, brain damage, heart disease, or even death.

Diagnosis

Syphilis is diagnosed with a history and physical exam, blood tests, and a microscopic examination of a smear (sample) taken from the sores or rash areas. Several blood tests may be necessary, as the bacteria may not show up on blood tests during the first one to two weeks after exposure to the infected person.

Treatment

Treatment of syphilis is accomplished with the administration of penicillin or other antibiotics if a penicillin allergy exists. Some cases of late syphilis are so advanced, however, that they will not benefit from treatment.

A person who has syphilis or any other sexually transmitted disease should abstain from sexual activity until all tests have confirmed that the disease is no longer present. Syphilis, as well as all forms of sexually transmitted diseases, requires that every sexual partner of the infected person be tested and treated if necessary.

Prevention

Syphilis can be prevented by avoiding sexual contact with someone who has the disease. However, since this is not always possible, it is important to remember that the chances of contracting this or any other sexually transmitted disease increase with the number of different sexual partners a person has, so limiting the number of partners can be beneficial in prevention.

Tetanus

Tetanus is an acute disease of infectious origin, commonly associated with improperly cleaned deep wounds, that causes severe muscle contraction.

Cause

Tetanus is caused by toxins (poisonous substances) that are produced by the bacteria *Clostridium tetani*. These bacteria usually enter the body through a wound in contact with material, such as soil, in which bacteria spores are present or by being present on the skin at the time of the injury. Puncture wounds seem especially vulnerable to tetanus infection since they are, by their nature, difficult to clean and medicate, and allow little air to reach the deep tissue (these bacteria cannot live in the air).

Symptoms

Tetanus symptoms are varied, depending on the extent of the infection and the body part that is affected. The most common symptom is called "lockjaw," in which the muscles of the jaw go into severe continuous contraction, thus rendering the jaw immobile. Symptoms also include a bowed or arched body (which is

rare) because of contraction of lower back muscles; back muscle spasms; and lethal throat spasms that can cause blockage of the airway. The affected body parts become immobile because of the simultaneous and continuous contraction of opposing muscles.

In severe cases, the contractions affect most of the cells in the affected muscle. The contraction is thus not merely a weak "twitch," but is instead an almost "complete" contraction, similar to what would be required in lifting a heavy weight or marshaling all the potential force of a muscle against a high resistance.

Treatment

Treatment consists of muscle relaxant drugs such as diazepam to ease the contractions. Antimicrobial drugs such as penicillin are used to fight the infection. Tetanus antitoxin is given intramuscularly in the hope of lessening the severity of the disease. However, the antitoxin does not counteract toxin already in the nervous system nor does it act to relieve symptoms already present.

Prevention

Immunization beforehand with the tetanus vaccine offers the best preventive against the disease. Also, wounds should be attended to immediately, especially puncture wounds. Tetanus "boosters" should be taken periodically, especially if small skin wounds are a common occurrence in the course of the workday.

FACTS ABOUT ALLERGIES AND THE IMMUNE SYSTEM

Immunity is the body's ability to defend itself against harmful substances. Essentially, it is a resistance to infection that may be inherited or acquired naturally or artificially.

Resistance occurs when foreign organisms called antigens enter the body, causing particular specialized cells to react either by attacking the antigen directly or by producing proteins (compounds essential to living cells) that neutralize the foreign agents. The most common types of antigens are forms of bacteria (one-celled organisms that have the potential to attack body tissues or secrete poisonous substances called toxins) and viruses (the smallest infective agents responsible for a variety of diseases).

Lymph system

The lymph system is the body's drainage system. It is composed of a network of vessels and small structures called lymph nodes. The lymph vessels carry away excess fluid collected from all over the body back into the blood circulation. Along the way, however, these fluids are forced to percolate through a lymph node so that they can be "filtered." Unwanted organisms are trapped and destroyed by the specialized white blood cells (lymphocytes) that are present in these nodes. Lymphocytes are also added to the lymph that flows out of nodes and back to the bloodstream.

Antibodies

The lymph system also manufactures antibodies. Antibodies are specialized proteins that the body produces in response to invasion of a foreign substance. The process of antibody formation begins when an antigen stimulates a lymph node into action. Antibodies then counteract invading antigens by combining with the antigen to render it harmless to the body. The antibodies coat the harmful organism so that the body's scavenger cells can destroy them more easily. The antibody molecule combines with the antigen molecule by matching com-

bining sites. They fit together like the pieces of a jigsaw puzzle. Other antibodies that neutralize toxins produced by bacteria are called antitoxins.

During periods of active antibody production, lymph nodes often enlarge and become tender to the touch. A vaccination — or injection of a natural or artificial antigen to stimulate the body to produce protective antibodies—in the arm can cause swelling under the armpit, while an influenza infection can affect neck glands. Enlarged nodes can be felt under the skin of the armpit, groin, or neck. The spleen, an organ located in the upper left part of the abdomen is also important in the manufacture of antibodies.

Immune reaction

Production of white blood cells and antibodies in response to an invading disease organism is called an immune reaction. This immune reaction is one of the body's primary and most efficient lines of defense. Once antibodies have been produced to fight a certain organism, that germ no longer poses a threat to the body. That is why one attack of a disease often prevents that same disease from infecting the body again. The first attack causes antibody production. In turn, these antibodies protect the body against subsequent attacks. With measles, for example, the antibodies created by having the disease or by being vaccinated with measles virus resist a second attack of the disease, thus providing immunity against its recurrence.

Antibodies are not always beneficial. For example, when tissue from another body, such as a transplanted heart, is introduced, antibodies are produced to destroy the "invader." Transplants usually are made possible only by means of drugs and occasionally radiation that act against the body's immune response. Also, when you have a blood transfusion, it must be of a matching type; otherwise your body will manufacture antibodies to destroy it.

Sometimes, the immune system causes reactions that make the body unusually sensitive to foreign material. When the immune response is disruptive to the body, it is called an allergic reaction.

Allergic reaction

An allergy is an extraordinary reaction or sensitivity to a particular environmental substance by the immune system.

Although it can be present almost immediately after exposure to the irritant, an allergy usually develops over time, while the immune system forms antibodies as a reaction to an invasion by a foreign substance. Under normal conditions, such antibodies work to protect the body from further attack. In the case of an allergy, however, the antibodies and other specialized cells involved in this protective function trigger an unusual sensitivity to the foreign substance (called an allergen). The antibodies then stimulate the special cells to produce histamine, a powerful chemical released from the cells that causes the small blood vessels to enlarge, the smooth muscles (such as those in the air passages or the digestive tract) to constrict, and hives to develop.

No one knows why allergies develop, but it is known that an allergy can appear, disappear, or reappear at any time and at any age. Allergic reactions rarely occur during the first encounter with the troublesome allergen because the body needs time to accumulate the antibodies. Also, a family history of allergies seems to be related to an individual's sensitivity to certain allergens. People who show a tendency to develop allergies are referred to as "atopic." This state of atopy frequently runs in families.

An allergic reaction can be so mild that it is barely noticeable or so severe that a person's life is threatened. Common symptoms of allergy are watery eyes, runny nose, itching or inflamed skin, or a swollen mouth or throat. Some allergic reactions may be accompanied by headaches, sinus stuffiness, a reduced sense of taste or smell, or difficult breathing.

Anaphylactic shock

An extremely severe allergic reaction, called anaphylactic shock, is characterized by breathing difficulties (caused by swelling of the throat and larynx and narrowing of the bronchial tubes), itching skin, hives, and collapse of the blood vessels, as well as by vomiting, diarrhea, and cramps. This advanced condition can be fatal if not properly treated.

Types

There are four categories of allergens: inhalants, contactants, ingestants, and injectants.

Inhalant allergens are breathed in, and include such substances as dust, pollen, feathers, and animal dander (small scales from the animal's skin). Hay fever is an inhalant allergy in which the mucous membranes react to various inhaled substances, usually the pollens associated with the changing seasons. Year-round hay fever may be a reaction to pet dander, feathers, mold, or dust. Hay fever symptoms include itching of the nose, eyes, and roof of the mouth; sneezing; headache; and watery eyes.

Contactant allergens are those that are touched and include such substances as poison ivy, cosmetics, detergents, fabrics, and dyes. Contact dermatitis is an example of an allergic-type reaction resulting from exposure to a contactant. Skin becomes inflamed, burning, and itching where it has come in contact with soaps, detergents, household cleaners, drugs, or chemicals found in food or cosmetics. Poison ivy and poison oak rashes are other examples of contactant allergic reactions.

Ingestant allergens are swallowed or eaten. A variety of foods and medications can act as ingestant allergens to persons overly sensitive to them. A food allergy usually occurs in children and is a reaction to an ingestant allergen, often milk, eggs, shellfish and other fish, peanuts, chocolate, strawberries, and citrus fruits. Symptoms of food allergies include abdominal cramps, nausea, vomiting, and diarrhea. Hives, rash, headache, nasal congestion, even anaphylactic shock can also accompany a food allergy.

Injectant allergens are substances that penetrate the skin, such as insect venom or drugs that are injected. For example, people who have severe allergic reactions to insect bites or stings are suffering from a reaction to an injectant allergen. Shortness of breath; strong, rapid heartbeat; coughing; wheezing; and light-headedness are common symptoms. The bite area swells and becomes tender or numb, and, in extreme cases, anaphylactic shock may occur.

Diagnosis

In any allergy case, identifying the offending allergen may be painful, time-consuming, and expensive, but it is necessary to avoid future allergic reactions. A medical history, a record of any recent changes in daily habits, and both skin scratch tests (in which small amounts of the suspected allergens are applied to tiny scratches in the skin) and intracutaneous skin tests (in which allergens are injected under the skin) are used to help detect the troublesome foreign substance. A blood test called RAST (radioallergosorbent technique) is often taken to measure the amount of antibodies in the blood that have been manufactured in response to an invading substance.

Treatment

Once the allergen is pinpointed, half the battle is won. Obviously, avoiding the troublesome allergen is a good start toward relieving an allergy problem. However, if the allergen cannot be avoided or removed, two treatments may be recommended: medication or immunotherapy. Three types of medication have commonly been prescribed: antihistamine drugs, which combat the effect of the histamines in the body; corticosteroids, which reduce inflammation and swelling; and bronchodilators, which ease breathing by opening bronchial tubes.

Allergy immunotherapy, or treatment by "desensitization shots," consists of the injection into the body of first small, then increasingly larger, quantities of the allergen. This allows the body to build up a form of resistance or immunity to the offending substance. Immunotherapy works best in controlling allergies to pollen (especially hay fever), insect venom, and dust.

A little common sense goes a long way in controlling allergies. Obviously, the offending allergen needs to be avoided, removed, or replaced. Natural fibers in the home can be replaced with synthetics; air conditioners or air filters can be installed for hay fever sufferers; those susceptible to insect bites can wear protective clothes and avoid bright clothing and perfumes, both of which attract insects; babies born into allergy-prone families should be breast-fed as long as possible to delay exposure to cow's milk, eggs, and citrus fruits.

Prevention

Allergies cannot really be prevented, but much can be done to help to control or diminish their effects on the overly sensitive body.

AIDS—acquired immune deficiency syndrome

Acquired immune deficiency syndrome (AIDS) is a condition in which the body's immunity, its natural defense system against disease, is somehow severely jeopardized thus enabling organisms that are normally fought off by the body quite effectively to become deadly.

Those at risk

The cause of the new disease discovered in 1979 is a virus. It is also known that male homosexuals, drug addicts who inject drugs, and hemophiliacs who receive blood transfusions for their disorder are all high risk groups. Homosexual practices (for example, rectal intercourse), use of nonsterile needles within a group, possible environmental factors, and multiple transfusions of pooled blood factors have all been respectively mentioned as possible means of transmission of an agent causing the syndrome. Of early known victims, 75 percent were male homosexuals, 12 percent intravenous drug abusers, and 0.5 percent hemophiliacs—but 6 percent were Haitian immigrants who were neither homosexuals nor drug abusers.

Symptoms

Symptoms include low-grade fever, swollen lymph glands, weight loss, fatigue, night sweats, long-standing diarrhea, and a general sick feeling. Up to one third of the victims develop a previously rare cancer known as Kaposi's sarcoma, which can appear as purplish bumps on the skin. Many come down with a severe form of pneumonia. The main problem, however, is the inability of the body to fight many diseases that come along, including various cancers, skin infections, fungus growths, and tuberculosis.

Individuals with AIDS almost uniformly have reduced numbers of lymphocytes. These are specialized white blood cells that are critical in combating infectious diseases, particularly those caused by tuberculosis, fungi, and viruses. Lymphocytes may also be instrumental in destroying malignancies in their early stages. There are two types of lymphocytes actively engaged in coping with infection: the T-cell and the B-cell. The T-cell is mainly concerned with direct cytotoxicity, that is, by a series of complex processes, it directly kills invaders. The B-cell, on the other hand, is concerned with the production of infection-fighting antibodies when stimulated. In AIDS the T-cells are greatly reduced; in fact, it is the "helper" T-cell (a further subdivision) that is most profoundly decreased. So far, this has been a constant finding in almost all AIDS victims and will possibly serve as a link toward the discovery of a treatment.

Treatment

Treatment to counter the effects of AIDS may involve the use of antibiotics, surgery to remove skin cancer, chemotherapy, and drugs to raise the body's resistance to diseases. No cure for the disease itself has been found yet. In addition, no specific means of preventing AIDS is known.

Anaphylactic shock

Anaphylactic shock, most correctly known as anaphylaxis, is a violent allergic reaction characterized by itching skin, hives, breathing trouble, collapse of the blood circulation system, and sometimes vomiting, diarrhea, and cramps in the abdomen. It can occur in a person who is extremely sensitive to a substance on first exposure and certainly can reoccur if the person then is exposed to the substance again. The result is an explosive over-reaction of the body's defense system to the foreign matter.

Causes

Often, the reaction is set off by an insect sting, such as that of a bee or wasp; by animal serum used in a vaccine; by desensitizing injections; or by one of various drugs. The allergen (the actual substance that sets off the reaction) is usually a protein, called an antigen. When it first enters the body, certain body cells treat it like an invading microorganism and create antibodies, which are protective substances that fight infection. On later exposures, the antibodies are ready for the "invader" and stimulate release of certain chemicals including that known as histamine, which causes smooth muscles such as those in the digestive and breathing systems to contract, resulting in symptoms in those areas such as cramps and wheezing, respectively. Histamine also causes the small blood vessels to enlarge and lose plasma (blood fluid) to surrounding tissues. The decreased blood in the vessels results in a drop in blood pressure that may lead to shock, or collapse of the blood circulation system.

Symptoms

Symptoms develop rapidly. Within one to 15 minutes, the exposed person becomes uneasy, upset, and red in the face. Rapid heartbeat, prickly and itching skin, throbbing in the ears, sneezing, coughing, and breathing difficulty are also likely. Vomiting, incontinence (involuntary release of urine and bowel contents), and even convulsions may occur. In another one or two minutes, shock may result, in which blood vessels collapse, the pulse becomes weak and rapid, and the person becomes cold, clammy, and faint. Without immediate medical aid, death may result.

Treatment

Medical aid should be obtained as fast as possible; call an emergency squad. Keep the patient's airway open. With the patient lying down, keep legs elevated. Immediate treatment with the drug known as epinephrine is critical. It counteracts the action of the histamines released in the blood that are causing the symptoms of anaphylactic shock. If a drug injection has caused the reaction, a tourniquet should be applied above the site of the injection and more epinephrine should be injected into the site. Antihistamine drugs should also be given. In extreme cases, especially when shock has occurred or there is great breathing difficulty, intravenous (IV) solutions of salt water are given to restore blood volume and raise blood pressure. Anyone with a severe reaction should be hospitalized for at least 24 hours to guard against a relapse.

Prevention

A preventive measure against possible anaphylactic shock is routine allergy skin testing before the use of substances about which there is a question of sensitivity or substances, such as animal serums in vaccines, that are commonly known to cause anaphylactic shock. In addition, anyone who has had an anaphylactic reaction to a stinging insect should carry a kit containing a filled syringe of epinephrine and also an epinephrine-filled nasal sprayer, for prompt self-treatment when stung again. Desensitization injections of the insect venom to allow the body to build up a resistance to the venom should also be considered, if your doctor feels that such injections will not trigger an anaphylactic reaction.

Anaphylactoid reactions

Somewhat similar to anaphylaxis are anaphylactoid reactions, which can occur on the first injection of certain drugs, including contrast media (used when taking X-ray pictures), histamine, and morphine. These are not allergic reactions in the pure sense, but are serious nevertheless.

Autoimmune diseases

Autoimmune diseases are disorders in which the body's immune (defense) system reacts against some of its own tissue and produces antibodies (protective substances) to destroy it.

Examples

Ailments believed to be autoimmune diseases include Hashimoto's thyroiditis and Graves' disease, disorders of the thyroid; systemic lupus erythematosus, which attacks connective tissue; myasthenia gravis, a muscular disease; and autoimmune hemolytic anemia, in which red blood cells are destroyed before the end of their normal 120-day life span.

Diseases that *probably* are autoimmune disorders include the joint disease rheumatoid arthritis; pernicious anemia, a blood disorder; Addison's disease, which attacks the adrenal glands; and some forms of diabetes mellitus, which is a breakdown of the body's ability to handle starches and sugars.

Possible autoimmune diseases are chronic active hepatitis, a liver disorder; some forms of vasculitis, an inflammation of blood vessel walls; and many other diseases that produce inflammation, degeneration, or wasting away of body tissue.

Causes

An autoimmune disease can begin in several ways:
• Some body substance that ordinarily never enters the bloodstream may do so because of injury. For example, a disease known as sympathetic ophthalmia occurs when tissue from the inside of an injured eye is released into the bloodstream. The tissue is recognized as "out of place" or "foreign" by the body's immune system and antibodies attack it — causing irritation in both the injured eye and in the noninjured eye. The reaction may be severe enough to cause blindness.
• Body substances may be altered by chemicals, sunlight, or a virus so that they become "foreign" to the body's immune system. The substance is then attacked by antibodies. This occurs in contact dermatitis, when, for example, metal in a bracelet causes chemical changes in the skin on one's wrist. The body reacts against the "different" skin and attacks it, causing a rash.
• Finally, infection of the body may cause the body to react with an immune response so strong that the body reacts against some of its own normal tissues.

There seems to be an inherited tendency to autoimmune diseases. Women are affected more often than men.

Contact dermatitis

Contact dermatitis is a type of allergy in which the skin becomes inflamed in the area where it has come in contact with an irritant.

Causes

Contact dermatitis can be caused by soaps, detergents, shaving materials, shampoos, hair colorings or sprays, solvents in household cleaners, chemicals in foods and cosmetics, and certain plants such as poison ivy or poison oak. Photodermatitis (a skin inflammation caused by light) is a type of dermatitis that develops when certain ingested drugs, such as some antibiotics, sensitize the skin in a manner that causes a rash to develop on those skin surfaces exposed to the sun (this can also be seen in some unusual systemic disorders and in people with "true sun allergy").

Symptoms

The major symptoms of contact dermatitis are burning, swelling, severe itching, and stinging sensations on the area of the skin that has been exposed to the allergen. Blisters may form that ooze a clear fluid; a cloudy or yellow foul-smelling fluid indicates a bacterial infection.

Diagnosis

Contact dermatitis is diagnosed by first identifying the allergen causing the trouble. In identifying this type of allergen, the process is somewhat simplified, because the location of the rash gives an important clue as to its identity. For instance, if the inflammation is on the scalp, the disorder may be assumed to be triggered by a shampoo, hair spray, or hair coloring. More specific identification of the allergen may be obtained from one of several tests available that pinpoint allergens in all types of allergies. These include scratch tests, in which a small amount of the suspected allergen is applied to a scratch on the skin; intracutaneous tests, in which a small amount of the allergen is injected in or under the skin; and the radioallergosorbent technique, a blood test in which specific antibodies produced by the body in response to the allergen are measured.

Treatment

Once the allergen is identified, the best treatment for contact dermatitis is to avoid or remove the allergen from the patient's environment. Common sense precautions can be taken to remove the allergen from the patient's surroundings, such as switching brands of soaps or shampoos, wearing rubber gloves when using harsh detergents, and using unscented or hypoallergenic cosmetics. If the use of a drug cannot be discontinued despite a case of photodermatitis, sunscreens or adequate clothing to shield the skin should be used when outdoors.

Steroid (cortisone) drugs, taken orally, help to relieve the itching of contact dermatitis; however, these are reserved for more serious cases. Topical (rubbed directly on the skin) steroids and antihistamines are more commonly used.

Prevention

There is no actual preventive treatment for contact dermatitis, but those susceptible to one or more contact allergens can usually prevent outbreaks by using common sense and avoiding exposure to the allergen or allergens as much as possible.

Food allergy

A food allergy is an allergic reaction to a specific food and most often occurs in children.

A food allergy needs to be distinguished from a food intolerance. A food intolerance exists when contaminants such as bacteria or chemicals are present in the food, or when the body lacks the certain natural chemicals called enzymes needed to digest the food. A food allergy exists when the body's immune system actually manufactures antibodies as a reaction to the food. This food then becomes an example of an ingestant allergen (an allergy-causing substance that is swallowed or eaten). Any food can become an allergen, but the foods most commonly found to cause allergic reactions are milk, eggs, shellfish and other fish, peanuts, chocolate, strawberries, and citrus fruits.

Symptoms

The symptoms of a food allergy most commonly occur in the digestive tract: cramps, nausea, vomiting, and diarrhea. Other signs may also be present: hives, rash, headache, nasal congestion, or even anaphylactic shock (a very serious reaction that can be fatal, characterized by breathing problems, hives, collapse of blood vessels, and sometimes vomiting, diarrhea, and cramps).

Diagnosis

Food allergy is diagnosed by having the patient maintain a detailed record of all foods eaten as well as of the times when symptoms appear. Elimination trials may also help diagnose the allergen; the patient eliminates one food at a time from the diet to see if the symptoms disappear. In addition, several tests are used to detect all types of allergens: scratch tests, in which a small amount of the suspected allergen is applied to a scratch on the skin; intracutaneous tests, in which a small amount of the allergen is injected in or under the skin; and the radioallergosorbent technique, in which specific antibodies in the blood are measured.

Treatment

There is no way to treat or prevent a food allergy other than to avoid eating the food. Fortunately, children usually outgrow these allergies.

Gamma globulin

Gamma globulin is a protein containing antibodies in the blood. Gamma globulin is developed by the body in response to invasion by harmful agents, such as bacteria, viruses and toxins. Its purpose is to react chemically with the invading agent and destroy it, thus providing immunity. Almost all antibodies produced in the body's defense system are gamma globulin molecules.

Prevention and treatment of diseases

Gamma globulin preparations are derived from the blood of another person or animal and contain preformed antibodies made by that person or animal. The preparations are widely used for the prevention, modification, and treatment of many kinds of infectious diseases. This type of gamma globulin is usually injected and contains almost all the known antibodies circulating in the blood. It can provide a passive (borrowed) immunity lasting up to about six weeks.

In cases of hepatitis, for example, gamma globulin injections are especially useful, since human blood gamma globulins do not transmit hepatitis. Gamma globulin is given not only to the hepatitis patient, but also to all household members and other persons who have been in direct contact with a case or cases of infectious hepatitis. Persons with a high risk of exposure to hepatitis, such as hospital staff members and persons traveling in areas where hepatitis is prevalent, should receive a dose of gamma globulin every four to five months to maintain the preventive effects.

Measles can be prevented in many cases by the administration of gamma globulin injections within five days of exposure. The injections are especially important for children under three years, for pregnant women, for tuberculosis patients, or for those with impaired immune mechanisms. Often even if measles is not prevented, a less serious case will result; however, gamma globulin is of no use once the symptoms appear. Similarly, chicken pox can be prevented or its seriousness modified if gamma globulin is given within five days of exposure.

Diagnosis of diseases

Gamma globulin can also be used as a diagnostic tool: one important symptom of multiple sclerosis, for example, is that the proportion of gamma globulin in the patient's cerebrospinal fluid is altered in about 60 percent of the cases, especially those that are long-lasting. This is an especially important finding, since this is the only definitive known lab test for multiple sclerosis.

Hay fever

Hay fever is a type of allergy in which the membranes of the nose react to an inhaled substance. For this reason, this substance is called an inhalant allergen.

Causes

Hay fever may be caused by a variety of environmental substances, but acute (short-lived), seasonal attacks are usually allergic reactions to pollen (the allergen). Most often, spring attacks are reactions to tree pollen; summer attacks are reactions to grass pollen; and autumn attacks are reactions to weed pollen. Chronic (year-round) hay fever may be an allergic reaction to a number of other substances, including pet dander (scales of dry skin on pets), fibers, feathers, dust, and molds.

Symptoms

The symptoms of hay fever are usually the same, regardless of the allergen causing the irritation. Common symptoms include itching of the nose and roof of the mouth; a thin, watery discharge constantly draining from the nose; itchy, watery eyes; sneezing; headache; irritability; a feeling of exhaustion; insomnia; loss of appetite; and, in advanced cases, coughing and wheezing.

Diagnosis

Hay fever, as well as other allergies, is diagnosed by identifying the allergen. This is done by taking a medical history and reviewing the patient's environment, daily habits, and recent changes in lifestyle. Skin tests and blood tests may also be taken. These include scratch tests, in which a small amount of the suspected allergen is applied to a scratch on the skin; intracutaneous tests, in which a small amount of the allergen is injected in or under the skin; and the radioallergosorbent technique, in which specific antibodies (developed in response to suspected allergens) in the blood are measured.

Treatment

A severe case of hay fever may be best treated by a change in environment, that is, removing or reducing the allergen causing the trouble. Those reacting to weed pollen may need to move to a more urban, less pollinated location; those allergic to household dusts may have to dust and wet mop more frequently; those reacting to pets or fibers in carpeting, stuffed furniture, or draperies may need to remove these allergens from the household. In addition, many hay fever sufferers would benefit from an air conditioner, which helps keep pollen and dust levels in the home to a minimum.

Several medications are available for the hay fever sufferer: oral antihistamines, which fight the histamine that is released by the body as a reaction to the forming antibodies; corticosteroids, which reduce swelling; eyedrops, which relieve itching and redness; and desensitization shots, which cause the body to develop its own tolerance of the allergen.

Prevention

There is no actual method of preventing hay fever, but precautionary measures such as those discussed above may help at least to relieve some of its discomfort.

Hives

Hives (also called urticaria) is a reaction of the skin marked by intense itching and, most noticeably, by the rapid development of raised smooth patches or welts (also called wheals). Hives is most often a sign of an allergic reaction.

During an allergic reaction, the body overreacts to a foreign substance (called an allergen) and causes special cells called mast cells to release a powerful chemical called histamine, which is instrumental in the development of hives.

Causes

Hives is often caused by an allergy to certain foods, particularly shellfish, tomatoes, strawberries, eggs, milk, and chocolate. It can also be a reaction to drugs, food dyes, molds, bacteria, and animal skin or hair. In addition, in a susceptible person, cold, the rays of the sun, and vigorous exercise have also been known to cause hives.

Symptoms

Hives is characterized by an outbreak of red and white welts appearing suddenly either in small areas or all over the body and varying in size. They often appear and disappear, lasting anywhere from a few minutes to a day or two, but the outbreak can last for weeks. Accompanying symptoms are intense itching; occasionally, fatigue, fever, and nausea; and difficulty in breathing if the allergic reaction has led to a swelling in the respiratory tract.

Diagnosis

Diagnosing the allergy and pinpointing the allergen that is causing the trouble can require extensive testing, especially when a food may be involved. Eliminating many suspected foods, then reintroducing them one at a time, sometimes helps to diagnose the cause of hives. This must be done under professional supervision and with extreme caution.

Treatment

Hives can be treated immediately by taking antihistamines. When taken several times a day at a specific, prescribed dosage, the correct type of antihistamine will help control swelling by preventing the released histamine from triggering the hives. Drowsiness is a common side effect of antihistamines, so the type and dosage may need to be adjusted periodically. Other drug therapies such as those involving corticosteroids, which reduce inflammation, may be used to treat serious hives.

Prevention

Hives can be prevented by avoiding contact with the allergen or stimulus once it is identified.

Immunization

Immunization is the means of producing immunity, or resistance by the body to a specific disease. Doctors employ two types of immunization: *active* and *passive*.

Active immunization

Active immunization is accomplished by injecting weakened or killed viruses or bacteria into the body. This stimulates the body's natural defense system. Certain specialized white blood cells—which are manufactured in the bone marrow, are circulated in the blood, and are stored in lymph nodes and elsewhere—produce substances known as antibodies, carried in the bloodstream, that are tailor-made to fight the invading organisms. They remain in the body for years, sometimes a lifetime, to protect it against that particular disease.

Passive immunization

Passive immunization involves injecting ready-made antibodies—usually extracted from the blood of animals that have been immunized solely for the purpose of producing antibodies to be used in passive immunization. Passive immunization is borrowed immunity and is only temporary but serves to protect a person who may already be infected until the body has time to create its own antibodies.

Immunization can provide protection against measles, mumps, rubella (German measles), polio, whooping cough, diphtheria, and tetanus.

Children's immunizations

To be completely protected against diphtheria, tetanus, and whooping cough (pertussis), a child needs a shot of the combination diphtheria-tetanus-pertussis (DTP) vaccine at two, four, six, and eighteen months and a booster shot upon entering school around age five years. When the child gets the DTP shots, he or she should also receive by mouth a drop of the oral polio vaccine (although since there are usually only four doses of polio vaccine, the child does not receive it at six months of age). At 15 months a child should have a combined shot for measles, rubella, and mumps. He or she should be tested for tuberculosis at the end of the first year and receive a tetanus-diphtheria booster shot between 14 and 16 years of age.

Parents who do not have a family physician can call their local public health department. It usually has supplies of vaccine and may give shots free.

Adult immunizations

Adults need a tetanus shot once every ten years. Otherwise, there are no routine immunizations necessary for adults in the United States, with the possible exception of influenza shots given annually (usually in the fall) to the aged and to patients with heart, lung, and other chronic diseases. (With the new purified vaccines, side effects are minor.) A vaccine for protection against 80 percent of serious pneumonias is available, to be given once every three to five years. HDCV, a new active immunization against rabies, is said to have only mild side effects for most people, with shots given on days 1, 3, 7, 14, 28, and 90 after a bite from a rabid animal (a passive vaccine is also given—once, on day 1). Immunization in advance against rabies is provided by a series of three shots of HDCV.

There are precautions to consider. Immunizations should not be given to pregnant women, nor in general to anyone whose immune system is weakened by leukemia, cancer, fever, or by prolonged X-ray or corticosteroid treatment.

Vaccination for foreign travel

Most persons traveling abroad in developed countries need no additional vaccination or medication. In general, in the United States, Canada, Australia, New Zealand, and Europe the traveler is safe without vaccinations. Travel in the less-developed countries of Africa, Asia, South America, Central America, Mexico, the South Pacific, Middle East and Far East may hold more risk, particularly in small villages or rural areas not usually visited by tourists.

In recent years no vaccination has been necessary for *direct* travel from the United States to most countries, nor to return to the United States. However, some countries require proof of vaccination from travelers who have passed through infected areas or countries, and it is best to get the shots before leaving home.

Any licensed physician can give immunizations, except that yellow-fever vaccinations must be given at an official "Yellow Fever Vaccination Center." Weeks before you plan to leave on your trip, call your local health department for latest information about vaccination requirements and recommendations for all of the countries you plan to visit. The vaccinating physician must fill out and sign an "International Certificate of Vaccination" that must be validated by a health department or by a physician with a "Uniform Stamp."

Vaccinations against cholera, which is transmitted by contaminated food and water, and against yellow fever, transmitted by certain mosquitoes, are the shots most often required for foreign travel. Because no cholera vaccine is very effective and because the risk of acquiring cholera is small, the United States Public Health Service does not recommend it for travelers unless the country visited requires it. However, yellow fever vaccinations are strongly recommended even if not required by law for travel to infected areas, usually parts of Africa and South America, and for travel in countries in "yellow fever endemic (ever-present) zones."

In no case should one be immunized for smallpox, which has been eliminated from the world. If a country still requires proof of vaccination, the United States Public Health Service recommends obtaining a written statement from a physician recommending against smallpox vaccination for health reasons (because serious complications can result for anyone). This will exempt the traveler.

Anyone not already immune to measles and mumps should receive vaccinations before traveling abroad, as should children not immune to rubella. Travelers to developing countries need diphtheria, polio, and typhoid immunizations, unless they are already immune, and a tetanus booster shot if they have not had one in the previous ten years.

Immunization cannot protect against malaria, a health threat in many developing countries. However, travelers to infected areas can take along protective medications, sleep in well-screened areas, wear protective clothing, and use chemical repellants to ward off the long-legged *Anopheles* mosquito, which transmits the disease.

Insect bite and sting

Insect bites and stings are minor inconveniences to most people, but to those who have an allergy to insect venom, the consequences can be serious.

Symptoms

Reactions to insect venom show themselves in various symptoms: shortness of breath, rapid heartbeat, coughing, wheezing, and light-headedness. The affected area swells and becomes tender or numb. In extreme cases, anaphylactic shock (a severe reaction that can be fatal, characterized by breathing problems; hives; collapse of blood vessels; and sometimes vomiting, diarrhea, and cramps) can occur.

Treatment

Serious reactions to bites and stings are treated by slowing the spread of the venom throughout the body and getting emergency medical treatment as soon as possible. The venom's progress can be slowed somewhat by applying an ice pack or a tourniquet (but not so tight as to stop the blood flow) to the affected area. Emergency medical treatment will consist of an epinephrine injection.

Prevention

Prevention of recurrent allergic reactions to insect venom is accomplished with treatments of desensitization shots; starting with an initially weak solution of insect extract, doses are gradually increased with each shot. This allows the body to build its own tolerance to the insect venom.

Currently, the serum in the shots is called whole body extract, meaning that the whole body of the insect is crushed and injected into the patient. Some scientists argue, however, that to be most effective, the serum should consist of only the insect's venom rather than the whole body. However, large quantities of insect venom are not available for this purpose, so whole body extract continues to be used.

THE BRAIN AND NERVOUS SYSTEM

The nervous system is a complex network of specialized tissue that regulates thoughts, emotions, actions, sensations, and basic body functions. The basic element of the nervous system is the neuron, or nerve cell. In combination, these neurons form nerve fibers that transmit impulses throughout the body. To protect neural function, myelin, a fatty substance, provides insulation for fibers of the nervous system.

There are two major divisions of the nervous system, the central nervous system and the peripheral nervous system. Distinctions between them depend upon function and location. The *central nervous system* consists of the brain and spinal cord. The brain lies within the skull (bony formation of the head). It governs body functions by sending and receiving messages through the spinal cord. Protecting the brain and spinal cord are bones, layers of tissue, and spinal fluid.

Once messages leave the central nervous system, they are carried by the *peripheral nervous system*. The peripheral system includes the cranial nerves (nerves branching from the brain) and spinal nerves (nerves branching from the spinal cord). These nerves convey sensory messages from receptor cells in the body to the central nervous system. They also transport motor impulses from the central system back to the body where muscles and glands can respond to the impulses.

The *autonomic nervous system*, which is part of the peripheral nervous system, regulates all activity that is involuntary but necessary for life, including activity of the internal organs and glands.

Working together, these divisions coordinate adjustment and reaction of the body to internal and external environmental conditions.

Brain

The brain is the control center for the entire body. The brain sends out to and receives stimulation from all body parts. Specifically, nerve cells from the brain transmit messages throughout the nervous system, the network of specialized tissue responsible for mental processes, sensations, actions, and emotions. More than ten billion interwoven brain cells regulate mechanisms during sleep and wakefulness.

Different areas of the brain control different body functions. The entire brain lies within the

Brain

Spinal cord

protective bony structure called the skull. At the back of the skull is the cerebellum. This part of the brain determines coordination of movements, balance, and posture.

Deep inside the brain is the thalamus, the center for pain, touch, temperature, and consciousness. In addition, the thalamus is the relay station for incoming impulses from the body, conveying these impulses to other parts of the brain.

Beneath the thalamus is the hypothalamus, which governs involuntary or automatic body operations such as heartbeat, blood pressure, and blood circulation. The master gland, or pituitary gland, of the endocrine system is attached to the hypothalamus by a thin stalk. Because the pituitary gland controls most of the hormones in the body, the hypothalamus is considered a major influence upon primary drives governed by hormones, such as sexual desire, hunger, and thirst.

Covering the inner parts of the brain is the cerebrum, which consists of two cerebral hemispheres. In these hemispheres are the nerve centers that regulate voluntary thought and action. Connecting the left and right cerebral hemispheres are bands of fibers called the corpus callosum. Because nerve fibers from the two cerebral hemispheres cross one another at the base of the brain (medulla) before progressing down the spinal cord, each hemisphere generally controls functions in the opposite side of the body.

The brain is the most complex part of the body. Although research has identified many of its capabilities for memory, reasoning, and creative thought processes, many functions of the brain remain a mystery.

Alzheimer's disease

Alzheimer's disease is a disorder in which there is a steady dete-

Cerebrum

Corpus callosum

Thalamus

Hypothalamus

Cerebellum

Pituitary gland

Spinal cord

Medulla

rioration of brain function resulting in continuing loss of memory, of recognition of friends and family, of personality, and of mental powers. Beginning as early as age 40 but most prevalent in the aged, it accounts for about half of all serious mental impairment in persons over age 65.

Changes in the brain

This disease has been studied extensively. As in any senile (characteristic of old age) condition, there is atrophy (shrinkage or wasting) of the cerebral cortex, which is the outer layer of the brain mostly concerned with intellectual and social functioning. In Alzheimer's disease, however, there are more specific abnormalities such as tangles or whorls of fibers within the nerve cells and senile plaques, deposits of a material, probably amyloid (a semisolid protein complex seen in many degenerative diseases). These abnormal changes are scattered throughout the cortex of an Alzheimer's victim and serve to distinguish the disease from other forms of senility. It is important to note that brain biopsies are not performed on individuals without very specific reasons and without intention of specific treatment. Therefore, these changes are only seen after death except in very unusual circumstances.

Causes

Theories abound as to the possible causes of Alzheimer's disease. Slow viruses (viruses acquired early in life that have taken many years to do their damage) have been considered as have been environmental factors and damage from previous disease(s). Recently, in some patients, a diminished amount of the enzyme choline-acetyltransferase — necessary to manufacture the critically important neurotransmitter acetylcholine (a chemical that promotes the passage of nerve signals in numerous brain functions) — has been found, and theories about replacement of the enzyme and/or neurotransmitter are being formulated. High levels of aluminum have also been found in the brains of Alzheimer's patients, and drugs that combine with the aluminum and draw it out of the tissues (a process called chelation therapy) have been tried —in order to slow the deterioration — with mixed results. Heredity seems to play some part, since a family member of an Alzheimer's victim is more likely than others to develop the condition. It is generally agreed that hardening of the arteries is not a cause. The disease does not appear to be contagious, nor is it caused by emotional upsets and stress.

Symptoms

Symptoms vary considerably from one person to another and may occur days or months apart. They begin with small memory lapses, almost always first involving loss of recall for recent events. This can happen to anyone, but in Alzheimer's disease they grow more serious in time. A man may forget his son's name or lose his way home from the office. A person may forget to turn off the oven, misplace articles, recheck to see if a task was done, or repeat questions already answered. Eventually the gaps in memory, and failure to recognize friends and family members, interfere with normal work and social life. The individual starts having trouble with figures when working on bills, with understanding what is being read, with organizing the day's work. As the disease progresses, the victim of Alzheimer's disease becomes confused, frustrated, and irritable. Although at first the person seems physically unaffected by the disease, as the condition advances the patient becomes restless, always moving about, and must be watched so that he or she does not wander away or into danger. Endless repetition of meaningless actions, such as the opening and closing of drawers, is another characteristic of the disease. Some victims of the condition may become extremely agitated with little provocation.

The course of the disease, which eventually can result in damage to the body and nervous system (apart from the brain) and in loss of control over bladder and bowels, may range from one to 20 years. It may cut life expectancy by as much as one-half by contributing to death from another cause such as pneumonia or heart or kidney failure.

Diagnosis

Other conditions can cause many of the symptoms of Alzheimer's disease, and many of these conditions are treatable. So it is very important for the patient to undergo a general medical examination with tests and extensive neurological and psychological studies. These involve computerized axial tomography (CAT scan — three-dimensional X-ray pictures), electroencephalography (EEG—a study of brain waves), blood tests, and often a sampling of spinal fluid. These procedures can rule out or identify possible causes such as a series of "little strokes," brain tumors or infections, pernicious anemia (curable with Vitamin B_{12}), overmedication with barbiturates or bromides, alcoholism, drug side effects, abnormal thyroid, or a blockage of cerebrospinal fluid in the head (hydrocephalus). Psychological depression is also an important — and treatable — cause of senile symptoms in the elderly and others, with symptoms of apathy, slowness of thought, inattention, and poor concentration. Death of a spouse or a shock such as moving to a nursing home could cause such symptoms temporarily.

Treatment

Medical science does not now know how to prevent or treat Alzheimer's disease. However, it is important to find a physician who is able to help the patient and family handle the many problems that are bound to arise. At times, tranquilizers can lessen agitation, anxiety, and undesirable behavior. Medication may also help improve sleeping patterns and treat depression.

It is important that the patient continue the daily routine, exercise as usual, and keep in touch with friends. Memory aids such as lists of daily chores, reminders about safety, and a large calendar can help in day-to-day living. As care of the patient becomes more difficult, it may be best for the patient and family alike to move the patient to a health facility where a professional staff can provide round-the-clock care. Families can find support and receive latest information about the disease from the self-help Alzheimer's Disease and Related Disorders Association, 360 North Michigan Avenue, Chicago, IL 60601.

Amnesia

Amnesia is the loss of memory and the inability to form new memories. It can be either temporary or permanent. The cause may range from brain damage to a psychological reason.

Retrograde amnesia

A certain type of amnesia (called retrograde) usually follows any severe head injury that produces unconsciousness. The patient is not able to recall what happened immediately before the accident causing the injury, the accident itself, nor some of the events of the recovery period. In most cases, this type of amnesia is not significant because no other memory is affected, and no treatment is needed.

Korsakoff's syndrome

An inability to record new memory along with a defect in memory of the past and usually accompanied by "confabulation" (storytelling of fabricated events) is known as Korsakoff's syndrome. It may be caused by head injury, stroke, encephalitis (inflammation of the lining of the brain), deficiency of Vitamin B, cancer of the brain, or poor blood supply to memory tissue or pathways in the brain. However, heavy drinking of alcohol, with resultant brain damage, is commonly the cause.

Although there may be little or no loss of memory or skills that were acquired before the disease began, the person with Korsakoff's syndrome cannot effectively learn new skills or remember recent events. To hide this loss, from self as well as others, the patient may describe imaginary or confused experiences to take the place of the missing experiences. Sometimes the stories are so convincing the patient appears normal.

Treatment of Korsakoff's syndrome is limited to treating the condition that caused it. Permanent brain damage, however, may make it incurable. Frequently, however, especially if it is caused by a brain concussion (a swelling in the head that puts pressure on the brain), it will disappear of its own accord.

Psychological amnesia

Amnesia of psychological cause is less common but more dramatic and newsworthy than other amnesias. A person disappears from home, job, and family, travels to a new place, assumes a new name, perhaps a new job, all without being aware that anything has changed. After days or weeks, the person "awakes," becomes his or her old self and wonders what happened. There is no memory of the period of amnesia.

Anxiety is the cause of this type of amnesia. The person is faced with an intolerable situation of high emotional stress or pain. To protect itself, the mind forgets the anxieties and everything related, including the person's identity.

Treatment may not be necessary, since most affected persons recover without help. However, if the problem that caused the amnesia still remains, it must be faced and solved. Family therapy and change of work or activities may help. Hypnosis may be used to bring back the memory of the "lost days" and unlock the ideas and feelings that caused the original flight from home and self.

Ataxia

Ataxia is a condition characterized by muscular incoordination, producing irregular and inaccurate movements of the body. The result may be a clumsy manner of walking with feet wide apart, a lack of balance, tremors of the arms, or slurring of speech.

Causes

Ataxia may be caused by anything that affects the motor control centers of the brain or the nerve pathways leading from them. Drunkenness can produce a temporary staggering ataxia. Permanent ataxia is caused by damage to the central nervous system (the brain, spinal cord, and spinal nerves).

Locomotor ataxia may be a late result of untreated syphilis. Its symptoms include sharp, stabbing pains, usually in the legs; an unsteady walk; and a feeling of walking on foam rubber. There may be an increased sensitivity of the skin, sometimes with burning, prickling, creeping, or crawling sensations.

Ataxia occurs in one case in ten of cerebral palsy, which is a group of movement disorders caused by damage to the brain or nerve pathways before or around the time of birth. Weakness, unsteadiness, clumsy walking, and difficulty with fine or rapid movements are typical. Physical and occupational therapy help patients handle daily life despite their condition.

Ataxia may also be caused by any one of a group of hereditary spinocerebellar diseases that attack the central nervous system. They cause degeneration of the spinal cord and cerebellum (the lower part of the brain, which controls muscle movements) and also frequently damage the brainstem and various nerves. Inherited disorders of body chemistry and body chemicals are believed to be involved, but little is known about them. Only one, Refsum's syndrome, can be treated—by reducing the excessive level of a body chemical known as phytanic acid.

Symptoms

Symptoms of the hereditary ataxias include unsteadiness in walking or tremor of the arms, muscle weakness, wasting away of muscle, and various other disorders depending upon the disease. For example, Friedreich's ataxia, the commonest, causes curvature of the spine (scoliosis) and damages heart tissue.

Treatment

All of these diseases continue throughout life and none can be treated effectively.

Bell's palsy

Bell's palsy is a sudden paralysis (loss of function or movement), total or partial, of one side of the face. It is believed to be due to inflammation of the nerve that controls the facial muscles. The inflammation, often of unknown cause but suspected to be the result of viral infection, causes the nerve to swell and to be compressed inside its bony passage in the skull. This reduces its blood supply and ability to function.

Symptoms

The disease can occur in someone of any age, but is most common from age 20 to 50. The first sign may be an aching pain behind or below the ear. Paralysis may develop in a few hours or more slowly, causing the entire side of the face to be flat and without expression (this is different from the facial paralysis caused by stroke or brain tumor, where the weakness is mostly below the forehead). The mouth droops on the weak side, with saliva drooling from the corner. Taste may be affected. The eyebrow cannot be raised. In most cases, the eye cannot be shut. When the patient tries to close the eye, it rolls upward (which happens in a normal person, but the movement is not seen). False tears may come from the affected eye.

Diagnosis

In diagnosing the case, the doctor must determine if the paralysis might be caused by other diseases affecting the facial nerve, including ear infections or skull fracture. The facial nerve can also be affected by many other conditions, cancers among them. However, other nerves are usually involved, and other signs and symptoms are frequently present. Head X rays may be taken.

Treatment

Primary treatment is aimed at reducing the inflammation of the nerve before any permanent damage is done to it. A cortisone hormone known as prednisone is given by mouth for this purpose. However, in many if not most uncomplicated cases, treatment with medication is unnecessary. After two weeks, if there has been no improvement in the ability of the muscles to move, the muscles of the weak side of the face may be stimulated electrically to maintain their condition.

The affected eye should be covered with an eyepatch, especially out of doors, and protected from dirt and wind. A facial sling is used to keep the mouth shut. Moist heat (not too hot) on the weak side of the face can reduce pain. Brief periods of upward facial massage help maintain muscle tone. So do facial exercises the patient can perform before a mirror. The patient needs help while eating, privacy to prevent embarrassment, and soft, easy-to-eat food (no hot food or drinks).

Fortunately, most Bell's palsy patients recover in one to eight weeks. Elderly patients may take much longer — up to two years. Complete recovery usually follows within several months if the paralysis is partial.

Cerebrospinal fluid

Cerebrospinal fluid (CSF) is a clear, colorless fluid that surrounds the brain and spinal cord and cushions them against injury.

CSF is made up of water containing small amounts of minerals and organic substances (especially protein). It is continually being produced from blood in networks of capillaries (tiny blood vessels) known as choroid plexi, which are located in the ventricles (chambers) of the brain. About one pint is produced every 24 hours; approximately five ounces is circulating at any one time. From the two lateral (side) ventricles, the CSF flows into the third and fourth ventricles of the brain. It then passes into the space between the innermost and second layers of the tissue covering the brain, bathing the entire outer surface of the brain in fluid before passing downward around the spinal cord. Eventually the fluid returns upward, is absorbed into special tissue between the linings of the brain, and passes into the blood vessels.

Samples of cerebrospinal fluid, drawn from around the spinal cord by a needle inserted in the lower back region (lumbar puncture), can be valuable in diagnosing disorders of the brain and spinal cord. The samples may indicate a hemorrhage or blood clot in the brain, various types of meningitis, a brain abscess, or a tumor of the brain or spinal cord.

Concussion

Concussion is a mild injury to the brain, resulting in unconsciousness, caused by a violent jar or shock such as a blow to the head. The force of the shock causes the brain to strike against the inside of the skull and produce temporary brain swelling and malfunctioning. However, the shock is not enough to cause cerebral contusion (bruising of brain tissue) or hemorrhage or hematoma (bleeding between the covering of the brain and the skull, or inside the brain covering), which are much more serious disorders.

A depressed or fractured skull and bleeding between the covering of the brain and the skull should always be ruled out in an individual with a head injury. Neither of these conditions occurs in a simple concussion.

Symptoms

Unconsciousness is the chief symptom of concussion, often lasting only a few minutes or as long as a few hours but never more than 24 hours (a longer period of unconsciousness or a deep coma indicates more serious brain damage). The patient may feel nauseous, irritable, "dragged out," dizzy, or suffer a severe headache, and these symptoms may continue for days or weeks after the accident and, on occasion, longer. Frequently, the individual cannot remember what happened just before the injury and later may not be able to recall anything that happened in the first few hours or on the day following the concussion.

An accident serious enough to cause more than a concussion — that is, a cerebral contusion (bruising of brain tissue), laceration (cutting and tearing of nerve tissue, blood vessels, and brain covering), or edema (fluid buildup within or around the brain)—often shows symptoms other than those accompanying a simple concussion. Signs of serious damage to the brain—much worse than concussion—include partial paralysis of the body; arms and legs extended rigidly, with the jaws clenched; and unequal or pinpoint pupils of the eye.

Diagnosis

A simple concussion usually requires no special care. The purpose of the doctor's examination is to determine if any more serious injury may have occurred. The patient is observed for level of consciousness, mental sharpness (if awake), and for proper nerve and muscle functions and reflexes. A head X ray may be taken to rule out a skull fracture (although most simple undepressed skull fractures are allowed to heal without treatment). If the patient acts strangely, out of character, or does not respond correctly to the tests, hospitalization and the services of a neurologist/neurosurgeon may be necessary.

Treatment

Once a doctor has determined that a patient has had only a simple concussion, the patient may be allowed to return home without hospitalization. For the next 24 hours, the person is advised to relax and to take nothing stronger than an aspirin substitute (acetaminophen). It is best not to eat solid foods, following any vomiting (which is common after concussion). A parent, roommate, or spouse is usually asked to wake the patient every two hours during the night, and ask three questions: "What is your name? Where are you? What is my name?" If the patient cannot answer these questions, will not awaken, or has convulsions, he or she should be rushed to the hospital. In addition, certain other danger signals should send the patient back to the doctor and hospital immediately: a continuing or worsening headache, blurred vision, extreme or constant vomiting, unusual eye movements, twitching, a staggering way of walking, or any change of personality.

If none of these symptoms develop, the patient can resume activities after a day or so of rest.

Encephalitis

Encephalitis is an inflammation of the brain. The term is usually used to describe an infectious process caused by bacteria, parasites, vaccines, and, most often, viruses. Noninfectious agents such as poisons (lead), metabolic abnormalities due to liver or kidney failure, and tumors can cause "encephalitis-like" conditions.

Causes

Viruses may cause encephalitis either as a primary disease or as a secondary complication of an infection. Some of these viruses are mosquito-borne and afflict humans only in warm weather when mosquitoes are in season. Many cases of encephalitis occur as complications of viral infections, such as measles, mumps, chicken pox, rubella (German measles), and other infections. These cases usually develop five to ten days after the onset of the original illness but can develop up to six weeks afterward.

Symptoms

Encephalitis may be associated with meningitis (infection of the layers of tissue that cover the brain and spinal cord) with evidence of brain disturbances such as alterations in mental state, personality changes, seizures, and paralysis. Edema (fluid buildup) in the brain is present and there may be petechial hemorrhages (small, red, bleeding spots) scattered throughout parts of the brain and spinal cord. As with meningitis, fever, headache, vomiting, and a stiff neck may be the first symptoms to appear.

Diagnosis

Prompt diagnosis and supportive treatment are essential in any case of encephalitis, or suspected encephalitis. Even patients who have been seriously or critically ill with encephalitis often recover. One problem of diagnosis is differentiating encephalitis from bacterial meningitis and other similar ailments. Even with ideal circumstances for diagnosis, the encephalitis virus is commonly not identified in many cases. Viruses can sometimes be isolated directly from cerebrospinal fluid or from the tissues. Since many forms of encephalitis, such as the mosquito-borne forms, have important public health implications, blood is often drawn whenever encephalitis is suspected and sent to local departments of health who can supply more precise diagnoses.

Treatment

With a form of encephalitis called herpes simplex encephalitis, early recognition and treatment with a medication that inhibits the reproduction of viruses reduce the chances of death and neurologic impairment significantly. However, the drug should be given before coma and/or paralysis set in for maximal effectiveness. There is no other known antiviral agent that is effective in cases of encephalitis. Supportive therapy involves bed rest and maintaining fluid balance to avoid dehydration (loss of body fluids).

Epilepsy

Epilepsy is a disorder characterized by sudden surges of disorganized electrical impulses in the brain, which lead to seizures.

There are several categories of seizures; they can be so mild as to go almost unnoticed or so severe that, if untreated, they can cause serious harm.

Causes

Epilepsy is usually divided into two categories: idiopathic (cause unknown) and acquired (cause —such as brain tumor or old injury—able to be determined). Up until the age of 35, idiopathic epilepsy is a very common cause of seizures. After age 35, however, a thorough diagnostic workup to exclude a cause is needed. Acquired epilepsy can be due to a multitude of causes, such as cerebral palsy, brain tumor, infection of the central nervous system, and malformations of blood vessels.

Idiopathic epilepsy, although by definition of unknown cause, has several consistent attributes. It occurs with highest frequency between the ages of two and five years and again at puberty and tends to run in families.

Symptoms

The symptoms of epilepsy vary according to the type of seizure experienced. A seizure is a term used to describe an attack of epilepsy. Not all seizures are convulsions. A convulsion involves the nerves that control movement and is characterized by jerking, spastic muscle movements. It is also marked by alterations in sensation and consciousness; in fact, loss of consciousness is common.

Seizures are classified according to the symptoms experienced. In the past, classifications were *grand mal* (big sickness), *petit mal* (little sickness), psychomotor, and focal. Current classifications separate seizures into partial or generalized types, depending on the extent of the brain's involvement.

The four current classifications and their symptoms:

- Simple partial seizures, confined to small areas of the brain, are experienced by feeling a tingling sensation in the arm, finger, or foot; perceiving a bad odor; seeing flashing lights; or speaking unintelligibly. The patient remains conscious.

- Complex partial seizures include episodes of "automatic behavior," in which the patient remains conscious but sits motionless or moves or behaves in a strange, repetitive, or somehow inappropriate way.

- Generalized convulsive seizures have a number of symptoms: the patient may cry out, stiffen and fall to the ground unconscious, lose urinary and bowel control, and have muscle spasms or thrashing movements that cause the limbs to jerk. Spasm of the jaw muscles can cause tongue biting. After the convulsion the patient falls into a deep sleep, and will awaken dazed, often with a headache and no recollection of the sei-

zure. Several warning signals (called the aura) may precede this type of seizure, among them headache, sleepiness, yawning, or tingling in the arms or legs.

- Generalized nonconvulsive or absence seizures, usually experienced by children, are characterized by periods of staring into space, rhythmic blinking, and what appears to be daydreaming. The patient remains conscious but is totally unaware of the seizure. This type of seizure may be mistaken for a short attention span or a learning disability in school.

Diagnosis

Epilepsy is diagnosed by observing the symptoms and by using an electroencephalograph (EEG), which measures the electrical activity of the brain and gives a visual record of brain impulses. In this way, abnormal electrical discharges can be detected if they are present in the brain. However, an abnormal EEG in the absence of symptoms is by no means proof of epilepsy, nor does a normal EEG rule it out.

Treatment

Non-medical treatment of an epileptic seizure should be limited to preventing injury and keeping the patient comfortable by loosening clothing or placing a pillow under the head. The patient should not be left face downward or in any position in which vomit can be swallowed or inhaled. *Never* should an attempt be made to pry open the mouth or insert any object into the mouth of a convulsing individual.

Anticonvulsant drugs are used to control epilepsy, and the majority of epileptics nowadays are well controlled. Patients who tend to have seizures following emotional or physical stress may also benefit from tranquilizers.

Epilepsy cannot be cured, but it can usually be controlled with a program of anticonvulsant drug therapy. After two to five years of drug control of idiopathic epilepsy, the dosage is sometimes decreased and, occasionally, when enough time has elapsed during which no seizures have occurred, medication can be discontinued.

Epilepsy cannot actually be prevented, but once the seizures are controlled by medication, epileptics can lead normal lives—hold jobs, raise families, drive cars, and so on—in the same way that victims of high blood pressure or diabetes can learn to live with their disabilities.

Headaches

A headache is a symptom, not a disease. A headache is rarely the symptom of a serious illness, but severe or frequent headaches can be exhausting and can affect daily life.

These blood vessels are the ones that are usually involved in a vascular-migraine headache.

There are three basic types of headaches. Vascular (pertaining to blood vessels) headaches occur when blood vessels in the head enlarge and press on nerves causing pain. The most common vascular headache is the migraine. Another common type of headache is the muscle contraction headache that results when the muscles of the face, neck, and/or scalp contract and tighten. A tension headache is an example of a muscle contraction headache. The third common kind of headache is the traction or inflammatory headache. These headaches are caused by pressure within the head, ranging from a minor condition like sinusitis to a more serious problem such as a brain tumor.

A more detailed description of each type of headache follows.

MIGRAINE HEADACHE

A migraine, or vascular headache, occurs when the blood vessels in the head enlarge and press on the nerves, causing pain. However, one theory about migraine headaches says that they result when the blood vessels first overreact to outside stimuli by constricting and thus blocking blood flow to parts of the brain; this may cause the visual impairment and numbness that often accompany a migraine. The blood vessels then become full of blood and press on surrounding nerves, causing pain.

Women are more prone to migraines than are men, and a certain personality type—compulsive, perfectionist, excessively neat, and very success-oriented—seems to be more susceptible to this kind of headache.

Causes

A number of physical and emotional factors may contribute to migraine headaches. Migraines may be triggered by a sharp reduction in caffeine intake or by allergies to certain foods or food additives (among them chocolate, fatty foods, alcohol, citrus fruits, monosodium glutamate, and nitrates). Emotional stress can also cause migraine headaches, as can drinking, smoking, or an interruption in routine eating and sleeping habits (all of which may be responsible for "week-end" headaches suffered by some patients). Cyclical, seasonal, or emotional factors, such as menstruation, for instance, may be associated with migraine. A tendency toward having this type of headache may be inherited.

Symptoms

The predominant symptom of a migraine headache is a sharp, pulsating, incapacitating pain on one or both sides of the head. Pale, sweaty skin; nausea; and sensitivity to light may accompany this pain.

Warning sensations (called an aura) may indicate an approaching migraine headache. Before the pain appears, some individuals may see flashing lights or "shooting stars," hear noises or smell fragrances, or feel a tingling sensation in the limbs.

Cluster headaches, a form of migraine most commonly experienced by men, occur in groups or clusters of up to six a day, lasting for weeks or months. Their symptoms are intense pain on one side of the head, teary eyes, and runny nose. Drinking and smoking may aggravate these headaches.

graines suffered by people who seem to react to certain foods or changes in eating and sleeping habits. In an elimination test, all the substances that are suspected to be causing the trouble are eliminated, then reintroduced one at a time, to determine the one causing the headaches.

Diagnosis

Vascular headaches are diagnosed by a careful review of the circumstances surrounding the headaches as well as by a physical exam to rule out any other disorder that may be causing them. Elimination tests may be done to identify the exact cause of mi-

Treatment

Treatment of a migraine already in progress usually consists of a drug therapy program chosen from a variety of painkillers, sedatives, and special drugs to combat migraine. For the occasional migraine sufferer, tranquilizers and sedatives may relieve some of

A muscular contraction headache usually involves these muscles.

the discomfort experienced during an attack.

Prevention

Prevention of migraines is possible with several types of medication. The most commonly prescribed is ergotamine, which constricts the blood vessels and thus prevents the swelling that causes pressure on the surrounding nerves. This drug is usually taken to stop an approaching migraine, so it has no effect on the "aura" symptoms some patients experience. Also, antidepressant drugs, taken in small doses, may prevent migraines in a patient who experiences them regularly.

A more recent development in migraine treatment is the use of the drug propranolol, a beta blocking drug. This drug works in the body to block what are called the beta effects, one of which causes blood vessels to enlarge. Because propranolol blocks the enlargement of blood vessels, it has been used to prevent, but not treat, acute attacks.

MUSCLE CONTRACTION HEADACHE

Muscle contraction headaches occur when muscles of the face, neck, or scalp contract and have spasms.

Causes

These headaches usually occur following a specific event that has caused the muscles to tense. The tension is then translated into physical discomfort in the form of a clenched jaw, aching neck, and squeezed muscles in the face and head.

Muscle contraction headaches can also be brought about by abnormalities in the eyes, neck, teeth, or jaws, or by poor posture—especially by holding the head at an awkward angle while reading, driving, or watching TV, for example.

Symptoms

The major symptom of these headaches is a tight, squeezing pain in the forehead, jaws, or around the back of the head or neck. This constant, dull pain usually occurs on both sides of the head.

Diagnosis

Diagnosis involves a review of the events that have led up to the headache as well as a physical examination to rule out any other disorder that may be causing it. A psychological examination may also be conducted to detect any emotional problems that may be contributing to the headaches.

Treatment

Eliminating the tension or correcting the physical problem that is causing the headaches is a good start in treating them. Painkillers, muscle relaxants, and tranquilizers may be used occasionally (although not on an everyday basis) to treat muscle contraction headaches. Also, antidepressant drugs may be effective in preventing these headaches in those persons who suffer from them regularly.

TRACTION OR INFLAMMATORY HEADACHE

Traction or inflammatory headaches occur when pressure within the head, stemming from a variety of disorders, causes pain.

Causes

Clogged sinuses or sinus infection are probably the chief cause of this type of headache. Sinuses are the cavities lined with mucous membrane within the facial bones. When mucus, which normally flows freely through the sinuses and drains out the nose, cannot properly drain, it collects in the sinuses and causes excess pressure on the surrounding tissues, leading to headache.

Other causes of traction or inflammatory headaches include aneurysm (a bulge in a blood vessel) or a brain tumor, both of which press directly on the brain; high blood pressure, which causes blood to rush through the vessels with too great a force, resulting in pressure in the head; infections, which inflame sensitive tissue; or fever, which may enlarge the blood vessels and cause excess pressure.

Symptoms

The symptoms of inflammatory headaches are a dull, aching pain, often occurring early in the day, accompanied by a feeling of pressure in the head. The pain is heightened by sneezing, coughing, bending over, or doing anything that increases the amount of blood in the head.

Diagnosis

This type of headache is diagnosed by determining first whether sinus problems are causing it; if not, the doctor may order X rays; a CAT (computerized axial tomography) scan, which shows a cross-sectional picture of the brain; or an EEG (electroencephalogram), which records electrical activity in the brain. These tests can detect the presence of a tumor, aneurysm, or abnormality in the brain.

Treatment

Inflammatory headaches are treated according to their cause. Those triggered by a sinus infection can usually be treated with painkillers or with antihistamines and decongestants, which dry out and help drain the sinuses. Headaches resulting from more serious disorders, such as brain tumor, brain abnormality, or aneurysm, will almost certainly require surgery.

Prevention

Prevention of these headaches is possible if the cause is as simple as a sinus infection. Of course, the correction of a more serious disorder that has caused the pain should also prevent future problems with traction or inflammatory headaches.

Hypothermia

Hypothermia is a condition in which the person's body temperature falls well below the normal temperature of 98.6°F. The lowering of the temperature can occur accidentally, or the temperature can be lowered in the course of medical treatment.

Accidental hypothermia

When hypothermia happens accidentally, the person's condition can become serious if the symptoms or signs are ignored. Among the causes of accidental hypothermia are the aging process, surgical procedures, certain drugs, and long periods of being exposed to the cold without having adequate clothing on. Hypothermia can occur easily in newborns and in infants, as well as in the elderly, as their heat-retaining mechanisms are, respectively, not fully developed and easily overtaxed.

The signs and symptoms of hypothermia include an altered level of consciousness, slow breathing, low pulse rate, listlessness, and mental confusion. The hands, feet, and abdomen of the hypothermic person will be cold to the touch.

Treatment

Basic treatment for hypothermia is the gradual or slow rewarming of the cold body. The rewarming must be gradual to prevent the sudden enlargement of blood vessels at the surface of the body, which may divert too much blood from some of the body's vital internal organs. Medical help should always be obtained for a person with hypothermia. While waiting for help to arrive, the cold person should be covered with blankets and, if alert, should be offered a warm non-alcoholic beverage. Alcoholic drinks do not help because they tend to reduce body heat. Also, briskly rubbing hands or feet to restore warmth is not recommended. Any other type of treatment depends on the underlying cause of the drop in body temperature. In severe cases where body temperature is critically reduced, warm intravenous (into the vein) fluids may be given. Peritoneal dialysis (injecting and withdrawing of fluid in the abdominal cavity) with warm fluids is also an excellent way of restoring normal temperature.

Intentionally induced hypothermia

The term "hypothermia" is also used to refer to a medical treatment technique. When this technique is used, the person's blood is gradually cooled, in order to lower the rate of the person's metabolism—that is, production of energy—so that the body's need for oxygen decreases. Once the need for oxygen decreases, the heart and brain can withstand a halt in the blood flow for short periods of time. Such interruptions make it possible for the patient to undergo delicate or painstaking surgery without hemorrhaging or severe bleeding. Intentionally induced hypothermia has been used, for example, in open-heart surgery.

Meningitis

Meningitis occurs when bacteria or viruses enter the spinal fluid and infect the meninges, the three layers of membrane that surround the brain and spinal cord. Meningitis can be fatal, although this is becoming less and less common because of the increased use of effective antibiotics.

Meningitis seems to strike males more often than females and is most commonly seen in children up to the age of four years and in adults over the age of 60. Swelling of the brain, as well as epilepsy, blindness, amnesia, and deafness, can result when meningitis is not properly and promptly treated.

The three layers of meninges are called the dura mater (the outermost layer), the arachnoid (the middle layer), and the pia mater (the innermost layer). A space between the inner two layers (called the subarachnoid space) is filled with clear fluid (called cerebrospinal fluid), which is produced in the brain. When bacteria or viruses invade this fluid and form pus, the surrounding membranes soon become infected, resulting in meningitis.

Causes

Meningitis is caused by an infection that enters the system through a serious head wound or through the bloodstream from a source of infection in another part of the body. The bacteria may also reach the meninges from an abscess (localized infection) of the brain itself, but this is quite rare.

A deficiency in the body's immune system, which can be either inherited or acquired over time, may lead to a greater chance of contracting this disease. Also, newborns may be at a greater risk if the mother had a genital infection such as herpes during the last week of pregnancy, if the membranes of the uterus ruptured prematurely, or if labor was prolonged.

Symptoms

The symptoms of meningitis are a "bursting" headache, high fever, rising pulse rate, irregular breathing, vomiting, and sensitivity to light. Pain extends down the neck, into the back and lower limbs; the neck may be stiff, and it will be difficult for the patient to bend forward. As the disease progresses, convulsions or coma may occur.

Diagnosis

If the doctor does not think there is increased pressure in the brain, meningitis may be diagnosed using a test called a lumbar puncture in which a sample of the cerebrospinal fluid is withdrawn and examined to see if it is clear (normal) or cloudy (pus-filled) and to identify the bacteria causing the infection. A physical exam, blood cultures, and cultures from the secretions of the respiratory tract may also be taken to determine the type of bacteria present. A viral infection, however, is much harder to diagnose; it may not show up on any tests.

Treatment

Immediate treatment is very important, so the doctor may prescribe medication for the meningitis patient even before the specific infecting agent is identified; once the cause is determined, an appropriate medication, most often an antibiotic, can be administered. The patient will be hospitalized where measures can be taken to reduce fever and control brain swelling.

Viral infections, again, are much harder to treat. There is no medication that will kill a virus that has entered the central nervous system. Treatment in this case is limited to hospitalization, where supportive therapy will be administered until the disease has run its course.

Prevention

Prevention of meningitis may be possible with some vaccines now available, which combat certain bacteria strains that cause meningitis. Research is still being done on vaccines for other bacteria strains.

Multiple sclerosis

Multiple sclerosis is a chronic disease of the central nervous system, consisting of the brain and spinal cord. Damage to the nerves results after the myelin sheath degenerates. The myelin sheath is the fatty substance insulating the nerve fibers of the nervous system. Once this protection disappears, body functions may become impaired. Ultimately, the patient may be wheelchair-bound or even die.

Causes

As yet, researchers have not determined the exact cause of multiple sclerosis. Some studies indicate that the disease follows exposure to a virus (contagious microorganisms attacking living cells). The virus may lie dormant (inactive) for some time before certain environmental factors, such as a second exposure to the virus or stress, trigger the disease.

Another theory suggests that multiple sclerosis affects people who have some defect in their immune system (the response of the body that attacks and inactivates disease-causing agents) that makes them more susceptible to the disease after exposure to the virus.

Symptoms

Initial attacks of multiple sclerosis are most common in people in their late 20s and early 30s. The disease begins with tingling and numbness in the arms and legs, muscle spasms, partial loss of vision, difficulty in walking, and impaired bladder control. After the first attack, there is usually a period of remission.

Subsequent attacks occur at irregular intervals and cause gradually increasing disability. Frequent episodes cause weakness, general incoordination, impaired speech, and a burning sensation in the affected areas. Sexual function lessens, and mood swings are common.

More extensive nerve damage may result in loss of muscle control and require the patient to use a wheelchair. Usually the earlier the onset of disease, the more slowly it progresses. Ten years after onset, less than half of these patients can continue regular daily activity.

Diagnosis

Physicians diagnose multiple sclerosis through physical examination and observation of symptoms. Often, diagnosis remains unconfirmed until a second attack occurs years later.

Treatment

Since there is no prevention or cure for multiple sclerosis, treatment concentrates on relieving the symptoms. Doctors prescribe muscle relaxants to help ease muscle spasms. Some patients find that corticosteroid drugs shorten acute attacks of the disease by reducing inflammation of the nerve tissue.

Besides drugs, many patients are more comfortable if they are well rested. Afternoon naps and adequate sleep at night offer some relief. In addition, cold temperatures sometimes improve symptoms, whereas heat makes them worse.

Myasthenia gravis

Myasthenia gravis is an uncommon disease of the nerves and muscles characterized by great fatigue and weakness in the muscular system, most notably in the face and throat, with slow and progressive paralysis, although the muscles do not atrophy (wither or waste away). It is most likely to strike adults, especially women between the ages of 18 and 25 and men older than 40, but it can affect any individual of any age.

Causes

Myasthenia gravis is sometimes associated with hyperthyroidism (overactive thyroid gland), excessive tissue in the thymus (a gland in the chest that is essential to the immune system), or tumors in the thymus.

The condition is a neuromuscular disorder; the muscles fail to receive messages from the nerves because of a lack of the important neurotransmitting chemical acetylcholine. Experts believe the problem originates in the autoimmune system, making the body fight against tissues instead of protecting them.

Symptoms

The muscular weakness first shows up in the face: eyelids droop, often causing squinting and double vision; there is an inability to move the mouth and lips, with subsequent difficulty in talking, chewing, and swallowing; cheeks generally droop or sag, resulting in a characteristic smile or stoical expression. Sometimes the arms and legs are afflicted, affecting basic motor movements like walking, standing, lifting a cup, and other simple tasks. It can also impair breathing. The degree of paralysis or weakness varies from hour to hour and day to day, although it tends to be minimal in the morning and worse at night. Blood tests and chest X rays aid in the diagnosis.

Treatment

Myasthenia gravis is usually not curable but drugs are available that restore nerve transmission to the muscles. The drugs neostigmine and pyridostigmine reestablish muscle strength and enable the patient with myasthenia gravis to live a more normal life. If it is determined that the problem originates in the thymus gland, it can be surgically removed.

Narcolepsy

Narcolepsy is a disorder in which the afflicted person is subject to a recurring, irresistible, uncontrollable desire to sleep, accompanied by muscular weakness and intense emotional reactions. The desire occurs during waking hours and often at inopportune times. Although the person falls into a deep sleep, it lasts only a few minutes. The person wakes up feeling refreshed but is likely to fall asleep again soon.

Causes

Narcolepsy is not necessarily related to a disease or condition, although it may be associated with cataplexy, a condition in which a person suddenly collapses to the floor at times of stress or unexpected emotional stimulus like laughter. It is thought that narcolepsy may be related to lesions or disturbances in the hypothalamus, a part of the brain, that cause a disorder in the endocrine system.

Treatment

Amphetamines, which are stimulants, are prescribed to treat narcolepsy.

Neuralgia

Neuralgia is pain that runs along the course of a damaged nerve. The condition ranges from mild and temporary to severe and chronic, but the pain itself is sharp and extreme, lasting only a few seconds at a time but tending to recur. The source of the injury to the nerve depends upon the type of neuralgia.

Trigeminal neuralgia

Tic douloureux or trigeminal neuralgia, the most common form, affects the faces of people over age 50 (except in cases of multiple sclerosis) and more commonly over age 70. The trigeminal nerve controls sensation in the face, teeth, mouth, and nasal cavity and triggers the muscles that move the jaw. The pain, usually excruciating, covers one side of the face and can be set off by eating, washing, or even by a gust of air. Eventually the stabbing pains occur closer together until they are constant. The cause is unknown, and, although not serious, it can become very disabling.

Sciatica

Sciatica pain is initiated by pressure on the body's largest nerve (sciatic) which runs from the spinal cord through the lower body and legs. The pressure is usually caused by a slipped disk between the vertebrae (backbones). The pain burns through the buttocks and along the back of the thighs.

Peripheral neuropathy

In peripheral neuropathy, impairment of the peripheral nerves, those outside the brain and spinal cord, occurs as a complication of other disorders—diabetes mellitus, alcoholism, a vitamin deficiency, anemia, tumors, or overexposure to certain chemicals and drugs (typical of farm and industrial workers). Symptoms begin as a tingling sensation in the hands and feet that slowly spreads up the limbs to the trunk; numbness follows in the same pattern, the skin becomes sensitive, and neuralgic pain ensues. Numbness in the hands leads to a loss of dexterity and susceptibility to accidents. A special risk is that a numbed part of the body can sustain an injury without the patient's awareness until it becomes infected or ulcerated.

Carpal tunnel syndrome

Carpal tunnel syndrome is compression of the large nerve that passes through the "tunnel" created by the wrist bones. It is fairly common, especially in pregnant women. Numbness, tingling, and a burning pain in the hand at first wake the patient at night and then begin occurring during the day.

Shingles

Shingles or herpes zoster is a viral infection characterized by intense pain and skin rash along the course of a nerve. Red blisters appear in a band usually along one side of the chest, trunk, or abdomen and can attack a nerve across the forehead. It occurs in adults during times of stress or after exposure to chicken pox, which is caused by the same virus.

Treatment

Treatment for the various types of neuralgia depends upon the location of the damaged nerves, severity of the pain, and the reason behind the impairment. Therapy may vary from cold or hot packs and aspirin to stronger prescription painkillers. For shingles, ointments may soothe and dry up blisters but, as with most viral infections, there is no direct treatment. A physician may refer a patient with neuralgia to a neurologist, a specialist in problems of the brain and nervous system. A neurologist may decide to sever a damaged nerve to eliminate the pain.

Prevention

There is virtually no way to prevent neuralgia, except to treat underlying diseases that may precipitate nerve damage and to avoid overexposure to chemicals and drugs.

Neurotransmitters

Neurotransmitters are chemicals that transmit nerve impulses from one nerve cell to another. The basic units of nerves are neurons, and their action is both electrical and chemical. At the ends of threadlike fibers extending outward from the core of each neuron are tiny sacs containing neurotransmitter chemical. After an electrical nerve impulse has traveled across a neuron, it reaches the nerve ending and stimulates the release of neurotransmitters from their sacs. The neurotransmitters travel across the gap (synapse) to the nerve ending of the next neuron and stimulate the production of an electrical charge that carries the nerve impulse forward. The process is then repeated until a muscle is moved or relaxed or a sensory impression is noted by the brain or a lower part of the central nervous system.

Paralysis

Paralysis is the loss of the ability to move a part of the body, usually brought on by damage to either the muscles or to the nervous system. Paralysis can vary in severity and degree from one small muscle to almost the entire body. Irreversible and permanent paralysis results when a nerve is completely severed and destroyed, whereas paralysis caused by some diseases that cause inflammation without actual destruction of nerve tissue may diminish as the condition is treated and the body recuperates.

Causes

There are numerous causes of paralysis. Brain damage resulting from disease or a stroke can lead to partial or total paralysis of various parts of the body. Such damage interferes with the transmission of nerve impulses from the brain to the muscles. Other diseases such as myasthenia gravis (a severe muscular weakness due to imbalances in the neurochemical transmission system) and poisons such as botulism or nerve gas sometimes also prevent nerve impulses from making contact with muscles, but do not necessarily cause complete loss of movement.

A spinal cord damaged or cut at mid to lower back can paralyze the legs and the lower part of the body, including the bladder and rectum; this condition is called paraplegia. A spinal cord that is injured around the neck affects both arms and both legs; this is known as quadriplegia.

Diabetes, cancer, alcoholism, vitamin deficiency, or drug reaction among others can injure peripheral nerves (those outside the brain and spinal cord) which then either weaken or totally immobilize the muscles they control, as well as cause loss of sensation in the areas they serve.

Treatment

Well-being and survival depend on the cause and extent of the paralysis. Obviously, paralysis that affects muscles involved in breathing is vitally significant because the very job of breathing has to be taken over by machines. However, artificial breathing may enable a patient to survive until the paralysis improves.

Patients whose paralysis does not require artificial measures for survival may benefit from physical or occupational therapy. These patients can learn to reuse a muscle or to develop other muscles to compensate for a disabled muscle. All patients with disabled muscles require special attention to prevent muscle atrophy (withering away), and ulcers (skin sores).

Parkinson's disease

Parkinson's disease is a progressive disorder characterized primarily by uncontrollable tremors in the limbs, a shuffling gait, and generalized muscular rigidity. It most often strikes people over the age of 60.

Parkinson's disease is usually not fatal, but it leads to changes in the entire body, making the patient more susceptible to other diseases. It can be present in a mild form for 20 or 30 years, but a severe case can lead to a serious disability within five to ten years.

Cause

The cause of Parkinson's disease is unknown, thus it is also not known why it strikes certain people. No inherited, medical, or environmental factors have been found definitely to cause the disease. The one exception to this is an epidemic of encephalitis (brain inflammation) that occurred some years ago following World War I. This disease produced a collection of symptoms and signs indis-

"Cogwheel rigidity" in a Parkinson's disease patient occurs when the arm is pulled straight and moves in a jerky fashion as if controlled by a rachet such as is found in a cogwheel.

tinguishable from true Parkinson's disease. However, since this is not true Parkinson's disease, the syndrome is referred to as "Parkinsonism."

It is known, however, that Parkinson's disease may be a reflection of a chemical imbalance in the brain. Those with the disease have been shown to have low levels of a neurotransmitter called dopamine. (Neurotransmitters are chemicals in the brain that transmit impulses across junctions between nerves; the balance of neurotransmitters in the brain is thought to be responsible for muscle control.) To date, no cause for this chemical deficiency has been found.

Symptoms

The symptoms of Parkinson's disease are uncontrollable shaking of the limbs, stiff muscles, drooling, reduced blinking, an expressionless face, stooping posture, and a shuffling walk. Tremors may worsen during rest periods and times of increased anxiety. Interestingly, the tremor may decrease when the patient reaches for an object or when he or she must act quickly under a great deal of stress.

As the disease progresses, speech slurs and sentences trail off into unintelligible muttering. Small muscle movement becomes increasingly difficult—reducing the ability to write, eat, chew, and swallow—and all movements seem overly stiff and slow. The term "cogwheel rigidity" is often used to describe the typical arm motion these patients may display; when pulled from a flexed position, the arm seems to jerk up and down as if controlled by a ratchet like that found in a cogwheel.

Excitement and tension can cause these symptoms to worsen, as can depression. Depression is common among Parkinson's disease victims, who are understandably upset by their loss of muscle control.

Diagnosis

Diagnosis involves a simple history, physical examination, and observation of the symptoms. If tremors are the only symptom displayed, the examination tests may be done to rule out the possibility that other disorders are causing the tremors, such as liver disease, multiple sclerosis (a debilitating muscular disorder), chronic alcoholism, or overactive thyroid gland.

Treatment

Treatment of Parkinson's disease consists of correcting the chemical imbalance caused by the dopamine deficiency. Dopamine itself cannot be absorbed directly into the brain from the bloodstream, so a substance called levodopa is prescribed to help the brain manufacture more of its own dopamine.

Levodopa has several undesirable side effects, among them nausea (which is decreased if the drug is taken with meals), an uneven "on-off" effect (causing symptoms to disappear and then reappear), and a loss of effectiveness over time. For these reasons and others, levodopa often is not prescribed or is given in smaller doses in combination with other types of drugs known as anticholinergics. These drugs decrease nerve to muscle transmission, thereby reducing tremor and rigidity. They also decrease drooling. Bromocriptine, a drug that enhances dopamine's effects, has also been successful, as have other drugs.

Physical therapy and exercise are also important in a treatment program for Parkinson's disease. In addition, emotional support and understanding are critical.

Rabies

Rabies (hydrophobia) is an acute infectious viral disease of the central nervous system of mammals, especially carnivores (meat eaters), which is characterized by central nervous system (CNS) irritation, followed by paralysis and, in some cases, death. Human infection usually follows the bite of a rabid animal (dogs, skunks, cats, foxes, coyotes, and so forth). In the later stages of the disease, it is marked by paralysis of the swallowing muscles and by throat spasms, which are set off by drinking or even the sight of liquids (hence, hydrophobia or "fear of water"). Convulsions, tetanus, and respiratory (breathing) paralysis are other symptoms of the last stages. Fortunately, because of animal immunization programs, there are now no more than about five reported cases of rabies per year in the United States.

Cause

Rabies is caused by a virus that is present in the saliva of rabid animals. Rabid animals transmit the infection by biting other animals or human beings. Rabies can also be acquired by exposure of a mucous membrane or of an open skin wound to infected animal saliva.

The rabies virus travels from the site of entry to the spinal cord and brain, where it multiplies. It then spreads to the salivary glands and into the saliva itself. In human beings the incubation period (the time between exposure to the virus and development of symptoms) may extend from ten days to one year, but the average incubation period is 30 to 50 days. The incubation period is shortest in persons who have been bitten on the head or trunk or those who have multiple bites.

Symptoms

The first symptom is a short period of mental depression, restlessness, and fever. In the next stage of the disease, the restlessness increases to an uncontrollable excitement and hyperactivity. There is excessive salivation ("foaming at the mouth") and painful spasms of the throat muscles. The spasms can be easily initiated — by a breath of air, a slight breeze, an attempt to drink water. Generally, the patient experiences overwhelming thirst, but cannot drink. In untreated cases, death occurs within three to ten days. However, patients often survive the disease if diagnosis and treatment are prompt.

Diagnosis

In human patients, diagnosis of rabies is usually suspected by a report of an animal bite or exposure to the saliva of a rabid animal. The diagnosis is confirmed by testing for the virus once the symptoms appear. A domestic animal with no symptoms, such as a cat or dog, that suddenly bites a human should be confined and observed by a veterinarian for ten days. If the animal still shows no symptoms, it was not infectious at the time of the bite and is usually released. However, if the animal is apparently rabid or is a wild animal, it should be captured. Local police or health departments should be notified so that they can capture and examine the animal. Only a professional should attempt to capture a suspected rabid animal.

Treatment

As soon as the bite or exposure of an open wound to animal saliva occurs, the contaminated area should be cleansed immediately and thoroughly with a 20 percent solution of medicinal soap. Deep puncture wounds should be flushed out with soapy water. It is not advisable to cauterize (seal by heat) or sew up the wound.

The next step is antirabies serum for passive immunization. This is followed by vaccine for active immunization. HDCV, a new active immunization, is said to have only mild side effects for most people. Both active and passive immunizing products should be used at once for best results.

HDCV injections are given on days 3, 7, 14, and 28 after exposure. The WHO (World Health Organization) recommends that a sixth injection be routinely done 90 days after the first injection.

Prevention

The best preventive measure for rabies is to minimize contact with rabid or suspected rabid animals. In many cases, persons with a high occupational risk of animal bites receive "preexposure" injections. This is especially helpful for zoo personnel and persons whose work or hobbies take them into areas where they are likely to encounter rabid animals.

As for domestic animals, restraining dogs and cats and impounding stray animals is the best preventive measure. Immunizing 70 percent or more of the dog population of major cities has helped to restrict transmission of rabies, even in areas where wild animals have the disease.

Controlling rabies in wildlife areas is more difficult, although rabies as a disease is self-limiting because it tends to kill off susceptible hosts in an area. Expensive control efforts are generally limited to areas where humans are apt to be exposed to wildlife—in campgrounds, parks, wildlife preserves, and so on.

Sciatica

Sciatica is a condition characterized by pain that extends along the entire length of the sciatic nerve (which runs down the lower back and outer side of the thigh, leg, and foot), radiating across the back of the pelvis through the buttocks and into the leg.

Area of lumbar vertebrae

Path of sciatic nerve

Sciatica is a condition in which pressure on the sciatic nerve causes pain to radiate along the path of the sciatic nerve as shown here.

Cause

Sciatica is most commonly associated with injury to or the rupture of a lumbar disk, one of the disks located between the lumbar (lower back) vertebrae. When the injured disk moves against the sciatic nerve, pain radiates down the nerve.

Symptoms

The symptoms of sciatica vary in intensity depending on the

extent to which the injured disk presses on the sciatic nerve and according to the individual's susceptibility to pain. In mild cases, the pain may be a slight discomfort in the lower back and along the leg. In severe cases, the pain is excruciating in the same areas and often completely immobilizes the victim. Furthermore, since the cause is usually a ruptured or "slipped" disk, it is difficult to know when an attack will begin. A sudden cough may cause the disk to move and press on the sciatic nerve, resulting in the pain that such pressure causes.

It is commonplace for sciatica patients to be free from pain one moment and in agony the next moment, depending on the position of the offending disk. Also, repeated problems with movements of the ruptured disk can cause a general inflammation of the sciatic nerve. In these cases, it is not a matter of the pain existing one time and disappearing another time. Instead, it is a matter of having less pain at one time than at another.

Treatment

In treating sciatica, the first line of attack is to make certain that the involved disk no longer presses on the sciatic nerve. Treatment to accomplish this may require placing the patient in traction, so that the spine is pulled from opposite directions, in the hope that the disk will slip back into place.

Physical therapy is also used to relieve the pain of sciatica. This treatment includes hydrotherapy, in which a stream of water is directed to the affected area, including the area of the ruptured disk. Also, many therapists advise their patients to overcome the effects of the ruptured disk by developing the core muscles—the four muscle groups that form the waist—in order to provide a supportive column of muscle that will help keep the disk in place.

In extreme cases, surgery is indicated. In this instance, the spine is fused in the area of the ruptured disk, and the possibility of further pressure against the sciatic nerve is eliminated.

THE SKIN

The skin is the outer covering of the body. This waterproof barrier affords protection from invasion of dirt, bacteria, and other harmful substances as well as helping to regulate internal body temperature.

Skin is the body's largest organ. The three layers comprising the skin cover about 18 square feet and weigh about seven pounds in an average adult.

Epidermis

The outermost layer of skin is the epidermis. The epidermis contains pigment cells that determine skin color and shield the skin against damaging sun rays. Specialized cells within this layer manufacture keratin, a tough substance found in hair and nails.

Epidermis cells continually reproduce and shed. This reconstruction is usually invisible, except when skin becomes irritated, such as in psoriasis, a disease that appears as scaly red patches.

Since the outer skin layer repairs itself quickly, any injury to the epidermis rarely causes injury to the body. However, damage which is severe enough to affect the middle layer, or dermis, can affect internal structures.

Dermis

The dermis is sometimes called the true skin because it contains blood vessels, nerve endings, hair follicles (tubes), sweat glands, and sebaceous (oil) glands. Damage at this level can send infection into the bloodstream and throughout the body.

Within the dermis, blood vessels and sweat glands help the body regulate heat. If the temperature of blood rises, the brain stimulates secretions from the sweat glands. Sweat then flows to the surface of the skin through ducts. Here, the liquid cools the skin by evaporating. Sebaceous glands in the dermis prevent excessive evaporation by coating the surface of the skin with an oily substance called sebum.

Subcutaneous layer

The innermost layer, the subcutaneous layer, is the layer in which the sweat glands originate. This layer also stores fat and supports the blood vessels and nerves that supply the outer layer.

Because the dermis and the subcutaneous layer are rich with nerve endings, the skin also serves as a sensory organ. Nerves throughout these layers transmit

This cross section of skin shows many of its structures.

tactile perceptions to the brain through the nervous system.

Acne

Acne is a condition of the skin that ranges in appearance from small raised bumps to pustules, large cysts and pimples on the skin surface. Acne is so common that more than 80 percent of the population can claim having had some form of it at some time.

Causes

Although there are several theories about what causes acne, authorities generally believe that acne is a by-product of hormonal changes in the body during pu-

berty—that period of life when a child develops the secondary sex characteristics (such as facial and body hair, deepened voice, and increased muscle mass in boys and breast development and menstruation in girls) of an adult. At this time, hormone production increases, particularly the male hormone testosterone, and stimulates the sebaceous (oil) glands that lie within the skin.

Most excess oil produced by these glands leaves the skin through a series of tubes called hair follicles that contain small hairs. Sometimes, oil clogs these tubes and creates comedones or blocked hair follicles. Comedones are what form the initial lumps in acne.

If comedones are open to the surface of the skin, they are called

When excess material produced by the sebaceous glands clogs the hair follicle tube, a blackhead results. A blackhead is open on the surface of the skin, but nevertheless blocks the normal release of material from the sebaceous gland to the skin's surface.

When a blocked hair follicle is not open on the surface of the skin, it may eventually rupture internally, discharging its contents into the surrounding tissues. This results in an inflammatory response that sets the stage for the development of acne.

blackheads. They contain oil (sebum) from the glands, bacteria, and any skin tissue that accumulates near the surface. Comedones that are closed at the surface are called whiteheads. Plugged follicles can rupture internally, resulting in a discharge of their contents into the surrounding tissues. This process sets up an intense inflammatory response that sets the stage for the development of acne.

The role of bacteria in acne is unclear. Bacteria may act by causing chemical reactions in the sebaceous fluid, leading to the release of very irritating compounds called "fatty acids." These in turn may cause inflammation that increases susceptibility to infection.

Authorities vary about emphasizing diet as a cause of acne. Diet alone does not cure acne, nor does acne stem from an allergic reaction to a specific food. However, some cases of acne improve after eliminating certain foods, particularly chocolates and fats. In addition, emotional stress seems to increase acne.

Symptoms

Acne causes raised swellings most frequently on the face, neck, back, chest, and shoulders. Severe acne may have pus-filled sacs that break open and discharge fluid. Soreness, pain, or itching may accompany the bumps. These symptoms could be acne, or they could indicate other skin reactions to such substances as cosmetics, medications, and grooming or cleaning products.

Since puberty plays a role in the onset of acne, the condition usually appears during teenage years. Nevertheless, it can extend to age 25 and over, particularly in women. Although acne is not life-threatening, it can be problematic. If untreated, comedones can leave permanent scars which can result in embarrassment and emotional stress.

Treatment

Acne has no prevention or cure, but there are several treatments. The simplest home remedy is to wash the affected areas thoroughly at least twice a day with warm water and mild soap. Washing gently will not dry or irritate sensitive skin. Regular shampooing also helps acne, especially if the hair is oily. Use of makeup should be limited. In addition, skin may heal with exposure to the sun. However, sunlamps or ultraviolet lamps should be used very cautiously under a doctor's supervision.

One form of treatment not recommended is picking or squeezing pimples, since more inflammation or scarring may result. Also, the risk of infection is increased.

Some over-the-counter acne medications, particularly lotions or creams containing benzoyl peroxide, can help troubled skin. However, most of these preparations tend to dry the skin if manufacturer's directions are not followed carefully.

For persistent acne, a doctor may prescribe a preparation that can be applied on the skin or oral antibiotics such as tetracycline or erythromycin. These antibiotics act to suppress bacteria that may cause the aforementioned chain of events.

Another drug, tretinoin (Vitamin A acid), has reduced acne in more than 50 percent of the people who have tried it. This drug can be taken independently or in combination with an antibiotic —all under a doctor's supervision. A newer drug, isotretinoin, is related to tretinoin and is used to treat severe cystic acne. It is usually not prescribed, however, unless all other acne treatments have failed. These drugs work by temporarily suppressing the activity of the sebaceous glands.

Athlete's foot

Athlete's foot (whose medical name is *tinea pedis*) is ringworm of the foot. A fungus infection of the skin between the toes and also of the skin on the soles of the feet, it causes itching, burning, and stinging sensations. The skin between the toes reddens, cracks open, and crumbles. In extreme long-lasting cases, the toenails may become infected, discolored, and overgrown. The fungus may spread to the underside of the foot, beneath the arch, producing groups of itching blisters and peeling of the skin.

Causes

It is important to rule out other causes of similar symptoms. For example, hot, tight shoes may produce sweaty feet in warm weather; the moisture and friction may cause softening and peeling of the skin on the soles. Dyes, adhesive cements, and other substances inside the shoes may cause irritation, as may powders and nail polishes. Eczema, psoriasis, and scabies are other sources of symptoms.

If sweaty feet are the cause, athlete's foot ointments should not be used. Instead, you should ask your doctor for suggestions about controlling the excessive sweating; there are ointments and solutions that can help this condition. Changing shoes may eliminate the problem if the feet are sensitive to chemicals inside the shoes.

Treatment

Most people can treat their athlete's foot condition at home using one of several good salves, powders, or liquids obtainable without prescription from the drugstore. These include compound undecylenic acid ointment, tolnaftate, and miconazole. Clotrimazole is another good medicine, but it requires a prescription from a physician. Directions usually call for application morning and night, to continue until one week after all symptoms have vanished. As long as loose skin remains, the feet should be soaked before the ointment is applied, and the loose skin removed carefully.

Severe cases of athlete's foot call for treatment by a physician. To relieve symptoms, the doctor may prescribe soaking the feet three times a day in a solution of aluminum sulfate and calcium acetate (often called Burow's solution) with an antiseptic solution added if a secondary infection is present. In extreme cases the antifungal drug griseofulvin may be prescribed, to be taken by mouth.

Prevention

Athlete's foot can recur despite any treatment, especially during the hot summer months. The organisms that cause athlete's foot thrive in a hot, moist setting. However, there are several things you can do to help prevent the disease. You can keep your feet clean, dry between your toes after bathing, and change socks frequently. Use dusting and drying powders to keep the feet dry. Separate your toes with small wads of cotton when you are sleeping. Wear wooden or rubber clogs in motel and community showers and sandals, open-toed shoes, or no shoes at all during hot weather.

Baldness

Baldness (the technical term is alopecia) is partial or complete loss of hair on the head. This may be caused by an inherited tendency and/or by aging, fever, infection, certain drugs, radiation, injury, or disease.

Male-pattern baldness

Male-pattern baldness is the most common form. There seems to be an inherited tendency toward it, and androgen, a male hormone, contributes to it. However, the exact way it occurs is not known. Hair loss is gradual, occurring at the forehead, on either side of the front (sometimes leaving a center tuft known as a "widow's peak"), and on the top of the head. It can begin as early as age 15 or 16, in which case it may indicate that considerable baldness is likely later (however, male-pattern baldness does not usually advance at a steady or predictable rate). Female-pattern baldness is fairly common in women of menopausal age and usually involves only the thinning of the hair in the area around the crown. It is also believed to be due to hormonal causes as is male-pattern baldness.

Temporary baldness

Temporary baldness sometimes occurs up to three or four months following a severe illness, especially one with fever such as scarlet fever. It can result from lowered activity of the pituitary or thyroid glands, from early syphilis, pregnancy, birth control pills, "crash" dieting or malnutrition, certain medications, or too much Vitamin A. When the cause is removed, the missing hair usually returns.

Spotty baldness

Spotty baldness (alopecia areata) may affect areas of the head and beard. The cause is unknown, but it often clears up after a few months if there are just a few spots and if it first occurs in adulthood. However, it may reoccur. The outlook is less favorable for spotty baldness that begins in childhood or if hair loss is widespread.

Occasionally, all body hair is lost. When this happens, and there is no readily apparent cause such as fever or severe illness, the hair is not likely to return.

Permanent baldness

Permanent baldness results when the scalp is scarred by burns, other injury, or disease. Diseases which can cause scarring baldness include severe bacterial infections, tuberculosis, ulcers, severe ringworm of the scalp, lupus erythematosus, and certain slow-growing tumors.

Treatment

There is no satisfactory medical treatment at this time to cure or prevent baldness. However, hair transplants can be effective. Scalp plugs containing active follicles (hair cells) to be transplanted are taken from the back of the head, which is not affected by male-pattern baldness. The transplanted follicles continue to grow hair just as before, despite the new location.

Boils

A boil, or furuncle, is a contagious bacterial infection and irritation of the skin and its underlying structures. It is a painful swelling in the skin that is easily detected by touch. When a group of boils interconnects below the surface of the skin, a carbuncle forms.

Causes

Boils develop when staphylococci bacteria enter the skin through a hair follicle and multiply in its warm, moist environment. Bacteria continue to grow while producing substances that invade surrounding cells. In the body's defense, white blood cells (whose job is to attack and kill invading organisms) travel to the infected hair follicle and enclose the bacteria. As more white blood cells gather, they eventually consume the bacteria and eliminate the infection. This counterattack by the white blood cells is what produces the pustule in the center of the boil, because of the buildup of white blood cells. When the pustule ruptures, pus and dead skin cells killed by the bacteria drain out, and the boil heals.

Staphylococci germs are often found in the nose and throat where washing cannot reach them. They spread to a hair follicle from there or another site on the body, by contact with another person or by contact with an infected article such as a washcloth or towel. In most cases, however, other people coming in contact with the bacteria do not get boils.

Those at risk

People with diseases such as anemia (deficiency of red blood cells), diabetes, or localized infections that weaken their natural defenses against bacteria seem more susceptible to boils. Others who are physically run down may also have greater difficulty fighting the infection. Often, those who work with greasy or oily substances are more likely to develop boils because these materials trap bacteria against the skin. Poor bathing habits, especially in summer months when sweaty skin provides the moist climate conducive to bacteria growth, also invite infection.

Symptoms

Boils can develop anywhere on the skin. They appear most frequently on the neck, face, and back, and they can erupt in several places at once. Although boils vary in size, they characteristically form white or yellow pustules. As the infection progresses, the pustule becomes red and hot. Excess fluid in the boil produces pressure on the nerves underneath that can result in considerable pain. When boils contain little pus, they are called *blind boils*. In this instance, the inflammation recedes slowly without rupturing, but sometimes it leaves a scar.

If boils are large or extensive, the person may also experience fever and a general weakened feeling. Sometimes, the infection gets into the bloodstream and spreads throughout the body. The same bacteria that cause the boil may also produce a toxin (poison) that causes blood clots, usually in the small blood vessels around the boil.

Treatment

Any treatment plan for boils and carbuncles emphasizes that they should *never* be squeezed, particularly if they are on the face. Squeezing may force the infection deeper into the skin and possibly into the bloodstream. Only a physician should lance a boil to encourage drainage. Afterwards, the doctor may prescribe an oral antibiotic such as penicillin or erythromycin to fight further infection.

Many boils will rupture and heal on their own. However, holding a soft cloth soaked with warm water against the boil for 15 to 20 minutes at least four times a day will speed the process. These warm compresses increase blood flow to the area and encourage pustule formation. Since bacteria from the boil is contagious, the cloth should be disinfected in boiling water or in the hot cycle of a washing machine.

When a boil bursts, the infected area should be washed thoroughly and covered with an antibiotic cream and sterile gauze. If the boil does not heal within a few days, or if the boil is located on or near the face, a physician should be consulted.

Prevention

To prevent new eruptions, the skin needs to be kept cool and dry. Sometimes, physicians advise washing the entire body with an antiseptic (germ-fighting) soap twice a day. If boils frequently recur, underclothing and bed linen should be changed every day.

Calluses

Calluses are thickened areas of the skin. They develop most often on the balls and heels of the feet and on the hands.

Causes

Skin buildup is the result of excessive friction or pressure against the surface of the skin. As pressure mounts, dead skin cells accumulate, and the skin thickens. Improperly fitting shoes or tightly held pencils can create the problem. Since calluses often follow blisters on the same site, they are considered to be the body's way of shielding the area against further injury.

People with flat feet have greater incidence of calluses. The reason for this is that because of the abnormal shape of the foot, the small bones in the front portion of the foot are forced downward against the skin of the sole with great pressure while walking. This creates pressure points, thus leading to callus formation. In addition, those who wear high heels promote growth of calluses by increasing pressure on the balls of their feet.

Symptoms

Calluses vary in size and shape depending upon where they grow and how much skin is affected. Sometimes, calluses grow so thick and irregular in shape that the skin becomes inflexible and cracks.

When pressure is relieved, calluses usually produce no pain. However, continued irritation, especially against split skin, can cause enough discomfort to interfere with physical activities.

Treatment

Immediate treatment involves removal of the pressure that caused the callus in the first place. Extremely persistent or painful calluses should be examined by a doctor. In rare instances, surgery may be necessary to alleviate intense pressure. In milder cases, calluses can often be eased by padding the exposed area to reduce further friction.

There are over-the-counter remedies that soften the callused tissue, making it easier to remove. Salicylic acid plasters, which are sold in medicated sheets, can be placed over the callus after bathing and secured with tape. The pad should be removed just before the next bath so that the softened skin can be gently removed with a pumice stone or other rough surface.

Home remedies should not be used by people who have diabetes, atherosclerosis, or other circulatory disorders because risk of infection is greater with these diseases. These individuals should consult their doctor before attempting any form of treatment.

Canker sores

Canker sores (technically known as aphthous ulcers) are inflamed tissue cavities or ulcers usually found in the mouth. They can be quite painful, often inhibiting eating ability. Even though up to one out of every four persons develops canker sores, they are not contagious.

Causes

Researchers differ about the cause of canker sores. One unconfirmed theory suggests that the sores are the result of an "autoimmune response," whereby the body develops antibodies to its own tissue. Other factors that have been said to trigger canker sores include fever, menstruation, fatigue, tension, or allergies. Some people get canker sores after eating certain foods. Poor dental hygiene, ill-fitting dentures, or injuries from stiff toothbrushes may also lead to the condition. All of the above may be contributing factors; however, the true cause of canker sores is unknown.

Symptoms

A canker sore begins as a small blister that occurs alone or in groups. It can be found almost anywhere in the mouth, such as inside the cheek and on the tongue, lips, or gums.

After the blister breaks, a small ulcer or cavity develops and enlarges until it becomes a bright red sore surrounding the whitish yellow cavity of the ulcer. This sore can last about 10 to 14 days before healing. Canker sores leave no scars. However, they often recur, sometimes every few weeks or months.

Treatment

Canker sores have no cure, but there are several treatments that may relieve pain. Some physicians prescribe the antibiotic tetracycline for canker sores. Treatment involves dissolving the capsule in an ounce of warm water and swishing the mixture in the mouth for five to ten minutes, three or four times a day for five to seven days. Sometimes, therapy includes soaking a cotton wad in the solution and applying it directly to the sores.

There are also various over-the-counter preparations designed to reduce discomfort. However, they are of uncertain value, and you should always check with your doctor before using them.

Prevention

People who have repeated attacks of canker sores should see a physician or dentist. Recurrence may be lessened by improving oral hygiene or by avoiding certain foods or other substances.

Corns

Corns are small, round mounds of firm, dead skin that form on or between the toes. Their hard,

Corns are small mounds of dead skin that form on or between the toes. Their cores, formed in the epidermis layer of the skin, bore down on underlying tissue and nerves in the dermis layer, causing pain.

waxy core, which bores down into the skin and presses on the underlying tissue and nerves, can cause extreme pain. At times corns are associated with bursae (fluid-filled sacs), which can become irritated and result in bursitis.

Causes

Corns are caused by a great deal of pressure or friction on the toes (as are calluses, their basis), usually from ill-fitting shoes or high heels. Since the skin acts as the body's protector from the outside environment, corns form when the body attempts to protect the troubled area from more pressure by building up a mass of dead skin cells and secreting a hard substance called keratin. Sometimes people who have abnormal bone structures in their feet or some types of arthritis tend to develop corns. Generally, however, those who avoid high heels or tight-fitting shoes should be able to avoid corns. Usually regular in shape, corns can be white, gray, or yellow, and usually form on the outside of the first or fifth toes, since that is where pressure most often occurs. Corns that form between the toes are called soft corns, since they are not as firm as other corns because of the moisture between the toes.

Treatment

Corns are best treated by first eliminating the cause of the pressure. Over-the-counter preparations are available. These include padding to reduce the friction on the area, ointments, and medicated pads, which will soften and blister the skin layers, making them easier to remove and reducing the pain. Severe or persistent corns must be treated by a doctor, but only rarely will they require surgery. Persons with diabetes, atherosclerosis, or other circulatory diseases should *never* treat a corn themselves, as the risk of infection is much greater for persons with these conditions.

Cyst

A cyst is a sac or membrane containing a fluid or semisolid material. In normal anatomy, the term literally refers to a bladder, including the urinary bladder (which is why inflammation of that bladder is called cystitis) and the gallbladder (which is why the duct leading from the gallbladder is called the cystic duct and the gallbladder itself is called the cholecyst). However, most cysts are not normal. Cysts may form around a foreign body, such as a particle in the lung or the skin, or around a parasite. They may entrap an escaping body liquid, such as blood hemorrhaging into tissue or fluid leaking from a bursa (a sac containing lubricant for a joint). In the intestine, they may develop in a fold or pouch lining the intestinal tract. They may be enlargements of natural fluid-filled sacs such as a bursa. They may develop on the ovaries; ovarian cysts are abnormal, sometimes painful, but usually harmless and self-healing entities of the ovaries that usually occur in response to changes in a woman's menstrual cycle.

Common types

Perhaps the most common cysts are those of the skin and mucous membranes. A *sebaceous cyst* occurs when a sebaceous gland, the tiny oil gland at the base of each hair root, becomes plugged. Ordinarily this plugging just results in a blackhead, or a pus-filled pimple if the blackhead becomes infected. Occasionally, however, the pimple does not break and the swelling becomes entrapped beneath the skin. Sebum (oil from the sebaceous gland) continues to flow into the sac that forms in the cavity, and the cyst grows to the size of a marble or larger. Sebaceous cysts—which can occur on any part of the body where there is hair, including the neck, scalp, and back—can easily be removed surgically if bothersome; however, if they become infected, they must be drained and removed. A type of tiny cyst known as *milium*, usually occurring on the scrotum, can simply be opened and drained. Larger cysts must be removed completely, or they will recur.

Mucous cysts which occur in the mouth, on the tongue, or on the lower lip are caused by plugged-up mucous glands and may grow to be the size of a pea or larger. They may be removed in the same manner as sebaceous cysts.

Traumatic epithelial cysts usually result from the trapping beneath the skin of a piece of skin, a blood clot, or foreign material because of some injury and may or may not need to be removed.

Dermatitis

Dermatitis is an inflammation of the skin. There are many different kinds of dermatitis, and a great variety of causes. Some of the more common varieties include the following.

Contact dermatitis

This is a skin inflammation caused by a substance that has touched the skin. This may be a harsh chemical or a detergent or soap that directly irritates. On the other hand, the substance may produce an allergic reaction that can appear five or six days after the contact or, less commonly, after years of repeated use. Common causes of allergic contact dermatitis are poison ivy, chemicals in shoes and clothing, metal watchbands and rings, antibiotic salves, and cosmetics. There are also cases in which a substance, such as a shaving lotion or cosmetic, produces a "photoallergic" reaction when the skin under the substance is exposed to sunlight.

Eczema

This inflammation of the skin is marked by blisters (when severe), redness, fluid in the tissue, oozing, scales, crusts or scabs, burning or itching, and sometimes dryness. There are several different forms of eczema. One of the more common types is atopic dermatitis. This is a continuing, itching skin inflammation whose victims often have a family history of allergic diseases such as asthma or hay fever. Typically, it begins in infancy, subsides by age three, and may reappear by age ten or 12. Foods such as wheat, milk, eggs, and substances such as pollen or fur often bring on symptoms and, if so, must be avoided.

Seborrheic dermatitis

This is a scaling and inflammation of the scalp and sometimes the face or other parts of the body. This is the cause of dandruff in adults and cradle cap in infants.

Nummular dermatitis

Coin-shaped patches of blisters that later ooze liquid and crust over mark this condition, which usually is accompanied by dry skin and itching. Most often it appears on the legs and sometimes the buttocks and trunks of middle-aged people.

Localized neurodermatitis

This condition is characterized by thick, sharp-bordered, scaly breaks in the skin, with little blisters. This is a temporary condition caused by habitual scratching of an insect bite or other irritation of the skin and is corrected by covering the area and stopping the scratching. In the case of an itch in the area around the openings of the vagina and colon, however, warts, pinworms, hemorrhoids, infections, or certain diseases may be the cause.

Chronic dermatitis

This often occurs on the hands or feet, and may simply be the result of continued irritation, especially by contact dermatitis. It is marked by thickened skin, inflammation, and scaling. Sometimes it is caused by excessive hand washing and by soaps or detergents accumulating under rings. Fungus infections of the feet occasionally spread to the hands, producing inflammation.

Exfoliative dermatitis

This condition produces a shedding of skin all over the body, together with hair loss. The entire skin surface is red, scaly, and thickened. The cause is unknown in most cases, but it sometimes occurs following a lesser dermatitis or as a side effect of a drug. Hospitalization is frequently necessary because the condition can threaten life. A first step is to consult a doctor about any medications and to ask about stopping or changing them.

Stasis dermatitis

This stubborn skin inflammation of the lower legs is usually the result of poor blood supply to the area. There is redness, mild scaling, and a brown discoloration of the skin. If the condition is neglected, the skin swells and may become infected or affected by ulcers (eroded skin sores).

Treatment

Because there is such a bewildering variety of skin diseases and because some can be dangerous if neglected, it is important to seek medical care for any dermatitis. In general, this care usually begins with very simple measures. Dry skins need lubricating agents, while moist or oily skins require powders or other drying substances. Inflamed skin is treated with creams; cool, wet dressings; or baths.

Hardened dried skin may be peeled off with strong substances. If possible, the cause of the dermatitis is sought out with the patient's help and eliminated. Cortisone creams are often used to make the patient more comfortable by reducing inflammation, although continuous use is not usually recommended. Antibiotics are employed promptly to eliminate any infections that arise, before they can spread to other parts of the body. Patients need to resist the constant temptation to scratch itchy areas or remove scabs, because that can simply prolong and even worsen the trouble. In addition, while cleanliness is desirable, some patients need to be told to reduce hand washing and the number of baths they take, because they are washing away natural oils designed to

protect the skin. Along the same lines, patients should not use more medication than the doctor recommends, or leave it on longer than directed. Overmedication of skin diseases is worse than undermedication.

Fever blisters

Fever blisters, also called cold sores, are fluid-filled blisters that appear on the border of the lips and on or around the nose. They are the result of a very contagious virus that has affected most of the population at one time or another.

Causes

The virus that causes fever blisters is a type of herpes simplex virus, and it enters the body most often in the mouth or nose areas where skin is easier to penetrate.

At first, characteristic blisters may or may not result. Antibodies (protective substances) in the body defend against the invading virus. When inactive, the virus withdraws to a nearby nerve, where it remains until stress to the body or a diminished capacity to fight off infection triggers a recurrence. When the virus reactivates, it overruns the body's protective system and progresses back along the nerve to the general area of original infection.

Factors that seem to favor the appearance of blisters include fever, colds, menstruation, skin injury from dental work, excessive sun and wind exposure, and emotional stress. Cold sores can return every few weeks for several weeks or not at all.

Symptoms

Initially, the virus may present no symptoms, so some people are unaware of infection. For others, the infection begins with numbness or tenderness in the affected area. Then small fluid-filled blisters appear. These blisters break, encrust, and heal within one to two weeks without leaving a scar.

Complications

Occasionally, excessive pain or swollen lymph glands develop. These symptoms may indicate a secondary bacterial infection that needs a doctor's attention.

Other complications can be more serious. *Herpes simplex keratitis* is a painful viral infection of the cornea (transparent covering) of the eye that can result in blindness if not treated. When inflamed eyes accompany fever blisters, a physician should be consulted immediately. In addition, steroid (cortisone) medication or cream should not be used near eyes during a herpes attack without consulting a doctor, since these preparations can encourage spread of the virus to the eye.

Other serious complications can occur in infants and extremely ill patients who contract herpes virus if the infection travels to the lungs, brain, or other internal organs.

Treatment

Treatment involves relieving symptoms since there is no known cure for fever blisters. Some over-the-counter remedies may relieve pain and help dry blisters. Topical corticosteroid creams, however, should not be applied unless prescribed by a physician; the possibility of spreading infection may increase if the corticosteroid depresses the immune response.

Healing time can be shortened by certain newer prescription drugs, if they are used early in the development of the disease.

Frostbite

Frostbite is damage to skin tissue resulting from exposure to low environmental temperatures. The condition can affect any part of the body, but more often those areas involved have the poorest blood circulation and greatest exposure to cold, such as the face, hands, or feet.

Causes

When exposed to cold, the body naturally tries to protect vital organs. Blood vessels near the surface of the skin constrict to preserve internal body heat. This tightening causes blood to be diverted away from the outside of the body, thereby reducing the supply of blood to skin tissues. As a result, skin tissue freezes from the lack of a warm blood supply and dies.

Frequently, frostbite develops after prolonged exposure to cold. Extremely low temperatures or forceful winds can also cause the condition. Insufficient or improper clothing increases susceptibility to frostbite. Contact with metal can freeze skin to the surface of an object and block circulation to the area. In addition, any health problem or damaged skin that may weaken the body or reduce circulation increases the likelihood of frostbite.

Stages of frostbite

Frostbite develops in three stages, and each stage can produce varying degrees of pain. First degree frostbite appears as white or slightly yellow skin accompanied by burning or itching sensations. In this stage, symptoms can be reversed if the affected area is warmed quickly.

Should exposure to cold continue, sensation in the affected area ceases. Disappearance of pain along with reddened and swollen tissue signals second degree frostbite. At this stage, warming the area may produce blisters and skin peeling. Blisters may persist for weeks, and tenderness may linger for months.

Skin with third degree frostbite becomes waxy and hard. By this stage, skin tissue dies and the affected portions may show edema (collection of fluid in tissues). Severe frostbite can damage muscles, tendons, and nerves. Blood clots may form in small blood vessels and inhibit circulation. In turn, blockage causes death of deeper tissue (gangrene).

Treatment

Initial treatment focuses on what *not* to do since there are many misconceptions about the proper course of action. Frostbitten tissue should not be rubbed with snow. In fact, the affected part should not be rubbed at all because further damage to tissue can result. Exercising the frostbitten area or walking on frostbitten feet aggravates the condition.

A good treatment plan includes going indoors as soon as possible to thaw the affected area. Frostbitten tissue should be immersed in lukewarm water rather than exposed to extreme heat of a radiator, stove, or fire. Ideally, water temperature should be between 100°F and 110°F. Any temperature above 110° can burn the skin that lacks sensation.

Rapid thawing produces pain, redness, and possibly blisters. However, these symptoms are part of the therapy necessary to reduce tissue loss and avoid complications. Patting the skin dry helps prevent additional injury.

If the patient remains outdoors, affected areas can be warmed by placing them in contact with warm portions of the body, such as under the armpit or between the thighs. The area can also be wrapped in a warm, dry blanket. Frozen parts need to be kept clean to prevent infection. Sometimes, warm nonalcoholic drinks aid circulation. Nevertheless, affected people should not smoke because smoking constricts blood vessels.

Once frozen tissue rewarms, the patient should elevate the extremity to promote increased blood circulation and maintain the skin at room temperature. Most cases of frostbite require a doctor's consultation. The physician may prescribe medication to prevent infection or formation of clots in blood vessels.

Prevention

The best prevention of frostbite is to wear adequate clothing to protect the skin. Feet, hands, and parts of the face need covering since these areas are likely to have the poorest blood circulation and are the most exposed. When weather is unusually cold or windy, remaining indoors or keeping outside trips short to limit exposure is recommended.

Heat rash

Heat rash, or prickly heat, is a mild skin condition that produces an itchy, burning sensation. It is found most often in infants and overweight people who have overlapping folds of fat.

When skin surfaces press together, sweat ducts that carry secretions from the sweat glands to the skin's surface become temporarily blocked. Normally, these sweat glands work along with blood vessels to regulate the body's heat. If the blood temperature rises, the brain triggers a reflex in the sweat glands to encourage secretion of sweat. Sweating reduces body temperature by releasing sweat to the surface of the skin where it evaporates and cools the skin. If sweat cannot reach the skin's surface, it may break through its duct wall and remain trapped in an inner layer of the skin where it can cause inflammation and a rash.

Causes

Heat rash can result any time the body needs to perspire. Most often, hot weather or exertion triggers the reaction. However, tight clothing or overdressing may compound the problem.

Heat rash in infants may be caused by immature sweat glands that cannot transport large amounts of perspiration to the surface of the skin. The sweat stays in the skin, thereby producing the same irritation.

Symptoms

Usually heat rash, or miliaria as it is known medically, appears on moist parts of the body where skin surfaces can touch, such as on the neck, under arms, or between legs. Infants can show the rash under a tight-fitting diaper. The rash looks like tiny, pinhead-sized red pimples, and it can cause itching and a prickling or burning sensation.

Heat rash is sometimes confused with a condition called chafing because the symptoms are similar. However, chafing is caused by friction between the two surfaces rubbing together and not by obstructed sweat ducts.

Under extreme conditions, the warm, moist areas where heat rash develops can become breeding grounds for microorganisms that cause secondary infection.

Treatment and prevention

Treatment and prevention of heat rash involve reducing or

Heat rash usually occurs in areas of the body where skin surfaces are close together or overlap. For example, folds of fat press together and may temporarily obstruct the opening of the sweat gland.

eliminating the stimulus for sweating. The affected person needs to stay in a cool environment and refrain from exertion. Cool showers followed by thorough drying can also help, as can wearing light, loose-fitting clothes. Once sweating stops, the rash may disappear in a few hours.

Babies who suffer from heat rash can be bathed in plain water and dried thoroughly. Cloth diapers are more likely to allow the natural evaporation process to occur than are paper diapers. If discomfort becomes prolonged or extreme, a doctor should be consulted.

Leukoplakia

Leukoplakia is a tough, fibrous lesion — most often in the form of a white patch — appearing on the lips, tongue, gums, and on other areas where there are mucous membranes (linings) such as the female genital organs. Leukoplakia is often referred to as smoker's patches or smoker's tongue. Although these lesions are generally not painful, they may cause difficulty and discomfort when the person talks or swallows, especially if the patches are on the lips, gums, or tongue.

Causes

The oral condition can be caused by badly fitted dentures, excessive smoking, overconsumption of alcohol, or a diet of highly spiced foods. Leukoplakia may also be a symptom of syphilis and may develop into a cancerous growth.

Diagnosis

If a person notices these persistent white patches, a physician should be seen immediately. A biopsy is often taken since the presence of cancer cannot be determined by merely looking at the lesion.

Treatment

After the physician examines the lesion, he or she may advise having dentures refitted or cutting down on smoking and the consumption of alcohol and excessive amounts of spicy foods. These patches should be examined by a physician frequently, since a cancer may develop in the future. In most cases, however, the physician will probably advise that the lesion be entirely removed.

If an unusual white patch appears on any skin surface, a physician should be seen immediately. One should never attempt to self-treat such a condition.

Mole

A mole is a cluster of cells, usually pigmented (colored), that appears on the skin. Moles are sometimes present at birth, but more often they appear during childhood, adolescence, or pregnancy. Although moles, which are commonplace, can become cancerous, they seldom do.

Types

Moles vary in size, shape, and color. They may be large or small, flat or raised, or smooth or warty. They may be skin-tone or their color may vary from yellow-brown to black. Some moles have one or more hairs in them.

The most common type of mole is the intradermal nevus, which forms in the lower layer of skin. It is a raised cluster of cells that ranges in color from skin-tone to black. Other types of moles include the (1) lentigo nevus, a flat, uniformly pigmented brown or black spot; (2) junctional nevus, a flat or slightly raised blemish that ranges in color from light brown to nearly black; (3) compound nevus, which is raised and is usually dark in color; and (4) halo nevus, a pigmented mole in the middle of a ring of depigmented skin.

Treatment

Moles are often removed for cosmetic reasons. However, any mole that enlarges suddenly, becomes darker, begins to bleed, or changes in any other unexplained way should be removed and the cells examined.

Onychogryphosis

Onychogryphosis (or onychogryposis) refers to unusual nail growth, to the extent that the nail begins to resemble a claw or horn. The nail becomes thick, long, horny or raised, and green or black in color with an opaque surface. It happens especially on the big toes.

Causes

Injury caused by going barefoot or wearing tight shoes is the usual cause of onychogryphosis, but the condition can also be hereditary. It may also be connected to congestive heart failure, in which there may be a shortage of blood circulation to the feet; peripheral neuritis, which affects nerves in the legs causing decreased sensation in the feet and therefore increasing the chance that the foot will be injured; dry, scaly skin; hormonal disorders; syphilis; and stroke.

Treatment

Properly-fitting shoes, hot baths, massage with warm oil or hydrogen peroxide, or treatment of the underlying disease should clear up the condition.

Onychomycosis

The most common of inflammatory nail disorders, onychomycosis is a fungal infection of the nails that is prevalent among those with a low resistance to infection (diabetics or patients taking corticosteroid, or hormonal, drugs), those who work with their hands in water and are prone to paronychia (inflammation of the skin around the nail) or those with ingrown toenails. Onychomycosis is caused by a number of fungi and is most often a result of paronychia.

Symptoms

Chronic but painless, the affected nails look dull, opaque, and brittle; are marked with grooves or ridges; and appear flaky. The surrounding cuticle may become red, tender, and swollen, and ooze pus if a bacterial infection accompanies the disorder. The fungi can be identified by examining nail scrapings in the laboratory.

Treatment

The condition is treated with griseofulvin, an antifungal drug that can be taken orally or applied topically. However, it may take months to cure. Furthermore, the condition may never clear up at all, especially if the toenails are affected. Cutting the nails short or removing the entire nail can help.

Prevention

To prevent onychomycosis, fingernails and toenails should be dried thoroughly after bathing; footwear should be changed often if feet tend to perspire. Thorough drying eliminates the moisture that fungi thrive in.

Photosensitivity

Photosensitivity is an abnormally increased sensitivity of the skin to the rays of the sun.

Causes

The causes of this condition are not fully understood, although it is known that certain substances when combined with ultraviolet light produce the reaction. Among those substances are: contraceptive pills; hexachlorophene, a skin antiseptic; sandalwood oil; coal tar; certain perfumes; and a variety of orally taken drugs. In these reactions, it appears to be the combination of ultraviolet rays with the agent that triggers the response.

Symptoms

The symptoms of photosensitivity range from burning reactions, similar to those ordinarily suffered after prolonged exposure to the sun, all the way to rashes; scaling; welts (raised areas) on the skin; and excessive burning, dizziness, nausea, and vomiting. The most common symptom is a rash.

Treatment

The most effective treatment is to discover the basic cause of the heightened sensitivity and to eliminate it. If, for example, photosensitivity is a reaction to a contraceptive pill, a different kind of pill or form of contraception could be prescribed. Treatment of photosensitivity symptoms duplicates that used for sunburn: ointments, topical anesthetics, and creams. It should be remembered that these treatments are standard topical therapy for the skin but do not eliminate the underlying causes of photosensitivity.

If it is impossible to isolate the cause of photosensitivity, the next best step to take is to avoid exposure to light by wearing light-colored clothing, white gloves, and broad-brimmed hats. Commercial sunscreen products are also helpful. Obviously, contact with the substances already listed should be avoided.

Psoriasis

Psoriasis is a persistent skin disease producing thick red eruptions — often covered by silvery scales — either in small patches or over large areas of the body. Although it is not contagious, psoriasis is fairly common, affect-

ing 1 to 2 percent of the population. The condition often first appears between the ages of 15 and 30 years and usually requires lifelong treatment.

Cause

The cause of psoriasis is unknown, but researchers believe the disease may be related to skin growth and regeneration (cell replacement). With normal skin, the epidermis, or outer layer, continually sheds old cells and replaces them with new ones formed in the skin's deeper layers. Cells live for about one month before they die and flake off. With psoriasis, the rate of cell growth accelerates. Skin cells may move to the surface and die in as short a time as four or five days. Increased cell growth causes buildup that can be extremely dry and irritating. While the normal shedding process is usually unnoticeable, psoriasis can produce very obvious blemishes.

Psoriasis seems to show a strong hereditary factor, although only one third of its victims can recall a relative who had the disease. There seems to be some relationship between the condition and arthritis, as well.

Once psoriasis develops, outbreaks of the disorder can be triggered in several ways. Injury to the skin, such as a cut or burn, may provoke a flare-up, usually eight to 18 days after the trauma. Seasonal changes may also affect psoriasis, with the disease worsening during winter months. Many patients have greater problems during periods of physical and emotional stress. Infections, too, such as upper respiratory infections, may aggravate psoriasis.

Symptoms

Psoriasis is characterized by reddened, raised patches of skin with silvery scales called plaques. These clearly defined plaques appear more on the elbows, knees, trunk, or scalp, although underarm and genital areas may also be involved. Patches on the scalp shed large silver-white scales at the hairline that resemble severe dandruff. Those patches found in moist areas, such as underarms, are usually less scaly and less red. All patches may itch. If fingernails are involved, the nails may be pitted or discolored. More advanced cases may show the nails separated from the nail bed.

Usually, psoriasis produces no general health problems. Sometimes, however, the disease becomes so severe that chills, painful reddening of the skin, cracking of the skin around joints, and shedding of large areas of scaled skin result. This condition is exfoliative psoriasis, and patients often require hospitalization for intensive therapy.

Treatment

As yet, there is no known cure for psoriasis, and treatment offers only temporary relief from symptoms. Cleaning the skin is important to prevent infection. Over-the-counter lotions and creams can cleanse irritated skin and reduce itching, as well. These preparations often contain small amounts of coal tar and other ingredients designed to remove scales. If the skin becomes sensitive after application, use of these preparations should be discontinued. Many patients find regular and controlled exposure to sunlight helpful. Where sunlight is scarce, a sunlamp is acceptable if used under a doctor's supervision.

More recently, various drugs have been shown to be effective in relieving psoriasis symptoms. Cortisone and newer steroids (hormonally-based medications) can clear plaques in about 50 percent of the cases when applied directly to the affected skin. Many physicians recommend covering the treated areas with a thin plastic wrapping in addition to the cream. This is called occlusive therapy.

Some drugs slow the growth rate of cells. The most commonly used of these drugs, methotrexate, reduces symptoms in severe cases. Because its side effects may be severe, however, the drug is prescribed only under close supervision of a physician.

Another form of treatment is called PUVA therapy. Here, the patient receives one dose of the drug methoxsalen followed two hours later by a dose of long-wave ultraviolet light. This procedure is repeated twice weekly until the psoriasis clears up (usually 20 to 25 treatments). More than 80 percent of the patients given this therapy report at least partial relief. However, these benefits need careful weighing against the premature skin aging and skin cancer that PUVA therapy may cause.

Purpura

The term purpura refers to a group of bleeding disorders that are all characterized by purplish or brownish-red discolorations, easily visible through the skin's outer layer, caused by hemorrhages (internal bleeding) into the tissues.

Types

Common purpura is the most widespread of such disorders and is marked by easy bruising and increased blood vessel fragility. It is an inherited condition occurring mostly in women, particularly following menopause. The result is simple, or senile, purpura, which often affects thigh tissue and produces large bruises rather than hemorrhages. The bleeding pattern is usually under the skin and may be intensified by surgery or injury.

Allergic purpura and anaphylactoid purpura are also known as Henoch-Schonlein purpura. This is a condition that is most often seen in children and can be associated with arthritis, gastrointestinal disorders, kidney failure, and erythema (skin inflammation). Purpura fulminans, a similar problem, is also seen in children, mainly after an infectious disease. It is marked by fever, shock (a dangerous, sudden lowering of blood pressure),

anemia, rapidly spreading symmetrical skin hemorrhages in the lower limbs, as well as by blocking of a blood vessel by a solid mass and tissue death.

Thrombocytopenic purpura is any form of purpura in which the platelet (the tiny elements in the blood that are vital to clotting) count is decreased, whether as a primary disease or as a consequence of another blood disorder. This form of purpura is characterized by anemia, side effects in the nervous system, and minor blood clots in tiny blood vessels.

Causes

Causes vary with the type of purpura. For example, common purpura, when it occurs in postmenopausal women, appears to result from decreased estrogen (female hormone) levels and thinning deep-layered skin tissues. Allergic purpura may result from the development of sensitivities that may follow an infection or allergic reaction. The secondary purpuras always accompany other diseases or disorders, and purpura sometimes is seen in the elderly because of the skin's fragility. There are also temporary forms of purpura in which vascular bleeding occurs as a result of fever, hypothyroidism (low output of thyroid hormone), generalized illness, defects in the small vessels, or a drug reaction to certain medications such as aspirin. Finally, purpura can sometimes stem from overly tight clothing or from injuries, such as a black eye.

Diagnosis

Laboratory testing is essential in the case of all the purpuras in order to exclude other primary causes if any. Perhaps the most difficult of the purpuras to diagnose is allergic (Henoch-Schonlein) purpura. Joint pain and bouts of abdominal pain in this disorder may mimic acute abdominal conditions or forms of arthritis. Later, kidney involvement during the course of this purpura may cause a misdiagnosis of kidney disease.

Treatment

In the case of allergic purpura it is advisable to eliminate the possible allergic cause. Corticosteroids (artificial hormones) are often prescribed but may produce disappointing results. Immunosuppressive therapy (artificial suppression of the immune system, often by means of drugs) is sometimes, though not always, useful. If the purpura is thrombocytopenic, the spleen, an abdominal organ tied into the circulatory system, may be removed if it is hoarding too many platelets. Milder cases of any form of purpura often improve spontaneously.

Prevention

Estrogen therapy has proved helpful in preventing or relieving common purpura in postmenopausal women. Other than preventive measures to avoid infections or allergic reactions, there is little that can be done to prevent purpura.

Sunburn

Sunburn is an inflammation of and damage to the cells of the skin caused by overexposure to sunlight or sunlamps. Sunburn can either be insignificant or serious, depending on the intensity of the sun's rays, the length of exposure, and the susceptibility of the individual to the sun's effects.

Causes

Sunburn is caused by prolonged exposure to ultraviolet solar radiation. Certain substances (such as deodorant soaps, perfume ingredients, cosmetics, and certain medications) may produce heightened sensitivity to ultraviolet radiation, with a corresponding increase in the severity of the burn. While light-skinned people usually burn more easily than swarthy or dark-skinned people, skin color is not always a dependable guide to individual susceptibility.

Symptoms

Irritation, a prickling sensation, and skin that is hot to the touch mark the onset of sunburn. Skin capillaries become congested, because of the release of certain inflammatory agents, thus producing the characteristic redness. Oral contraceptive users may develop irregularly shaped dark splotches, and some sensitive individuals may develop allergic reactions in the form of rashes or welts.

As the burn progresses in severity, the skin will feel tight and swollen, dry or brittle, and may become hypersensitive to touch. Overheating and loss of fluids through the damaged skin may also produce dizziness, nausea, vomiting, hyperventilation (rapid breathing causing loss of carbon dioxide from the blood), impaired vision and hearing, irregular heartbeat, and loss of consciousness.

The aftermath of severe sunburn often includes blistering and peeling, as well as permanent freckling, splotching, or scarring of the skin. Long-term effects may include premature skin aging, marked by chronic dryness, wrinkling and leathery texture, and loss of elasticity. In some cases, melanomas, or skin cancers, may be induced by chronic overexposure to sunlight.

Treatment

Minor sunburn can be effectively treated by a wide variety of commercially distributed, nonprescription ointments, oils, powders, creams, and sprays that restore fluids and prevent further drying, relieve discomfort, and promote healing. Many over-the-counter medications contain mild anesthetics to relieve stinging and suppress the desire to scratch itching areas. One of the most common complications is the infection of blistered and peeling areas of the skin. This condition should be treated by a physician.

In the case of severe sunburn, care should be taken not to become overheated or dehydrated (lose too much fluid). Above all, the victim should be taken out of the sun immediately, and placed in a cool, shaded area until a physician can be summoned. Cool, not cold, wet clothes can be applied to the arms, the head, and the legs. Care should be taken not to chill the sufferer. Iced water or other cold drinks may trigger unwanted responses. Commercial mineral and electrolyte mixtures at room temperature will replace lost fluid faster and more safely than water taken alone. If the victim is perspiring profusely, a fan may help evaporate the water on the skin's surface, thus aiding a natural cooling process.

Prevention

The best prevention of sunburn is simply to avoid prolonged exposure to the direct rays of the sun or a sunlamp. When this is not possible, the first line of defense is to cover the skin completely, preferably with cool, loose-weave, loose-fitting, light-colored clothes. Wide-brimmed hats, long sleeves, white cotton gloves, caps with sun visors, and lightweight scarves for the neck will help.

The second line of defense is a sunscreen: an oil, cream, paste, lotion, or liquid. Most sunscreens are intended to block ultraviolet rays. Many common preparations contain para-aminobenzoic acid.

This compound may affect some individuals adversely, particularly those with photosensitivity (abnormal sensitivity of the skin to light) because of certain drugs. For these people, opaque (light-blocking) creams, pastes, and lotions are available as well as other chemical sunscreens known as benzophenones.

Anyone with a question as to possible adverse effects of sunlight with their medication should contact their doctor before exposure to sunlight.

Warts

Warts are infectious swellings or tumors in the outer layer of skin. Because they are contagious, they can spread from person to person or from one site to another on the same person. Most frequently, warts appear on hands, fingers, and soles of feet. However, they can emerge anywhere on the skin, including the genital and anal areas.

Cause

Common warts are caused by exposure to a virus called the human papilloma virus. The virus can remain inactive for up to six months after contact before erupting into abnormal skin masses.

The virus transfers to another person or another site on the body by direct contact. For example, brushing or combing the hair can spread the virus from a wart on the scalp. Shaving or scratching a given area on the body and then touching another spot will also carry the virus. In addition, moist parts of the body, such as the soles of the feet, provide a breeding ground for growth of the virus.

As people become older they seem to develop an immunity or resistance to wart virus. For this reason, children acquire warts more frequently than adults. Nevertheless, warts can occur at any age.

Symptoms

Usually, warts appear as firm gray masses that feel tender or itchy. Their size and shape vary depending upon the location and severity of the virus. Children develop flat warts most often, particularly on the face. This variety looks smooth, flat, and yellow-brown.

Plantar warts grow on the soles of the feet, where they can become as large as two inches in diameter. These warts cause considerable pain because the tissue swelling pushes inward with the pressure from walking. Discomfort from plantar warts feels like stepping on a pebble in the shoe.

Most warts are not health threatening. However, they can be so extensive in number as to cause extreme sensitivity or pain.

Treatment

Studies report that two out of every three warts disappear on their own within two years. Consequently, physicians usually recommend leaving warts alone unless they cause discomfort or obstruction.

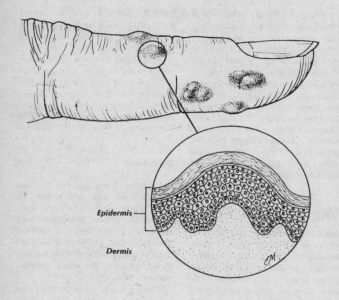

Epidermis

Dermis

CM

Warts, infectious swelling or tumors in the outer layer of skin, are caused by a virus.

Sometimes, doctors treat one or two warts and find that other warts on the same person also clear up. In this situation the original treatment stimulates manufacture of antibodies (protective substances) that fight the virus in other warts.

There are over-the-counter preparations to aid removal of warts. Most of these remedies contain a form of acid, which is dangerous if not used according to directions. Although some of these drugs are effective, only a doctor should remove a wart. Home care could scar tender skin by pulling or cutting.

Physicians may try a variety of topical preparations to loosen the warts. A solution containing cantharidin, a substance that causes blistering, may be applied directly on the wart. About one week after application, the doctor should be able to remove the wart with a knife or scissors. Corn plasters with salicylic acid placed over the tissue softens the wart so it can be scraped away.

When a wart persists, physicians may advise surgery to remove affected tissue. Electrosurgery dissolves wart tissue with electric current. Cryotherapy freezes the area and allows the wart to be lifted off easily.

BONES AND MUSCLES

Our body's frame is an intricate structure of interconnecting parts. Every voluntary movement is the result of the coordination of the bones and muscles, as well as the tendons and ligaments.

Bones

Bones are hardened masses of living tissue that have several functions. They collect calcium for the entire body, storing 99 percent of this mineral that is required to keep all bones firm and strong. In addition, bones produce large numbers of red and white blood cells within their softer tissue center called marrow.

There are 206 bones in the body. Together they form the skeleton or framework for the body. The total structure maintains the body's shape and protects internal organs from injury. For example, bones in the skull shield the brain while bones in the rib cage encircle the lungs and heart.

The place where two bones meet is called a joint. This juncture usually allows movement of the bones that are involved. However, movement is governed by ligaments (bands of fibrous tissue) attached to the bones and cartilage (elastic tissue) lining the ends of bones. Ligaments connect one bone with another. Cartilage

cushions and protects bones with the aid of various joint fluids and bursae (small sacs containing lubricating fluid located within the joints). Other bands of connective tissue called tendons attach bones to muscles. Muscles are specific kinds of tissues that have the ability to contract. This contraction and pull on the tendon are what actually create movement of the bones. In order to move any part of the skeletal structure, coordination of ligaments, tendons, and muscles is necessary.

Muscles

Body movement is affected by three different types of muscle: striated, smooth, and cardiac. Striated, or striped, muscle consists of layers of connective tissue divided into bundles of interwoven fibers running parallel to each other. These layers are attached to the skeleton, and they aid the body in voluntary movement.

Smooth, or organic, muscle lines most of the internal organs of the body, including the intestines, bladder, and blood vessels. Therefore, this type of muscle assists all functions controlled by the autonomic nervous system which governs functions under involuntary control. For example, smooth muscle helps circulate blood and

Skull

Collarbone
(clavicle)

Shoulder
blade
(scapula)

Shoulder
joint

Breastbone (sternum)

Rib

Vertebra

Radius

Pelvis

Carpus

Ulna

Metacarpus

Phalanges

Thighbone
(femur)

Hip joint

Kneecap
(patella)

Tibia

Fibula

Tarsus

Metatarsus

Phalanges

gland secretions throughout the body, move material through the digestive tract, and regulate breathing in the lungs. Smooth muscle contains elongated spindly cells arranged parallel to one another that are often grouped into irregular size bundles. Under a microscope, this muscle appears smooth.

Cardiac muscle is the muscle of the heart, and its job is to pump blood within and from the heart. The unique characteristic of this muscle is that its fibers are striated, but they are controlled by the autonomic nervous system.

Arthritis

Arthritis is an inflammation of the joints, the junctures where the ends of two bones meet.

Types

Inflammation develops in one of two ways. With *osteoarthritis*, there is gradual wearing away of cartilage in the joints. Healthy cartilage is the elastic tissue that cushions the joints and prevents the bones from touching. When this cartilage deteriorates, the bones rub together causing pain and swelling. Although osteoarthritis can result from direct injury to the joint, it commonly occurs in adults over the age of 55 because of long-term wear and tear on the joints.

Rheumatoid arthritis, on the other hand, can attack at any age. This form of arthritis affects all the connective tissues in the body. The precise cause of rheumatoid arthritis is unknown. Some researchers believe that a virus may trigger the disease, causing an autoimmune response whereby the body develops a sensitivity or allergy to its own tissues. However, evidence for this theory is inconclusive as yet. What is confirmed is the progression of the condition. First, the synovium, which is a thin membrane lining and lubricating the joint, becomes inflamed. The inflammation eventually destroys the cartilage. As scar tissue gradually replaces the damaged cartilage, the joint becomes misshapen and rigid.

Those at risk

Arthritis is not an inherited disease. Nonetheless, people who have arthritis in their family are more prone to develop the disease. Women have a greater tendency to develop arthritis than men, although the reason for this is unclear. In addition, excess body weight may promote osteoarthritis because of increased load on the joints. Constant joint abuse from strains of sports or employment may encourage arthritis, but inactivity can also cause the problem.

Symptoms

Symptoms of arthritis include swelling, tenderness, pain, stiffness, or redness in one or more joints. For many patients, pain is greater in the morning, and it subsides as the day advances. Damp weather and emotional stress do not cause arthritis, but they can

In osteoarthritis, the cushioning cartilage at the ends of bones wears away or erodes, possibly causing the bones to rub together which results in swelling and pain.

Rheumatoid arthritis is characterized by a swollen and inflamed synovium, the membrane that lines the joint and produces lubricating fluid.

make symptoms worse.

With rheumatoid arthritis, these symptoms may be accompanied by more generalized feelings of fatigue and fever. Often, this form of arthritis goes into periods of remission when symptoms disappear. When symptoms return, however, they can be more severe. If left untreated, rheumatoid arthritis may damage heart, lungs, nerves, and eyes, whereas complications of osteoarthritis can cause permanent damage and stiffness of the joints.

Diagnosis

To diagnose arthritis, a physician observes the symptoms and administers a standard physical examination. X rays and laboratory tests may be recommended for confirmation of joint swelling.

Treatment

The most effective treatment program for arthritis consists of drug therapy, exercise, and rest. Treatment should begin early after diagnosis to prevent permanent damage.

Of the drugs administered for arthritis, aspirin is the most common. Doctors prescribe two to three tablets several times a day to relieve pain and reduce inflammation. To prevent stomach irritation, they suggest taking aspirin after meals or in a coated tablet form.

Often nonaspirin pain relievers and nonsteroid anti-inflammatory drugs (for example, ibuprofen, naproxen, tolmetin, or sulindac) may be prescribed. Corticosteroids also relieve inflammation, but they can cause adverse side effects. Sometimes, a doctor needs to try several different drugs before finding an effective one that produces no side effects.

Moderate daily exercise, such as swimming, walking, or perhaps physical therapy, is critical to maintaining mobility in arthritic joints. A supervised exercise program interspersed with rest periods helps to reduce joint inflammation. To lessen pain while increasing movement, moist heat often helps. In addition, maintaining correct posture and body weight eliminates extra burden on sore joints.

Some severe cases of rheumatoid arthritis may require surgery to remove inflamed synovial tissue. With either form of arthritis, artificial joints may be implanted to replace those damaged beyond repair.

Backache

A backache is generally a gripping pain near the inward curve of the back above the base of the spine. It is one of the most common physical ailments, affecting about 80 percent of the population at some time in their lives.

Causes

Pain results from a variety of causes. Strains are especially common when overworked or underexercised back muscles perform beyond their normal capacity. Muscles will then contract or go into spasm and become a tight mass of tissue. Meanwhile, the body transmits a sharp pain signal as nearby muscles tighten in an effort to protect strained muscles and prevent further damage. Strain of back muscles can be due to sports, a sudden jerking motion such as a car braking, or reflex actions like sneezing.

Overweight is a leading cofactor of backache, since excess pounds increase stress on back muscles. Similarly, pregnancy can produce back pain because of the weight or position of the unborn child. For some women, menstruation results in back discomfort.

Many people develop back pain as they age and joint tissues deteriorate or shift. Psychological tension, stress, or anxiety about everyday problems can also lead to backache. In addition, back pain can result from diseases of the kidneys, heart, lungs, intestinal tract, or reproductive organs.

Occasionally, backache stems from a congenital (present from birth) malformation. In this case, pain usually results from unusual stresses the deformity imposes on surrounding muscular structures rather than from the abnormality itself. For example, having one leg shorter than another forces the neighboring muscles out of alignment and may cause back pain.

Symptoms

Backaches can appear abruptly after physical activity or develop slowly. The pain may feel like a sharp jab or a dull ache. Sometimes, pain becomes so piercing that a person who is bending over may not be able to straighten up. Severe back pain may also be accompanied by pain or numbness radiating down the leg(s). Most muscular back pains disappear within a week or two of their onset, while some will last one to two months, but pain may recur unless preventive measures are taken.

Diagnosis

Sufferers of prolonged back pain (more than two to three weeks) should consult a physician to check for underlying disorders such as kidney or lung problems that may be causing the backache. Once other medical causes have been ruled out, an ortho-

pedic physician specializing in bone and muscle conditions may be able to determine the cause of the discomfort.

During the examination, the physician asks questions about the type of pain and its location, general health, previous illnesses, and physical activity routines. The patient walks, sits, stands, and performs exercises while being observed. If an X ray is recommended, it may or may not reveal adverse changes in the bones of the spine since not all problems can be revealed on film.

Treatment

If there are no physical causes for the backache, physicians usually recommend an exercise program to strengthen weak muscles. Losing weight can also relieve unnecessary pressure on the back.

For immediate symptoms, hot pads at the site of the pain will reduce soreness. Over-the-counter preparations in the form of a rub containing menthol salicylate (oil of wintergreen) or similar ingredients may produce a soothing heat sensation when applied to the pain site. Physicians may also prescribe muscle relaxant drugs.

When backache is the result of some deformity, surgery may be necessary to correct the problem. Sometimes, braces, corsets, or shoe lifts improve the condition. Specific exercises strengthen participating muscles and counter stress caused by the malformation. Almost all types of musculo-skeletal backache respond well to complete bed rest that allows muscles to relax and inflammation to subside. Here, time is the best healer, especially in extreme situations.

Prevention

To prevent back pain, stress to the spine should be avoided. Good posture when awake and asleep relieves tension on the spinal column. Properly-fitted shoes encourage good posture, as does a semi-firm bed. Contrary to popular belief, a hard mattress distorts alignment of the spine and causes back problems as much as a soft mattress does. A semi-rigid mattress is recommended because it conforms to the arch of the back and maintains spine alignment.

Good posture is also important when performing daily activities. Kneeling, rather then bending from the waist, when lifting objects keeps the weight of the object on the legs, leaving the back straight. Avoid sitting for long periods of time at a desk looking down or watching television with the chin on the chest.

Bunion

A bunion is a swelling on the foot usually at the joint of the big toe. Often, a bony protuberance is found at the joint of the big toe, which gives the bunion its bulging appearance.

Causes

Bunions are most often caused by poorly fitting footwear, but they can also be the result of inherited deformities in bone structure. In a normal foot, the two main bones of the big toe must align to fit together. However, some people have loose bone joints in the foot that allow their big toe to point outward toward the other foot. This inherited condition causes problems when footwear encloses the foot. Shoes force the big toe inward and the big toe joint outward so that the joint rubs against the inner surface of the footwear. Friction from such rubbing produces a bunion. The same action results when pointed-toed or tight shoes put pressure on the joint — whether or not the genetic tendency exists.

Symptoms

A bunion is characterized by swelling at the big toe joint that may be accompanied by pain and tenderness. Bunion formations can be acute or chronic. Acute bunions are a type of bursitis, which is an inflammation of the bursae. A bursa is a fluid-filled sac that cushions the juncture where two bones meet. With an acute bunion, the bursa covering the big toe joint becomes inflamed from friction at the joint, often producing considerable pain. Chronic, or long-term, bunions develop an inflexible bony protrusion.

Complications

Complications can develop if the bunion grows and increases pressure on the big toe. This pressure may force the other toes to overlap, encouraging corns (mounds of dead skin found on toes) or other problems that could result from friction on the skin of the distorted toes.

Diagnosis

A physician diagnoses a bunion by general physical examination. To verify bone problems, X rays may be necessary.

Treatment

Surgery is the only permanent cure for bunions. It can entail simple removal of the excess bone or more complex realignment of the bones, muscles, and tendons that led to formation of the bunion. Sometimes a doctor can remove a bony protrusion in the office with local anesthetic. Pain is minimal, and the incision is probably only about an inch long. With this treatment, the patient has full use of the foot in about six weeks.

For more extensive surgery, the patient goes to a hospital and requires longer recuperation time. Usually, an orthopedic surgeon performs this type of surgery. Nonsurgical devices can relieve the pain and discomfort of bunions. Padding can be used to shift the weight of the foot in the shoe, lessening friction. Protective shields can also prevent contact between the bunion and the inside of the shoe.

Prevention

Wearing properly fitting footwear is the best prevention of bunions. Even a child's first shoes should have a sturdy sole and be wide enough to accommodate all toes without cramping, since early childhood is when most foot problems begin.

When buying shoes, the width and length of each foot needs to be measured separately. If one foot is larger than the other, shoe size should correspond to the size of the larger foot. A one-inch gap between the big toe and the tip of the shoe allows enough moving space. Even more room is needed with pointed-toed shoes. Shoes should be comfortable from the first wearing—without requiring a breaking-in period.

Women who wear stylish high-heeled or pointed-toed shoes may be damaging their feet. Heels about one inch in height are actually best for feet. However, if higher heels are chosen, open-toed styles cause fewer problems. Similarly, narrow-toed shoes are less damaging with low heels.

Nothing is better for feet than walking barefoot on unlittered sand or grass. Sandals or thongs are the next best kind of footwear to avoid the cramping effects of shoes. For some people, wooden clogs provide the same relief.

Bursitis

Bursitis is an inflammation of the bursae, the sacs or pouches located at the ends of the bones in the joints. Bursae contain lubricating fluid and normally eliminate friction in the area and maintain smooth muscle movement over the bones.

Bursitis seems to be more common in males than females, possibly because of greater physical activity. Continual stress on a joint increases the probability of injury and inflammation. In advanced cases, swelling and calcium deposits within a joint may render it immobile.

Causes

The inflammation can result from either sudden extreme pressure or from continuous strain. Some occupations and sports that require constant use of certain joints contribute to acute or chronic bursitis. For example, "typist's shoulder" and "baseball pitcher's elbow" are forms of chronic bursitis. Acute bursitis can develop suddenly and may be triggered by a chill or draft.

Symptoms

Inflamed bursae produce tenderness and swelling near the affected joint. Pain from bursitis can be very disabling. At times, it is so severe that movement becomes impossible. Any joint in the body can be the site of bursitis, but shoulders, knees, and elbows are most commonly affected.

Diagnosis

To diagnose bursitis, your physician may suggest an X ray to determine if there are calcium deposits in the bursae. For bursitis that is stress-related, however, X rays only show bursae that are swollen.

Treatment

Acute bursitis may heal with time if the joint is immobilized. Patients may consider using a sling, crutches, or complete bed rest to relieve pressure on the affected area.

Applying moist heat directly to the inflamed joint frequently reduces the discomfort of bursitis, although some patients find cold compresses more effective. Aspirin and other over-the-counter pain relievers may also alleviate pain. In some cases, anti-inflammatory corticosteroid drugs may be injected directly into the inflamed area, but these drugs should be used judiciously since they have been known to cause adverse side effects.

For severe cases of bursitis, a doctor may recommend surgery by an orthopedic surgeon to remove calcium deposits or free the area from chronic inflammation by removing the bursa.

Carpal tunnel syndrome

Carpal tunnel syndrome is weakness, pain, tingling, numbness, or burning of the palm part of the thumb, the index finger, third finger, and inner part of the ring finger caused by an entrapment of the median nerve in the wrist. The condition most often affects women in their 30s, 40s, and 50s. It may develop or become worse because of work, such as scrubbing, that requires repeated grasping, twisting, or turning of the hand and wrist.

The condition, like any syndrome, is not a disease in itself but a collection of symptoms. The carpal tunnel consists of the bones

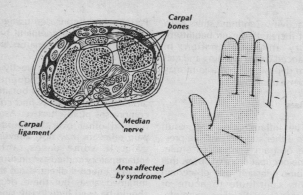

Carpal tunnel syndrome is weakness, pain, tingling, numbness or burning in the palm part of the thumb, and the index, third, and inner part of the ring fingers caused by entrapment of the median nerve within the carpal tunnel of the wrist. The carpal tunnel consists of the carpal bones of the wrist overlaid by the tough band of connective tissue called the carpal ligament.

of the wrist ("carpal" means "wrist") overlaid by a tough band of connective tissue known as the transverse carpal ligament. Inside the tunnel are the median nerve, its artery, and tendons that flex the fingers and thumb. Any swelling or thickening of tissue within the tunnel can cause the median (middle) nerve to be compressed between the tough band of carpal ligament and the tendons or other contents of the tunnel. The squeezed nerve, which controls the thumb, index finger, and third finger, cannot work as it should, and the symptoms of carpal tunnel syndrome result.

Causes

Pregnancy and other conditions that produce generalized swelling of body tissues may be a cause of carpal tunnel syndrome.

So can localized swelling caused by a dislocation, sprain, or fracture of the wrist. Rheumatoid arthritis can cause inflammation of the sheaths (coverings) of the tendons, causing compression. Other possible causes include inflamed wrist joint, benign (noncancerous) tumor, myxedema (tissue swelling caused by lack of thyroid hormone), tuberculosis, amyloidosis (a disease characterized by abnormal deposits in body organs of the protein amyloid), acromegaly (overgrowth of connective tissue), and diabetes mellitus.

Symptoms

Aching pain may travel up the forearm and even into the shoulder joint, neck, and chest (this particular pain can usually be relieved by shaking the hand vigorously or dangling the arm loosely from its socket; occasionally such pains are caused by a compression of the median nerve in the forearm or upper arm). Other signs include an inability to make a fist, deteriorating nails, and dry and shiny skin over the involved surfaces. The pains may occur in both hands at the same time. They may be constant or may come and go and are increased by manual work or movement that flexes the wrist or palm. Weakness of the fingers occurs later than other symptoms and accompanies a wasting away of the muscle. Symptoms are usually worse at night and in the morning.

Diagnosis

Diagnostic tests include tapping the wrist, which causes tingling in the area of pain if carpal tunnel syndrome is present, and forced flexion of the wrist, which may also reproduce the pain. X rays may be taken to reveal abnormalities of the wrist bones. Tests made to detect a delay in the conduction of nerve impulses are the most specific means of diagnosis.

Treatment

Treatment is aimed first at relieving pressure on the median nerve. If soft tissue swelling is a cause, elevating the hand may eliminate the symptoms. It may help to keep the forearm in a splint at night, which holds the hand upward extending the wrist. If an inflammation (other than infection) inside the wrist is at fault, the carpal tunnel may be injected with cortisone. Other causes of the disease are treated appropriately.

The definitive treatment, to prevent permanent damage to nerves and muscles and to relieve symptoms, is surgery that releases the carpal tunnel ligament, relieving the pressure on the nerve. Muscle strength gradually returns following such surgery, but if the surgery has been delayed too long and muscles are severely deteriorated, full strength does not return. Symptoms usually disappear permanently shortly after the operation.

Fracture

A fracture is a break in a bone or a cartilage, and it can be one of several different types.

Types

The most common fractures are the closed fracture, the comminuted fracture, the complicated fracture, the composite fracture, the greenstick fracture, the impacted fracture, and the open fracture.

- Closed fracture—one in which the skin is not broken
- Comminuted fracture—one in which the bone is broken into several pieces
- Complicated fracture—one in which significant injury has been done to internal organs, blood vessels, or nerves
- Composite fracture—one in

Impacted   Composite   Comminuted   Greenstick

Artery

Complicated

Open

Closed

A fracture is a break in a bone and can be one of several types as shown here.

which there are multiple breaks in the bone
• Greenstick fracture—one in which only one side of the bone is broken and the bone is not severed
• Impacted fracture — one in which the ends or fragments of bone are jammed together

• Open fracture—one in which the broken end(s) of the bone pierces the skin.

Those at risk

Fractures are common among children and older people. Children have relatively soft, elastic bones. For this reason, their breaks may be incomplete, that is, they may be on only one side of the bone. Older people have brittle bones that tend to break easily. Hip fractures are particularly common among the elderly.

Complications

Among the more serious consequences of fractures are the possibility of infection and the possible damage done to the nerves, blood vessels, and internal organs near the fracture.

Causes

Most often, fractures are caused by direct violence, such as a blow from a heavy object. They can, however, be the result of an indirect cause. A fall on a hand, for example, may result in a fractured collarbone. There are also pathological fractures, in which disease softens the bone and leads to a break.

Symptoms

Among the symptoms of a fracture are pain, swelling, loss of strength, abnormal movement, and a grating sound caused when the broken pieces of bone rub together. Shock may also occur with a severe fracture if large amounts of blood are lost.

Treatment

Bone fractures are treated by closed (nonsurgical) or open (surgical) reduction. Reduction is a procedure in which the broken bone is manipulated, for example, by pulling or bending, so that the ends will be in the best position for healing. The pieces of bone are often held together by pins, metal plates, and rods, some of which are left in the body and others of which are removed after healing has taken place. Most fractures are treated through closed reduction. However, open reduction may be required when damage to bones, joints, ligaments, tendons, or other internal parts is severe or extensive.

Gout

Gout is a form of recurrent acute arthritis whose underlying cause is a defect in the body's processing of uric acid, a chemical normally found in the blood and urine. If the body does not properly process uric acid, resulting in high blood levels of uric acid, the uric acid may crystallize and become deposited in and around the joints and their tendons. An acute attack of gout is caused by the affected joint's inflammatory response to the deposits of crystals.

The high levels of uric acid can also lead to deposits in areas of the body other than the joints, most notably the skin and the kidneys. Uric acid deposits in the skin take the form of white lumps under the skin, most often appearing in the rims of the outer ear, the hands, the feet, and the elbows. Uric acid deposits in the kidneys may lead to the formation of kidney stones and perhaps even kidney failure (if the kidneys are blocked with numerous stones). About 20 percent of those with chronic gout also have kidney stones.

Most gout victims are middle-aged men. Rarely does the condition affect young women, although it can appear after menopause when the uric acid levels in the blood tend to increase.

Symptoms

Gout usually first appears as a sudden and extremely painful attack in a single joint, usually the big toe. Later attacks can involve several joints, such as the ankle, knee, wrist, and elbow. The pain commonly begins at night during sleep and may occur without warning or may be preceded by excessive alcohol consumption or unusual exercise earlier in the day. The pain grows in intensity and is often described as throbbing or crushing. Inflammation follows with swelling, warmth, redness, and tenderness over the affected joint. Sometimes the pain is so severe that the individual cannot tolerate the weight of a sheet over the joint. Other symptoms that may accompany the joint pain and swelling include fever, rapid heartbeat, chills, and an overall feeling of being unwell.

The first attacks usually last only a few days, but if the disorder goes untreated, later attacks may last for weeks. Symptoms eventually disappear, and joint function returns to normal between attacks. As the disease progresses, the periods of remission become shorter and shorter as more and more attacks occur each year.

Treatment

The treatment of gout is twofold: (1) to relieve the symptoms of an acute attack and (2) to prevent attacks from occurring. The drug colchicine has traditionally been used to relieve a gout attack, but now — although colchicine is still used — nonsteroidal anti-inflammatory drugs are more often prescribed to relieve the inflammation and pain. These drugs are quite effective. However, they do have side effects so they should be used only under close and continuous medical supervision.

Once the acute attack is under control, prevention of future attacks is the main goal. This can be done with the drug allopurinol, which interferes with the formation of excess uric acid and thus prevents the deposits of uric acid crystals in the body. Allopurinol usually has to be taken for long periods of time to maintain normal blood levels of uric acid. There are also other drugs, called uricosurics, that speed up the excretion of uric acid by the kidneys. These drugs, however, cannot be used if there is known kidney damage.

Lupus erythematosus

Lupus erythematosus is a degenerative disorder of the skin and of the connective tissues. The disorder occurs in two different forms — discoid lupus erythematosus and systemic lupus erythematosus.

Discoid lupus erythematosus

Discoid lupus erythematosus is a chronic disease of the skin that is characterized by a red rash that appears on the cheeks and nose, as well as on other parts of the body. It often appears for the first time after the skin has been exposed to sunlight. Discoid lupus erythematosus is usually treated with drugs commonly used in the treatment of malaria. Even though discoid lupus is not at all related to malaria, the use of these drugs may improve the rash.

Systemic lupus erythematosus

Systemic lupus erythematosus is a widespread disease of the blood vessels and connective tissues affecting the joints, skin, and numerous other organs in the body including the heart, lungs, liver, intestine, and kidneys. Red patches appear on the cheeks and nose that resemble an open-winged butterfly. Symptoms may also include severe pain in the joints, an intermittent fever, and unusual fatigue. The inflammation may involve many other parts of the body and cause severe and irreversible damage to the blood vessels and to the kidneys.

Cortisone and other steroids are used to control the inflammation in the joints and in other parts of the body; aspirin and other analgesics are used to control the pain. As with discoid lupus erythematosus, antimalarial drugs are used in the treatment of the rash.

This disease may be mild or it may progress rapidly to affect many organs seriously. Death may result in severe cases.

Osteoporosis

Osteoporosis is a common disorder characterized by a decrease in the calcium content of bone tissue that leaves the skeletal system thin and susceptible to fracture.

To date, the cause of osteoporosis is unknown. However, chances of acquiring the disease seem to increase dramatically with age, especially for women. One prevailing theory maintains that osteoporosis results from a loss of the female hormone estrogen, which affects the calcium content of the bones. Menopause (cessation of menstruation or periods) often leads to osteoporosis because the body's production of estrogen is reduced at this time. Almost one third of all women over 60 years of age have the disease to some extent.

For reasons not entirely known, white and Oriental women are likelier to develop osteoporosis than black women. In addition slender females, especially those with fair skin, run a higher risk than stouter, darker-skinned women.

Besides developing spontaneously, osteoporosis can also appear as a result of other conditions. Surgical removal of both ovaries (the female sex glands that produce estrogen), chronic arthritis (inflammation of the joints), or Paget's disease (a disorder of unknown origin that results in bone destruction) may lead to osteoporosis. People who are inactive, either by choice or because of confinement from illness, seem more susceptible to the disorder. In addition, a diet without various nutrients, especially calcium, that promote bone development may also contribute to osteoporosis.

Symptoms

Depending upon the strength of the bones, osteoporosis may initially cause either no symptoms or extreme pain, commonly in the lower back. The disease is not life-threatening, but it may lead to serious fractures which, for the elderly, can result in serious complications. Initially, sudden back pain may follow fracture of the vertebrae, bones in the spine. Pain from the fracture itself may subside but discomfort from os-

Normal vertebrae

Vertebrae with osteoporosis

Osteoporosis, a condition in which the bones weaken and break easily, may lead to compression of the vertebrae (backbones) because of the pressure of the body's weight on the weakened vertebrae.

teoporosis may continue. This pain may lead to further inactivity which may weaken additional vertebrae. Hence, a vicious cycle develops whereby pain leading to inactivity encourages osteoporosis which, in turn, increases bone fragility.

As the disease progresses, the spinal column may become reduced in length or may become curved due to the pressure of body weight—hence, the term "widow's hump" or "dowager's hump." As osteoporosis progresses, the individual may actually lose several inches in height.

Diagnosis

Often, osteoporosis progresses undetected until a fractured bone develops and an X ray is taken. At this time, a physician may notice that bone thinning has become a generalized condition throughout the body.

Treatment

Physicians urge patients with osteoporosis to follow an exercise program that will strengthen the muscles supporting weakened bones. To protect bones in the spinal column, however, lifting heavy objects should be avoided. For advanced cases, a back brace may be necessary to support body weight while sitting or standing. Crutches, walkers, or a cane may assist walking.

Sometimes, physicians prescribe the female hormone estrogen to women to decrease bone loss. Women taking these medications need careful supervision as the hormones may cause adverse side effects. Anyone receiving estrogen therapy should have a physical examination and a Pap test (examination of cells scraped from the vagina and cervix to detect cancer) every six months because of a suspected link between estrogen supplements and uterine and breast cancer. Men may be given the male hormone testosterone, which stimulates growth of body tissues, to treat osteoporosis.

For people prone to injury from osteoporosis, a balanced diet is an important factor in preventing or controlling the disease. Foods rich in vitamins and minerals, particularly calcium and Vitamin D, encourage bone formation. When the diet is deficient in these ingredients, vitamin and mineral supplements may be prescribed by a doctor.

Otosclerosis

Otosclerosis is a condition in which an abnormal spongy overgrowth of bone in the middle ear leads to totally or partially muffled hearing or deafness. The excess bone grows at the entrance to the middle ear where it immobilizes the base of the stapes, a tiny stirrup-shaped bone that is one of three interconnected bones transmitting sound waves to the inner ear. As a result, sound-conducting vibrations are diminished and impaired hearing results. In most cases, both ears are affected. The cause of otosclerosis is unknown, but the condition tends to be hereditary.

Symptoms

Hearing loss generally begins in the late teens or early 20s; the rate of deafness may accelerate and stabilize several times, but ordinarily the loss is complete within ten to 15 years, sooner if the disease began in childhood. In some cases, the hearing loss stops just short of deafness and the affected person still can hear loud sounds. Otosclerosis usually affects one ear before the other and is preceded by tinnitus (ringing in the ear). Special hearing tests aid in diagnosis.

Treatment

The only way to halt or reverse otosclerosis is surgery—treatment that is successful about 70 percent of the time. Although a hearing aid can help, most doctors prefer to operate. In a procedure called a stapedectomy, a surgeon folds back the eardrum, removes the affected stapes and replaces it with a synthetic or wire substitute that restores the conductive vibrations of the inner ear. Because the bones involved are the tiniest in the body, the surgery is very delicate and carries a 2 to 5 percent risk of failure. However, in most cases the operation is only done on one ear at a time, thereby reducing the risk.

After surgery, the hearing of most patients is greatly improved within two to three weeks. Sometimes a residual blood clot at the site of the surgery temporarily blocks hearing until it dissolves. Patients with advanced otosclerosis in both ears are usually advised to undergo the stapedectomy as soon as possible.

Paget's disease of the bone

Paget's disease (osteitis deformans) is a disorder in which the normal turnover (breaking down and reforming) of bone is greatly accelerated. The disease develops in three stages. In the first stage (destructive), bone tissue breaks down but is replaced with blood vessels and dense fibrous tissue making the bones very vascular (having a great deal of blood flowing through them). During the following stage (mixed), new bone formation takes place at a rate geared to the breakdown process. In the third stage (sclerotic), the breakdown process slows, allowing for the hardening of new bone which becomes quite dense.

Although any bone can be affected, Paget's disease most commonly invades the pelvis, skull, thighbone, shin, vertebrae (backbones), collarbone, and the ribs.

The condition normally affects 1 to 3 percent of the elderly, especially males. Its incidence is higher in some European countries than in others and rare in Asia, Africa, and South America. The cause is unknown.

Symptoms and complications

Bone pain is one of the most prevalent symptoms. Sometimes complications develop. The thickened, enlarged bones are susceptible to fracture, particularly during the destructive phase of the disease. When the disease attacks the skull bone, it can compress the auditory nerve that relays signals from the ear to the brain and cause deafness. Heart failure can result from stress of the increased blood flow through the bones. Malignant bone tumors are another complication, but fortunately are uncommon. The disease can affect appearance if it enlarges the head, bends the back, or bows the legs. In some severe cases particularly if the person is immobile, calcium levels in the blood and urine increase and may lead to formation of urinary stones.

Diagnosis

A history and physical examination, blood tests, and particularly X rays confirm the diagnosis of Paget's disease.

Treatment

Although there is no cure, analgesics (painkillers) like aspirin offer some relief. Severe pain or other complications are sometimes managed with chemotherapy (drug therapy) or corticosteroids (cortisone). Injections of calcitonin, a hormone normally produced in the thyroid gland that promotes calcification of bone, may help block bone breakdown.

Slipped disk

A slipped disk is a back problem involving the disks of elastic carti-

lage tissue located between the vertebrae, the bones of the spine. The bones are loosely strung together by bands of tissue called ligaments that allow the body movement and flexibility. The function of each disk is to cushion any friction between the bones as the body moves.

When this intricate spinal structure experiences strain and over-exertion, the rim of the disk weakens and tears, rather than "slips," causing part of the gelatinous center of the disk to be forced out of position. In its new position, the protruding material presses against an adjacent spinal nerve and causes pain along the path of the affected nerve.

Causes

Most often, a slipped disk occurs when bending and straightening the back to lift heavy objects results in strain or injury. Damage to the disk may not be realized for many months, however. People with the problem frequently have a history of damage to the same area.

Disks also seem to disintegrate with age. They lose some of their fluidity and become more compressed. This form of degeneration usually results in only mild pain with intermittent backache and stiffness.

Symptoms

Symptoms of slipped disk may vary with the location of the disk. The most common slipped disk is the lowest movable disk in the

Disks of cartilage lie between the vertebrae to cushion the friction between the bones. If the rim of a disk weakens or tears, part of the jelly-like center becomes pushed out. This protruding material presses on a nearby spinal nerve causing pain along the path of the nerve. This is referred to as a slipped disk.

small of the back. Injury to this disk causes pain along the sciatic nerve, a condition called sciatica. Mild or disabling pain and tenderness may result. Any straining, such as coughing or moving, can aggravate the discomfort. Weakness, tingling, or numbness in parts of the arms, legs, or feet may also result from damage to a particular disk.

Diagnosis

To determine the source of back pain, a physician requests a current medical history; observes the patient sitting, walking, and bending; and explores for sensitive areas by maneuvering the patient's legs in different positions, checking ankle and knee reflexes, and testing muscle strength. If needed, X rays reveal any structural changes in bones, joints, or disks.

For locating particularly problematic disks, or with a recommendation of surgery, special tests are necessary. A myelogram is an X ray taken after dye is injected into the space surrounding the spinal cord and nerve roots. The protruding disk is detected at the point where the flow of dye is interrupted or distorted. Discography gives much the same information; but before this X ray, dye is injected directly into the disks.

Treatment

The first course of treatment for slipped disk involves complete bed rest on a firm mattress. Rest relieves pressure of the disk on the nerve and may shrink the protruding material. For moving about, some form of back support may improve comfort, but under no circumstances should a patient lift heavy objects.

For severe pain, a physician may prescribe a pain reliever. As pain subsides, an exercise program may be recommended to gradually strengthen muscles.

Most people find partial or complete relief of slipped disk from nonsurgical therapy. However, in some cases, removing the disk surgically provides the only remedy.

There is a new treatment still being investigated that offers the same results of eliminating or reducing the disk without major surgery. With this method, the drug chymopapain is injected into the damaged disk after the patient receives local anesthetic. This drug acts by slowly dissolving the part of the disk that is pressing on a nerve. Treatment is fast and relatively painless, but pain reduction occurs slowly, maybe in a couple weeks, if at all.

Tendonitis

Tendonitis is an inflammation of a tendon, a band of fibrous tissue connecting muscle to bone. The condition appears most often as a result of physical activity. It also can be a symptom of a more generalized inflammatory disease such as rheumatoid arthritis.

Causes

Improper activity, lack of conditioning, and poor equipment encourage the development of tendonitis. Nonathletes who suddenly begin long distance jogging or other athletic activity or athletes who resume strenuous sports after intervals of passive activity have an increased likelihood of the condition. In addition, people who wear shoes with rundown heels put needless tension on the Achilles tendon, which joins the two major muscles on the back of the legs to the back of the heel bones. Similarly, women who wear high-heel shoes may have problems with inflamed Achilles tendons because the angle created by the shoes considerably shortens the tendons.

Symptoms

A tendonitis attack causes pain in the affected tendon worsened by activity. The tendon may grow thicker than normal and be tender to the touch. Sometimes, the tendon can be very painful. When minor injuries are continually placed under stress, an already inflamed tendon could rupture and become a greater problem.

Diagnosis

Physicians diagnose sports-related problems by first acquiring an exercise history to determine the patient's normal activity, and if there have been any changes in routine. A doctor also checks muscle lengths to find unusually short or inflexible muscles which may be producing the problem.

Treatment

Treatment for tendonitis involves resting the affected area. Pain relievers and anti-inflammatory drugs are used to ease immediate symptoms, but these preparations will not by themselves cure the condition or keep it from recurring.

In rare cases, tendonitis patients require surgery to remove damaged tendons. Fortunately, surgical procedures have advanced in the past few years. Previously, tendons were replaced with artificial tissues that never assumed the strength and flexibility of natural tissues. Now, newer techniques and materials are being developed.

Prevention

People participating in sports can prevent tendonitis by taking time for warmup prior to exercise. For example, leg and calf muscle stretching before and after running may help prevent inflammation of the Achilles tendon.

Supports in shoes worn during physical activity can correct instability of the foot and lessen pain when tendonitis occurs.

Tic

A tic is a spasmodic movement or twitching that is usually a brief, repetitive, purposeless, semivoluntary or involuntary muscle contraction, most commonly seen in the face, shoulders, or arms. A typical "nervous tic" is a twitching of the corner of the eye or the mouth, grimacing, blinking, or making repetitive motions with the arms or shoulders.

Tics in children often occur between the ages of five to ten years and may gradually disappear as the child grows older; however, they can also persist into adulthood. Nervous tics, when the first arise, can usually be voluntarily controlled, but persistent tics often become automatic after a period of time.

Causes

Some tics are associated with nerve or brain damage. However, most tics are of unknown origin.

With the exception of the tics that develop as a result of other conditions, the physiological basis of ordinary tics is largely unknown. They often, but not always, accompany tension, emotional upset, or some hidden psychological problem. Such conditions as hereditary tremors and organic disorders such as Parkinson's disease also often worsen with emotional stress.

Types

There are several different kinds of specific tics: *facial tic,* or spasms of the facial muscles, and *Gilles de la Tourette's syndrome,* a childhood disorder marked by multiple tics and compulsive use of profane language, are two examples.

Facial tic, the simplest, is marked by simple spasms of the facial muscles. These may be simple twitches, such as twitching of the corner of the eye, twisting or grimacing of the mouth, or raising of an eyebrow.

Gilles de la Tourette's syndrome, the most complicated of the types of tics, may be marked by single or multiple tics (blinking, grimacing, shrugging of the shoulders, repetitive arm movements) that gradually worsen in extent, severity, and frequency. In many patients, vocal tics such as sniffling, grunting, shouting, or barking noises also occur. About half of all patients develop coprolalia, or compulsive swearing.

Tourette's syndrome is the only type of tic associated with a definite syndrome. The other tics are at the beginning hard to distinguish from many neurologically-based illnesses.

Treatment

For mild childhood or adult tics, minor tranquilizers or muscle relaxants may be prescribed. Tourette's syndrome has been known to respond to the major tranquilizer haloperidol. Psychotherapy as treatment for tics may be ineffective, but it may help to relieve some of the emotional stress that precipitates attacks or intensifies symptoms.

Prevention

No preventive measures for tics are known at present.

Trichinosis

Trichinosis is a condition caused by the parasitic infestation of the body by the *Trichinella spiralis,* a worm commonly found in pork.

Cause

Trichinosis is most commonly caused by eating pork that has not been cooked for a sufficient length of time or at a sufficiently high temperature to kill the *Trichinella spiralis* worms. The worms are encapsulated in the meat itself. When the meat is eaten the worms emerge from it and begin their life cycle in the human host. This begins in the small intestine, where the worms' larvae mature within two days after they emerge from the meat. The adults breed, the males die, and the females give birth to other larvae that invade the tissues of the bowel and are then dispersed to the body's muscles where they lodge.

The muscles around the eyes, the tongue, and the diaphragm (the muscle separating the chest cavity from the abdomen), and the muscles between the ribs are the most common sites of larvae attachments.

Symptoms

Quite often, the infested patient is entirely unaware of the presence of trichinosis. When large infestations do occur, however, they are accompanied by symptoms. Soon (one to two days) after consumption of the contaminated meat, a severe flu-like illness consisting of fever, nausea, vomiting, diarrhea, and abdominal pain occurs. After about a week, severe symptoms such as rash, swelling of the eyelids, and neurologic disorders may develop. Myocarditis (inflammation of the heart muscle) can also be seen in this stage. Eventually the larvae in the muscles die and become calcified; tenderness and swelling around the muscle tissue are common.

Treatment

Since there is no way to get the larvae out of the muscle tissue, treatment is aimed at relief of discomfort. Analgesics, such as aspirin, are administered for pain, and anti-inflammatory steroids (cortisone drugs such as prednisone) are administered for allergic symptoms, myocarditis, and/or central nervous system involvement. Thiabendazole (which tends to kill worms, such as the trichinella) is often given with good results. A close watch is kept for drug fever, abdominal pain, vomiting, and dermatitis (inflammation and/or rash of the skin).

Prevention

The only real preventatives are keeping the hogs from becoming infected by thoroughly cooking their food, and making sure that pork is sufficiently cooked to kill the larvae (30 minutes for each pound of meat, to an internal temperature of at least 185°F).

THE EYE AND VISION

The eye is the organ of sight. This complex structure works by capturing light and transforming it into impulses that the brain can interpret as images. These visual images give individuals information about their environment.

In order to understand visual perception, it is important to know the functions of various parts of the eye. The eye includes the eyeball (globe) and all structures within and surrounding its almost spherical mass. To guard the eye, the bony socket of the skull nestles the delicate organ. A layer of fat cushions the socket while the eyebrow, eyelashes, and eyelid provide a barrier against incoming irritants. Lining the inside of the eyelid and continuing over the exposed surface of the eyeball is the conjunctiva, a thin protective membrane. Tears (watery secretions) released from the lacrimal (tear) glands moisten the conjunctiva and keep the eyeball clean.

Light first enters the eye through the three outer layers of the eyeball. The cornea is a transparent covering over the area that admits the light. The sclera is the white of the eye (actually the tough, outer covering of the globe), and the choroid membrane contains blood vessels to nourish the eye.

Light enters the eye first through the cornea. Behind the cornea is a pigmented (colored) structure called the iris. The iris surrounds an opening known as the pupil. The iris changes the size of the pupil depending on the amount of light present in the environment. If the surroundings are relatively dark, the pupil is enlarged to admit more light; if the environment is bright, the pupil is made smaller. Behind the iris is the lens, a transparent body held in place by elastic muscular-type tissue. The shape of the lens is changed to focus on objects at varying distances.

Between the cornea and the lens is a space, the anterior chamber, filled with a substance called aqueous humor (fluid). Aqueous fluid contains nutrients that nourish the cornea and the lens. The fluid also allows light rays to pass through easily.

Another chamber of the eyeball behind the lens holds vitreous humor. This clear jelly is surrounded by the retina, the innermost layer of the eyeball. In the retina are the sensitive nerve endings that convert light focused from the lens into electrical impulses. These impulses are then transmitted to the brain by the optic nerve, which extends from the rear of the eyeball to the brain.

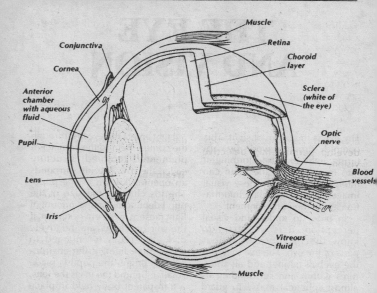

Astigmatism

Astigmatism is a type of distorted vision caused by a defect in the curvature of the eye. This prevents all the rays of light entering the eye from being properly focused on the retina at the back of the eye. Some rays are misplaced, causing the image to be partially out of focus.

Types

Most people with astigmatism can see clearly those objects directly in front of them. However, their peripheral vision is imperfect. They may have vertical astigmatism, in which the scene above and below their direct gaze is imperfect. They may have horizontal astigmatism in which the right and left sides of their field of vision are warped; for example, a straight horizontal line may appear curved to the right and to the left. The astigmatism may also be diagonal.

Treatment

Fortunately, the defect in the curvature of the eye is usually uniform and can be easily corrected by eyeglasses or contact lenses. The fault is usually in the shape of the cornea, the clear "window" in front of the iris and pupil, which may be slightly flattened vertically or horizontally. The eyeglass or contact lenses do not bend rays entering the band of clear vision but are curved to adjust the angle of rays entering from either side or top and bottom, depending upon the prescription.

Although most people with astigmatism were born with a tendency toward the condition, a few cases are caused by eye disease or injury. These may be more difficult to correct. Regardless of the cause, astigmatism — as with any vision problem — should be corrected as early as possible. A child, in particular, with an uncorrected vision problem may develop permanently defective vision.

Blepharitis

Blepharitis is an inflammation of the edges of the eyelids, with redness and thickening. Scales and crusts or shallow ulcers (eroded areas) may also appear. The disease is common, especially in children, and often affects both eyes and upper and lower eyelids.

Causes

Bacterial (*Staphylococcus aureus*) infection of eyelash follicles and oil glands causes blepharitis with ulcers. The non-ulcerous variety may be the result of an allergic reaction, or it may be linked with seborrheic dermatitis, an inflammatory scaling of the scalp, eyebrows, and sometimes ears. Occasionally the non-ulcerous form is caused by lice on brows and lashes, which irritate lid margins.

Symptoms

Symptoms of blepharitis include itching, burning, "red-rimmed" eyes; swelling of the lids; loss of eyelashes; and irritation of the underside of the lid, as if dirt or sand were underneath. The eyes may tear and be sensitive to light. In blepharitis with ulcers, tough dry crusts form that leave a bleeding surface when removed. Greasy, easily removed scales appear on the edges of the lids in the non-ulcerous variety.

Treatment

Blepharitis caused by a bacterial infection can be treated with an antibiotic ointment, such as erythromycin or bacitracin, specially formulated for use around the eyes. The salve is applied three times a day to the eyelash margins with a cotton-tipped swab, after the margins have been softened with warm compresses for ten minutes and the crusts removed. Sulfacetamide-corticosteroid drops are often used to combat irritation or other types of bacterial infection and may replace the second application of ointment.

If an allergy is the cause, a cosmetic may be at fault and should be removed. If there is scaling on the eyebrows and scalp — that is, seborrheic dermatitis — the doctor is likely to recommend a special shampoo, such as a sulfur or tar shampoo to control the dandruff, and to prescribe a cortisone lotion or cream to be rubbed into hairy areas. Absolute cleanliness of hair, scalp, eyebrows, and eyelid margins is necessary during treatment.

If the blepharitis is caused by lice, nits (lice eggs) are carefully removed with tweezers and steps

204 THE EYE AND VISION

are taken to keep the patient free of lice.

Both of the principal varieties are difficult to cure and often recur. Blepharitis without ulcers causes no permanent damage. However, ulcerous blepharitis, if it recurs often enough, can cause scarring of eyelids, loss of lashes, and even ulcers of the cornea (the transparent covering across the front of the eyeball).

Complete cleanliness may help prevent the disease. If it is treated promptly when it occurs, permanent damage can probably be prevented.

Cataract

A cataract is a clouding of the lens of the eye that results in obscured vision. Because people with cataracts see their environment as if they were looking through a waterfall, the condition is called cataract from the Greek word for waterfall.

Normally, the lens is clear. Its function is to direct light into the eye so that the eye can focus on objects at various distances more distinctly. However, if the lens becomes hazy, incoming light scatters and vision blurs.

Causes

The exact cause of cataracts is unknown. Aging may play a role in development of cataracts, but newborns whose mothers contracted German measles during pregnancy and some young people may also develop the condition.

Such conditions as diabetes (inability to use carbohydrates), glaucoma (increased pressure within the eyeball), or detachment of the retina (innermost layer of the eye) may lead to cataracts. In addition, injury to the lens, prolonged use of certain drugs, or high dosages of radiation (for example, prolonged exposure to X rays) may trigger the condition.

Although usually the condition is curable, in rare cases, cataracts can cause blindness. In addition, the shadowy lens prohibits a clear view of the interior of the eye. Because of this obstruction, a physician may not be able to detect other potentially serious eye disorders such as changes in the retina (innermost light-sensitive layer of the eyeball) or damage to the optic nerve (which transmits messages from the eye to the brain).

Symptoms

The main symptom of cataracts is painless blurring of vision, occurring most often in only one eye. During initial stages of development, cataracts can cause the person to experience glare in bright light since the clouded lens scatters rather than focuses incoming light. As the condition progresses, the lens becomes milky white, and vision worsens.

Treatment

Successful treatment involves surgical removal of the affected lens followed by the wearing of special eyeglasses or contact lenses. With the aid of a micro-scope, a surgeon opens an area in the front of the eye and with-draws the lens. Local anes-thetic eyedrops make the proce-dure relatively painless. After a few weeks of recuperation, an eye specialist prescribes special cataract eyeglasses or a contact lens to help correct the vision resulting from the removed lens. These aids are by no means perfect and require an adjustment period.

More recently, many doctors recommend an intraocular lens (IOL) to be implanted in the eye after the cataract lens is removed. This lightweight plastic is relatively free from distortion and closer to normal vision than eyeglasses or contact lenses because it occupies the exact position of the natural lens. Nevertheless, not everyone can benefit from an intraocular lens. Doctors advise patients with glaucoma, detached retina, or eye disorders caused by diabetes to wear eyeglasses or contacts to restore vision.

Ninety-five percent of the surgery for cataracts is without complication. Restoration or sub-stantial improvement of vision results after surgery in the majority of the cases. When vision remains unimproved, other disorders that were undetected because of the cataract may be causing the con-tinued problem. Generally, how-ever, cataracts can be successfully removed and the patient can resume a normal life.

Color blindness

Color blindness is an inability to identify certain colors. By far the most common type is inherited red-green color blindness, which affects 8 percent of men and boys but only 0.5 percent of women and girls. Total color blindness, which is very rare, and pastel-shade blindness are believed to be inherited. Others, including blue-yellow blindness and red blindness, can be either inherited or acquired. Disease or injury of the retina, the light-sensitive tis-sue at the back of the eye, some-times causes color blindness.

Description

Color blindness results from a defect in the cone-shaped light-sensitive cells of the fovea, the tiny yellowish pit at the rear of the eye that is the eye's center for color and for close work. The cone cells — seven million of them — are much different from the 130 million rod-shaped cells in the rest of the retina, which register only in black and white. The cones are believed to contain bleachable pigments for red, green, and blue, colors which can combine to pro-duce all of the colors of the spec-trum. The pigments become more vivid or fade in response to colors that the eye sees. The changes of pigment produce tiny flashes of electricity that are carried by means of the optic nerve to the visual center of the brain. There, the electrical signals are com-bined into a full-color picture. In the color-blind person, for unknown reasons, the cones are effective in other ways but the process for one or more color pigments simply does not work right. No cure for the condition is known.

Inheriting red-green color blindness

Why is red-green color blindness inherited by boys more often than by girls? The reason is that the defective gene for color blindness is carried in the pair of chromosomes which determines the sex of the child. In the female, who has two X sex chromosomes, the defective gene is almost always counteracted by a normal gene in the matching sex chromosome. In the male, with an X and Y sex chromosome, there is no matching normal gene in the paired chromosome to block the defect, and the boy is born color blind.

Red-green color blindness cannot be passed from an affected father to his sons. Nor will his daughters be color blind, unless the mother carries the same defective gene. However, all of the daughters are carriers of the defective gene, and the daughters' sons will have a 50 percent chance of inheriting it and being color blind.

Conjunctivitis

Conjunctivitis, or pinkeye, is an inflammation of the conjunctiva. The conjunctiva is a delicate membrane that lines the inner surface of the eyelid and covers the exposed surface of the eye.

Causes

Most cases of conjunctivitis result from disease-causing microorganisms such as bacteria, fungi, or viruses. Allergies, chemicals, dust, smoke, or foreign objects that irritate the conjunctiva may also lead to conjunctivitis. Swimming may also irritate the conjunctiva — either from chlorine in the pool or from contaminated water. Occasionally, a sexually transmitted disease can cause pinkeye if the eyes are rubbed after touching infected genital organs.

Children contract conjunctivitis most often. Measles, a viral disease, may be accompanied by the eye inflammation. In addition, those people, both children and adults, who have allergies, such as hay fever, or who work and live in areas where they are exposed to chemicals or other irritants are more susceptible to noninfectious conjunctivitis.

Symptoms

Conjunctivitis causes redness, a grating sensation, burning, itching, and perhaps light sensitivity. Sometimes, tearing or a discharge containing pus occurs. Symptoms can last a few days or up to two weeks.

Usually conjunctivitis produces no permanent damage. However, if left untreated, the infection can lead to more serious eye problems. Ulcers, or eroded areas, may form on the cornea (the transparent covering across the front of the eye). Should these ulcers persist, they can scar the eye and interfere with vision.

Treatment

Treatment depends upon the cause and resulting symptoms of

THE EYE AND VISION   207

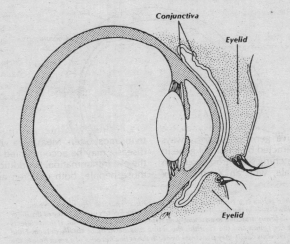

The conjunctiva is a delicate membrane lining the inner surface of the eyelid and covering the exposed surface of the eye.

the conjunctivitis. If the inflammation is environmentally caused, simply removing the irritant may be sufficient to eliminate the condition. For more difficult cases, a physician may prescribe antibiotic, steroid, or combination eyedrops to be used several times a day as directed. Frequent use is necessary because drops tend to be washed away by the natural cleansing action of tears.

Sensitive eyes should be rested and shielded from bright lights. When the discharge glues the eyes closed, bathing them with warm water and wiping with a clean cloth will loosen eyelids.

A most important fact about conjunctivitis is that its infectious form is highly contagious. Individuals with infectious conjunctivitis should not share handkerchiefs, towels, or washcloths. If one eye becomes infected, you should not touch the clear eye after rubbing the infected eye since the second eye can then become infected.

Detached retina

A detached retina is a condition in which the retina separates from its attachment to underlying tissues in the eye. Normally, the retina — the delicate, light-sensitive lining of the inner eyeball — is firmly attached to an underlying structure called the choroid. If fluid collects between the retina and the choroid, the retina may partially or totally detach. Fluid from the vitreous cavity — the fluid-filled space within the eye — may penetrate beneath the retina because of a small hole in the ret-

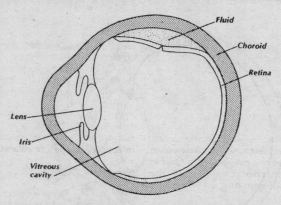

A detached retina is a condition in which the retina separates from its attachment to underlying tissues in the eye. Normally, the retina—the light-sensitive lining of the inner eyeball—is firmly attached to an underlying structure called the choroid. If fluid collects between the retina and the choroid, the retina may partially or totally detach. Fluid from the vitreous cavity may penetrate beneath the retina because of a small hole in the retina. Fluid leaking out of certain blood vessels in the eye may also penetrate beneath the retina to cause detachment.

ina. Fluid leaking out of certain blood vessels in the eye may also penetrate beneath the retina to cause detachment.

Causes

Cataract surgery, severe myopia (nearsightedness), and injury can cause retinal detachment. Although injury can be the primary cause of this condition, it is more likely to accelerate a detachment that has already begun. Conditions that increase susceptibility to retinal detachment are inflammation or tumors of the eye, high blood pressure, and vitreous hemorrhaging.

Symptoms

Symptoms of detachment — at the onset—include seeing floating dark spots or flashes or streaks of light, or experiencing a blurring of vision. As the condition progresses, a curtain or veil seems to fall over the field of vision.

Treatment

The detached retina can be treated by using a laser to fuse the retina to the choroid. It can also be treated through the use of diathermy (repair using heat), cryotherapy (repair using extreme cold), or microsurgery (surgery using a microscope). Left untreated, the detachment will enlarge and can, in extreme cases, lead to the loss of sight.

Glaucoma

Glaucoma is an eye disorder that results from increased pressure within the eyeball. The pressure builds up because fluids within the eyeball are unable to circulate and drain normally.

Cause

Although glaucoma is understood to be a problem with the eye's fluid-regulating mechanism, its precise cause is unknown. In the healthy eye, aqueous fluid in the anterior chamber of the eyeball remains under gentle pressure. When the delicate fluid balance changes, internal pressure rises in the eye. This buildup produces damage to the sensitive structures and nerve endings within the eye.

Forms of glaucoma

Depending upon the type of defect in the fluid-regulating system, one of two primary forms of glaucoma results. *Chronic*, or *open angle*, glaucoma develops when pressure elevates gradually and normal fluid drainage slows but is not obstructed. *Acute*, or *closed angle*, glaucoma occurs when pressure mounts suddenly and forces the iris (colored portion of the eye) into an angle joining the cornea (transparent covering across the front of the eyeball that helps focus light), thereby blocking fluid drainage from the anterior chamber of the eye.

Those at risk

Both forms of glaucoma are more common in adults over 40 years of age. Statistics show that people with glaucoma in their families have greater risk of acquiring the condition, but inheritance has not been proven. Some evidence suggests that glaucoma may be linked to long-term use of certain drugs, especially steroids that can alter body fluid levels. Glaucoma can also follow other eye disorders such as infections, injuries, or cataracts.

Symptoms

Chronic glaucoma begins with no noticeable symptoms. Vision deterioration is so gradual and painless that this form of glaucoma has been termed the "sneak thief of sight." Sometimes, peripheral, or side, vision loss slowly progresses as central vision remains normal. As the disorder advances, other symptoms that may be intermittent or constant include foggy or blurred vision; difficulty in adjusting to brightness and darkness; and slight pain in or around the eye, usually on one side. The one symptom indicative of chronic glaucoma is the perception of a faint white circle or halo surrounding a light. This halo is most visible in the dark while looking at a distant light.

Acute glaucoma brings sudden and severe symptoms of extreme eye pain and abrupt vision blurring. Frequently, the pain can be so intense that it causes nausea and vomiting. Fortunately, acute glaucoma is rare, but when it does occur, medical attention is needed immediately to prevent permanent blindness. Usually, however, the symptoms are so severe that medical help is promptly sought.

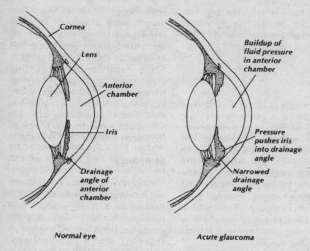

Normal eye   *Acute glaucoma*

In acute glaucoma, normal drainage may be obstructed by a sudden elevation of fluid pressure which pushes the iris into the angle of the eye where the iris joins the cornea.

Diagnosis

If left untreated, glaucoma can lead to partial or complete vision loss. However, if diagnosed early, treatment can usually halt the problem. Because chronic glaucoma gives no warning signs, it is particularly important that persons over the age of 40 be tested for glaucoma every two or three years. In addition, physicians recommend that people with family history of the disease be screened every year and possibly before the age of 40.

Glaucoma testing is a simple procedure. First, eyedrops anesthetize the eyeball. Then, the doctor places a pressure gauge on the front surface of the eye to measure the amount of pressure within. In addition, the doctor inspects the interior of the eye through a special instrument that allows a view of the angle where the iris and cornea meet. This part of the examination shows whether there is blockage in the drainage system or damage to the optic nerve. Side vision is also tested by measuring the point where objects enter the patient's field of vision.

Treatment

Glaucoma treatment is usually effective if started early in the course of the disease. Acute glaucoma needs surgery to quickly restore the eye's draining system. Chronic glaucoma responds well to medications. Oral drugs work by decreasing production of eye fluid, while daily applications of eyedrops promote fluid drainage. Some medications constrict pupils of the eye, which can be misconstrued as a symptom of drug overdose. Consequently, many glaucoma patients carry an ID card with their medical history in case of emergency.

There is a new type of eyedrop called beta blocker which reduces production of eye fluid without altering the size of the pupil. However, beta blockers can affect heart rate and narrow breathing passages, making these drugs unsuitable for patients with heart or lung disease.

Although chronic glaucoma responds to medication, some patients (less than 5 percent) require surgery to open new pathways for fluid drainage. Laser therapy is the most current surgical technique under investigation. Here, the laser, or intense light beam, generates enough heat to alter tissues and cells in order to stimulate better fluid drainage.

Prevention

The best way to prevent serious complications of glaucoma is periodic screening for early diagnosis. If glaucoma is diagnosed, attention to prescribed treatment procedures is required.

Keratitis

Keratitis is an inflammation of the cornea—the transparent covering over the iris and pupil of the eye— which commonly produces redness, tearing, tenderness, sensitivity to light, and blurred vision.

Herpes simplex keratitis

The most common type of keratitis is caused by herpes simplex virus, the same virus that produces cold sores. Although herpes simplex keratitis is not painful, at first there is a sensation that foreign matter may be present. If left untreated, all feeling in the cornea is eventually lost. Like cold sores, the infection tends to come and go, but it should be taken care of when the first sign—a whitish lesion on the cornea—appears. Treatment usually consists of applying eyedrops or ointment, but some specialists prefer to scrape the cornea, after which they cover the affected eye temporarily.

Traumatic keratitis

Traumatic keratitis occurs when a corneal injury leaves scar tissue after the injury itself has healed. If the scar tissue covering the pupil is considerable, blindness may result. This condition can be cured by corrective surgery.

Interstitial keratitis

Interstitial keratitis is most often caused by congenital (present at birth) syphilis in children or by tuberculosis. This type of keratitis produces deep deposits of scar tissue, which cause the cornea to become hazy and give it a ground-glass appearance. There is little that can be done for this condition, although the inflammation and redness usually diminish after a month or two. Vision may or may not be impaired thereafter.

Macular degeneration

Macular degeneration is the deterioration of the macula, a yellowish depression in the back of the retina of the eye. The retina, which is sensitive to light, is the innermost of the three coatings of the eyeball. The other coatings are the choroid, which encircles the retina, and the sclera (white of the eye), which covers the choroid layer. These coatings surround the inner globe of the eye, called the vitreous cavity.

The macula is located on the retina near the optic nerve at the very back of the eye. The function of the macula is distinguishing fine detail in the central vision field. Thus, the macula is that part of the eye with the sharpest vision. As light enters the eye, any image that is focused on the macula is the one that is most accurately perceived in the brain. Consequently, degeneration of the macula leads to blurring of central vision.

Causes

Macular degeneration is often secondary—that is, a result of other conditions of the eye — and is usually hereditary. However, one form is not hereditary and occurs primarily in persons over 60 years of age. In many of these cases, the blood vessels of the eye narrow, possibly as a result of atherosclerosis, and the macula's blood supply is diminished. Since the macula requires a plentiful blood supply, any deficiency causes degeneration of the macula.

Symptoms

Macular degeneration develops slowly and painlessly. Therefore, the blurring of central vision is gradual. If both eyes are affected — as is almost always the case — activities requiring sharp vision, such as reading or driving, usually have to be curtailed. Eventually, all central vision disappears, although peripheral vision is unaffected.

Treatment

There has been no treatment for macular degeneration until recently. It has now been found that about 5 percent of affected individuals may be helped by treatment with laser beams. Early in the course of the condition, vision may be improved by special powerful eyeglasses.

Myopia

Myopia, also called nearsightedness, is a very common optical defect in which the eyes can see close objects clearly but faraway objects look blurred. About one in every five people is myopic; it tends to be hereditary, developing around age 12 and progressing until about age 20.

Cause

The defect is caused by an eyeball that is too long from front

Myopia — nearsightedness — is a vision defect in which the eye can clearly see close objects but distant objects appear blurred. It is caused by an eyeball that is too long front to back causing incoming light to fall short of the light-sensitive retina. This results in a fuzzy image.

to back. Normally, the eye's cornea (the curved transparent tissue that covers the front of the eye) and lens (the disk-shaped structure just behind the front of the eye responsible for focus) refract or bend light coming from the viewed distant object so that the image focuses on the retina (a layer of light-sensitive nerve cells that line the back of the eyeball). In myopia, the focused image falls short of the retina because of the greater length of the eyeball, resulting in a fuzzy image.

Types

There are several kinds of myopia. Curvature myopia refers to an excess curve of the refractive surfaces of the eye causing light to enter the eye in an abnormal path. The curvature is either in the front surface of the cornea or the lens. In index myopia, there is an increase in the light-refracting properties of the lens. It is sometimes associated with future development of cataracts or iritis (inflammation of the iris). Progressive myopia is an uncommon form in which the eyeball continues to elongate throughout a person's life, eventually leading to degeneration of the retina or a detached retina.

Diagnosis

Blurred or fuzzy vision should be examined by an ophthalmologist (physician who is an eye specialist) who will look inside the eyes with a special instrument (ophthalmoscope), diagnose any disorders, and test the acuity (sharpness) of vision.

Treatment

Nearsightedness is easily corrected with a concave (inwardly curved) lens that pushes the images back to the retina and focuses them clearly.

A surgical procedure known as radial keratotomy corrects myopia but is considered controversial. It involves cutting 16 "spokes" in the cornea coming out from the center; as the cornea heals, it flattens and counteracts the problem.

Myopia rarely progresses after age 30. In fact, the onset of middle age sometimes lessens the condition.

Night blindness

Night blindness—or nyctalopia—is a condition in which a person can see well in good light but not in dim or fading light.

Photoreceptors (nerve-end organs sensitive to light) in the retina make the adjustments that govern the eyes' ability to adapt to varying degrees of light. The retina is a layer of light-sensitive nerve cells that lines the interior of the eyeball; it acts as the film for images the eye sees. The nerve cells are either cones or rods. Cones, concentrated in the center of the retina, distinguish fine detail and color while rods, which are around the edges of the retina, are sensitive to the intensity of light and do most of the work of

seeing in dim light. Rods contain the pigment rhodopsin or visual purple that becomes temporarily bleached out by bright light. The speed at which rhodopsin adjusts to darkness depends upon a sufficient supply of Vitamin A in the body.

Causes

Night blindness is caused by either a severe deficiency of Vitamin A or by retinitis pigmentosa, an inherited degenerative disorder of the retina. In cases of extreme Vitamin A shortage, the cornea may soften or start to dissolve (keratomalacia) or the eyes may become excessively dry (xerophthalmia).

Treatment

The Vitamin A deficiency can be treated with doses of the vitamin but there is no cure for retinitis pigmentosa.

Prevention

The only way to prevent night blindness is to include enough Vitamin A in the diet.

Nystagmus

Nystagmus is the involuntary, rhythmic, and rapid movement of the eyeballs in a horizontal, vertical, or rotary direction. A person who sits in a moving vehicle and watches the scenery flashing by demonstrates normal nystagmus.

Abnormal nystagmus

Abnormal nystagmus is brought on by one of three problems: defective vison in which the eye does not receive enough stimulation for it to concentrate on one object; disturbances in the elaborate mechanisms in the ear responsible for balance; and diseases of the nervous system, especially those affecting the parts of the brain responsible for eye movement and coordination. Generally, the only symptoms are double vision or vertigo and dizziness. Treatment depends on the underlying cause.

Retinitis

Retinitis is an inflammation of the retina, the innermost layer of the eye that is sensitive to light. There are several types of retinitis, each one dependent on the cause.

Types

Toxoplasmic retinitis, which is either acquired or present at birth, is caused by a microbe from outside the body. (If it is present at birth, the microbe was passed to the unborn baby through the placenta, the temporary organ in the uterus that nourishes the unborn baby.) A similar retinitis is caused by blood infection that settles in the eye. Exudative retinitis stems from unknown causes, but results in detachment of the retina from the eyeball.

The most common form of retinitis, however, is retinitis pigmentosa. It is an inherited disorder in which excess amounts of a substance called phytanic acid accumulate in the system and cause extensive damage to the retina. Phytanic acid is a form of phytol, a compound found in green vegetables.

Symptoms

The symptoms of retinitis pigmentosa are night blindness, inflammation of the retina, pronounced limitation of the field of vision (tunnel vision), loss of kinesthetic sense (sense of where the body is), shrinkage of the retina, clumping of retinal pigment and dislodgement of the retina's blood vessels.

Many of the same symptoms are found in the other forms of retinitis. Sometimes, they are accompanied by a cloudiness in the liquid filling the eyeball (called vitreous fluid). This can be seen by a physician examining the interior of the eye.

Treatment

In the case of retinitis pigmentosa, there is little that can be done except to avoid foods containing phytols. If the retina is detached, a condition often caused when a hole in the retina allows the eye's fluid to seep in and create a pocket, surgery is usually the treatment. The pocket is eliminated either by freezing or by heat, sometimes with a laser. If the retinitis is the result of blood infection, the obvious course to follow is removal of the underlying problem.

Prevention

There are no clear-cut preventive measures against retinitis.

Retinopathy

Retinopathy is a condition in which deterioration of the retina — the light-sensitive, image-receiving innermost lining of the eye — is caused by damage to or overproduction of its blood vessels.

Causes

The vast majority of retinopathy cases stems from diabetes. Although fewer than 5 percent of all diabetics completely lose their sight because of retinopathy, that figure still means diabetes is one of the leading causes of irreversible blindness today. Other condi-

tions that increase susceptibility to retinopathy include high blood pressure (in which the retinal veins and arteries are either constricted or entirely blocked); hemorrhaging resulting from the sudden appearance of a blood clot, fat globule, or cholesterol plaque; and chronic kidney failure.

If retinopathy is triggered by sudden hemorrhage, total blindness in the eye can strike swiftly, so the victim is advised to seek immediate medical attention. In cases of high blood pressure or diabetic retinopathy, vision usually worsens over time.

Treatment

Controlling diabetic or high blood pressure retinopathy is best achieved by strict control over glucose (blood sugar) levels or blood pressure, either through

Retinopathy is a condition in which the light-sensitive innermost lining of the eye, the retina, deteriorates because of damage to or overproduction of its blood vessels.

diet or medication depending on the severity of the condition. If diabetics chronically allow their glucose levels to exceed normal bounds, retinal damage can be extensive and may require laser treatments to burn and seal off leaking blood vessels. In cases where these excess or weakened veins and arteries have clouded the eye's normally clear vitreous liquid, doctors can siphon off the fluid and simultaneously replace it with a harmless salt water solution.

Sty

A sty is an inflamed or infected swelling of the sebaceous (oil-producing) glands in the eyelid.

Causes

The infection is commonly caused by staphylococcus, a type of bacteria. An external sty appears on the surface of the skin at the edge of the eyelid. An internal sty is due to inflammation, infection, or obstruction of a sebaceous gland on the inner surface of the eyelid. This type of sty is often seen as a protrusion or lump on the eyelid without visible pus or redness.

Symptoms

Initially, a sty feels like a foreign object is in the eye. Tearing, redness, swelling, and tenderness in or around a particular area of the eye soon follow. The eye may be sensitive to light and touch. In addition, small, yellow bumps filled with pus may develop. These growths often burst, release the pus, and begin to heal. Once the pressure releases, the pain usually subsides.

Treatment

Treatment for a sty often involves putting antibiotic eye-drops and/or ointments into the eye. Warm, moist compresses applied to the eye three or four times a day for about ten minutes may encourage the sty to burst. In some cases, particularly in internal sties, surgical opening may be needed to cure the condition. Never should one attempt to open a sty on his or her own, as the risks of spreading and worsening the infection would be quite high.

EAR, NOSE, AND THROAT

The ear, nose, and throat are interconnected, and for this reason they are often grouped together in the field of medicine. Because they are joined, infection in one structure may spread into one of the others.

Ear

The ear is the organ of hearing consisting of three parts: the external ear, middle ear, and inner ear. The pinna, or external ear, traps sound waves and directs them into the ear canal through the eardrum into the middle ear.

In the middle ear, sound waves vibrate through three tiny bones called the hammer, anvil, and stirrup. Vibrations continue into the inner ear, where the cochlea transforms the sound waves into nerve impulses. These impulses then travel to the brain through the auditory nerve.

A eustachian tube in the middle ear connects the ear with the nasopharynx, the upper part of the throat opening into the nose. This tube allows air pressure in the middle ear to equalize with pressure outside the body, thus helping to prevent a ruptured eardrum. However, the eustachian tube also provides a passageway for infecting microorganisms to enter the middle ear from the nose or throat.

Besides functioning as the organ of hearing, the ear also provides signals to the brain about the position of the body. Semicircular canals (or labyrinth) within the inner ear serve as the organ of balance by detecting motion of the head and feeding this information to the brain.

Nose

The nose is a specialized structure with two nostrils, or external openings. The nose serves dual functions as the organ for the sense of smell and as an entry to the respiratory system.

When the nose works as the organ of smelling, nerve receptor cells within the nose detect odor and transmit signals to the brain through the olfactory nerve. The sense of smell also enhances the sense of taste. The ability to smell is more refined than the ability to taste; therefore, when a cold blocks nasal passages, food may seem bland and tasteless.

As an organ of breathing, the nose moisturizes incoming air and filters out any foreign materials. Small glands within the lining of the nose secrete mucus, a sticky substance that lubricates the walls of the nose and throat.

The ear is a complex structure that is responsible for the sense of hearing and for the body's sense of balance.

Mucus humidifies the incoming air and traps bacteria, dust, or other particles entering the nose. Many disease-causing bacteria are either dissolved by chemical elements in the mucus or transported to the entrance of the throat by tiny hairs called cilia. In the throat, any remaining bacteria are swallowed and killed by acids and other chemicals produced in the stomach. This efficient line of defense protects the body against the billions of bacteria continually entering the nose.

Connected to the nose are sinuses. Sinuses are cavities lined with mucus-secreting glands and filled with air located in certain facial bones. There are four groups of sinuses — frontal, sphenoid, ethmoid, and maxillary. Their purposes are to resonate the voice and lighten the weight of the skull.

Throat

The throat, or pharynx, is a passageway connecting the back of the mouth and nose to the esophagus, the tube between the mouth and stomach, and to the trachea, the tube between the mouth and the lungs. Because air and food pass through the throat, the throat is considered a part of both the respiratory and the digestive systems.

Three sections comprise the five-inch throat tube. The nasopharynx is the upper part of the throat that opens into the nose, and the oropharynx is the middle portion that opens into the mouth. The lower section of the throat, or laryngopharynx, connects the other sections with the larynx, or voice box.

Within the throat are two small

The ear, nose, and throat are interconnecting structures.

tissue masses called tonsils. Tonsils help fight disease by destroying bacteria that enter the throat. This can be a formidable task, since disease can easily spread from the nose and ears to the throat.

glands containing the specialized white blood cells that help localize and destroy harmful bacteria and viruses. They thus provide an important defense against diseases of the respiratory (breathing) system.

Adenoids

Adenoids are masses of protective (lymphoid) tissue located in the lining of the nasopharynx, the cavity above the throat and behind the nose. Like the tonsils located below them, the adenoids (technically known as the nasopharyngeal tonsils) are lymph

Enlarged adenoids

It is normal for adenoids to become enlarged during throat infections, just as the tonsils do, and then diminish in size after the infection passes. Sometimes, however, as a result of continuing infection or allergies the adenoids remain enlarged. The resulting obstruction of the nasal passage may cause mouth breathing, the characteristic "nasal" voice, and continuing drainage down the throat of pus-filled mucus. It may also cause a blockage of the two eustachian tubes, which connect the throat to the inner ears, resulting in retention of fluid in the middle ear, impaired hearing, earache, and sometimes serious recurring ear infections.

Treatment

Treatment of infected adenoids is with antibiotics, taken by mouth. Surgery may be recommended when the infected or enlarged adenoids themselves are the source of the disease (usually the tonsils beneath are infected as well and are removed in the same operation). This would be the case when there is recurrent or continuing infection of the adenoids that cannot be eliminated with antibiotics, when the adenoids cause repeated ear infections, or when there is cancer or an abscess (a mass of pus in a cavity surrounded by decaying tissue). When chronically infected adenoids may increase susceptibility to a condition like rheumatic fever or nephritis (a kidney disease), your doctor may consider surgical removal of the adenoids. However, surgery should not be performed during an acute attack of tonsillitis, because it may worsen the infection.

Surgery may not be the answer to prevent snoring, mouth breathing, or "nasal" voice caused by enlarged adenoids, since the enlargement usually diminishes after childhood.

An adenoid is a mass of lymphoid tissue, located above the throat and behind the nose, whose function is to trap and destroy harmful bacteria and viruses.

Prevention

Adenoid infection and enlargement cannot always be prevented. In fact, enlarging in order to trap and fight infecting organisms is a normal function of the adenoids. Good general health measures can help, however, as can the use of doctor-prescribed antibiotics when the adenoids become infected and enlarged.

Common cold

A simple, common cold is a collection of familiar symptoms signaling an infection of the upper respiratory tract, which includes the nose, throat, and sinuses.

Colds are self-limiting diseases, meaning that their symptoms last a certain length of time (or "run their course," as is often remarked) and then disappear without leaving lasting ill effects. A cold is a mild but commonplace disease, one contracted by adults about two to four times a year and by children six to eight times. Adults with children at home are more likely to catch colds than are those who do not live with children. Children are especially susceptible to colds because they have not yet developed immunity or resistance to the many viruses that can cause colds. Small children gradually build up immunity to viruses in their homes; then, when they go to school and have close contact with many other children, they have to combat new viruses. Similarly, adults who

travel frequently or have a high number of close contacts outside their community are more likely than those leading more isolated lives to contract colds or encounter new cold viruses to which they are not immune.

Complications

A cold can be a minor irritation, but it can increase susceptibility for more serious conditions, especially in children, the very old, and the very weak. Pneumonia, an infection of the lungs, is probably the most serious. Ear infections, sinus infections, and bronchitis are other possible complications. Children sometimes develop croup, a few days after a cold, recognized by its harsh, barking cough that signals a swelling of the airways to the lungs.

Causes

At least five major categories of viruses cause colds. One of these groups, the rhinoviruses, includes a minimum of 100 viruses. A different combination of symptoms and possible complications can develop from each of these viruses. It is not known exactly how viruses spread, but it seems to be a combination of physical contact and the presence of both virus particles and moisture in the air. So a virus can spread from hand-to-hand contact, for example, or from the infected person's nasal passages and throat (by droplet) into the air or onto the skin of another person. Colds have an incubation period of 48 to 72 hours, meaning that it takes that long after the virus enters the body for early symptoms to appear.

Symptoms

Early symptoms of the common cold include stuffy or runny nose, sneezing, sore or scratchy throat, cough, and occasionally a mild fever. Usually, as the cold progresses, other symptoms may appear: burning or watery eyes, loss of taste or smell, pressure in the ears or sinuses, nasal voice, and tenderness around the nose.

Symptoms vary in type and severity among the various viruses, so a cold can begin with any symptom or combination of symptoms. Most colds last about a week, but about 25 percent of all colds last two weeks. Smokers and those with chronic respiratory diseases tend to display more severe symptoms, have longer-lasting colds, and develop complications more readily than do those who do not fall into these categories.

Diagnosis

Since common colds are mild diseases, the physician, in diagnosing a cold, will actually be looking for symptoms indicating a complication more serious than the common cold. Material from the patient's throat or nasal passages may need to be tested for bacterial infections; a blood test

may be recommended to check for mononucleosis, characterized by a long-lasting sore throat and swelling glands; or an X ray of the sinuses may be necessary if an infection of the sinuses (called sinusitis) is suspected.

Treatment

Getting plenty of rest, drinking lots of fluids to prevent dehydration, and using a humidifier or vaporizer can help relieve the irritating symptoms of a cold. Nevertheless, the common cold cannot be cured, and no known treatment will actually hasten recovery. Many over-the-counter medicines and preparations are available that will at least ease the discomfort of a cold. However, it is best to take specific medicine only for the symptoms actually present and to carefully follow directions on the medication package. Overuse of an otherwise effective remedy can backfire and actually make the symptoms worse, and treating symptoms that are not there can complicate matters. For example, the overuse of an antihistamine or other drying agent for nasal congestion can make a cough more uncomfortable; or the use of a nasal decongestant for more than three days can cause more congestion because the blood vessels in the nose which have been constricted by the decongestant tend to relax in a rebound fashion after a few days' use of a decongestant, causing even more congestion. Anyone who is pregnant or has a chronic disease should check with a doctor before using cold preparations, even seemingly harmless over-the-counter drugs.

Prevention

There is no known prevention for the common cold. Vitamin C has been said to help prevent colds, but many studies have shown that it has no measurable effect in this area. Avoiding exposure to viruses, when possible, may be the only means of avoiding the common cold.

Deafness

Deafness is a term to describe complete or partial loss of the ability to hear. There are four main types of deafness.

Types

Conductive deafness. This type of deafness is caused by a defect in the external or middle ear, which prevents normal transmission of sound. It may be present at birth as the result of an inherited defect, an accident in development, or an infection of the baby in the womb. It may be produced by an injury that perforates the eardrum or that breaks up the linkage of the three tiny bones — hammer, anvil, stirrup — that normally transmit sound from the eardrum through the middle ear to the inner ear. Inflammation of the middle ear, a condition known as otitis media, is another important cause of conductive deafness.

Infection from an upper respiratory (breathing) tract ailment such as strep throat or flu can produce a buildup of pus in the middle ear so great that it ruptures the eardrum. Also, a plugged-up eustachian tube (the tube leading from the back of the throat to the ear) may trap fluid in the middle ear, creating temporary deafness. Conductive deafness in the middle and later years is most often caused by otosclerosis. In this inherited condition, new spongy bone grows over the stirrup bone, preventing it from vibrating when sound travels to it through the hammer and anvil bones.

Sensorineural deafness. This type of hearing loss, known less accurately as nerve deafness, occurs because of damage to the bony structures of the inner ear, to the auditory nerve carrying sound messages to the brain, or to the hearing center in the brain itself in the temporal lobe. It may be due to a head injury during birth, the effects of a woman's rubella infection on her unborn baby, a skull fracture affecting the inner ear or the auditory nerve, fever, bacterial or viral infections such as mumps or meningitis, tertiary (final stage) syphilis, Meniere's disease, cancers, multiple sclerosis, a hemorrhage or blood clot occurring in the inner ear, drug side effects, normal aging, prolonged or repeated exposure to intense noise, or edema (fluid buildup) caused by a thyroid deficiency. Most sensorineural deafness is not nerve deafness, the popular term for it. It is usually sensory deafness, caused by defects not in nerves but in the structure of the inner ear, especially in the fluid-filled cochlea and its organ of Corti which contains sensory cells that code sound waves into electrical impulses to be transmitted to the brain.

Mixed deafness. This is a combination of conductive and sensorineural deafness and is common.

Functional deafness. This form of deafness is that which occurs without any organic defect of the hearing system or of the brain.

People with pure conductive deafness simply need louder volume to hear all sounds. Those with defects in the inner ear can hear low sounds more easily than high sounds, and some sounds may be distorted. When there is damage to the temporal lobe, the hearing center in the brain, the person may be able to hear sounds, but has trouble recognizing them and understanding words (this problem can also occur with the other types of deafness).

Diagnosis

When hearing loss is suspected, a complete examination of the ear, nose, and throat is necessary to identify any infections or abnormalities which might be involved. Infected adenoids or tonsils, as well as sinus or nasal infections may be linked to ear infections.

Testing for hearing loss is important for all ages, but especially for infants. Many times, partial deafness in a baby is not discovered until the child fails to learn to talk—a direct result of the hearing loss. Babies who have been born prematurely or ill, or whose mothers had certain viral infections such as rubella during pregnancy, are in special need of testing.

Treatment

Although at present inborn hearing defects usually cannot be corrected, deaf children can be helped to deal with their handicap. Starting very early, they may be fitted with hearing aids, may be instructed in lipreading or sign language, and are taught to speak although they cannot hear.

Surgery to correct conductive hearing loss includes middle ear operations to replace the stirrup bone or all three tiny bones with tissue or synthetic material, to repair a punctured eardrum, and to clean out a chronic middle ear infection.

A hearing aid can help to restore hearing loss in many people. It should only be purchased, however, after thorough testing of the hearing by a specialist in audiometry, who can advise on the need for a hearing aid and on the type to buy. Classes in lipreading and listening can also be helpful.

Prevention

It is far easier to prevent deafness than to cure it. Antibiotics have made it possible to eradicate most of the middle ear infections that have been the major source of conductive hearing loss in children. Sometimes the middle ear problems are eliminated by treating allergies that cause the eustachian tubes to close up, or by removing infected adenoids. Nerve deafness caused by continued exposure to intense industrial noise, gun shots, rock music, or aircraft engines may be avoided by wearing ear plugs or other ear protectors. Some lost hearing may return after several months of relief from intense sound. Drugs that can cause hearing loss, including some antibiotics and certain drugs that remove water from the blood, need to be used with care, and signs of hearing loss should be noted.

Ear infections

The ear, which is responsible for both hearing and the body's sense of balance, can become infected in any one of its three parts—the inner ear, middle ear, or outer ear. However, most commonly, ear infections settle in the middle ear. The medical term for middle ear infections is otitis media.

Ear infections are much more likely to affect children than adults; those most susceptible range from ages six months to six years. Children who contract ear infections in their first year are more likely to have chronic (long-term) ear infections later in life, and by the age of eight, almost every child has had at least one ear infection.

Inner ear infections

Inner ear infections are rare, but they may result from middle ear infections and can lead to permanent ear damage. The inner ear has two parts: the labyrinth, the semicircular canals that act as the organs of balance; and the cochlea, which converts sound into nerve impulses and transports them to the brain.

Outer ear infections

Outer ear infections are basically skin infections, are seldom serious, and can be treated by cleaning, sometimes, with antibiotic or steroid ointments or drops. The outer ear includes the pinna (the visible ear), and the outer ear canal.

Middle ear infections

Middle ear infections usually clear up quickly, but the more serious or persistent infections can lead to a variety of serious complications: temporary or permanent hearing loss, infection of the semicircular canals in the inner ear, facial paralysis, brain abscess, meningitis (infection of the covering of the brain), and infection of the mastoid bone, located behind the pinna. The middle ear includes the eardrum and the three tiny bones — the hammer, anvil, and stirrup—that vibrate and convey sound into the inner ear.

Middle ear infections develop when viruses or bacteria in the nose or throat travel to the ear through the eustachian tube, which connects the middle ear to the nose and throat. The middle ear also can become infected when infection spreads from a severe outer ear infection or injury.

Symptoms

Middle ear infections can be recognized by severe throbbing pain in the ear; fevers up to 104° or 105°F (101° or 102°F in adults); hearing loss; and possibly dizziness, nausea, vomiting, or sore throat. Eardrums may bulge out or may even burst, oozing blood and pus into the outer ear and relieving the pain. Symptoms may worsen over hours or days. A child too young to talk may seem ill or feverish or may pull on an ear.

Diagnosis

Ear infections are diagnosed by an inspection of the eardrum. If it is red and swollen or bulging out, middle ear infection can usually be confirmed.

Treatment

Middle ear infections are usually quickly eliminated when they are treated with an antibiotic, often a form of penicillin, as well as with, at times, decongestants. If a virus infection is present, however, antibiotics are not used, since viruses do not respond to antibiotics. If the eardrum is bulging out and the pain is severe, the doctor may make a small cut in the eardrum (called a myringotomy) to relieve the pressure. If the eardrum bursts, the outer ear must be kept clean to prevent infection from spreading.

Improved antibiotics have lessened the need for surgery, but the infected tissue, in rare cases, may need to be surgically removed.

However, it should again be emphasized that this is seldom necessary because of modern, improved antibiotics.

Glossitis

Glossitis is an acute or chronic inflammation of the tongue. It may exist either as a primary disease or as a symptom of another disease or disorder.

Causes

The causes of glossitis can be either *local* or *systemic*. Local causes include immediate irritants such as jagged or broken teeth; badly-fitting dentures; poor oral habits; biting of the tongue (such as during convulsions); irritants such as alcohol, tobacco, hot or spicy foods; or even mouthwashes, toothpastes, or breath fresheners. Local infections, burns, and injuries may also produce glossitis symptoms. Systemic causes may include certain vitamin deficiencies (especially Vitamin B deficiencies, such as in pellagra), anemia, generalized skin diseases such as erythema (redness of the skin because of capillary congestion), and syphilis.

Symptoms

Glossitis symptoms vary widely, ranging from simple redness of the tip and edges of the tongue (if the cause is pellagra, anemia, or irritation from smoking or a tooth with a rough surface) to painful ulcers and whitish patches. In the later stages of pellagra, the entire tongue may be fiery red, swollen, and ulcerated. In iron deficiency and pernicious anemia, the tongue is pale and smooth. Painful ulcers on the tongue may indicate herpes lesions, tuberculosis, a streptococcal infection, or other diseases. White patches suggest candidiasis (a type of yeast infection), syphilis, or simple mouth breathing (which dries out the mucous membrane of the tongue). Very smooth and painless areas may be what is called geographic tongue, or "benign" glossitis. Hairy tongue usually has no symptoms and often follows antibiotic therapy, a high fever, excessive use of certain mouthwashes, or a simple reduction in saliva secretion. Tiny brown growths on the tongue usually come from tobacco stains or from certain bacteria; the treatment is to stop smoking or otherwise correct the underlying cause and also to "brush" the tongue with a toothbrush.

Severe acute glossitis, which can result from local infection, burns, and injury, can cause tenderness and pain sufficient to make the tongue protrude from the mouth into the back of the throat—creating the danger of airway obstruction and even suffocation. In severe cases, the patient may not be able to chew, swallow, or speak. Steroid drug treatment usually reduces the swelling and helps relieve symptoms.

Patients may also complain of a painful burning tongue without other symptoms of inflammation. This is a common complaint among postmenopausal women. Diabetes, anemias, nutritional deficiencies, and malignancies should all be considered as possible primary causes.

Treatment

When the cause of glossitis can be correctly determined and corrected, the response is usually prompt. The patient should be reassured to know that redness and lesions of the tongue are usually harmless and respond well to treatment. Such complaints as ulcers and "hairy tongue," however, often recur periodically; ulcers that do not respond to treatment after a week or so should be biopsied (have a sample of tissue taken to be examined under a microscope).

In treating glossitis, specific causes, such as jagged teeth or ill-fitting dentures, should be corrected. Irritants, including hot or spicy foods, tobacco, alcohol, mouthwashes, and toothpastes, should be avoided once they are identified as the source of the trouble. A bland or liquid diet, preferably cool or cold, will often have a soothing effect. Good oral hygiene is indicated in all cases.

Symptomatic relief for large lesions includes rinsing the mouth with a medicated mouthwash before meals. Topical anesthetics, such as lidocaine and benzocaine, applied to the lesions, can give relief. Patients with complaints of painful burning should be tested for Vitamin B_{12} deficiency and to rule out more serious ailments, such as diabetes and anemias.

Prevention

Prevention of glossitis involves avoiding all irritants to the tongue and mouth as well as correcting nutritional and vitamin deficiencies and treating all primary infections that produce glossitis as a secondary symptom.

Laryngitis

Laryngitis is an inflammation of the mucous membrane (or lining) of the voice box (larynx), located in the upper part of the respiratory tract. It causes hoarseness and even possibly a temporary loss of speech.

Causes

Laryngitis may result from a bacterial or viral infection, such as a cold or flu; from an irritation of the mucous membrane of the larynx, such as that caused by smoking; or from overuse of the voice.

Chronic or persistent laryngitis is most often caused by smoking, air pollution, dust, or smoke. It may also stem from tonsillitis, tuberculosis, early cancer, or paralysis of the vocal cords. Because laryngitis may be a symptom of a more serious condition, persons who consistently suffer from it should consult a physician.

Symptoms

Symptoms of this condition — other than hoarseness or loss of voice — include dryness and scratchiness of the throat, coughing, and pain from speaking.

Treatment

Laryngitis is best treated by totally resting the vocal cords. Pain may be eased with throat sprays, steam inhalations, and mild pain relievers such as aspirin or acetaminophen.

Mastoid infection

A mastoid infection is a bacterial invasion of the mastoid air cells, small air-filled cavities located in the mastoid bone. The mastoid bone is the bulge in the skull behind the ear. A mastoid infection is most often a complication of a middle ear infection.

Symptoms

Mastoiditis is characterized by ringing in the ear, a discharge of pus from the ear canal, and, very often, fever. Other indications include swelling and tenderness of the mastoid bone.

Complications

In severe cases, an abscess may develop in the mastoid bone. This is a serious complication because it carries the risk of spreading to the interior of the skull and infecting the meninges, membranes that cover the brain. This is called meningitis.

Treatment

Since antibiotics are so effective against ear infections and

A mastoid infection is an infection of the air cells—air-filled cavities—in the mastoid bone, which is the protrusion of the skull immediately behind the ear.

mastoid infections, mastoiditis is fortunately now rare. Sometimes, however, surgery is required to remove the infected cells if antibiotic treatment is started too late or is not effective.

Meniere's disease

Meniere's disease is the result of an increase in pressure in the inner ear because of a buildup of fluid in the labyrinth—the part of the inner ear that controls body balance and equilibrium. This buildup of pressure distorts and sometimes ruptures the lining of the labyrinth wall.

Causes

Meniere's disease is an uncommon disease, and its cause is unknown. However, it is thought that the pressure changes may be brought on by an infection, a small hemorrhage in the ear, or an allergic response. It occurs most commonly in men aged 40 to 60.

Symptoms

Symptoms of Meniere's disease include recurring and violent attacks of vertigo or dizziness, ringing in the ears, muffled or distorted noises, and nausea that is sometimes accompanied by vomiting. Deafness in one or both ears may eventually develop.

Mild attacks of Meniere's disease may last from a half hour to several days before fading away naturally. They may recur regularly at intervals of weeks, months, or years. Severe attacks may last for several weeks, requiring the person to be confined to bed. In such cases, almost any movement of the head will result in bizarre and disturbing sensations that the floor and the furniture in the room are spinning around. Severe cases may also be accompanied by anxiety attacks and migraine headaches.

Treatment

The use of certain drugs such as diuretics and antihistamines may help to relieve severe and recurrent attacks. In severe cases, surgical destruction of certain nerves in the ear may be necessary.

Nosebleeds

A nosebleed occurs when there is a break in the blood vessels in the inner lining of the nose, causing bleeding from the nose. Nosebleeds seldom require medical attention, but it is possible, although relatively rare, for nosebleeds to be symptoms of serious illnesses.

Causes

Nosebleeds can be caused by an injury to the nose; breathing dry air for long periods; repeated blowing or picking of the nose; tumors in the nose; or high blood pressure or other blood diseases.

Treatment

Very persistent or frequently occurring nosebleeds will require the attention of a doctor who may

cauterize (use heat or the application of the chemical silver nitrate to seal off) the blood vessels in the back of the nose.

However, occasional nosebleeds can be treated by simply sitting up and leaning forward, so as not to swallow the blood, and pinching the entire soft portion of the nose between the thumb and forefinger for ten minutes. If the bleeding does not stop, cold packs can be applied to the bridge of the nose for 15 to 20 minutes. If bleeding still persists, a doctor should be notified.

Frequent nosebleeds from dry air may be relieved by the use of a humidifier. Also, those who have frequent nosebleeds should not blow the nose too harshly nor blow through one nostril.

When nosebleeds occur along with colds or other respiratory infections, a nasal decongestant may help to shrink the blood vessels in the nose. However, these decongestants should not be used by anyone with high blood pressure, heart disease, diabetes, or thyroid disorders, because decongestants also shrink blood vessels in parts of the body other than the nose, which can lead to complications for these patients.

Sinusitis

Sinusitis is an infection of one or more of the sinuses, usually caused by bacteria and more commonly occurring in adults than in children.

The sinuses are air-filled cavities within the facial bone structure, connected to the nose, and lined with mucous mem-

The sinuses are air-filled cavities within the facial bone structure that are connected to the nasal passages. The four major groups are the frontal, ethmoidal, sphenoidal, and maxillary. The sphenoidal sinuses are located behind the ethmoidal.

brane. There are four major groups of sinuses: frontal, ethmoidal, sphenoidal, and maxillary sinuses.

Sinuses are normally kept clear and free when mucus drains through them into the nasal passages. If they are obstructed for any reason, such as from the congestion present during a cold, they are not able to drain properly, and infection of the sinuses can result.

Complications

It is rare but possible for long-lasting sinusitis to lead to more serious disorders. A persistent infection may travel to the brain, causing meningitis (inflammation of the membranes surrounding the brain), or to the bone, resulting in osteomyelitis.

Causes

A sinus infection can be triggered by anything that prevents the mucus in the sinuses from draining properly into the nasal passages. Possible causes can include swimming and diving, injuries, abnormal structures in the facial bones, congestion from flu or colds, allergies such as hay fever, even an abscess (inflamed pocket of pus) in a tooth, which may penetrate the sinuses and allow bacteria to enter them. Many different bacteria can cause sinusitis, including some of the same strains that lead to pneumonia, laryngitis, and middle ear infections.

Symptoms

Sinusitis is characterized by pain and tenderness above the infected sinus, felt in the face, forehead, behind the eyes, in the eyes, near the upper part of the nose, even in the upper teeth (but not in a single tooth). This facial pain may be accompanied by headache, slight fever, chills, sore throat, nasal obstruction, and a pus discharge from the nose.

Sinusitis usually lasts about two weeks, with the pain often subsiding in the morning and worsening as the day goes on, or fluctuating as the patient moves about and changes positions.

Diagnosis

Sinuses cannot be seen directly by a doctor, so diagnosis may include X rays to check for fluid present or abnormalities in the sinuses and to identify exactly which sinuses are infected. To identify the bacteria the doctor may need to perform a sinus puncture, in which a needle is inserted into the sinus through the upper jaw above the molar teeth and a sample of the bacteria is removed from the sinuses. This procedure may be necessary because the nasal discharge may contain different bacteria from those in the sinuses.

Treatment

Sinusitis is treated by draining the sinuses and thereby removing the bacteria that are causing the infection. Nasal decongestants, hot compresses, and dry heat all work to aid sinus drainage. An antibiotic is usually prescribed that will kill one of the two most common bacteria that trigger sinusitis.

If these treatments bring no relief, the doctor may perform a sinus puncture to determine exactly which bacteria are present, then prescribe another antibiotic. In severe cases, codeine may be prescribed to dull the pain, and the doctor may clear the sinuses by injecting a salt water solution through the nose to flush out the bacteria.

In very rare cases, surgery may be necessary to remove a nasal polyp (a mass of swollen tissue), repair abnormal bone structures, or remove infected sinus tissue.

Prevention

There is some evidence that smokers are more likely to suffer from sinusitis than are nonsmokers. In addition, those who frequently have colds are more susceptible to sinusitis. Precautions may be taken along these lines to prevent sinus infections by avoiding smoking and colds.

Tonsillitis

Tonsillitis is an infection and often enlargement of the tonsils, occurring most commonly in children ages five to 15 years, and rarely in those under the age of two.

The tonsils are two small, almond-shaped lumps of tissue located in the throat at the back of the mouth. They are barely visible in infants, increase in size during the preschool and early school years, and shrink by adulthood.

The function of the tonsils has not been exactly pinpointed, but scientists believe that they perform at least two vital jobs: they release an antibody, or protective agent, into the throat to prevent infection from spreading into the lungs (a useful service to children, who are highly susceptible to ear, nose, and throat infections); and they attract bacterial infection and thereby stimulate the production of antibodies, which accumulate in the body in order to prevent future, and much more serious, infections. Antibodies normally do not develop unless infection is present.

If the tonsils do indeed perform these two functions, then each attack of tonsillitis may help immunize a child from disease, and once this resistance is developed, the function of the tonsils is complete.

There are two types of tonsillitis: acute tonsillitis, in which the infection flares up, then disappears in a short time; and chronic tonsillitis, in which the tonsils seem to be permanently engorged and have abscesses (pus-filled cavities) on them.

Complications

Complications resulting from tonsillitis seldom occur today because of effective and fast-acting antibiotics, but rare cases of rheumatic fever (a disease affecting the heart valves) and infections of the sinuses, ears, or kidneys are possible.

Causes

Tonsillitis is caused by many different infectious agents, both viral and bacterial, the most common bacteria being streptococcus bacteria. Acute tonsillitis is usually a "strep" infection. Chronic tonsillitis, however, is more of a mystery; it is not known why chronic tonsillitis occurs in certain people or what causes it.

Symptoms

The symptoms of acute tonsillitis are a sore throat, fever up to about 101°F, chills, headache, and muscle aches. These symptoms worsen for one to three days, then subside. In addition, nausea, vomiting, stomachache, and swelling of glands located in the neck may also occur and may last for about a week.

The symptoms of chronic tonsillitis include a persistent or recurrent sore throat, difficulty in swallowing or breathing, and foul breath.

Diagnosis

Tonsillitis is diagnosed by an examination of the tonsils, to check for redness, swelling, and a gray or yellow infectious material deposited on them. The doctor will take a sample of this material with a cotton swab in order to identify the bacteria causing the infection.

Treatment

Bed rest or reduced activity and the use of antibiotics, often penicillin, are recommended to treat tonsillitis if the inflammation is due to bacteria. Gargling with warm salt water can help relieve sore throat.

Surgical removal of the tonsils (called a tonsillectomy) is performed only if the tonsils are abscessed (filled with pus) or greatly enlarged, thus blocking the air passages. Tonsillectomies are seldom performed today, because research has found that even when tonsils are enlarged, they almost always shrink over time. Furthermore, removing the tonsils does not necessarily prevent recurrent sore throats or colds, as was once believed.

Prevention

Since it is not known why some people suffer from chronic tonsillitis, preventive measures are also uncertain. Because episodes of acute tonsillitis may help build up immunities in the body, prevention of such episodes may not be of vital importance until more research is completed in this area.

THE LUNGS AND RESPIRATORY SYSTEM

The respiratory system includes the nose, the throat, the larynx, the trachea, the bronchi, and the lungs. Breathing is the process by which air flows through these structures to the lungs and by which waste gases exit from the body. The respiratory system's function is to supply the blood with necessary oxygen and relieve the blood of the waste product carbon dioxide. This exchange of oxygen and carbon dioxide occurs in the lungs. Air from the outside enters through the nose where it is warmed, moistened, and filtered before it passes through the throat into the trachea (windpipe). The trachea divides into two bronchi, passageways leading into each lung. Within each lung the bronchi divide and subdivide until the smallest bronchial tubes end in small cup-shaped sacs called alveoli. It is in the alveoli that the oxygen/carbon dioxide exchange takes place. Each alveolus is served by numerous tiny blood vessels called capillaries. Oxygen in the alveolus crosses the alveolar and capillary walls to enter the blood while carbon dioxide passes from the blood through the capillary wall into the alveolus. The oxygen is then carried by the blood to the body's cells and the carbon dioxide is released by the alveolus into the outside environment on exhalation.

During inhalation and exhalation the lungs expand and contract. However, they have no muscle tissue and are expanded and contracted by the ribs and the diaphragm, the large muscle separating the chest and abdominal cavities. During inhalation the diaphragm contracts which causes it to descend and the chest cavity to expand. At this point the air pressure inside the chest cavity is less than that of the air outside the body; consequently, air from the outside rushes into the lungs. During exhalation, the diaphragm relaxes and moves up, reducing the chest capacity and pushing air out of the lungs.

The friction caused by expansion and contraction of the lungs is eased by the pleura, a thin, moist membrane that covers the lungs and lines the chest cavity. The pleura permits the surfaces of the lungs and chest cavity to slide and glide past each other as the lungs expand and contract.

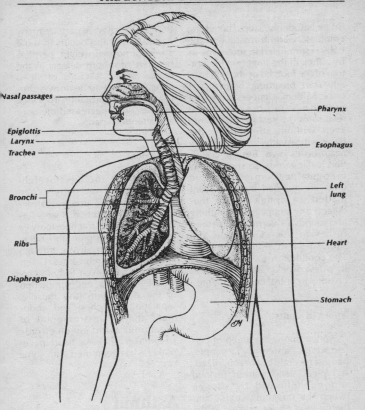

The respiratory system's function in the body is to supply oxygen and to remove carbon dioxide.

Apnea

Apnea is an interruption in breathing that occurs in some very premature babies and also during the sleep of some adults. The usual cause in infants is immaturity of the brain centers that regulate breathing. In adults, most often the cause is obstruction of the upper airway; the second most common cause is malfunction of the breathing control centers of the brain.

Apnea in infants

Apnea in a tiny baby appears frightening. From time to time, the infant suddenly stops breathing completely and turns blue. If the baby is stimulated in some way, as by a flick of the finger on the bottom of the foot, he or she will usually start breathing normally at once. Seldom is it necessary to use first-aid measures or a mechanical respirator to restart breathing. Even without stimulation, the baby will usually start to breathe again on its own. But the condition is dangerous, so such babies in hospital newborn intensive care units are guarded by equipment (called an apnea alarm) that detects any stoppage of breathing and sounds an alarm. A nurse then rushes to the baby's side and stimulates it to resume breathing. The condition usually disappears in a few weeks after the baby's breathing control centers mature.

Apnea in adults

Apnea during the sleep of certain adults, particularly fat people, has just recently been recognized. A typical sleep pattern is loud snoring, followed by silence (when the breathing stops), and then a loud choke or gasp as the sleeper partially wakes, clears the air passage, and resumes breathing. This may occur many times within an hour for a number of hours during the night. In some sleep-apnea patients such as those with severe emphysema, during the apnea, carbon dioxide in the blood builds up, occasionally to a dangerous level. The reason for the closure of the airway is not fully known, but obesity is thought to play a part in many cases. Apnea also occurs in some adults of normal weight, perhaps because of inborn defects in the upper airway. Victims of sleep apnea are likely to be drowsy during the day and irritable, from lack of sleep, with decreased memory and attention span.

Treatment

Treatment includes weight reduction for fat patients. In extreme cases of airway obstruction, the only solution is for a surgeon to create a tracheostomy—a hole in the windpipe and neck, below the upper airway, through which the patient breathes. Drugs are sometimes given to help correct sleep apnea, and stimulation of the diaphragm (the muscle, separating the chest and abdomen, that is instrumental in breathing) with an electronic pacemaker — like a heart pacemaker—has been tried with some success.

Asthma

Asthma is a respiratory disease characterized by unpredictable periods of acute breathlessness and wheezing. Asthma attacks can last from less than an hour to a week or more and can strike frequently or only every few years. Attacks may be mild or severe and can occur sporadically, at any time, even during sleep.

The difficult breathing occurs when the small respiratory tubes

Trachea (windpipe)

Excessive mucus production

Constriction of bronchiole

Swollen membrane

Right lung

Blocked airway

Alveoli (air sacs)

The difficult breathing characteristic of asthma occurs when the small respiratory tubes (bronchioles) constrict or become clogged with mucus, or when the membranes lining the tubes become swollen. Stale air is trapped in the air sacs and less fresh air can be inhaled.

(called bronchioles) constrict or become clogged with mucus, or when the membranes lining the tubes become swollen. When this happens, stale air cannot be fully exhaled but stays trapped in the lungs, and so less fresh air can be inhaled.

Causes

Asthma attacks can result from the bronchial system's oversensitivity to a variety of outside substances or environmental conditions. About one half of all attacks are triggered by allergies to such substances as dust, smoke, pollen, feathers, pet hair, insects, mold spores, and a variety of foods and medications. Attacks not related to allergies can be set off by environmental conditions such as ear, nose, or throat infections, strenuous exercise, breathing cold air, or even emotional stress. Heredity may play a part in the tendency to develop asthma; children with one or both asthmatic parents have a 50 percent chance of developing the condition.

Asthma is rarely fatal, but it can be a very serious condition, especially in young children. Nevertheless, attacks often become less frequent and less severe as children grow up.

Symptoms

Common symptoms of an asthma attack include tightness in the chest, difficult breathing, coughing, and the characteristic wheezing that is caused by the effort to push the flow of air through the narrowed bronchioles. As the attack progresses, muscles surrounding the bronchioles constrict further, breathing becomes even more difficult, and mucus collects.

Diagnosis

Diagnostic procedures may include a complete medical history, physical examination, chest X ray, and allergy and skin scratch tests.

Treatment

Asthma cannot be cured, but it can be controlled with a variety of drugs. An epinephrine (adrenaline) injection or an adrenaline aerosol may be administered during an acute attack in order to enlarge the bronchioles; however, these drugs may overstimulate the heart and so cannot be used for long periods of time (they, therefore, are usually used only in an emergency). Adrenaline-like drugs, taken orally, can be administered for longer periods because they lack this stimulating effect on the heart since they affect only the muscles of the airways. However, these drugs are usually recommended to be taken for only a few days after an attack, because constant use may result in the body's building a tolerance to the drugs, thus making the next attack more difficult to treat.

For long-term therapy, the drug theophylline can be used to keep the bronchioles constantly cleared. Its prescribed dosage, however, must be closely supervised because its rate of absorption into the body can vary widely among patients; some persons eliminate the drug so quickly it is almost ineffective while in others the drug accumulates in the body at times to toxic levels. Also, nausea, vomiting, and agitation are common side effects.

Corticosteroids can control asthma, but patients may become dependent on them and they may have such undesirable side effects as weight gain, ulcers, high blood pressure — even a stunting of growth in children.

Cromolyn, a drug that actually prevents attacks, acts to inhibit the release of histamines, the chemicals manufactured by the body during an allergy reaction. Cromolyn, however, cannot relieve an attack already in progress and is usually only for mild cases.

Regardless of which drug is prescribed, all asthmatic patients should drink plenty of water to keep the bronchial tubes moistened and to replace fluids which may be depleted by the use of drugs.

If an allergy is causing the attacks, the troublesome foreign substance (called an allergen) must be removed. If this cannot be accomplished, allergy shots to reduce the patient's sensitivity to the allergen may be beneficial. The use of antihistamines may also bring some relief.

Prevention

Several precautions can be taken to reduce the possibility of an asthma condition developing. Since the tendency to develop asthma is inherited, babies of asthmatic parents should be fed breast milk or soy protein formula, since these are less likely than cow's milk to cause allergic reactions. Smoke and pet hair, as well as rugs, drapes, and overstuffed furniture, which tend to attract dust, can be removed from the home. Moderate exercise is a good preventive method, although strenuous exercise may cause an attack.

One additional note: asthmatics who also suffer from angina or heart problems should take beta blocker drugs only with extreme caution, as these drugs may cause spasms in the airways.

Bronchiectasis

Bronchiectasis is a lung condition in which some of the small and medium-sized bronchi (air tubes) have lost their elasticity and have expanded and filled with fluid.

Causes

Most often, bronchiectasis follows pneumonia, whooping cough, tuberculosis, or other lung disease or is the result of an obstruction. (Fortunately, the use of antibiotics has reduced the number of cases.) Other causes include the hereditary disease cystic fibrosis, with its thick secretions of mucus; a rare inherited condition in which the little air sacs at the end of the bronchi are not developed completely; and a condition in which the cilia do not work properly (the cilia are hair-like projections that line the bronchial walls and wave mucus, pus, and dirt upward).

Symptoms

Bronchiectasis is a chronic condition that persists for life. The individual almost always has some symptoms that will at times worsen if an acute infection occurs. The most typical symptom is a chronic cough, producing a thick white or green sputum (discharge). In older cases the sputum may be foul-smelling and abundant and may settle into three layers if placed in a cup: a thick film of pus on the bottom, green or brownish fluid in the middle, and froth on top. It may also contain blood. The individual generally coughs up large amounts of sputum after changing position, for example, after rising from bed.

Diagnosis

The doctor, listening to the chest with a stethoscope, can hear abnormal sounds inside the lungs as the patient breathes. An X ray, made with the use of dye injected into the bloodstream or directly into the bronchi, will show up the characteristic appearance of the disease. Chronic bronchitis (continued inflammation of the mucous membrane in the bronchi) must be ruled out as a cause, along with tuberculosis, certain fungus infections, cancer or other tumor, and objects that the patient may have inhaled that are lodged in the bronchi.

Treatment

Treatment of an active case of bronchiectasis includes fighting the infection with antibiotics, such as penicillin or tetracycline, and eliminating the fluid with postural drainage. In this procedure, the patient lies face down in bed with pillows elevating the hips as a therapist strikes the back over the chest area with cupped hands to loosen mucus. The treatment, which can be taught to a family member, requires two to four 10-minute sessions a day. Inhaling warm mists may also help to loosen sticky fluids in the lungs. The patient should avoid anything that can irritate the lungs, such as smoke (especially cigarette smoke), fumes, and dust.

Most attacks of bronchiectasis can be handled well with the above methods. However, in a few cases in which the infection is progressing despite antibiotics and is confined to a small part of the lung, it may be best to remove the portion of the lung that contains the bronchiectasis with surgery.

Prevention

You can prevent repeated attacks by being immunized against flu and pneumonia, avoiding anyone with a cold or cough, and stopping smoking. Prompt treatment with antibiotics can help to control new infections.

Bronchitis

Bronchitis is a respiratory disease characterized by an inflammation and swelling of the main breathing tubes (called the bronchi) that connect the windpipe and lungs. When these tubes develop inflammation in their inner linings or mucous membranes, the mucous glands located in the membranes will expand and release more mucus. The bronchi, already narrowed by the swelling, become further clogged with the excess mucus. This mucus must then be coughed up in order to keep the breathing tubes free for normal air flow into the lungs.

When the excess mucus is produced and coughed up, the patient has what is known as a productive cough. A short period of productive coughing is called acute bronchitis; when the coughing lingers for six months, or when it occurs for three months a year and for two years in a row, it is called chronic bronchitis. In either case, the coughing stops only when the source of inflammation has been removed or overcome and the inner linings of the bronchi have returned to normal.

Complications

Bronchitis alone can be fatal, but more likely it will lead to another condition that proves to be fatal. For example, in some severe long-standing cases, bronchitis-damaged lungs can deprive the heart of adequate oxygen, resulting in death from heart failure. Also, bronchitis can be very serious when combined with other respiratory diseases. Such is the case for people who suffer from a category of respiratory conditions called chronic obstructive pulmonary disease (COPD). Bronchitis, emphysema, and several other diseases are included in this category, and patients may suffer from two or three of the COPD conditions, or one may lead to another.

Causes

Bronchitis occurs when the bronchial tubes are infected or irritated. A cold, flu, or strep throat may lead to acute bronchitis, or even chronic bronchitis, if these infections occur often enough. However, chronic bronchitis is more commonly triggered by the constant irritation of environmental substances such as cigarette smoke, air pollutants, or occupational dusts.

Cigarette smoking is the predominant cause of chronic bronchitis. Seventy-five percent of all those who suffer from bronchitis are cigarette smokers. When tobacco smoke reaches the bronchial linings, it stops the action of the cilia, the hair-like projections whose job it is to sweep mucus out of the lungs, mucus that normally carries with it dust and bacteria. Once the cilia are stilled by smoke, these irritating particles remain trapped in the stagnant mucus, aggravating the delicate bronchial tubes and eventually creating a breeding ground for infection.

Some degree of bronchitis occurs in about 90 percent of all smokers who live in polluted environments or who are exposed to occupational dusts. Babies and young children with chronic bronchitis usually overcome the condition, but are more likely to contract it later in life. People who are undernourished, inadequately housed, or often fatigued are more likely to contract bronchitis. Also, this disorder tends to occur within certain families, but the reason is not yet known.

Symptoms

Bronchitis can be recognized by its major symptom, the persistent cough that brings up the lung's excess mucus. Acute bronchitis may be accompanied by hoarseness, chest discomfort, slight fever, wheezing, and shortness of breath. In children, the productive cough may establish itself after several short-term infections and chronic bronchitis will set in. In adults, the beginnings of chronic bronchitis can be recognized by regular coughing and clearing of the throat the first thing each morning; the coughing will become more persistent and the mucus more plentiful as the disease progresses, and these symptoms may be accompanied by wheezing, shortness of breath, chest infections, and heavy panting after exercise.

As the years pass, chronic bronchitis may cause the bronchial tubes to become severely obstructed and the breathing irreversibly impaired. The heart will pump harder to get its needed oxygen and sometimes become enlarged. Nails, lips, and skin may even develop a blue tinge from lack of oxygen.

Diagnosis

To diagnose bronchitis, the doctor will take a medical history, physical examination of the chest with a stethoscope, and perhaps a chest X ray. Special machines can measure the amount of air flowing in and out of the lungs, and others can measure how well oxygen is being transported from the lungs to the bloodstream.

Treatment

Bronchitis is treated by removing the troublesome outside irritants, clearing the lungs of mucus, and trying to prevent infections. A chronic bronchitis patient will need to quit smoking and to avoid constant exposure to pollutants or hazardous dusts. Humidity plays a large part in treating bronchitis; patients should drink plenty of water and hot liquids, breathe warmed and humidified air from a vaporizer or humidifier, or even inhale steam from hot water or hot liquids, like chicken soup, a popular home remedy. Humid air and steam will act to loosen trapped mucus in the lungs.

A drug that relaxes the air passages, called a bronchodilator, may be prescribed, to be used along with the humidity treatments. Also, mucus may be more easily loosened and the bronchial tubes drained when the head is lower than the chest, so lying on a bed with the head hanging off the edge may bring some relief.

Prevention

Bronchitis can best be prevented by avoiding the irritants that cause it, namely cigarette smoke, air pollutants, and dusts. Chronic bronchitis patients can prevent further irritation by maintaining good health and eating habits to avoid infections. Antibiotics, flu shots, and pneumonia inoculations can help to prevent infection.

Dyspnea

Dyspnea is a sensation of "air hunger." It is usually accompanied by difficult, labored breathing and discomfort. Dyspnea is a symptom that may occur in a variety of different diseases and conditions.

Causes

Dyspnea may be caused by lack of oxygen being delivered to the tissues, as in severe anemia; by failure of the heart to keep up with the needs of the body, as in heart failure; as well as by extreme exercise. It may also be the result of obstruction of the airways, such as the narrowing of air passages that occurs in asthma, or by restricted capacity of the lungs, as in chest deformities. Emphysema (in which many of the lung's small air sacs have been weakened or destroyed) is also commonly associated with dyspnea. It can also occur because of fluid in the lungs, as in pneumonia or congestive heart failure. Here, the access of oxygen into the air exchange units of the lungs (alveoli) is blocked by the fluid, thereby preventing oxygenation of the blood.

Types of dyspnea

A nighttime form of dyspnea is called paroxysmal nocturnal dyspnea, in which the patient awakens gasping for breath and can only breathe by sitting up or standing. Usually this is caused by congestive heart failure.

Another type of dyspnea is psychogenic (originating in the mind) or hysterical hyperventilation (excessive breathing), caused by anxiety. This excessive breathing leads to exhaling too much carbon dioxide, which makes the blood too alkaline. This produces light-headedness, numbness and tingling of the hands and toes, and sometimes fainting. (Breathing into a paper bag restores the carbon dioxide balance.)

Symptoms

Signs of dyspnea include noisy breathing; an anxious, distressed expression; dilated nostrils; gasping; protruding abdomen; expanded chest; and blue lips and fingertips.

Treatment

Treatment involves treating the condition causing the dyspnea, including the anxiety responsible for psychogenic hyperventilation.

Emphysema

Emphysema is a chronic, progressive lung disease. Emphysema

develops when the small air passages leading to the air sacs (alveoli) in the lungs become distended and the walls dividing the sacs themselves are injured or destroyed. Spaces form where alveoli had been, and lung tissue becomes nonfunctional. Emphysema is commonly associated with chronic bronchitis, which is a condition in which the airways become inflamed, causing specialized cells within them to secrete a great deal of mucus. The inflammation and swelling, along with mucus plugging, result in a great deal of obstruction to air flow and cause air to become trapped.

Effect on the body

As the disease progresses, many complex changes take place, ultimately leading to a diminished amount of oxygen in the blood, frequently associated with an increased amount of carbon dioxide. Also, as the lung tissue deteriorates and loses its elasticity, changes also occur in the blood vessels carrying deoxygenated blood to the lungs for a fresh supply of oxygen. The net effect of all of this is that the right side of the heart, which is responsible for collecting deoxygenated blood from the veins of the body and pumping it through the lungs, must now work much harder. As the process continues, the right heart muscle is weakened by this extra work and becomes less able to pump blood into the lungs. The blood "backs up" causing

increased back pressure in the veins. This, in turn, causes the exodus of fluid into the tissues, and the result is severe swelling of the feet, ankles, and legs. If this right-sided heart failure (also known as cor pulmonale) is very severe, distention of the abdomen with fluid will also occur.

Causes

External factors that irritate the lungs, such as tobacco smoke and air pollutants, are commonly linked to emphysema, but no one single cause has been determined. Emphysema does not stem from viruses or bacteria, as do some respiratory diseases. However, it is often aggravated by a case of bronchitis (an inflammation of the bronchial passages) or any lung infection.

In a minority of cases, emphysema may result from a genetic deficiency or an inherited lack of a blood protein that may lead to loss of elasticity in the lung's air sacs.

Those afflicted with emphysema are usually white males over the age of 50, although females are becoming equally susceptible because of increased smoking among women during recent years.

Symptoms

Emphysema is characterized by one major symptom: shortness of breath. Patients may also have a persistent, racking cough, which

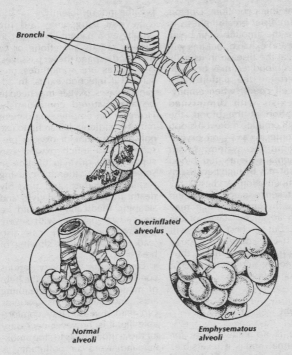

Normal
alveoli

Overinflated
alveolus

Emphysematous
alveoli

Emphysema is a chronic disease in which the tiny air sacs (alveoli) of the lungs become overinflated with trapped air.

either brings up mucus or is overly dry. Patients experience difficulty in breathing, often taking twice as many breaths as others to get enough oxygen. It has been found that advanced emphysema sufferers exert tremendous amounts of energy just to breathe. They also tire quite easily and require more calories to maintain their weight than does a normal individual. Many patients may develop an enlarged, rounded "barrel" chest from over-inflated lungs and over-developed chest muscles used in breathing. Lips, ear lobes, skin, and fingernails may become tinged blue from lack of oxygen in the blood.

Diagnosis

Emphysema is usually diagnosed by several procedures, since no one single test exists to pinpoint the condition. Doctors may administer breathing tests to measure the amount of air being inhaled and exhaled, but this will not reveal the disease in its early stages. A blood test may be given to determine the patient's red blood cell count; when emphysema exists with diminished oxygenation of the blood, the body will produce more red blood cells in order to carry more oxygen throughout the system, so an emphysema patient's red blood cell count may be high because of this compensation. A chest X ray may be taken to search for specific changes in the lungs that may point to advanced stages of the disease, but a chest X ray will not actually diagnose early emphysema. Emphysema is thus diagnosed by putting together a collection of findings.

Treatment

There is no known cure for emphysema, nor is it reversible. However, the progress of the disease can be checked by removing irritants, particularly cigarette smoke. Patients are encouraged to drink large amounts of fluids to help thin out the mucus that is blocking the airways. Adequate rest, a balanced diet, and moderate regular exercise are recommended. Vaporizers, humidifiers, and air conditioners help to moisturize and filter the air. Patients can learn to use their chest and abdominal muscles (with the help of a therapist) to breathe more efficiently.

Several drugs may aid the emphysema patient. They act to loosen mucus secretions or to relax and expand the air passages. Antibiotics are sometimes prescribed if infection exists. In advanced cases, oxygen may need to be administered continuously. However, an emphysema patient must be particularly careful to use only the amount of oxygen prescribed. Too much oxygen can suppress the drive to breathe in some patients, thereby causing respiratory failure and possibly death. In addition, sedatives and sleeping medications should be avoided by patients with severe emphysema as these can also lead to a dangerous slowing of breathing.

Emphysema is a very serious condition. However, with the help of modern treatments, breathing aids, and medications, patients can lead a reasonably comfortable life. It is, however, necessary for these individuals to stop smoking and avoid air pollutants as much as possible.

Pleurisy

The term pleurisy is another name for pleuritis and refers to any inflammation of the pleura, the membrane that covers the outside of the lungs and lines the chest cavity. It is a complication that generally develops from other upper respiratory tract infections such as pneumonia or tuberculosis.

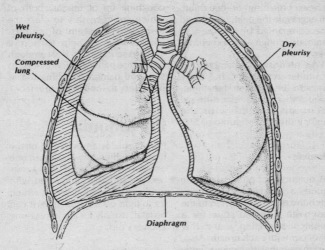

Pleurisy is an inflammation of the pleura, the membrane covering the lungs and lining the chest cavity. A simple inflammation is called dry pleurisy; if fluid is produced by the inflamed pleura, the condition is called wet pleurisy. This fluid may compress the lung.

Types

There are two types of pleurisy: dry pleurisy, the more common inflammation; and wet pleurisy, a similar condition except that fluid oozes from the inflamed tissue into the space between the lungs and the chest wall. Compression of the lungs by this fluid may occur, making breathing difficult.

Dry pleurisy is caused by an infection already in the lungs, often viral or bacterial pneumonia or acute bronchitis (inflammation of the air passages). It can arise as a complication of tuberculosis or because of a tumor. Wet pleurisy can also develop from an infection, tuberculosis, or a tumor, as well as from an injury or a liver disease. Certain liver diseases can inflame the diaphragm (the muscle separating the organs from the chest region from those of the abdomen) and also the part of the pleura that covers the diaphragm. People highly susceptible to respiratory infections are more likely to develop pleurisy.

Symptoms

The major symptom of dry pleurisy is a sharp, stabbing pain toward the side and lower part of the chest. The pain also may be felt along the shoulders, neck, and abdomen. Any action in the chest, such as breathing or coughing, will aggravate the pain, which will be accompanied by shortness of breath, dry cough, and sometimes fever.

Wet pleurisy is characterized by similar symptoms, but there may also be difficult breathing, chills, and often a blood-tinged mucus discharged with the cough, indicating pneumonia.

Diagnosis

A diagnosis of pleurisy usually requires a physical exam during which the doctor will listen to the chest with a stethoscope for a low-pitched, grating sound that will occur with each breath. Also, the skin near the affected area may be tender. Wet pleurisy also calls for an analysis of the fluid that is oozing from the pleura. A tuberculin skin test may be taken to rule out tuberculosis, and an X ray may be ordered if the pleurisy does not seem to be caused by another respiratory infection.

Treatment

To treat pleurisy, the doctor will first need to treat the underlying infection or disease that has triggered it, often with antibiotics. The symptoms of pleurisy can be relieved somewhat by bed rest, by use of a humidifier or vaporizer to add moisture to the air, or by strapping the chest with a tight binder. The latter is not always recommended, however, as it may prevent deep breathing and coughing up of mucus, both of which are necessary to clear the respiratory system of mucus. Painkillers may help to relieve chest discomfort at least enough so that the patient will not need to stifle the painful coughing that is necessary to loosen the mucus.

Pneumonia

Pneumonia is an infection of the lungs in which tiny air sacs in one or more sections of the lungs become inflamed and filled with fluid and white blood cells, which try to fight off the infection. It can be fatal, usually for the very young and very old.

Types

There are several types of pneumonia, distinguished by the part of the lung that is infected. Lobar pneumonia is an infection in only one section, or lobe, of the lungs. Double pneumonia is an infection in a lobe or lobes of both lungs. Bronchial pneumonia, a complication of acute bronchitis, is the term used to describe an infection in the section of the lungs near the bronchi (the airways connecting the windpipe and lungs). Walking pneumonia is a general term people often use to describe the condition of someone who has pneumonia but is not aware of it and has not sought treatment.

Pneumonia most often strikes the person whose resistance is lowered, often by another upper respiratory tract infection or a systemic (bodywide) disease. It is often a secondary disease stemming from inadequate defense mechanisms, from cold or flu, or from long-term diseases, such as chronic bronchitis, emphysema, asthma, diabetes, cancer, or sickle-cell anemia.

Causes

Viruses, bacteria, fungi, or other microorganisms may cause pneumonia. Also, it may develop if a person inhales certain chemicals or if food, vomit, or a foreign object passes through the trachea (the windpipe) instead of the esophagus (the passageway from the mouth to the stomach) and settles in a lung. Smoking, excessive drinking, a prolonged period in bed, anesthesia, sedatives, and immune-suppressing drugs may make an individual more likely to develop pneumonia if exposed to an infectious organism. Pneumonia is most common during flu and cold epidemics and during the winter months when people are indoors where bacteria and viruses are easily spread.

Symptoms

All types of pneumonia are characterized by four major symptoms: chest pain, a sudden rise in temperature, coughing, and difficult breathing. Viral pneumonia, more common and generally less serious than other varieties, is recognized by coughing and other cold symptoms, as well as by general fatigue. Also, fever, chest pain, and difficult breathing may signal the presence of this disorder. Bacterial pneumonia generally comes on suddenly with shaking chills and a rapid, steep rise in temperature; shallow breathing; and a cough that brings up a bloody, dark yellow, or rust-colored sputum. An oxygen shortage that sometimes accompanies bacterial pneumonia will be indicated by other symptoms such as headache; nausea; vomiting; and cyanosis, a blue discoloration of the lips and fingertips.

Diagnosis

Pneumonia is diagnosed by listening to the chest with a stethoscope in order to detect the presence of fluid in the lungs; X rays and an analysis of the discharge that is coughed up may also help to identify pneumonia.

Treatment

Viral pneumonia is usually treated with commonsense remedies: staying in bed; drinking lots of fluids; maintaining a light diet; and using pain relievers to combat discomfort and, sometimes, oxygen to ease breathing difficulties.

The more serious bacterial pneumonia, however, requires antibiotics such as penicillin. Patients also need to stay in bed, or, if the case is serious enough, enter the hospital for care and supervision. If breathing difficulty worsens, oxygen may be administered.

Prevention

There are vaccines that may help in preventing some types of pneumonia. Bacterial pneumonia caused by certain bacteria can possibly be prevented with a vaccine and it is especially recommended for the elderly or for those with chronic diseases that may weaken the respiratory system. Viral pneumonia caused by certain flu viruses may be prevented with a vaccination against influenza A, a virus which often leads to pneumonia.

The very young, the very old, and the chronically ill are the most likely to contract pneumonia, so care must be taken to protect those who fall into these categories from respiratory infections.

Psittacosis

Psittacosis (parrot fever or ornithosis) is a rare form of pneumonia caused by bacteria that are transmitted to humans by certain birds. The disease was first observed in parrots and later in other birds and domestic fowl. It is often accompanied by fever, coughing, and enlargement of the spleen.

Causes

Psittacosis is found principally in such birds as parrots, parakeets, lovebirds, and less often in poultry, pigeons, and canaries (in which the disease is often called ornithosis). Human infection usually takes place when a person inhales dust from feathers or excrement of infected birds. It can also be transmitted directly to a person by a bite from an infected bird or, rarely, by cough droplets of infected persons. Person-to-person transmission is rare.

Symptoms

After a one- to two-week incubation period (the time between exposure to the illness and the appearance of symptoms), the disease usually begins with fever, chills, headache, muscle aches, and loss of appetite. The patient's temperature continues to rise and a dry cough develops that brings up mucus and pus in the later stages. Chest X rays made during the first week of noticeable symptoms will show inflammation of the lungs. During the second week, the typical symptoms of pneumonia develop. The patient's temperature will remain above normal for at least two to three weeks and then slowly will begin to fall. A steady increase in pulse and respiratory (breathing) rates may be potentially serious. About 30 percent of untreated cases end in death. Recovery in those people who receive treatment may be gradual.

Treatment

The most common drug to treat psittacosis is tetracycline, an oral antibiotic. Strict bed rest is necessary in most cases. Cough preparations with codeine are also advised. In severe cases, tetracycline may be given intravenously (through the vein).

Prevention

Infected flocks of pigeons or other birds, dust from feathers, bird cage contents, and any sick domestic birds or fowl should be avoided. Specially treated feed is often used to prevent the spread of infection among imported parrots, parakeets, and lovebirds, as well as among turkeys raised for market.

Tuberculosis

Tuberculosis is an infection that causes small nodules called tubercles to break down healthy tissue and form pus. Tuberculosis usually affects the lungs, but it can travel to other parts of the body, such as the spine, kidneys, digestive tract, and lining of the heart. It also may be complicated by a streptococcal (a type of bacteria) infection.

Inactive tuberculosis

Eighty percent of all people who contract tuberculosis will never experience its symptoms. This happens because the tuberculosis bacteria usually lie dormant in the body, never developing into an active disease; instead, the body surrounds the offending bacteria with closed sacs, or cysts. This acts to contain the bacteria

and prevent the spread of infection; yet, the body cannot kill the bacteria, only contain them.

Of the remaining 20 percent who do develop an active case of tuberculosis, only half of them will become sick within three months of contracting the infection, and the other half will suffer from the disease some time in their lives, perhaps years later. The bacteria often lie inactive until some other disease weakens the body's defenses.

Causes

Tuberculosis is contracted when a person breathes in droplets containing bacteria, called *Mycobacterium tuberculosis,* that have been coughed or sneezed into the air by an infected person. Tuberculosis can be contagious, especially for people living in crowded conditions. Also highly susceptible to this disease are those who are undernourished, in poor health, living in poor urban areas, as well as the very young and very old, and people in the medical professions. Anyone who has been in close contact with a tuberculosis patient should be tested for the disease.

Symptoms

The symptoms of tuberculosis are similar to those of many other diseases, and its true symptoms do not appear until the disease is in its advanced stages. For these reasons, coupled with the fact that the incidence of tuberculosis has been declining in recent years in the United States, this disorder often remains untreated or misdiagnosed for some time before the patient is finally tested for it.

Early signs include fever, as well as fatigue, loss of appetite, and weight loss. Its later signs include coughing up of a blood-tinged discharge called sputum, chest pain, and shortness of breath.

Diagnosis

Patients can be tested for tuberculosis with a tuberculin skin test. If the bacteria are present, whether active or inactive, the patch of skin that has been treated with dead tuberculosis bacteria will swell. Chest X rays or an analysis of the patient's sputum may also help to pinpoint the infection.

Treatment

Tuberculosis is treated with a variety of antibacterial drugs simultaneously so that the body will not become immune to one particular medication. The drugs are usually prescribed for a long period of time, perhaps nine to 18 months, but after two weeks the patient is no longer contagious and can resume normal activities.

With this type of treatment, the disease is rarely fatal any longer, and the biggest problem with such drug programs is that the patient discontinues the medication too soon. Also, severe side effects, such as liver or hearing damage, can result from some antituberculosis drugs.

Prevention

An active case of tuberculosis can be prevented in some persons who are considered to be high risks by the administration of certain antituberculosis drugs, but these are likely to have undesirable side effects. (High risk cases include persons under the age of 35, especially children, who have been exposed to the disease, as well as those with chronic diseases that may weaken their respiratory systems enough to make them more likely candidates for the disease.) Liver damage from the drugs is more likely to occur in those over the age of 35, so people in this age group seldom receive these drugs.

Regardless of age or physical condition, anyone who has been in close contact with a person with active tuberculosis should be tested for the disease.

THE HEART AND CIRCULATORY SYSTEM

The circulatory system, which includes the heart, the blood vessels, and the blood, nourishes every part of the body.

Heart

The heart is a hollow, muscular organ that is the basis of the circulatory system, which maintains blood circulation throughout the body. The organ lies behind the sternum, or breastbone, between the lungs; and its size in most adults approximates that of a clenched fist. A normal heart can beat from 60 to 90 times per minute. A heartbeat is the rhythmic contraction of heart muscle pumping blood.

Blood passes through four chambers in the heart separated by valves. Valves control movement of blood among these compartments. First, blood flows from the veins into the right atrium or upper right chamber. The fluid continues down to the right lower compartment, or right ventricle. From this chamber, the blood is pumped into the lungs to exchange carbon dioxide (waste product from cells) for oxygen (element necessary for cell life).

This rejuvenated blood then returns to the heart into the upper left chamber, or left atrium, which pumps the blood down into the lower left chamber, or left ventricle. From here, the left ventricle forces blood away from the heart through the aorta (main artery or passageway that extends through the chest and abdomen) to arteries that carry the blood to all the tissues of the body.

Blood vessels

Blood vessels comprise the network of passageways transporting blood throughout the body. This complex system consists of various types of blood vessels that are defined according to their size, function, and physical properties. Arteries can be large and elastic, medium-sized and muscular, or small (called arterioles). Their job is to receive blood from the heart and move it out to body tissues.

In the tissues, smaller subdivided arteries, called capillaries, exchange nutrients for waste products. Then, veins carry the "used" blood back to the heart to be recirculated through the

Aorta

Vein

To lungs

Left atrium

From lungs

Right atrium

Valve

Valve

Vein

Left ventricle

Right ventricle

The heart is a hollow, muscular organ that is divided into four chambers. Valves between the chambers control the movement of blood between the chambers. The heart acts as a pump to maintain the circulation of blood.

lungs and then back through the heart and arteries to the body.

Blood

Blood is the fluid that travels in blood vessels throughout the body transporting oxygen and other nutrients to the tissues and carrying waste products away from the tissues. It consists of plasma, a faint yellow liquid comprised of protein and water. Within the plasma are three formed elements—red blood cells, white blood cells, and platelets—that are visible only under a microscope. These elements are manufactured by the soft tissue, called bone marrow, in the center of bones.

Red blood cells carry oxygen from the lungs to various body tissues. Oxygen travels attached to hemoglobin, a pigmented substance in red blood cells that contains iron. When the amount of hemoglobin or the total number of red blood cells falls below a specified amount, anemia develops. Normally, there are about 27 million red blood cells in one teaspoon of blood.

The job of the white blood cells is to protect the body from invading organisms. Whenever the body becomes wounded or infected, white blood cells attack and kill disease-causing agents in the affected area. In addition, certain white blood cells produce antibodies. These substances counteract harmful agents by destroying or inactivating them so they are powerless. Because the body produces more white blood cells in response to infection, any change in their number signals disease. From 25,000 to 50,000 white blood cells exist in one teaspoon of blood.

Platelets are small colorless disks numbering between 750,000 to 1,750,000 in a single teaspoon of blood. They work to help the blood clot.

Anemia

Anemia is a general term referring to a shortage of red blood cells or a reduction of their hemoglobin content. Hemoglobin is the pigment (colored agent) in the blood that carries oxygen in the blood cells. Therefore, a shortage of red blood cells or hemoglobin means that the blood will be unable to carry enough oxygen to the body.

Types

There are many types of anemia, such as iron deficiency anemia, folic acid deficiency anemia, pernicious anemia (Vitamin B_{12} deficiency), aplastic anemia, and various hemolytic anemias (in which red blood cells are broken up) including sickle-cell anemia. Each type has its own cause and therefore its own methods of treatment, but all types of anemia are the result of an excessive loss or destruction of red blood cells or an inadequate production of red blood cells and hemoglobin.

Causes

Anemia can be caused by vitamin deficiencies or the body's inability to absorb certain vitamins, the destruction of red blood cells, inherited abnormalities in the blood, or the bone marrow's failure to manufacture red blood cells. Such diverse conditions as bleeding ulcers, drug allergies, cancer, and exposure to radioactivity can lead to anemia.

People with poor diets or histories of alcoholism are more likely to develop one of the anemias caused by vitamin deficiencies. Women are particularly susceptible to iron deficiency anemia (a shortage of the mineral iron, which is necessary to produce hemoglobin) because of regular loss of blood during menstruation as well as depletion of iron during pregnancy by the unborn baby. A tendency toward anemia can also be inherited, in the form of sickle-cell anemia, for instance.

Anemia can range from a severe case which may lead to extreme exhaustion or even death, to a mild condition which may be recognized only by a persistent tiredness.

Symptoms

The symptoms of anemia are fatigue, shortness of breath, pounding and increased heartbeat, headaches, loss of appetite, dizziness, ringing in the ears, and weakness or faintness. Burning of the tongue, and/or a change in its appearance, may also be a clue. A

Heart

Kidney

Veins

Arteries

This illustration of the circulatory system shows the heart, the kidneys, and the major arteries (left side of the body) and major veins (right side of the body).

physical sign of anemia may be paleness in the creases of the palms, under the fingernails, and in the lining of the eye. Very severe cases may be signaled by swollen ankles and other signs of heart failure, and shock.

Diagnosis

Diagnosis includes a physical exam as well as tests of the blood and often the bone marrow to detect shortages of red blood cells or hemoglobin.

Treatment

Each type of anemia has different causes and therefore different treatments. Iron deficiency anemia is caused by a shortage of the mineral iron, which is necessary to produce hemoglobin. This shortage can be caused by a variety of conditions: a drastic blood loss, such as from an accident, or a chronic blood loss, such as from a bleeding ulcer or excessive menstrual flow; hookworm; a diet lacking in dark green vegetables and organ meats, which are good sources of iron; and pregnancy. This type of anemia can be treated with iron supplements (ferrous sulfate or ferrous gluconate tablets).

Folic acid deficiency is caused by insufficient folic acid in the diet, also necessary for hemoglobin production. This deficiency may be caused or aggravated by malnourishment and alcoholism. Some disorders of the small intestine, such as inflammatory bowel disease, may also cause it. It is

treated with folic acid and sometimes additional vitamin supplements.

Pernicious anemia is caused by the body's inability to absorb Vitamin B_{12}, necessary for the production of red blood cells in the bone marrow. A substance called the intrinsic factor, which helps to absorb Vitamin B_{12}, is lacking in the stomach of someone suffering from this condition. Pernicious anemia is treated with Vitamin B_{12} injections directly into the bloodstream, bypassing the stomach completely. Inability to absorb Vitamin B_{12} can be caused by some parasites, inflammatory bowel disease, and other diseases of the small intestine.

Aplastic anemia is caused by the bone marrow's inability to produce blood cells. This deficiency affects the production of white and red blood cells, as well as the platelets (the blood cells that work to coagulate or clot the blood). The bone marrow's ability can be inhibited by cancer or exposure to radioactivity, hazardous chemicals, or some drugs. This variety of anemia is treated with blood transfusions and bone marrow transplants. It is a serious condition.

Hemolytic anemias are caused by the destruction of red blood cells. These anemias can be either acquired (developed over time) or congenital (present at birth).

Acquired hemolytic anemias can be caused by mismatched blood transfusions, a drug allergy, cancer, or a serious infection. Treatment of the source is necessary to treat the resulting anemia; blood transfusions can treat the condition temporarily.

Congenital hemolytic anemias are caused by an inherited abnormality in the red blood cells. The most common type is sickle-cell anemia, a disorder that strikes mostly black people, in which the red blood cells, sickle-shaped instead of disklike, cannot carry enough oxygen throughout the body. These cells are also very fragile and break easily (or hemolyze). This disease is characterized by crisis period bouts of severe joint or abdominal pain and can lead to complications such as kidney disease, gallstones, and heart failure. Sickle-cell anemia is treated with painkillers, oxygen, and transfusions. Avoiding situations in which oxygen may be scarce, such as high altitudes, is advisable.

Prevention

There are no specific methods to prevent anemias other than a balanced diet to prevent anemia caused by vitamin and mineral deficiencies.

Aneurysm

An aneurysm is a bulge in a blood vessel, usually an artery, due to a weakness in the vessel wall particularly in the elastic, muscular layer of the artery wall. An artery has three layers: the intima, which is the smooth inner layer; the media, composed of the elastic and muscular fibers; and the adventitia, the tough outer layer. A true aneurysm involves all three layers, whereas a "false" aneurysm is a disruption and/or clot in one or two of the layers causing a bulge in the vessel. A dissecting aneurysm occurs when blood enters the layers of the media, causing it to become separated from the other layers, thereby creating an extra channel through which blood flows and is diverted from the organs. This dangerous condition can develop rapidly, in hours or days. Once between the media layers, the blood keeps creating a new channel that may finally extend the full length of the artery.

The main danger of most untreated aneurysms is that they may rupture or dissect causing death from loss of blood. If death does not occur, blood loss may so decrease blood flow to the heart that the heart cannot work properly.

Causes

There are various causes of aneurysms. Those occurring in the arteries of the brain are often due to a genetic (inherited) defect —a weakness in or lack of elastic tissue in the media. If they rupture, a stroke can result.

Aneurysms in the small arteries may be caused by blood infections that weaken the vessel wall. Penetrating wounds occasionally can cause aneurysms. The sexually transmitted disease syphilis may also be a cause of aneurysms. Syphilis can cause an inflammation of the microscopic arteries that feed a large one (this is called vasculitis). When this occurs,

Adventitia layer of artery wall (outer)

Media layer (middle)

Intima layer (inner)

An aneurysm is a bulge in an artery because of a weakness in the vessel wall. A true aneurysm involves all three layers of the vessel wall, whereas a "false" aneurysm, shown here, is a disruption in one or two of the layers causing a bulge in the vessel.

these small arteries are lost, thereby causing a loss of nourishment to and a dying off and scarring of parts of the large arterial wall. This process leads to weakness of the wall and consequent formation of an aneurysm.

Dissecting aneurysms usually occur in the aorta (the main blood vessel leading away from the heart through the chest and abdomen), with atherosclerosis (hardening and scarring of the arteries) the most common cause, especially in the elderly. However, when dissecting aneurysms occur in the young, the cause is usually an inherited condition that results in damage to the media.

Symptoms

Symptoms of dissecting aneurysms of the aorta, if in the chest, include sudden, severe pain in the area of the aneurysm, often resembling a heart attack. There may be pain under the breastbone or in the back of the neck, difficulty in swallowing, shortness of breath, hoarseness, or a heavy cough. An aneurysm in a neck artery may create a pulsating swishing sound that the patient can detect.

Evidence of an aneurysm can be a tender, pulsating mass in the abdomen, or a painful, tender mass at the back of the knee (the latter can lead to blood clots that can travel downward and may result in death of tissue and gangrene in the toes). Symptoms of dissection or rupture in the abdomen can include sudden, severe central or low abdominal pain radiating to the back; a loss of blood flow to the legs; and shock — collapse of circulation with fainting, pale and clammy skin, and rapid weak pulse. Death can result quickly.

Diagnosis

X-ray and ultrasound pictures are taken of affected areas and used to locate aneurysms and determine their extent. The most reliable test is called an arteriogram or angiogram. In this test an X-ray dye is injected directly into the aorta providing an excellent visual picture on an X ray.

Treatment

Treatment of most aneurysms, especially dissecting aneurysms, should begin as soon as possible. Patients with dissecting aneurysms belong in an intensive care unit. Drugs are given to lower high blood pressure (which worsens a dissecting aneurysm) and thus to reduce the chances of rupture. Occasionally, under lessened pressure, a dissecting aneurysm heals itself. Long-term medication which keeps blood pressure low is standard treatment for those who cannot be operated on. Surgery, however, is by far the most satisfactory solution where it is possible. The damaged portion of the blood vessel is removed and replaced with a synthetic or natural vessel. Patients with ruptured aortic and, in most cases, dissecting aneurysms need emergency surgery. Rapid replacement of blood is necessary, as is intensive monitoring. Surgery for aneurysm is usually long and difficult. However, with newer methods of diagnosis, many more people are being spared the risks of surgery by correction of the aneurysm before it becomes a problem.

Angina pectoris

Angina pectoris, usually referred to simply as angina, is a warning signal in the form of chest pain, commonly dull and pressure-like, indicating that the heart muscle is getting insufficient blood and therefore insufficient oxygen. Angina occurs when the heart is using oxygen beyond what its blood supply can provide and is a sign that the body needs to slow down to permit the heart to catch up.

An angina attack is not a heart attack. Its pain is usually not as severe or as long-lasting as that experienced during a heart attack, and it does not destroy the heart muscle, as does a heart attack. However, those who suffer from this condition are probably more prone to heart attack than are those who do not.

Causes

Angina can be caused by any number of factors that prevent the heart muscle from getting enough blood from the circulatory system. By far the most common cause of angina is coronary artery narrowing due to atherosclerosis. The coronary arteries supply the heart muscle itself with blood. When an increased demand is placed upon the heart by the body, for instance, by exercise, the heart must work harder to supply blood (and

Although anginal pain is most often felt in the chest, it can also be felt below the breastbone near the uppermost part of the abdomen and along the neck. Pain and numbness may also extend down the arm and wrist to the little finger.

thereby oxygen) to keep the muscles and organs nourished. This increased work effort causes the heart muscle itself to require more blood. When narrowing of the coronary artery is present, the areas of heart muscle supplied by that part of the coronary artery cannot get enough blood in time to keep up with the demand. When this occurs, the muscle reacts by causing pain — angina pain. Exercise, stress, or even cold weather can trigger an attack.

This pain usually occurs during or after physical exertion or emotional stress, lasts only three to five minutes, and is relieved by resting or relaxing. If the pain does not go away within five minutes or if the pain increases in severity, the condition causing it may not be angina. It may be another disorder unrelated to the heart or it may be a heart attack.

Overeating and smoking can also trigger and aggravate angina: overeating by drawing much needed blood to a full stomach to aid in digestion, and smoking by causing the coronary arteries to contract thus reducing the oxygen-carrying capacity of the arteries.

Risk factors

Several so-called "risk factors" are associated with the development of coronary artery disease and angina. Family history of heart attack, smoking, high cholesterol levels, and high blood pressure are among the best-known. There is much controversy in medicine regarding the degree of impact these factors have. It is not yet clearly established whether alteration of one or more of these will definitely prevent or delay the onset of heart disease. However, there is much evidence favoring reduction of any and all of these factors. Furthermore, common sense would dictate that one attempt to do this.

Symptoms

The major symptom of angina is a dull pressure or a sensation of squeezing or burning in the center of the chest behind the breastbone. This dull pain in the chest is often compared to that accompanying indigestion. Angina pain can also be felt in the uppermost part of the abdomen and along the neck, and numbness may extend down the arm and wrist to the little finger. The bodily location and severity of the pain vary among angina patients, but the same symptoms usually reoccur for the same patient with each incident.

Diagnosis

Angina is diagnosed by first eliminating the possibility that the pain is originating from some other disorder, such as gallbladder disease, rib injury, muscle spasm, or pleurisy (an inflammation of the membrane that covers the lung). The doctor will take a complete medical history, physical exam, and probably an exercise or stress test using an ECG (electrocardiograph) which measures the heart's electrical impulses during exercise. This test can indicate abnormalities in the arteries that are preventing sufficient blood to flow to the heart. Also, radioactive isotopes or X-ray opaque fluids can be injected into the bloodstream to monitor the flow of blood through the heart. The most definitive test for the diagnosis of coronary artery disease is the cardiac catheterization or angiogram. In this test, a radiopaque (able to be seen on X rays) dye is injected through a tube (catheter) placed directly into the heart through an artery in the leg or arm. Once the dye is injected, X-ray films are taken, and the areas of obstruction to the dye within the coronary arteries can be clearly seen. During this procedure, other important information, such as the overall condition of the heart muscle, can also be obtained.

Treatment

Angina is often treated by recommending changes in the patient's lifestyle, to reduce the strain on the heart, and by administering medication, to modify the supply-demand relationship of the heart muscle and its blood supply.

A change in lifestyle will be necessary for patients who smoke, overeat, or overexert themselves. Certain types of exercise may be too stressful, but regular exercise is necessary to improve collateral circulation (the natural development of a system of small blood vessels that detour obstructions in the arteries and supply blood directly to the heart).

The medication most often used to treat angina attacks is nitroglycerin, which may act by expanding blood vessels to increase blood flow and/or by altering the distribution and volume of blood in the heart. Nitroglycerin is taken in the form of a tablet that is dissolved under the tongue. Pain should stop within three or four minutes; if it does not, the pain may not be due to simple angina. Nitroglycerin can also be prescribed as an ointment. This is used for the prevention of attacks, not for the treatment of an acute episode.

Surgery to bypass the obstructions in the arteries is performed only when angina cannot be controlled with medication or when its pain is becoming increasingly severe. There has been much controversy surrounding bypass surgery, mainly centering around the question of whether this procedure can increase life expectancy in those with coronary artery disease and angina. At present, there is no question that the surgery relieves pain and allows for greater exercise tolerance in the majority of patients who undergo it for severe angina. In certain patterns of disease such as obstruction of the "left-main" coronary artery, the operation definitely prolongs life expectancy. In other patterns such as "triple vessel disease" where branches of all three coronaries (except for the left-main) are involved, the surgery most likely allows a longer life. In still other patterns, the question is unsettled. Whether or not the surgery will prevent a heart attack is also an unsettled issue.

Prevention

Incidents of angina pain can be prevented with several drugs: nitrates and calcium antagonists (drugs such as nifedipine and verapamil that act by blocking the constricting actions of calcium on arterial muscle), which have a longer lasting effect than plain nitroglycerin and may be taken on a regular basis; and beta blockers, which also effectively prevent angina, since they decrease the work of the heart, thereby lessening its oxygen needs and making it less likely that angina will occur. (One additional note: beta blockers should be used with caution if at all by asthma patients, as these drugs may cause spasms in the breathing tubes and subsequent breathing difficulties.)

Atherosclerosis

Atherosclerosis is a slow, progressive disease of the arteries in which various fatty deposits partially clog or, eventually, totally

Atherosclerosis occurs when the normally smooth, firm linings of the arteries become roughened and thickened with deposits of fat, calcium, and cellular debris. Developing into a hard film called plaque, this deposit eventually may build up and block the artery.

block the blood flow. It is often called "hardening of the arteries."

Complications

This blockage of various arteries can result in serious complications when the arteries involved lead to vital organs: heart attack can result when an artery to the heart is totally blocked, and angina pectoris (chest pain) can be caused by partial clogging of an artery; stroke occurs when an artery to the brain is blocked; kidney disease can develop from obstruction in the arteries leading to the kidneys; blindness or diseases of the extremities can result from blockages of the arteries supplying these areas of the body.

Descriptions

Atherosclerosis occurs when the normally smooth, firm linings of the arteries have become roughened, thickened, and clogged with deposits of fat, fibrin (a clotting substance), calcium, and cellular debris. This condition develops over time, in a step-by-step procedure. Fats (called lipids), necessary for the production of certain hormones and tissues, are constantly present in the bloodstream. When the level of these fats is greatly increased, however, fatty streaks form along the artery walls. These streaks, harmless in themselves, can cause small nodules of fatty deposits (cholesterol) to jut out from the normally smooth linings of the artery walls. Fibrous scar tissue grows under these nodules and further attracts calcium deposits; accumulated calcium develops into a hard, chalky film called plaque that cannot be removed. This permanent coating inside the arteries hampers their ability to expand and contract properly and slows the blood flow through the now narrowed channels. Clots may now easily form, totally preventing the blood from traveling through the artery.

Causes

The exact cause of this process has not been pinpointed, but the initial increase of the blood's fat content may be triggered by diets high in saturated fats (fats that are usually solid at room temperature, including all animal fats such as those found in butter and meats). Also, the body's inability to absorb these fats from the bloodstream may lead to their increased build-up in the arteries.

Hypertension (high blood pressure) can increase the risk of atherosclerosis because it puts constant strain on the arteries, thus speeding up the clogging and hardening process. Smoking narrows the arteries, thus restricting blood flow and inviting atherosclerosis to set in.

Symptoms

Atherosclerosis alone has no visible symptoms. In fact, the disease often remains undetected until the arteries are totally blocked, and strain or damage to the affected organs produces symptoms. For example, if an artery supplying the heart is afflicted with atherosclerosis, chest pain may be felt; if atherosclerosis affects a head artery, the patient may experience dizziness, blurred vision, and faintness.

Diagnosis

Diagnosis of atherosclerosis involves several methods: an exercise tolerance or stress test using an ECG (electrocardiograph), which measures the electrical impulses generated by the heart and which will indicate damaged heart tissue or blocked arteries; ultrasound, which records blockage in the arteries, abnormalities of the heart chambers and valves, and the movement of blood through the heart; and radioactive isotopes or X-ray opaque fluid, which, when injected into the bloodstream, can be traced through the circulatory system to indicate obstructions or areas insufficiently supplied with blood.

Treatment

Treatment of this disorder aims at reducing the strain on the heart and preventing further artery damage. Changes in lifestyle and eating habits along with the administration of medication can accomplish this. Currently there are no available medications that will actually dissolve the deposits that have clogged the arteries. Delicate surgical procedures, however, may be performed to remove those deposits that are blocking arteries to vital organs. These procedures, called endarterectomies, are performed on relatively large vessels such as those entering the brain, heart, kidneys, and legs. Surgery cannot remove deposits in small blood vessels of these organs.

Lifestyle changes include cutting out smoking; reducing cholesterol intake; perhaps losing weight (obesity puts a strain on the heart); and maintaining a moderate, but not overly strenuous, exercise program (exercise helps develop the collateral circulation, a system of small blood vessels that can bypass the partially blocked arteries and directly supply organs with blood).

Anticoagulants may be prescribed to thin the blood and prevent clotting. If atherosclerosis has led to angina, several other drugs may help to suppress chest pain by expanding the arteries and increasing blood flow; they are nitroglycerin, nitrates, and calcium antagonists. If high blood pressure contributes to the problem, two other types of drugs may be prescribed: diuretics, which lower the resistance in the blood vessels, and beta blockers, which reduce both the heart rate and the amount of blood pumped from the heart with each beat. Note: asthma sufferers should use beta blockers only with extreme caution, as these drugs can cause spasms in the respiratory passages.

When medication is not sufficient and the individual suffers from severe and recurrent chest pain, surgery may be performed to bypass the major obstructions.

Bypass surgery

Coronary bypass surgery is performed on one or more of the three great blood vessels, the coronary arteries, that lie on the outer surface of the heart and supply heart muscle with the oxygen and nutrients it needs. In coronary artery disease, a section or sections of the arteries gradually become obstructed with a buildup of cholesterol, calcium, and scar tissue. The purpose of the operation is to bypass the blood around the obstruction using a section of blood vessel (usually a vein taken from the leg) that is sewn into the artery in front of and behind the blockage. This permits free blood flow again. Without it, heart muscle below the obstruction is starved for blood and oxygen, especially during exercise. This creates the chest pains known as "angina." If one or more of the coronary arteries become completely obstructed, the result may be a heart attack, in which a portion of heart muscle becomes so starved for blood that it dies.

Usually if there is one obstruction in the coronary arteries, there

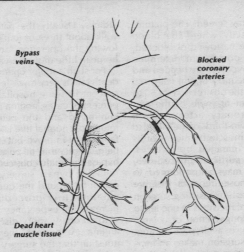

Bypass veins

Blocked coronary arteries

Dead heart muscle tissue

In coronary artery disease, a section of the coronary arteries gradually becomes obstructed with a buildup of cholesterol, calcium, and scar tissue. The coronary bypass operation bypasses the blood around the obstruction in the coronary arteries using a section of blood vessel—usually a vein taken from the leg—that is sewn into the artery in front of and behind the blockage. This permits free blood flow again.

are others (there may be two in the same artery). A "double bypass" operation means that two vessels are bypassed, a "triple bypass" means that three vessels are bypassed, and so forth.

Bypass surgery is usually considered when a person suffers frequent chest pains from angina. However, not all persons with angina need bypass surgery. Advances are being made in medication to control angina. Furthermore, some angina is caused by spasms (sudden, violent contractions) of the coronary arteries, which bypass surgery may not prevent or help. In the future, obstructions in the coronary arteries may be eliminated by methods that do not require cutting open the chest, perhaps by a cutting or crushing instrument that is threaded to the site of the obstruction through the blood vessel. Even without outside help, and given enough time, the heart creates its own partial bypass, by developing blood vessels that detour the blood around the obstruction; this is known as "collateral circulation."

Diagnosis. If you have severe chest pains often and they cannot be controlled by medication, your doctor may decide to order that X-ray motion pictures of your heart be taken. Through a thin woven plastic catheter (tube) entering at the arm or leg and passing through large blood vessels to your heart, X-ray contrast medium is injected so that it flows into the coronary arteries, outlining them on the X-ray screen. The pictures show exactly where the blood vessels are narrowed or blocked. Thus the doctor can determine whether bypasses are needed and where. The most urgent reason to operate is the obstruction, of 50 to 70 percent or more, of the left-main coronary artery, which supplies two-thirds of the blood to the heart muscle by means of its two lower branches.

Procedure. The bypass surgery operation takes about four hours or more depending on the number of bypasses. An assisting surgeon cuts several incisions in one leg to obtain a long section of a large vein for use as bypass tubing. Next, the surgeon makes an incision down the middle of the chest, divides the breastbone with an electric saw, and separates the two sides of the rib cage enough to expose the beating heart. The heartbeat is then stopped using either electric shock, ice water, or certain drugs. A heart-lung machine, connected to large vessels carrying blood from and to the heart, takes over the job of adding oxygen, removing carbon dioxide, and pumping the blood through the body.

The surgeon cuts through the pericardial sac (a bag of tissue around the heart) to expose the coronary arteries outlined on the heart surface. On either side of each coronary artery blockage, the surgeon cuts open the artery and sews in either end of bypass tube—a piece of vein taken from the leg. Thereafter, blood will flow freely around the obstructed portion to nourish the heart muscle and thereby protect the patient against chest pains and heart attacks. Usually the patient can walk about three or four days following the operation, and return home in little more than a week.

For such a major operation, the death rate is very low—less than 1 percent in some hospitals. In 80 percent of cases, angina pains are eliminated and the patient can return to a normal life. Life expectancy may improve but it cannot be guaranteed in all cases. There has been much controversy surrounding bypass surgery, mainly centering around the question of whether this procedure can increase life expectancy in those with coronary artery disease and angina. At present, there is no question that the surgery relieves pain and allows for greater exercise tolerance in the majority of patients who undergo it for severe angina. In certain patterns of disease such as obstruction of the "left-main" coronary artery, the operation definitely prolongs life expectancy. In other patterns such as "triple vessel disease" where branches of all three coronaries (except for the left-main) are involved, the surgery most likely allows a longer life. In still other patterns, the question is unsettled. Whether or not the surgery will prevent a heart attack is also an unsettled issue.

Congestive heart failure

Congestive heart failure, often simply called "heart failure," is a condition in which the heart weakens and fails to keep the blood moving adequately. As a result, the supply of blood to the body's tissues decreases, lowering body efficiency and endurance. With poor circulation, the kidneys fail to remove enough water, salt, and wastes from the blood. In addition, the kidneys, as a result of the decreased blood flow presented to them, also try to increase blood volume by retaining even more salt and water. As a result, blood volume increases, making more work for the already overworked heart, which may enlarge and beat faster in an attempt to satisfy the body's hunger for oxygen-rich blood. Veins distend with fluid and the balance of pressures between fluids inside and outside the veins shifts, which causes fluid that normally stays in the bloodstream to leak into surrounding tissue. This fluid leakage, the reduction of forward blood flow, the backflow of blood, and other factors are responsible for the accumulation of fluid in the lungs (called pulmonary edema) as well as for the swelling of the abdomen and legs often seen in patients with congestive heart failure.

Causes

The usual cause of congestive heart failure is a diseased heart that just cannot pump enough blood. The most common reason for that is severe coronary artery disease that decreases the flow of blood to the heart muscle. Coronary artery disease is largely responsible for a heart attack, which leaves non-working scar tissue that lowers the efficiency of the heart as a pump. However,

other heart conditions can also cause congestive heart failure. Leaky or narrowed heart valves, due to a birth defect or rheumatic fever, can lead to heart failure. A large cardiac aneurysm, a bulge caused by the thinning of the wall of the lower left heart chamber (ventricle) that pumps blood out of the heart into the body, may weaken the heart's pumping ability.

Less frequently, the root of the problem is one of several different heart muscle diseases. Some are caused by poisons like alcohol (liquor), some by viruses, and others by the deposit in the heart tissue of iron or an abnormal body substance known as amyloid. Disturbances of the normal rhythm of the heart may also lead to failure.

Symptoms

Early signs of possible heart failure include unexplained rapid heartbeat, unusual fatigue during exertion, shortness of breath during stair climbing or other mild exercise, and inability to withstand cold. Attacks of shortness of breath and coughing when lying in bed that are relieved by sleeping with pillows under the back to tilt the chest are also early symptoms. Sometimes, a person is actually awakened by "air hunger" and must sit or stand to breathe more easily. These symptoms are caused by increased fluid pressure in the lung circulation. The relief obtained by assuming a more erect position is due to a shift of fluid (blood) volume to the lower half of the body, easing the burden of the heart. In advanced congestive heart failure, shortness of breath and, frequently, a severe cough with rusty or brownish-colored sputum (from blood) are common. There may also be swelling of the ankles and a feeling of fullness in the neck or abdomen.

Diagnosis

Usually congestive heart failure can be diagnosed after a physical examination and on the basis of symptoms. However, a chest X ray is commonly taken to determine how much the heart has become enlarged by its overload and to see if fluid has accumulated within the lungs. In addition, an electrocardiogram (ECG), a tracing on a graph of the electric current produced by the contraction of the heart muscle, may reveal past heart attack damage and irregularities in the heart rhythm.

Treatment

Treatment for congestive heart failure includes rest, oxygen, drugs (like digitalis) to strengthen the pumping ability of the heart, and medicine to prevent irregular heart rhythms. Diuretic drugs are given to help the kidneys remove more salt and water from the blood and thus decrease the amount of volume the heart must pump, and a low-salt diet is prescribed to prevent water buildup in the blood and tissues (salt tends to cause fluid to accumulate in the body). In more severe or chronic cases, a drug may be given to expand the blood vessels and thus make it easier for the heart to pump blood through them.

In some cases the original cause of the congestive heart failure can be corrected. Thus, bypass surgery may be performed on the coronary arteries to improve blood supply to the heart muscle. Surgery is also done to replace or correct a faulty heart valve, or to repair an aneurysm. Contributing factors to be controlled or eliminated may include high blood pressure, anemia, excess salt or alcohol intake, fever, overactive thyroid, and stress due to overexertion.

Prevention

Congestive heart failure usually results from an already damaged heart; thus, the prevention of congestive heart failure rests on those good health habits that help prevent heart disease in general: a well-balanced diet with moderate or low intake of fats; weight control; plenty of exercise, rest, and sleep; avoidance of tobacco and excess alcohol; and periodic medical checkups to detect conditions such as high blood pressure that might eventually overload or injure the heart and thus lead to congestive heart failure. In people who already have congestive heart failure, control of the condition is much helped by eliminating salt and highly salted foods, avoiding overexertion, and adhering strictly to the prescribed program of medication.

Cor pulmonale

Cor pulmonale is the enlargement and failure of the right ventricle (the lower right chamber) of the heart, due to poor functioning of the lungs.

The right ventricle is affected because its main job is to pump blood returning from the veins of the body into the lungs, through the pulmonary artery. When the lungs are not working properly — for example, when many of the capillaries (tiny blood vessels) in the lungs have been destroyed or constricted by disease — not enough blood can get through the lungs. The blood backs up, its pressure rises, and it enlarges both the pulmonary artery and the now harder-working right ventricle. Blood pressure also rises in the veins leading to the heart.

In addition, because not enough blood is getting to the appropriate areas of the lungs and because of disease or destruction of the oxygenating units of the lungs called alveoli, the oxygen content of the blood decreases. This causes the bone marrow to produce more oxygen-carrying red blood cells, which in most circumstances would allow the blood to carry more oxygen. However, in this case it only makes matters worse, by thickening the blood which is then harder to pump. The result of the whole process is failure of the right ventricle to perform well.

Causes

In nearly six cases out of seven, the lung condition that has led to cor pulmonale is chronic obstructive pulmonary disease (COPD), which is a breakdown in breathing resulting from emphysema, chronic bronchitis, asthma, or a combination of these diseases. Some of the other causes are cystic fibrosis, recurrent blood clots in the blood vessels of the lung, loss of lung tissue because of surgery or injury, extreme obesity that prevents proper breathing, diseases of the nerves controlling the breathing muscles, or insufficient oxygen from living at high altitudes (chronic mountain sickness). Almost always the cause of cor pulmonale is a chronic, lifelong condition. One exception is acute (sudden and severe) cor pulmonale resulting from a massive blood clot in the lungs; the clot can sometimes be removed by surgery. More often, an acute worsening cor pulmonale results from a severe infection of the breathing tract in someone with a chronic lung condition. Proper treatment usually can bring this under control.

Symptoms

Symptoms of right heart failure include increasing fatigue, drowsiness, fainting on exertion, ankle swelling, fullness in the neck and abdomen, enlarged neck veins, and an enlarged and tender liver. As in the more common left ventricle failure, the patient may wheeze; cough; find breathing difficult and painful (however, in pure right ventricle failure, there is no fluid in the lungs); and may at times be blue in the lips, nails, fingertips, and even the face from lack of oxygen.

Diagnosis

X-ray or ultrasound pictures reveal the enlargement of the right ventricle and pulmonary artery. A markedly increased number of red blood cells that exceeds 50 percent of the blood volume is a telltale clue. Heartbeat patterns indicating right ventricle failure can be seen on the electrocardiogram (ECG)—a visual record of the heart's electrical impulses.

Treatment

Treatment for cor pulmonale is twofold to treat the heart failure and the lung condition at the same time. Heart failure therapy includes oxygen to make the patient more comfortable, to reduce the high blood pressure in the pulmonary artery, and to prevent a high red blood cell count. Salt and water restriction and diuretics can reduce excess fluid in the tissues. Bed rest reduces the load on the heart.

In general, treatment of the underlying lung condition is much the same as it was (or should have been) before cor pulmonale occurred. The patient should not smoke. In most patients, smoking helped to cause the original condition, and smoking worsens the present condition. Once home from the hospital, the individual should regularly prac-

tice breathing exercises and may need oxygen and suction treatments to relieve symptoms. The patient should rest frequently, watch for signs of ankle swelling or other fluid buildup, avoid people with colds, and report early signs of infection.

Prevention

You can help to prevent the lung condition leading to cor pulmonale by not smoking; by having periodic physical examinations including a test of lung function; and by seeking prompt medical treatment by a physician for any chronic cough or recurring respiratory (breathing) infection. It is especially important to observe these precautions if you come from a family that has an inherited tendency to certain chronic respiratory diseases.

Cyanosis

Cyanosis is a bluish coloration of the skin and mucous membranes. The abnormal coloration is easily seen in these areas, both because of their rich blood supply and their relative transparency. Usually it is a sign that the tissue is getting too little oxygen from the blood.

Blood rich in oxygen from the lungs is bright red. This is because of the red iron-containing pigment known as hemoglobin found in the erythrocytes, the disk-shaped red blood cells which carry oxygen. When blood passes through the blood vessels of the lungs, oxygen from the air in the lungs combines with the hemoglobin, which causes it and the blood to turn a very bright red. After the blood releases its oxygen to the cells of the body and picks up carbon dioxide and other waste products, the hemoglobin fades and the blood turns dark. However, if the lungs are not working well or if for some other reason the red blood cells are not being oxygenated, the blood appears bluish, producing cyanosis.

Cyanosis is a sign of reduced air supply that can be due to such conditions as asthma, choking, pneumonia, and lung collapse. It can also be a sign of certain inborn heart defects, of severe heart failure, or of abnormally excessive production of red blood cells. It is seen most frequently in cold weather when lips, toes, and fingers turn blue from extreme cold, the result of sluggish surface circulation of the blood. This can be a normal phenomenon and does not indicate disease.

Defibrillation

Defibrillation is a technique to correct the fibrillation of the heart, a disorder marked by very rapid disorganized twitching or trembling of the heart muscle in place of the normal beat. Fibrillation produces a condition called cardiac arrest, in which no heartbeat, pulse, or blood pressure can be detected. Death or permanent brain damage follows within a few minutes unless this condition is corrected, or unless first aid measures maintain blood circulation

and breathing until help can arrive.

Causes of fibrillation

The most common cause of fibrillation of the heart is heart attack. When this happens, certain parts of the heart will start contracting independently of the normal heartbeat. Other causes of fibrillation are severe electric shock and prolonged exposure to extreme cold.

Defibrillation treatment

Correction is by means of an electric defibrillator. A pair of metal paddles is placed on the patient's chest and a single jolt of direct-current electricity from the defibrillator is directed into the heart to shock it back into its regular rhythm. The shock stops the independent action of individual muscle fibers and allows the natural pacemaker of the heart to take over again. Once the heartbeat is restored, other measures are taken. A drug such as lidocaine is injected to prevent further fibrillation. An intravenous tube is inserted to drip sodium bicarbonate (to neutralize acids in the blood) and defibrillating medication into a vein. A breathing tube is passed down into the lungs, attached to a mechanical pump that forces air in and out of lungs. Then the patient is taken to a hospital cardiac intensive care unit, where electric instruments constantly keep track of the patient's condition and sound an alarm if danger threatens. An electric defibrillator is close at hand if needed in an emergency.

Electric defibrillation is also used to restart a heart which has been stopped for purposes of heart surgery.

Embolism

An embolism occurs when some part of the circulatory system is either partially or completely blocked by some obstructing mass that has traveled through the system. The occurrence of an obstruction is called an *embolism* while the mass causing the embolism is called an *embolus*.

Types

Emboli (the plural of embolus) are classified in three major groups:
- Solid emboli, which are made up of a variety of substances, such as clumps of tissue, tumor cells, or pieces of blood clots
- Liquid emboli, which are made up of globules of fat or amniotic fluid (fluid in which the fetus is bathed during pregnancy)
- Gaseous emboli, which are made up of the different constituents of air.

Common locations

Emboli are further categorized according to the location of the blockage:
- Arterial emboli, which originate either from the heart or the artery itself, travel downstream, and prevent the flow of fresh blood to whatever area or organ is being supplied
- Paradoxical emboli, which originate in the venous system and pass over into the arterial system (this usually occurs because of defects in the walls separating the chambers of the heart)
- Pulmonary emboli, which block vessels in the lungs
- Coronary artery emboli, which block coronary arteries of the heart
- Cerebral emboli, which usually originate in the heart or the carotid arteries in the neck leading to the brain (these are a major cause of stroke).

Causes

Emboli have a variety of causes, depending on the specific type. The most common cause is the breaking away of a blood clot from within the heart or blood vessels. Arterial emboli commonly originate in the heart itself, because of plaques or accumulations on the heart's valves, from blood clots on the walls of the heart, or within an aneurysm. An arterial embolus can also originate from a plaque or clot within the artery itself. Fat emboli can develop from injury to the bones (particularly the long bones of the leg) or from damage to cells in fat tissue. Air emboli can develop (rarely) if a very large amount of air is admitted during an intravenous (into the vein) infusion or as a complication of surgery, espe-

An embolus is a piece of a clot that has broken off and traveled through the circulatory system. The embolus will usually lodge downstream causing loss of blood flow and death of tissue in the area nourished by that vessel.

cially in operations on the neck or the chest. In these cases, air enters vessels that are open because of the surgery. However, the oxygen in air is not the only gas involved in gaseous emboli. When divers ascend from high pressure levels in the water to normal pressure levels too quickly or when aviators (in planes without cabin pressurization) climb from normal pressure levels to low pressure levels, there is always the possibility of nitrogen bubbles arising in the bloodstream because of too rapid decompression. If any of these gaseous emboli find their way into the central nervous system, the result can be catastrophic.

An arterial embolism deprives the affected area of its blood sup-ply, which can cause damage or death of the area. An embolism in a brain artery may produce the symptoms of a stroke. In an embolism in the leg, the area beyond the blockage—if totally or nearly totally deprived of blood—becomes white and painful. If the obstruction is not relieved, death of tissue will ensue.

Treatment

Emboli resulting from blood clots are often treated with a variety of anticoagulants (agents that inhibit normal clotting mechanisms in the blood). Common anticoagulants such as heparin and warfarin do not actually dissolve clots, but instead prevent additional clots from forming and embolizing. There are newer drugs that do dissolve clots, but their use is restricted to special situations. If an embolism is in an available location, such as in an artery in a limb, and tissue is threatened, surgery to remove the clot is the preferred method of treatment to save the limb. In cases of a massive embolism to the lung (usually from deep veins in the legs) where life is threatened, surgery can also be attempted. In addition, if an individual has clots in the deep venous system of the lower half of the body and for some reason (for example, a recent hemorrhage in the brain or other vital organ) anticoagulants cannot be prescribed, blocking devices such as clips can be placed on or in the main vein (inferior vena cava) receiving blood from the lower body to prevent emboli from reaching the lungs.

Endocarditis

Endocarditis is the term used to describe an inflammation of the endocardial layer of the heart. The heart is made up of three cellular layers: the endocardium (innermost layer), myocardium (middle, muscular layer), and epicardium (the outermost layer). The endocardium lines all of the chambers and valves of the heart, and its cells are continuous with those of blood vessels leaving the heart. Endocarditis is divided into two forms, infectious and noninfectious.

Infectious endocarditis

Infectious endocarditis usually occurs in people with congenital (inborn) or acquired defects in the walls and/or valves of the heart. An example of the former would be a hole in the wall between the different chambers of the heart. Examples of an acquired defect are heart valves damaged by rheumatic fever and damage that may result from the use of nonsterile needles by drug addicts who inject intravenously. For complex reasons, these anatomic or structural abnormalities are more susceptible to infection. Bacteria probably circulate through the bloodstream of all people at some time or another. However, certain procedures such as dental work (fillings, extractions, cleaning, gum surgery) lead to significant bacteremia (the presence of large amounts of bacteria traveling through the bloodstream). The bacteria somehow rest on these abnormal areas in the heart and cause inflammation and/or infection that serve as a foundation for the collection of platelets, strands of clotting material (fibrin), and other debris of the circulatory system. The clump of material that forms is referred to as a "vegetation."

Abnormal heart valves or walls can be infected with microorganisms from any site in the body that contains a high amount of bacteria. People with abnormal heart valves, prosthetic (artificial) valves, and other structural abnormalities must be given antibiotics before and after any procedure (dental work, surgery of the urogenital or large intestinal tract, opening of an abscess) likely to disperse bacteria. Fungi and yeast (candida) can also cause endocarditis but usually in people with other serious diseases and depressed immune function. The antibiotics serve either to prevent or at least lessen the number of microorganisms passing through the bloodstream, thereby lessening (significantly) the chance of developing endocarditis.

Symptoms

Infectious endocarditis is a serious systemic disease with a wide spectrum of symptoms and signs. Patients may complain of fevers, weakness, and weight loss. Anemia (deficiency in red blood cells) may also be present. Pieces of the vegetations may break off and embolize to (travel to and lodge in) other areas of the body, for example, the brain causing a stroke, or to the kidneys causing microscopic blood in the urine, among other problems. If the infection of a valve is particularly intense or if a prosthetic valve is involved, the valve may actually have to be surgically replaced.

Diagnosis

The diagnosis of infectious endocarditis is made by the history and physical examination along with appropriate laboratory data. Blood cultures (taking of blood and placing it into special materials designed to support bacterial or fungal growth) are the mainstay of diagnosis.

Treatment

Once the infectious agent is isolated, appropriate antibiotics can be administered. Antibiotic administration is by the intravenous route (at least at first) and usually for long periods up to six to eight weeks.

Prevention

Prevention of infectious endocarditis involves having knowledge of abnormalities in one's heart and taking the proper antibiotics prior to and after dental and many surgical procedures.

Noninfectious endocarditis

Noninfectious endocarditis can be associated with many different diseases. Endocardial inflammation with consequent changes causing some loss of function of the heart is one form. Another is the formation of valvular vegetations that are sterile, but nonetheless can embolize and cause serious damage. Treatment of these conditions depends on the underlying disease process.

Extrasystole

An extrasystole is a contraction (beat) of the heart caused by a stimulus or impulse somewhere in the heart other than in the sino-atrial node, the natural pacemaker of the heart. In some ways, the condition is like a "stray" signal or "static" in an electrical circuit.

While physicians have for years debated the importance of extrasystoles, recent thought on the subject has led to a reassessment of the seriousness of the phenomenon. Many sudden deaths may be attributed to severe cardiac arrhythmia that was itself triggered by ventricular extrasystoles in patients with severe underlying heart disease.

Causes

While the immediate cause of an extrasystole is a "stray" signal telling the heart muscle to contract, the real causes lie elsewhere. For example, strenuous activity, especially if there are existing heart problems, can trigger extrasystoles, which, in turn, may trigger an episode of heart arrhythmia (abnormal rhythm and rate of the heart beat) that leads to more serious complications. Coffee, nicotine, and certain drugs, as well as anxiety and sudden shocks or frights, are thought to play a role in extrasystoles. It is important to note, however, that extrasystoles also occur in normal hearts and, in these cases, are quite harmless and do not necessarily indicate underlying heart disease.

Symptoms

The symptoms of extrasystoles are familiar to anyone who has ever been startled and found that his or her heart "skipped a beat." The extrasystole sometimes presents itself as an extra beat and sometimes as two extra beats. On other occasions, there will be a beat followed by a long silence, then a couple of quick beats. Some people experience a feeling of giddiness, shortness of breath, and weakness, with momentary feelings of blacking out. These symptoms, if prolonged and particularly if associated with a loss of consciousness, usually indicate that a sustained arrhythmia (alteration of the normal rhythmic contraction of the heart) is occurring, which should be reported to a doctor.

Diagnosis

One method of documenting the occurrence and nature of extrasystoles is continuous ambulatory electrocardiographic monitoring. The patient in whom arrhythmias are suspected is hooked up to a monitor the size of a portable cassette tape recorder which he or she carries for a certain period of time. A diary is furnished so that the patient can record his or her activity and symptoms. The patient is usually told to perform the normal routine activities during the test. After a specified time period, usually 24 hours, the monitor is taken off and the tape translated into a continuous electrocardiographic record. This record allows a definite diagnosis to be made as to the presence and type of arrhythmia. Treatment can then be prescribed

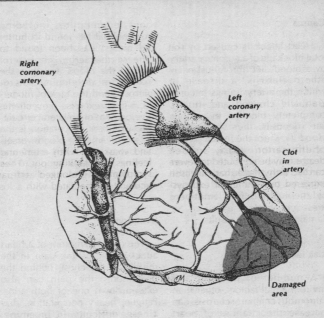

A heart attack occurs when an area of the heart is damaged or dies because of a reduction in the blood supply to that area. The reduced blood supply results when the coronary artery supplying the area is blocked by a blood clot or advanced atherosclerosis.

on the basis of concrete evidence.

Heart attack

A heart attack (or myocardial infarction) occurs when an area of the heart muscle is damaged or dies because a coronary artery has been blocked and the oxygen-rich blood supply to that area of the heart has been drastically reduced. The damaged muscle tissue of the heart is replaced with scar tissue, which affects the heart's future performance.

Although the chances of surviving a heart attack are now better than ever and complete recovery is common, heart attack or another form of circulatory disease is still the number one cause of death in the United States. Heart attacks that do not result in death often lead to serious complications: shock; cardiac arrhythmia, marked by an irregular heartbeat; or congestive heart failure, in which the heart cannot pump enough blood to meet the body's needs and fluid accumulates in the lower parts of the body.

Causes

Heart attack is caused by the total blockage of a coronary artery by a blood clot (thrombus) or by atherosclerosis, a disease in which the artery linings become gradually clogged and, finally, completely blocked by various fatty deposits, thus shutting off blood flow to the heart. Other healthy arteries that are not clogged may be much narrower and therefore unable to deliver the extra oxygenated blood needed by the heart during emotional stress or physical exertion. So damage to the heart results.

Risk factors

A number of physical and environmental factors, other than a thrombus or atherosclerosis, can increase the chances of heart attack: hypertension (high blood pressure) increases the resistance in the blood vessels, making the heart pump harder to push blood through; excessive cholesterol in the blood increases the likelihood of developing atherosclerosis; and birth control pills, especially those taken by women over the age of 35 or by smokers, have been linked to the increased incidence of heart attack.

Smoking, stress, improper diet, and lack of exercise have also been associated with the increased risk of heart attack. Smoking acts to constrict the arteries and reduce the blood flow to the heart muscle; stress puts an extra demand on the heart's need for blood; a diet high in saturated fats (fats that are usually solid at room temperature, including those animal fats found in butter and meats) has been found to increase the serum cholesterol level in the blood and thus the chances of developing atherosclerosis; and the lack of moderate, regular exercise prevents the development of collateral circulation. Collateral circulation is the system of smaller blood vessels that bypass a blocked artery and increase the blood supply to the area that the blocked artery serves.

Symptoms

The major symptom of a heart attack is a crushing pain in the middle of the chest, behind the breastbone; the pain can also extend down one or both arms. Fatigue, heavy perspiration, dizziness, difficulty in breathing, and, occasionally, fever, may accompany this pain. The pain may be somewhat similar to that experienced from angina pectoris (chest pain), but the pain of a heart attack is more intense, will not be relieved by nitroglycerin, and will not go away within a few minutes, as angina pain will. Also, a heart attack may take place during sleep, which is rare for angina pain.

Heart attacks range from very mild, signaled only by a slight discomfort, faintness, and nausea, to very serious, which can be accompanied by cardiac arrest (when the heartbeat completely stops) or ventricular fibrillation (when the normal, steady heartbeat is reduced to a useless quivering that prevents blood from being pumped through the body).

Diagnosis

Heart attack is diagnosed by the electrocardiograph (ECG), which measures the electrical impulses produced by the heart; a diseased heart will show a record of disturbed patterns because the impulses must travel around the damaged area. A test for an increased white blood cell count may also be done, as the body's immune system will increase its number of white blood cells in order to carry away dead tissue from the damaged heart. Other blood tests may be taken to measure certain proteins in the blood that signal damaged heart muscle, although these tests may not show results until 24 to 72 hours after the attack.

Treatment

The best and only treatment for heart attack is to rush to a hospital for emergency medical treatment as soon as an attack is suspected. More deaths could be prevented if heart attack victims did not delay going to a hospital. Studies have shown that, on the average, heart attack victims wait three hours before seeing a doctor.

In almost every case, hospitalization will be necessary following a heart attack. Treatment in the hospital will probably include care in the cardiac care unit (CCU), with limited physical activity at first and a gradual return to normal activities. In some cases, surgery to bypass the major obstructions in the arteries may be necessary.

A variety of medications are used to treat heart attack patients: anticoagulants, which thin the blood and prevent clots; digitalis, which establishes a steady heartbeat; anti-arrhythmics, which inhibit irregularities in the heartbeat; diuretics, which reduce strain on the heart by removing excess water from the blood; anti-anginals, which diminish chest pain; sedatives, which relax the body; and beta blockers, which ease the strain on the heart by decreasing its work. Beta blocker drugs have been found to be especially effective in preventing additional heart attacks in those who have survived the first heart attack. (Nevertheless, beta blockers should be used only with great caution by asthma sufferers, as these drugs can cause spasms in the air passages and subsequent breathing difficulties.)

Lifestyle changes will also help heart attack victims. Patients will be expected to stop smoking, perhaps lose weight, and partake in regular, moderate exercise.

Prevention

Prevention of heart attack begins with sensible health and dietary habits. Those who do not smoke, do not overeat or overindulge in saturated fats, and do not take birth control pills, but do exercise regularly and eliminate as much stress as possible from their lives are much less likely to become heart attack victims. Those who have already suffered one or more heart attacks can possibly prevent further attacks by changes in their living habits along these lines.

In the event of an attack, obtaining immediate medical attention can prevent death. A person with a suspected heart attack should not hesitate in going to the nearest hospital.

Heartbeat irregularities (arrhythmia)

Heartbeat irregularities (called arrhythmia) are defined as any deviation from the normal, steady beating of the heart, which is responsible for regular circulation of the blood throughout the body.

Minor irregularities in the heartbeat are common, but more serious arrhythmias can lead to fainting, angina (chest pain), or heart attack. The most devastating heartbeat irregularity is called ventricular fibrillation. This occurs when the normally steady pumping of the heart is reduced to a useless quivering, preventing the heart from pumping sufficient blood throughout the body. Ventricular fibrillation often occurs after a heart attack or some other serious injury, such as a severe electric shock, and it must receive immediate emergency medical attention or it can be fatal.

Causes

Arrhythmias are usually caused by damage to the heart muscle or to a small mass of specialized heart tissue called the sinus node. The sinus node, the natural pacemaker of the heart, is responsible for establishing and maintaining a healthy, steady heartbeat.

Heartbeat irregularities can also be caused by improper use of drugs (drugs prescribed for arrhythmia can actually cause it if dosage is too high); excessive smoking (the nicotine in cigarettes slows the heartbeat); or consumption of large quantities of caffeine (the high amounts found in coffee, tea, chocolate, cola, and some cold medicines may overstimulate the heart).

Heartbeat irregularities may also develop as a result of congenital damage (present at birth) to the heart; a poorly functioning left ventricle (the lower chamber of the heart that pumps blood into the arteries); high blood pressure; or a previous heart attack in which the resulting scar tissue interferes with the nerve impulses governing the heartbeat.

Symptoms

Some heartbeat irregularities have no noticeable symptoms. Others will be signaled by lightheadedness, fainting, a pounding heart, dizziness, and chest pain.

Diagnosis

Arrhythmias are diagnosed primarily with the electrocardiograph (ECG), which records the electrical impulses made by the heart's beating. A normal heart will produce a record of regular peaks and valleys; an arrhythmic heart will show an uneven pattern. Another method of diagnosing heartbeat irregularities is the injection of radioactive isotopes or X-ray contrast dyes into the bloodstream; in this way, the regular or irregular movement of blood through the heart can be traced.

Treatment

Occasionally, an arrhythmia is so mild that no particular treatment is required. But most irregularities are treated with medication, defibrillators, or pacemakers. All of these methods act to steady the irregularities and maintain a healthy, steady heartbeat.

Medications commonly used include digitalis, which slows the heartbeat; beta blockers, which correct extra beats originating in the lower chambers of the heart; and various antiarrhythmics, which act on specific problems of the heartbeat.

A defibrillator is a device applied to the chest which electrically jolts the quivering heart that is suffering from ventricular fibrillation back into a normal pattern of beating.

For those whose arrhythmia is caused by a faulty sinus node, an artificial pacemaker may be implanted in the heart. A pacemaker is a tiny electrical device powered by a small generator which, when implanted in the chest, acts to steady an abnormal heartbeat. Once inserted under the skin and threaded through a vein into the heart, it takes over the job of regulating the heartbeat by sending out electrical impulses similar to those emitted by the heart. Some pacemakers only go into action when the heart fails to beat after a specified time period; others completely take over the heart's job and are set to beat at a constant rate, usually about 72 times per minute.

Lifestyle changes will probably be recommended to patients suffering from heartbeat irregularities; they may need to quit smoking, lose weight, exercise more regularly, and reduce their caffeine intake. These precautions may also be taken in an effort to prevent arrhythmias.

Heart murmurs

Heart murmurs are extra whishing sounds — over and above the regular "lub-dub" sound of the heartbeat — made as blood flows through heart chambers and valves.

Innocent heart murmurs

Heart murmurs can be heard in many healthy people, especially children, teenagers, and pregnant women, and in these cases are considered innocent or functional because they are a normal sound caused by the blood rushing through the heart.

Abnormal heart murmurs

On the other hand, heart murmurs can be a symptom that first alerts a doctor to the possibility of a heart condition or disease. These abnormal murmurs come from vibrations or turbulence in the bloodstream. They are called organic or structural heart murmurs and can be caused by blood being forced through narrowed or obstructed heart valves, a defect in the heart walls; or valves that do not close completely and allow blood to seep back into the upper or lower heart chambers.

Causes

Heart murmurs can be congenital (existing at birth but not hereditary) or acquired because of rheumatic fever, atherosclerosis, syphilis, or other ailments.

Symptoms

Heart murmurs can be detected only by physical examination. A doctor listening to the heart, either directly or through a stethoscope, can usually distinguish any extra sound and identify whether or not it signifies a serious problem by its quality, intensity, location, and timing.

Diagnosis and treatment

A person with a functional or innocent heart murmur can live a completely normal life. If the heart murmur is organic or structural, the doctor will order tests (chest X ray, electrocardiogram, ultrasound, cardiac catheterization, echocardiogram, or fluoroscopy) to evaluate the extent of the condition and prescribe appropriate treatment.

Hemoglobin

Hemoglobin is the pigment (colored agent) in the blood that carries oxygen in the blood. The blood is made up of plasma (the liquid portion), various elements, white blood cells, and red blood cells. The white blood cells help the body fight infection, while the red blood cells carry oxygen throughout the body. The red blood cells are enabled to do this task by the presence of hemoglobin, which is formed when the red blood cells are developed in the bone marrow.

Functions

Each hemoglobin molecule is made up of a protein molecule (called *globin*) and four pigmented molecules made up of a compound called *heme*. Each heme molecule has one atom of iron; there are four heme molecules in a single molecule of hemoglobin, hence a single molecule of hemoglobin has four atoms of iron. This structure makes it possible for one hemoglobin molecule to join with four oxygen molecules to form a substance called *oxyhemoglobin*. This reaction is also reversible, thus enabling hemoglobin to pick up oxygen while the blood is in the lungs and deposit oxygen in the cells after the heart has pumped oxygenated blood into the circulatory system.

Anemia and other disorders

The blood of males usually has more hemoglobin per unit volume than that of females (14 to 16 grams per 100 milliliters of blood for men, but only 12 to 14 grams per 100 milliliters of blood for women). If the blood contains less than 12 grams of hemoglobin per 100 milliliters, it is considered below normal and the person with such blood is diagnosed as being anemic.

Hemoglobin disorders occur when there is a change in the chemical structure of the hemoglobin, thus reducing its oxygen-carrying or oxygen-releasing capabilities. One condition, called Bart's disease, for example, occurs when the internal composition of hemoglobin has a high attraction for oxygen, so that the hemoglobin can pick up and carry oxygen, but cannot readily give it up and release it to the body cells. Cancer of the bone marrow can also cause changes in hemoglobin, either in its composition or in its production. Because the pigmented portion of hemoglobin is made up of iron, a lack of iron in the diet also affects hemoglobin functions.

In addition to hemoglobin deficiencies, there are also conditions in which there is too much hemoglobin in the blood. For example, while an anemic person has less than 12 grams of hemoglobin per 100 milliliters of blood, a person suffering from polycythemia often has counts of more than 17.5 grams of hemoglobin per 100 milliliters of blood. It should be noted that the anemic person may or may not have a shortage of red blood cells, and (although the name implies differently) a person suffering from relative polycythemia does not necessarily have too many red blood cells. The problem is in the amount of hemoglobin the red blood cells carry, not in the number of red cells.

Hemorrhage

Hemorrhage is the technical term for bleeding, often referring to substantial blood loss or uncontrollable bleeding, either externally or internally. The effects of and damage from hemorrhage depend on the part of the body that is bleeding and the total amount of blood that is lost. Hemorrhage can be a symptom of a number of serious, sometimes fatal, disorders.

Causes

Hemorrhage occurs when blood vessels are torn or broken. In normal situations, blood clots within seconds or minutes, stopping the blood flow. However, when serious injuries or other disorders are involved, the body's normal blood-clotting function may be inadequate or malfunctioning; if blood loss is not quickly stopped, death may result.

When the blood-clotting mechanism is temporarily inadequate (usually caused by some kind of serious injury) or when the blood-clotting mechanism has been disrupted as a result of some disorder (including hemophilia, thrombocytopenia, peptic ulcer, cancer, or diseases involving the stomach, kidney, or urinary tract), internal hemorrhage may result.

Symptoms

Severe external hemorrhage displays the following symptoms: rapid pulse; dizziness or faintness; collapse; shock; a drop in blood pressure and a rise in pulse rate; and pale, cold, clammy, or sweaty skin.

Internal hemorrhage may also show symptoms, even if the bleeding is slight. Black, tarry stools may signal bleeding in the intestinal tract from a peptic ulcer or cancer of the colon; blood in the vomitus indicates bleeding in the stomach; and blood in the urine means bleeding is occurring in the kidneys or urinary tract.

Blood in the stool, urine, or vomitus should always be reported to a doctor at once, as should external bleeding that occurs frequently or that cannot be stopped within minutes or hours, depending on the severity of the wound.

Treatment

Treatment for internal hemorrhage involves correcting the cause of the bleeding, possibly with surgery. External hemorrhage is treated by applying pressure to the wound with a sterile bandage (or, in an emergency, just pressing it with the fingers) until the bleeding stops. If bleeding cannot be stopped, the patient will almost certainly be hospitalized, where lost blood can be replaced with blood transfusions or damaged blood vessels can be surgically tied off and sealed.

Hypertension

Hypertension, or high blood pressure, refers to persistently elevated pressure of blood within and against the walls of the arteries, which carry blood from the heart through the body. This excessive force being exerted on the artery walls may cause damage to the arteries themselves and thereby to body organs such as the heart, kidney, and brain, leading to heart attacks, kidney failure, and strokes.

Causes

Although many people believe hypertension is a condition caused by extreme activity or tension, this theory has not been proven. Actually, high blood pressure may have no known cause, or it can be associated with other diseases. When no underlying cause is discovered, the disease is called primary or essential hypertension. If another disease, such as kidney or heart disease, causes the elevated blood pressure, the condition is labeled secondary hypertension.

Those at risk

Contrary to popular belief,

there is no typical hypertensive person. However, there are some people more susceptible to developing high blood pressure. Persons with either one or both parents who are hypertensive are at greater risk of acquiring this condition since heredity may play a role in the development of hypertension. In the past, hypertension has been attributed to aging, but current evidence shows that age is not a primary factor. Blacks, both children and adults, have at least twice the incidence of hypertension as whites.

Overweight, prolonged stress, smoking, drinking, and excessive sodium (salt) in the diet causing fluid retention may increase blood pressure, especially in people prone to hypertension. There are also indications that oral contraceptives may contribute to increased blood pressure. However, this is more likely to occur with women who are overweight, whose parents are hypertensive, or who have other hypertensive risk factors.

Symptoms

Hypertension has been called the "silent disease," because it often has no obvious symptoms. A person may have high blood pressure for years without noticing any symptoms. What symptoms do occur may include headache, fatigue, dizziness, flushed face, ear ringing, thumping in the chest, or possibly frequent nosebleeds. However, these symptoms may result from other conditions.

Diagnosis

To diagnose hypertension, a simple, risk-free, painless test using a stethoscope and a sphygmomanometer, an inflatable arm cuff attached to a graduated mercury manometer (device measuring the tension of fluids), is used. Blood pressure is measured in a main artery of the arm by first shutting off and then releasing the flow of blood in the artery with the cuff and listening to the artery pulse with the stethoscope.

The blood pressure measurements are read as the systolic pressure (the first beat of the pulse after release of the cuff) over the diastolic pressure (the pressure at which the last beat is heard)—for example, 120/80 is considered normal in the average adult. The systolic pressure essentially measures the pressure of the heart during a contraction or heartbeat. The diastolic pressure is that which exists when the heart is filling between beats. Although diastolic pressure is considerably lower than systolic, there is still pressure in the body when the heart is filling. Therefore, both numbers count. An unusually high systolic pressure may mean the heart is pumping too hard or the arteries are stiff; a high diastolic pressure means that the arteries have an abnormally high tone or resistance.

Normal blood pressure is about 80/46 at birth and climbs as age increases. The normal adult pressure is around 120/80. Female hypertensives seem to do better than males; however, their risk of cardiovascular disease is still greater than that of normal females.

Treatment

Fortunately, hypertension responds well to treatment. When the condition is mild (systolic around 140 and diastolic 90 to 94) and there is no indication of other disease, doctors may suggest lifestyle changes before prescribing medication. These changes may include weight loss for the overweight; a regular exercise program; and strict limitation of salt (sodium) intake, which affects fluid balance and volume and therefore blood pressure. Controlling salt in the diet requires restriction of table salt as well as careful scrutiny of food and drug labels .

If medication is indicated, a physician may prescribe one drug or a combination of drugs as part of a "stepped care" program. Step one may start with a diuretic, a drug that promotes water loss. Step two may be a beta blocker, a medicine that reduces the work of the heart, or a "centrally acting" drug that lowers blood pressure by affecting the blood pressure center of the brain. Step three could be a vasodilator, a drug that dilates or opens narrowed blood vessels that contribute to hypertension by increasing resistance to flow. If none of the first three steps proves effective, a combination of two or more steps may be repeated or other still more potent drugs may be used—all under the physician's close supervision.

While tension and stress do not directly cause hypertension, these factors do affect the condition. Persons with hypertension are urged to avoid high-pressure situations and learn to deal with stress. Since techniques such as biofeedback, self-hypnosis, and meditation have proven useful for reducing stress, they may help someone with hypertension. Blood pressure can be monitored at home by purchasing a special kit and learning to use the sphygmomanometer. Children of hypertensive parents especially need to have their blood pressure measured early in life on a regular basis. If three separate elevated readings (above 140/90 in adults) are detected, a trip to the doctor is in order.

Hypotension

Hypotension is low blood pressure. Unlike chronic high blood pressure, which can be a serious health problem, low blood pressure is usually not a problem and need not be reason for concern.

Causes

Blood pressures vary depending on such factors as age, race, sex, and environment. On rare occasions, individuals may have medical problems that, themselves, cause low blood pressure. Among such conditions are some types of heart disease, hormonal deficiencies, and malnutrition. In these cases, the hypotension will be corrected by the treatment of the medical problem.

Postural hypotension

In addition, one form of low blood pressure called postural hypotension can cause dizziness or a feeling of faintness when a person stands up abruptly from a sitting or reclining position. Normally, when an individual stands up, the blood vessels contract and otherwise act to maintain normal blood pressure in the new position. However, in those persons with postural hypotension this mechanism probably does not work properly, and upon standing these people experience a temporary reduction in the blood flow to the brain that leads to dizziness. Also, if a person stands in one position long enough, blood pools in the veins of the legs, decreasing the amount of blood returned to the heart and therefore the amount pumped to the brain.

Sometimes postural hypotension results from medication for high blood pressure; in these cases, reducing the dosage or changing the medication will correct the problem. Often, postural hypotension is no cause for concern. Arising slowly will usually prevent the symptoms.

Ischemia

Ischemia is an inadequate flow of blood to a specific part of the body caused by an obstruction of the blood vessels supplying that part of the body. The obstruction is the result of the narrowing, compression, or destruction of arteries and is due to such factors or conditions as a blood clot or hardening of the arteries (atherosclerosis). In the latter condition, the hardened arteries gradually narrow to a point where not enough blood can pass through them.

Ischemia in the brain

An ischemic attack in the brain occurs when the supply of blood to the brain is reduced. This type of attack resembles a stroke. If the brain is deprived of blood, and thereby life-giving oxygen, for more than four minutes, the result is irreversible brain damage and often death.

Ischemia in the heart

When the blood supply to the heart is reduced, angina pectoris results. When the blood supply to the heart is cut off, a heart attack occurs. The less blood that gets through to the heart, the greater the severity of the attack. If a weakened heart is unable to pump an adequate supply of blood to other parts of the body, the other organs will work at less than capacity, and the whole system may break down.

Treatment

Occasionally, ischemic attacks can be controlled by medications called vasodilators that dilate or enlarge blood vessels. Angina pectoris is often managed in this way. For more serious cases, surgery to remove or to bypass the obstruction is recommended.

Lymphocytes

Lymphocytes are a type of white blood cell produced in the bone marrow and lymph nodes and stored in the thymus gland, spleen, and lymph nodes (which are found throughout the body; the most easily felt lymph nodes are found in the neck, armpits, and groin).

Function

Lymphocytes play an important role in the body's immunity. Divided into T and B cells, lymphocytes make their way through the lymph channels into the bloodstream, where they identify and "memorize" the characteristics of foreign elements called antigens. B cells manufacture antibodies, which are protein-based substances whose job is to destroy the antigens—also essentially proteins—by combining with them. T cells, which are 70 percent of the lymphocyte total, regulate antibody production and oversee immune responses.

Proportion in blood

Lymphocytes normally constitute between 22 and 28 percent of the white blood cells in an adult's circulation. In cases of infection, specifically those caused by viruses, the percentage of lymphocytes in the blood may increase to above 50 percent.

Lymphocytes are normally the second most numerous type of white blood cells in the body. The most common white blood cells are called polymorphonuclear leukocytes. These white blood cells act by engulfing bacteria and killing them.

Necrosis

Necrosis is the death of individual cells, groups of cells, or localized areas of tissue or bone while the surrounding tissue remains alive and healthy.

The tissue or bone dies because it has not survived the ravages of an infection or because it has been cut off from its blood supply by any one of several diseases or conditions. Necrosis can occur in tumors that outgrow their blood supply; in any area of the body where the nurturing blood vessels have been blocked by fatty deposits (atherosclerosis), clots, or emboli; in small areas of the heart following a heart attack; or in bones where osteomyelitis (inflammation of the bone due to infection) chokes off the arteries supplying the bone.

The symptoms and management of necrosis vary widely depending upon the underlying infection or blockage.

Pericarditis

Pericarditis is an inflammation of the membranous bag surrounding the heart, known as the pericardium. Often with pericarditis, a great deal of fluid collects between the membrane and the heart (an effusion), which may lead to complications.

Causes

The inflammation commonly stems from an infection, such as pneumonia or tuberculosis. Viral infections are also common causes of pericarditis. Pericarditis can also be seen in noninfectious diseases such as diseases of the connective tissues and chronic kidney failure. Occasionally, pericarditis can occur after a heart attack or chest injury.

Symptoms

Although mild pericarditis occurs commonly in conjunction with a viral infection, serious pericarditis is unusual. Pain in the center of the chest (and possibly the shoulders, neck and upper arms) that worsens with coughing, lying flat, or breathing may signify pericarditis. Since this type of pain is a symptom of several serious illnesses, a doctor should be consulted about any severe chest pain that lasts more than a few minutes.

Diagnosis

A chest X ray, electrocardiogram, and blood tests, along with the history and physical exam, will usually identify pericarditis and, often, its cause.

Treatment

When a large effusion exists, the motion of the heart may be restricted, thereby preventing it from filling and pumping effectively. This can be life-threatening and must be corrected as soon as possible. The fluid may be drained by inserting a needle through the chest into the pericardial sac. This is done either to diagnose the condition or to relieve the effusion. Once the cause is diagnosed, the doctor will treat the underlying cause (such as using dialysis in kidney failure or antibiotics for bacterial infection).

Constrictive pericarditis

Occasionally, long-term pericarditis arises from a chronic condition, most notably tuberculosis, but also from many other causes of pericarditis. The chronic inflammation causes thickening and contraction of the pericardium to the point that it restricts the heartbeat. Called constrictive pericarditis, this condition is not quite as common anymore because of the decrease in reported tuberculosis cases, but it is a severe condition calling for immediate attention.

With constrictive pericarditis, the legs and abdomen swell and, without surgery, this cannot be corrected. In this case, a pericardectomy to remove the scarred pericardium is the appropriate surgical procedure.

Platelets

Blood platelets (also called thrombocytes) are tiny disk-shaped cells that play a critical role in the process of blood coagulation, or clotting. They are manufactured in the bone marrow, and usually live for about ten days.

Proportion in blood

The number of platelets per unit volume of blood plays an important role in proper platelet function. The normal number ranges between 200,000 and 500,000 platelets per cubic millimeter of blood. Platelets initiate the coagulation process by aggregating (or clumping) together, and the usual amount of time for adequate coagulation is five minutes or less.

Blood coagulation is a complex process requiring the presence of many substances in the blood besides platelets. However, without platelets, coagulation would be impossible.

Low count

A low platelet count may be seen with many different diseases including certain liver diseases, uncommon forms of anemia caused by vitamin deficiencies, and certain cancers (such as leukemia) of the blood-forming organs.

The most common cause of a low platelet count is destruction of platelets by the body's immune system. For an unknown reason, the bodies of some individuals may recognize platelets as foreign, and these platelets will be destroyed by antibodies.

Treatment

When a lack of platelets prolongs bleeding time, several types of treatment may be attempted, depending on the cause of the low platelet count. If the platelet count is too low, prolonged bleeding results. If the platelet count is too high, emboli (clots or clumps of blood materials that obstruct vessels) may develop. Neither condition is desirable, so increasing platelet counts must be done with care.

The usual method to increase the number of platelets in the blood is by transfusion. These transfusions are normally reserved for patients with severe platelet deficiencies.

Care should be taken by any patient whose platelet count is low, since bleeding will be prolonged and coagulation will not occur within normal time limits. For this reason many physicians recommend that, until normal platelet counts are attained, patients should (in severe cases) avoid anything that may cause bleeding such as toothbrushes, abrasive foods, and enemas. They should also avoid any kind of contact sports and accidental hard contact with objects such as furniture or automobile doors.

Polycythemia

Polycythemia is a chronic disorder characterized by an increase in red blood cell mass and in concentration of hemoglobin (the substance in red blood cells that carries oxygen). Polycythemia literally means "many blood cells."

The exact cause of polycythemia remains unknown. The average age of the patient at onset of the disease is 60 years, but 5 percent are under 40 when the ailment first appears. It is more often seen in males and people of Jewish descent, but others are also affected. Its occurrence is rare; about seven per one million persons.

Symptoms

The initial symptoms include fatigue, difficulty in concentration, headache, drowsiness, forgetfulness, and dizziness. Half of its victims complain of itching, especially after a hot bath. Reddish skin color, or flushing, may be observed. On the other hand, patients may have completely normal skin color, with redness only of the mucous membranes, especially the inner lids of the eyes. Patients may complain of blurred vision, ringing in the ears, and circulatory disturbances.

Later symptoms include abnormal increase in all bone marrow material, abnormal increase in the body's blood volume, strain on the heart, and impaired blood flow.

Treatment

Phlebotomy—incision of a vein and withdrawal of blood to counterbalance the overproduction of red blood cells—is probably the safest treatment since it does not interfere with the functions of bone marrow. Usually, three to six separate phlebotomies are needed for red blood cell and hemoglobin levels to return to normal. Iron deficiency anemia often develops after a phlebotomy is performed. However, supplemental iron must not be given and foods with very high iron content should be avoided since they will raise the hemoglobin to abnormal levels. Phlebotomy followed by radiation therapy to suppress bone marrow activity produces positive results in most patients.

Pulmonary embolism

A pulmonary embolism is a clump of matter that blocks a blood vessel in the lungs. Emboli are composed of a variety of materials, and when they travel, they eventually come to vessels too tiny for them to pass. When this happens in the lungs, these clumps are called pulmonary emboli.

Causes

Emboli develop from a variety of causes. They may break off venous thrombi (blood clots that originate chiefly in the lower extremities, especially the thigh), which may be caused by an increase in number and clumping of platelets (the blood elements that help in clotting), as the result of injury, surgery, and peripheral

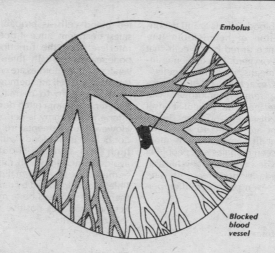

Pulmonary embolism occurs when the blood vessels of the lungs are blocked by a clump of matter. The blood supply in the area behind the blockage is thus cut off.

vascular diseases. Also, venous thrombi are sometimes the result of an increase in the thickness of the blood (as would occur in polycythemia—a chronic disorder characterized by an increase in the total number of red blood cells in the blood).

Other types of emboli may consist of either pieces of matter that have broken loose from their points of origin (as in pieces of tumors or whole tumors) or the clumping of blood cells around a foreign body such as a catheter particle or a foreign protein (for example, venom or other poisonous substances).

Emboli may be classified as solid (detached blood clots, clumps of tumor cells, or bits of foreign objects); liquid (globules of fat); or gaseous (air). Emboli may also be either bland (non-poisonous) or septic (poisonous or infectious). Any one or more of these types of emboli may find its way into the lungs and become a pulmonary embolus.

Symptoms

The sudden development of the following symptoms may indicate the presence of a pulmonary embolus: wheezing; dyspnea (labored or difficult breathing); chest pains; hemoptysis (spitting up blood); unexplained low oxygen levels in arterial blood; and right heart strain, as indicated on an ECG (electrocardiogram).

Diagnosis

Diagnostic procedures for

detection of pulmonary embolism may include a test of arterial blood (blood pumped out of the heart), an ECG, and a lung scan with X rays. The definitive diagnostic procedure is pulmonary angiography, which consists of an X-ray scan of the lungs after the introduction of a dye into the bloodstream. This will show the embolus in relief against the contrast dye and can pinpoint its location. As serious as pulmonary emboli potentially are, only a small number are lethal.

Treatment

In the event of pulmonary embolism, oxygen is administered, and blood pressure as well as heart functions are supported by medication or manual resuscitation, if necessary. Anticoagulant medication (to slow blood clotting) is administered, in order to prevent the development of additional emboli. The drugs usually given are heparin and warfarin.

In about 20 percent of pulmonary embolism cases in which a venous thrombus is determined to be the origin, the inferior vena cava (the main vein for the lower limbs and the pelvis) may be deliberately blocked by an "umbrella filter" or a clip in order to keep a venous thrombus from traveling farther.

Sometimes the embolism must be removed surgically. This is done only when the patient demonstrates low blood pressure as a side effect of the embolus, and when surgery can be done only a few hours after the embolism has occurred.

Prevention

The best prevention of pulmonary emboli is early detection and treatment of venous thrombosis.

Raynaud's phenomenon and disease

Raynaud's phenomenon and disease involve a spasm or spasms of the arterioles (small artery branches), especially in the fingers and hands and occasionally in other parts, such as the nose and tongue. It is often accompanied by intermittent paleness or cyanosis (bluish discoloration) of the skin.

Causes

Raynaud's phenomenon may be of unknown cause, in which case it is called Raynaud's disease, or it may be a secondary symptom of conditions such as connective tissue disorders (scleroderma), nerve disorders, drug reactions, pulmonary hypertension, and myxedema (a dry, waxy swelling of the skin sometimes called "non-pitting edema"). If it is caused by another condition, it is called Raynaud's phenomenon.

For whatever reason, Raynaud's disease is most common in young women. Often, the attacks are precipitated by exposure to cold or by emotional upsets or stress.

Symptoms

The color changes in the skin

may come in three stages—pallor (extreme paleness), cyanosis, and then extreme redness, called reactive hyperemia. On the other hand, the color changes may go through only two cycles: cyanosis and then redness. Normal color and sensation are restored when the hands are warmed. Color changes in the hands do not affect the joints and seldom affect the thumb. Pain is usually not present, but numbness, tingling, or burning are common complaints.

Raynaud's disease differs from secondary Raynaud's phenomenon in that both sides of the body are involved. Raynaud's disease also tends to continue for at least two years with no progression of symptoms.

If Raynaud's phenomenon is associated with diseases such as scleroderma, there can also be tightness and thickening of the skin of the hands, arms, and face; difficulty in swallowing; painful open sores on the fingertips or along the nails; blood vessel lesions on the hands, wrist, and lips; and sometimes, blockage of an artery in the wrist.

Treatment

Therapy for secondary Raynaud's phenomenon depends chiefly on diagnosing correctly and then treating the underlying disturbance.

Mild cases of Raynaud's disease can be helped substantially by protecting the body and extremities from extreme cold. Also mild sedatives, taken orally, can be of help. The patient is always advised to stop smoking, since nicotine acts as a constrictor of blood vessels. Reserpine, an antihypertensive and tranquilizer, may be useful but there are side effects, such as depression.

A more extreme measure is regional sympathectomy (an interruption of some part of the nerve pathways). This operation is reserved for patients with progressive disability; while it abolishes the symptoms, the relief may last for only a year or two. Results of the surgery are usually better in patients with Raynaud's disease than in those with the secondary phenomenon.

Restless legs syndrome

"Restless legs" syndrome (also called Ekbom syndrome, "jimmy legs," or "jitter legs") is a feeling of uneasiness, shakiness, twitching, and restlessness that affects the legs after a patient has gone to bed for the night. Insomnia is almost always a result of the syndrome.

Causes

Precise cause of the syndrome is not known, although some authorities consider it to be brought about, or intensified, by poor blood circulation. It is most common in neurotic (mildly psychologically disturbed) individuals, but is also seen in normal persons. Some physicians claim that it is more common in hyperactive patients; others say that it can be brought about by intense activity, especially physical activity, just before bedtime.

Treatment

Since the syndrome has been connected with circulatory disorders, drugs that increase the circulation to the lower extremities may prove helpful. A mild sedative at bedtime is also useful in preventing insomnia.

Rheumatic fever

Rheumatic fever is the result of a bacterial disease characterized by inflammation, swelling, and soreness of the joints—especially the ankles, knees, and wrists — and inflammation of the heart. Commonly occurring in children and adolescents, it is a serious illness that can result in permanent damage to the heart. The attacks of fever may recur over a period of years and last from a few weeks to several months.

Cause

The disease is considered to be a late stage of a streptococcal infection such as a "strep throat," even though in some cases the earlier infection may have been so minor that it cannot be recalled. The body's immune system, by which antibodies are formed to attack infecting bacteria, apparently becomes disordered and the antibodies turn on healthy tissues such as that of the joints and the heart. The disease is more prevalent in some families than in others; but whether this indicates a hereditary factor or is due simply to sharing the same environment and living habits is not clear. Only 1 percent of all cases of streptococcal infection in children and adolescents are followed by rheumatic fever, so it is believed that a special susceptibility may be involved.

Symptoms

Rheumatic fever should immediately be suspected when a child or teenager develops an unexplained fever with joint inflammation a few weeks after an untreated (or unrecognized) throat infection or tonsillitis. Other joints then become inflamed one after another, and a peculiar skin rash develops, lasting a day or two. Nodules may emerge over the elbows, kneecaps, and other bony prominences; they may even form within the heart. Chorea, a spasmodic jerking and twitching of the limbs and facial features, may be among the symptoms if the infection spreads to involve the brain. Fortunately, it leaves no lasting brain damage and passes off after sometime, even without specific treatment.

Effects on the heart

The acute stage of joint involvement leaves no permanent deformity or crippling, but damage to the heart is permanent when it involves destruction of heart valve tissue. Scar tissue is then eventually formed on the valves, so that they cannot open and close properly. The heart,

Fever

Inflammation of brain

Initial symptoms: tonsillitis or sore throat

Skin rashes

Inflammation of heart valves

Nervous system attacked

Inflammation of joints

Nodules over joints

Rheumatic fever begins with a sore throat or tonsillitis that progressively leads to other symptoms.

unable to carry out efficiently its function of pumping blood through the circulatory system, must work harder and becomes enlarged. Blood clots may form on its inner lining and be carried in the blood throughout the body, often lodging in a blood vessel and blocking it.

Treatment

The chief treatment for rheumatic fever is the use of antibiotics over an extended period of time—long enough to eliminate all bacteria. Aspirin is commonly used to bring down fever and relieve inflammation and pain. Hormones such as cortisone are usually given if there are signs of heart involvement, and sedatives may be prescribed if chorea becomes severe. The long periods of immobilization in bed once recommended are now believed to be unnecessary, although bed rest during acute attacks may be prescribed. Seriously damaged heart valves can often be repaired surgically or even replaced by artificial valves.

Prevention

The only form of prevention of rheumatic fever is prompt diagnosis and adequate treatment of all streptococcal infections in children and young people, especially those involving the throat and ears. Since dental procedures can sometimes be a source of bacterial infection, it has been suggested that special precautions be taken during dental treatment (such as the administration of antibiotics).

Rheumatic heart disease

Rheumatic heart disease consists of a variety of abnormal cardiac conditions, including heart valve scarring, and endocarditis (inflammation of the lining of the heart).

Cause

This disease is a potential aftermath of rheumatic fever, once one of the prime killers of children. Rheumatic fever is an inflammatory disease that primarily affects the heart, tendons, joints, and arteries. Rheumatic fever may cause an inflammation of the heart valves that reduces their ability to close. This allows oxygenated blood that should be pumped out to the body from the heart's left ventricle (lower chamber) to seep back into the left atrium (upper chamber), thereby reducing the total amount of oxygenated blood in the circulatory system. This, in turn, causes a chronic feeling of tiredness on the part of the patient, which is unrelieved when the primary rheumatic fever symptoms finally disappear.

The heart tends to enlarge drastically during this phase of the disease in order to meet the system's demands for fresh blood. As the heart grows larger, it sometimes grows less able to supply itself with blood. As a result, a point of diminishing returns is reached, and the patient's activities sometimes become permanently restricted, leading to a completely sedentary life.

Chronic effects

Among the chronic effects of rheumatic heart disease are: heart "murmur," caused by the backflow of blood from the left ventricle into the left atrium; the formation of microscopic blood clots in the heart, which can break loose, enter the bloodstream, and find their way into the vessels of the retina (the light-sensitive tissue lining the back of the eye), causing hemorrhaging (internal bleeding) and possible impairment of vision; kidney dysfunction in middle or later life; shrinkage of muscular tissue from underactivity; irregular pulse, shortness of breath, and fainting spells; and lack of muscular or cardiovascular endurance.

Treatment

Presently, rheumatic fever is treatable by a number of antibiotics. Penicillin has been used for 30 years as a preventive against recurrences. Many victims of rheumatic heart disease, even those who contracted it in the late 1930s, have gone on to live extremely active lives, despite heart murmurs, heart enlargements, and damaged valves. Although rheumatic heart disease is a serious matter, regular exercise, a sensible diet, and quiet determination can mean the difference between a sedentary and an active life.

Supervision by a physician is a must for anyone who suffers from rheumatic heart disease and wants to embark on a regular exercise program. In some cases, however, it may be impossible for a patient to participate in vigorous physical activity, especially if the heart damage is advanced or severe. For some of these individuals, surgery to implant an artificial valve can offer relief.

Rh factor

Rh factor refers to a characteristic of blood in which it can be classified as either Rh positive or Rh negative. Rh positive blood has the Rh (named for the Rhesus monkey, in whom it was first discovered) antigen on its red cells; Rh negative blood does not. An antigen is a substance that can provoke an immune, or protective, response to the presence of foreign bodies. An estimated 85 percent of the population has Rh positive blood, that is to say, they possess the Rh antigens.

Blood consists of several components: plasma (the liquid portion), erythrocytes (red blood cells, which contain hemoglobin, their oxygen-carrying element), platelets (tiny cells which play a critical role in the coagulation process), white blood cells, and various other elements. Yet it is the antigens that induce the production of antibodies whose action is crucial to the functioning of the body's immune system.

Antigens and blood types

Each antigen causes the manufacture of antibodies that will interact only with that antigen. These antibodies will treat blood not of its type as a foreign substance. Transfusions of blood of different blood groups (Types A, B, AB, or O) will not be successful:

the blood of the person receiving the transfusion will reject the blood being transfused.

Each of the lettered blood groups has different antigens, hence different antibodies. They are as distinctive as fingerprints. Within this classification, Type A has antigen A on its red cells, Type B has antigen B on its red cells, Type AB has both antigen A and antigen B on its red cells, and Type O has neither antigen A nor antigen B on its red cells.

Blood of different types and different Rh factors literally do not mix. Type A blood plasma, for example, does not contain any anti-A antibodies. It does, however, contain anti-B antibodies. If Type B blood is transfused, the anti-B antibodies in the plasma will destroy the type B red cells that have type B antigens on them.

Blood normally has no anti-Rh antibodies. But these anti-Rh antibodies can develop in the Rh negative blood if Rh positive blood is introduced into the bloodstream. This can come about in two ways: if a person with Rh negative blood receives a transfusion of Rh positive blood, or if a woman with Rh negative blood conceives a baby with Rh positive blood (inherited from the father) and some of the Rh positive substance from the unborn baby finds its way into the bloodstream of the mother.

Dangers of anti-Rh antibodies

In either of these cases, the Rh positive red cells will stimulate the person's body to form anti-Rh antibodies. If this happens, the blood will form clumps and a potentially lethal situation will develop: the clumps may block the blood vessels, leading to death.

If difficulties do not appear with the formation of these antibodies during the first transfusion or the first pregnancy, they will surely appear if any Rh positive blood is ever again introduced into the person's bloodstream. The antibodies are already present, and the introduction of additional Rh positive blood will result in a mobilization of existing antibodies and the production of even more. In addition to clumping of blood, other problems will arise. For example, hemolysis (the liberation of hemoglobin from the red blood cells) will make it impossible for the red cells to carry oxygen, thus producing the symptoms of anemia and lack of oxygen.

There are potential dangers to an unborn baby if the mother's blood contains anti-Rh antibodies. If the unborn baby has Rh positive cells, anti-Rh antibodies may pass through the placenta from the mother's bloodstream to cause hemolysis of the baby's blood cells. Once born, the baby may have to have massive, possibly total, transfusions of Rh negative blood to prevent clumping, as well as hemolytic anemia. Nowadays, this situation is relatively rare following the introduction of injections given to the Rh negative mother after the birth of her first Rh positive baby. These injections inhibit the formation of the potentially dangerous antibodies.

Stroke

Stroke is an interruption of the blood supply to a group of brain cells, damaging those cells and causing malfunction or lack of function in those parts of the body that the damaged cells control. Generally speaking, each side of the brain controls the motor and sensory functions of the opposite side of the body, so damage to cells on the left side of the brain, for instance, will impair function on the right side of the body.

Stroke can have a wide range of consequences; it may, among other conditions, cause temporary or permanent loss of memory and difficulty in speaking, walking, and controlling emotions.

Causes

Stroke can be caused by several conditions. One is called cerebrovascular embolism, which occurs when a "wandering" blood clot, formed elsewhere in the body (usually in the heart or in one or both carotid arteries in the neck that carry blood from the heart to the brain), lodges itself in an artery leading to or within the brain. Interruption of blood flow also occurs when a similar clot is formed in the arteries because of the presence of atherosclerosis (a narrowing and clogging of the arteries by various deposits).

Stroke can also be caused by cerebral hemorrhage, in which a diseased artery in the brain bursts, depriving the cells that are normally nourished by that artery, as well as flooding the surrounding tissue with blood. This accumulation of blood forms a clot which displaces and compresses brain tissue and thus interferes in the brain's functioning. This type of stroke often strikes people who have both hypertension (high blood pressure) and atherosclerosis.

A third condition that can lead to stroke may be an aneurysm (a bulge in an artery because of a defect in its wall) that ruptures and interrupts blood flow to an area of the brain as well as flooding the area with blood. The formation of aneurysms is sometimes associated with hypertension, but is often congenital (present at birth). Thus aneurysms are often the cause of cerebral hemorrhage in young people.

Those at risk

People who have both hypertension and atherosclerosis are the most likely to suffer a stroke, since both diseases weaken and damage the arteries. Hypertension probably encourages hemorrhage. Heredity may play a role in stroke, since the tendencies to develop both hypertension and atherosclerosis appear to be inherited. Black people are more likely candidates for stroke because high blood pressure is at least twice as common among blacks as among whites.

Smoking, diabetes, and high blood cholesterol may also contribute to stroke. Furthermore, stroke is more likely to victimize anyone with a history of mild stroke-like episodes called TIAs (transient ischemic attacks). TIAs are essentially strokes that clear up within 24 hours, that is, an individual may develop paralysis of one side of the body as in a classic stroke, but the symptoms clear within 24 hours, leaving no residual effects.

Symptoms

A stroke can present itself in many ways, but some of the more common symptoms are a sudden weakness or numbness in the face, arm, and/or leg on one side of the body; loss or slurring of speech or difficulty in understanding others speak; unexplained unsteadiness, and persistent falling to one side. It is possible, however, to suffer a mild stroke and experience minor degrees of these symptoms.

Diagnosis

Stroke is diagnosed mostly by the history and physical examination. Sophisticated X-ray techniques are also employed. For example, arteriography (the injection of X-ray opaque dye into a main artery) will show damage or clots in the arteries leading to or within the brain, and a computerized axial tomography (CAT) scan produces a cross-sectional picture of the area, which can provide the physician with crucial information such as whether the stroke was caused by a hemor-

rhage or by blockage of blood flow. Tumors, which can cause symptoms identical to that of stroke, are also frequently diagnosed by these means.

Treatment

Treatment of stroke begins with immediate hospitalization. Blood pressure is normalized and drug therapy to prevent further damage as well as to reduce swelling of the brain tissue is often instituted. Also, depending on the cause of the stroke and other factors, anticoagulants (agents that inhibit the normal clotting of blood) are sometimes administered in the hope of limiting the progress of the stroke or preventing additional strokes. After the acute period, rehabilitation is begun by speech, physical, and occupational therapists.

Prevention

For those who have experienced TIAs or other warning signs of stroke, precautions can be taken to prevent an actual stroke. Usually after a TIA, some form of arteriography is performed to locate obstructions or ulcerated areas of the carotid arteries. Depending on the results of the arteriogram along with the general condition of the patient and many other factors, the decision of whether to operate (to "clean out" the arteries) or to treat with anticoagulants is made.

Prevention of stroke mainly involves control of high blood pressure and other risk factors such as smoking and high cholesterol intake.

Thrombocytopenia

Thrombocytopenia is a disorder characterized by a decrease in the number of platelets in the blood. Platelets are tiny components of the blood that act to promote clotting when there is an injury or other problem that requires bleeding to be stopped. Normally there are about five to ten times the number of platelets needed for clotting circulating in the bloodstream; this amounts to about 200,000 to 500,000. Thrombocytopenia is present usually when platelet counts are less than 100,000. Abnormal bleeding commonly does not occur, however, until the count is less than 50,000, and serious or unprovoked bleeding usually does not occur with counts above 20,000.

Causes

There are basically two mechanisms whereby thrombocytopenia occurs: decreased production and increased destruction of platelets. In the former, the elements in the bone marrow responsible for the production of platelets may be severely diminished (as in aplastic anemia where all of the blood-forming elements are diminished or absent) or may malfunction. Increased destruction of platelets occurs in diseases such as essential or idiopathic (of unknown cause) thrombocytopenia. In this

disorder, which is common in children, antibodies are made against the individual's own platelets thereby causing their destruction. Drug-induced thrombocytopenia can be due to this same mechanism or others. Severe, overwhelming infection can also cause increased destruction of platelets. In pregnancy, platelets from the fetus can sometimes escape into the circulation of the mother causing antibody formation and the consequent destruction of fetal platelets with abnormal bleeding at birth.

Symptoms

Signs and symptoms of thrombocytopenia include reddish to reddish-purple spots on the skin, seen as a rash. These are due to bleeding within and underneath the skin. Abnormal or easily provoked bleeding is the most dangerous symptom of thrombocytopenia. This bleeding can be minor such as oozing from the gums while brushing the teeth, or bruising caused merely by leaning on or brushing up against something. The bleeding can also be major as in spontaneous internal bleeding that may go unrecognized until shock appears.

Treatment

Treatment depends on the cause. If infection is present, this must be remedied and the platelet count will usually return to normal on its own. In essential or idiopathic thrombocytopenia, corticosteroids (cortisone or prednisone) are the first line of treatment. In drug-induced thrombocytopenia, the first move is to discontinue the drug. This will usually result in improvement; if not, corticosteroids may be helpful in some cases. In immune thrombocytopenia of the newborn, if severe, exchange transfusion (where all or most of the blood is exchanged with transfused blood) may be necessary. If the platelet count in any of these conditions is dangerously low (around 20,000), transfusion of platelets until the disease process is controlled is indicated.

Prevention

Thrombocytopenia may not be preventable in most cases, but early recognition of symptoms and signs such as rash and easy bleeding may lead to prevention of serious complications.

Thrombophlebitis

Thrombophlebitis is a condition in which both inflammation and blood clots exist in a vein. This can be caused by a number of factors. Commonly, when a person is immobilized, blood stagnates in the veins of the legs; this induces clotting which in turn prevents blood from returning to the heart. The blood below the clot remains there, causing a buildup of pressure that forces fluid into the tissues thus resulting in swelling. Also, simultaneously, the vein(s) and surrounding area may become quite inflamed and tender. This condition is most often found in the deep veins of the legs, but it can also occur in veins of the pelvis and arms.

Thrombophlebitis itself may not be too serious, but it can lead to a life-threatening condition called pulmonary embolism (a blood clot lodged in the lung). This develops when a clot formed in a deep leg vein breaks loose, travels through the bloodstream, and becomes lodged in the vessels of the lung. A pulmonary embolism can lead to chest pain, shortness of breath, coughing up of blood, and even death.

Causes

The development of thrombophlebitis is favored by any condition that inhibits the free flow of blood through the veins. These include prolonged bed rest or inactivity, perhaps following illness or surgery; congestive heart failure, which affects the heart's ability to pump blood throughout the body; and injury or infection that damages a vein. Other factors that may lead to an increased tendency toward thrombophlebitis are the use of birth control pills in susceptible individuals, as well as pregnancy itself; occupations that require long periods of standing or sitting; obesity; old age; and chronic infections. In addition, thrombophlebitis, in some cases, may indicate the presence of a tumor in the pancreas or lung, since these disorders might produce or release a substance that affects blood clotting.

Symptoms

Common symptoms (which often appear only in advanced cases) of deep thrombophlebitis are swelling, aching, and a feeling of heaviness in the leg or affected area; the skin may appear white and will be painful to the touch. If the veins of the leg are affected, the condition is characterized by increased pain when walking or when the foot is flexed backward or forward.

Diagnosis

Thrombrophlebitis of a surface vein (known as superficial thrombophlebitis) can be diagnosed by a simple physical examination usually revealing a red, warm, tender cord-like vein. Superficial thrombophlebitis rarely, if ever, leads to pulmonary embolism.

Diagnostic tests for thrombophlebitis include the Doppler (a technique used to detect obstructions by changes in sounds made by flowing blood), nuclear scans, a test to measure the resistance to flow in the veins, and venography. Venography involves the insertion of X-ray contrast dye into the veins so that the X ray will visualize a clot. This is the most sensitive and specific test for thrombophlebitis.

Treatment

Treatment of superficial thrombophlebitis consists of bed rest with elevation of the leg. Warm compresses are also helpful as are anti-inflammatory drugs.

Deep vein thrombophlebitis, because of the potential for pulmonary embolism, is treated much more aggressively. The patient is usually hospitalized and put on bed rest with the leg elevated. The anticoagulant (an anticoagulant is an agent that inhibits the normal clotting mechanisms of the blood) heparin is given intravenously, usually for about seven days and up to ten days if pulmonary embolism has occurred. The patient is also usually placed on the oral anticoagulant warfarin for about six weeks or three to six months if pulmonary embolism has occurred. It is important to note that these drugs do not dissolve an existing clot, but serve to prevent new clots from forming while the old ones are resolving. Newer drugs do dissolve clots, but are still used only in special situations.

Prevention

Prevention of thrombophlebitis is a controversial subject. In hospitalized patients who are immobilized for long periods or about to undergo major surgery, leg exercises along with long support stockings and increased activity as soon as feasible may be helpful. So-called "mini-heparin" (low doses of heparin given by injection under the skin two to three times a day) has also been beneficial in preventing deep vein thrombophlebitis in certain patients. For nonhospitalized patients who are susceptible to this condition, regular exercise of the legs along with elevation of legs when lying down and support hose are probably helpful. Self-injected heparin and warfarin are also used.

Transient ischemic attacks (TIAs)

Transient ischemic attacks (TIAs) are sudden, neurologic deficits (such as loss of vision in one eye, inability to speak, paralysis, or weakness of one side of the body) that last for less than 24 hours. Although they are similar in appearance to minor strokes, they do no discernible lasting damage to the brain's functions.

Causes

TIAs are probably due to an interruption in blood flow to an area of the brain. They can be caused by a narrowing in the carotid arteries (the arteries in the neck that supply the brain with oxygenated blood). This narrowing is usually due to the presence of atherosclerosis. Blood vessel spasms and showers of tiny emboli (clots that travel to the brain) are also possible causes.

Symptoms

The symptoms of transient ischemic attacks are both varied and frightening to the victim. They can include weakness of the side of the face; numbness in various parts of the body; blindness in one eye; weakness in the arms or legs on one side; difficulty in speaking and/or understanding

speech; and prickling or "pins and needles" sensation in parts of the body. Vertigo (sensation of spinning) combined with any of these symptoms and others can also be due to TIAs. Fainting spells alone and dizziness (light-headedness) are usually not due to TIAs.

The major importance of transient ischemic attacks is their use in the diagnosis of stroke. Any such attack may be a predictor of stroke. Often, when a person describes a "light stroke," he or she is really talking about a transient ischemic attack. If left unattended, TIAs can indeed lead to major strokes, with permanent damage to all parts affected, as well as to the possibility of sudden death.

Diagnosis

The first line of attack in diagnosis is a complete examination, including history and physical, neurological, and eye exams. "Bruits," noises caused by narrowing in an artery, can be heard in a carotid artery. Detailed testing, commonly with arteriography (injection of X-ray contrast into the artery with subsequent X-ray pictures taken), is performed to determine the problem.

Treatment

Treatment of TIAs is aimed at preventing stroke. There are two basic methods of treatment: medical with anticoagulant drugs, and surgical with the opening and "cleaning out" of the artery (arteries). Which one of these methods is more effective in preventing further TIAs and/or stroke is dependent on many factors and is presently a subject of considerable controversy. TIAs can be an indication of serious problems and, if experienced, must be brought to the attention of a physician immediately.

Varicose veins

Varicose veins are swollen, stretched veins in the legs, close to the surface of the skin, caused by pooling of blood.

Blood from the legs needs to return uphill, against the force of gravity, to the heart, so the veins in the legs are lined with one-way valves to prevent blood from flowing back down toward the feet. When pressure on the veins stretches them, the valves cannot close properly, and some blood travels back down. This blood accumulates in pools, which stretch the veins even more. The result is varicose veins, highly visible bluish lines that bulge from the legs and that can be very painful.

Varicose veins alone are not too serious, but they may lead to other conditions: a leg ulcer (an eroded patch on the skin); phlebitis (an inflamed vein); or a blood clot (a thrombus).

Causes

Varicose veins are caused by a number of factors that put excess pressure on the veins in the legs: prolonged standing; prolonged sitting, especially with the legs crossed; lack of exercise; confining clothes; a diet low in fiber (hard stools and the pressure needed to excrete them put extra stress on the veins); obesity (which puts excess pressure on the legs and contributes to the muscles' inability to push blood upward); heredity (a tendency toward weak vein walls and valves seems to be inherited); and even height (tall people may be more likely to develop this conditon because their blood needs to travel farther in its return trip to the heart).

Pregnancy greatly contributes to the development of varicose veins because female hormones, especially those released at this time, tend to relax the walls of the veins. Thus, the condition is more commonly seen in women than in men. Varicose veins often appear during the last few months of pregnancy due to the increased strain from the weight of the growing uterus. These veins may recede, however, after the baby is born.

Symptoms

Varicose veins are very noticeable since they form close to the skin. They appear as bulging, bluish, cord-like lines running down the legs. Symptoms that accompany varicose veins are feelings of achiness, heaviness, and fatigue in the legs, especially

Normal

Varicose vein

At top, the illustration shows the interior of a normal vein, in which blood returning to the heart is not allowed to drop downward by the action of the valve. In the bottom drawing, the vein's valve has been weakened and cannot completely close, thus resulting in an accumulation of excess blood in the vein. The result is a varicose vein.

at the end of the day; itchy, scaly skin covering the affected areas; and, in advanced cases, swollen ankles, pain shooting down the leg, and leg cramps at night.

Treatment

Varicose veins are usually treated by wearing elastic stockings, which act like muscles to help push the blood upward. Severe cases may require a surgical procedure called vein stripping, in which the afflicted veins are tied off and removed; other healthy veins in the area will take over the job of pushing blood toward the heart. A chemical can also be injected into the veins, closing them off and forcing the blood to find other channels to the heart. However, this procedure can cause more complications, so it is not performed as often as surgery.

Those with varicose veins may need to lose weight, increase the fiber in their diets, exercise regularly, and stretch their legs or put their feet up whenever possible. Exercises to improve circulation in the legs may help relieve pressure.

THE DIGESTIVE SYSTEM

Digestion is the process whereby the body converts food into basic substances that can either be absorbed in the bloodstream as nutrients or passed out of the body as waste. This breakdown and assimilation occurs within the digestive tract, a convoluted tube over 30 feet long lined by a mucous membrane that aids in absorbing nutrients. The tract includes several hollow organs — mouth, esophagus, stomach, small intestine, and large intestine (colon)—each of which has a specific function in digestion. Muscles of these organs move the food through the system while mucus lubricates the tract and prevents irritation. Solid organs—the liver, gallbladder, and pancreas — also are critical in digestion.

Food first enters the digestive tract through the mouth. In the mouth, the jaws and teeth chew the food into smaller pieces that are mixed with saliva, a secretion of the salivary glands in the mouth. Saliva moistens food for easier swallowing and contains an enzyme (a special protein) that begins breakdown of starches.

From the mouth, food passes down the throat and into the esophagus (a muscular tube) through which it is conducted to the stomach. The stomach is a large pouch or sac in the abdominal cavity where food is combined with acid and digestive juices secreted by gastric glands within the stomach. The food becomes semifluid so that it can pass into the small intestine.

In the first ten inches (duodenum) of the small intestine, food is broken down further with additional digestive juices from the liver and pancreas. This process further separates nutrients and allows for their absorption into the bloodstream, which takes place in the remainder of the small intestine.

Aiding digestion is the liver, an accessory organ of digestion. The liver produces bile that is necessary for absorption of fat in the small intestine. The liver also functions to purify and remove some wastes from the blood, as well as to produce and store glucose and to process many drugs.

The gallbladder on the underside of the liver is another organ that provides an indirect digestive function. The gallbladder stores the bile manufactured by the liver. As bile is needed, the gallbladder contracts and releases the fluid into the small intestine.

Other digestive juices required by the small intestine to digest and absorb food, particularly fats and starches, come from the pancreas, an organ located just under the

Salivary gland
Mouth
Teeth
Esophagus
Liver
Gallbladder
Stomach
Pancreas
Bile duct
Duodenum
Small intestine
Large intestine (colon)
Appendix
Rectum
Anus

The digestive system includes the mouth, esophagus, stomach, small intestine, large intestine, liver, gallbladder, and pancreas, each of which plays a specific role in digestion.

stomach. The pancreas also secretes insulin and other hormones into the blood. Insulin is the hormone responsible for aiding absorption and use of glucose (sugar).

Whatever substances are not assimilated into the bloodstream through the small intestine move into the large intestine. Within the large intestine, waste material is processed into stool (feces). At this point, too, water is absorbed to preserve the body's balance of fluids.

The left colon then stores the fecal matter until its transfer to the rectum, its lower part. Once in the rectum, waste is ready to be passed out of the body through the opening at the end of the digestive tract (anus).

Appendicitis

Appendicitis is an inflammation of the appendix that results from a bacterial infection.

The appendix is a small worm-like portion of intestinal tissue located at the juncture of the small and large intestines. Although it may have had a function at some point in human development, the appendix serves no purpose now.

Causes

Nevertheless, despite its uselessness, the appendix can cause problems when it becomes inflamed. Inflammation occurs when the hollow tubular structure clogs with masses of waste matter, intestinal worms, or other material that can prevent normal drainage. The blockage provides a fertile environment for bacteria to grow and multiply, thereby causing infection and inflammation.

Symptoms

In the beginning, appendicitis may produce a dull or sharp pain in the navel area of the abdomen. Any movement, coughing, or sneezing can intensify the pain. Patients in early stages may also feel nauseous and be unable to eat. Constipation usually accompanies appendicitis; nonetheless about 10 percent of the patients may have diarrhea instead. Adults may run a mild fever (up to 102°F), but children generally experience higher fevers. Occasionally, pulse rates accelerate to about 100 beats per minute.

Within hours, the pain becomes continuous and moves to the lower right side of the abdomen over the appendix. Because the location of the appendix may vary depending upon the individual, pain may emanate from the back, side, or pelvis, or even the opposite side of the abdomen. The entire appendix area becomes extremely tender as abdominal muscles tighten.

If fever rises and pain grows more intense, chances of rupture become greater. Rupture results when the appendix becomes so swollen and filled with pus from bacteria that it bursts, spreading infection to surrounding organs. Infection spreads so quickly that gangrene of the appendix may occur within hours after the first symptoms. One serious complication of rupture is peritonitis, an inflammation of the lining of the abdominal cavity.

Any fever with nausea and abdominal pain should be reported to a physician. More severe pain is an immediate medical emergency that must be diagnosed to prevent potentially fatal complications. Appendicitis can affect anyone but the disease is more prevalent among people between ten and 30 years of age.

Diagnosis

When confirming appendicitis, the doctor checks for tenderness over the appendix. A blood test determines whether or not there is a high white blood cell count (with an infection, the body produces extra white blood cells to help fight the disease). Morever, the doctor may perform additional tests to rule out other diseases sometimes mistaken for appendicitis, such as gallbladder attack, kidney stones, or kidney infection. In women a twisted ovarian cyst (growth on the female sex organ) or a ruptured ectopic (tubal) pregnancy may produce symptoms similar to those of appendicitis.

Treatment

Although appendicitis cannot be prevented, prompt diagnosis can lead to effective treatment. Patients who suspect appendicitis should not eat food or drink water, or take drugs to relieve pain until a doctor is consulted. Eating or drinking any substance, including laxatives, may cause the appendix to rupture by stimulating activity in the intestine.

A mild case of appendicitis may subside by itself, but some people may have recurrent attacks. The most common cure for acute appendicitis is surgery to remove the inflamed organ and to avoid complications. To insure against further infection, antibiotics may also be prescribed.

Bile

Bile is a fluid produced by the liver and discharged into the small intestine, where it helps in the digestion of food, particularly fats. Yellow-green or golden in color and bitter to the taste, bile is made up of water, salts, bile acids, cholesterol (a fatlike substance), and lecithin (a fatty acid).

Functions

Bile acts like a detergent to break down fat in the intestine into tiny globules that can be dissolved and suspended in water so that they can pass through the walls of the small intestine's cells into the bloodstream (to provide fuel for the body). The bile "detergent" (known as bile salts) is also absorbed through the walls of the intestine but is returned to the liver to reform new bile. The color of bile is due to pigments known as bilirubin and biliverdin. Bilirubin is a yellow pigment derived from decomposed red blood cells. Biliverdin is a green pigment derived from conversion of bilirubin by a chemical reaction. These pigments are also responsible for some of the coloration of body wastes, in which the pigments are passed out of the body.

Bile is continually produced in the liver and passes through ducts to be stored in the gallbladder, a hollow organ located just beneath the liver, until mealtime when it is emptied into the duodenum, the entrance to the small intestine just below the stomach. Digestive disturbances result if the flow of bile is stopped or reduced, either because of a liver disorder or because a duct has been blocked by inflammation or a gallstone (a solid chunk of deposited material, usually calcium, cholesterol, bilirubin, or combinations thereof, formed in the gallbladder). Any of these conditions can also cause jaundice, in which the pigments bilirubin and, to a lesser extent, biliverdin accumulate in the blood. Jaundice is a symptom of trouble, not a disease in itself, and shows up as a yellow staining of the skin, eyes, and body fluids.

Cholecystitis

Cholecystitis is an inflammation of the gallbladder. The gallbladder is a small pear-shaped organ that stores bile, produced by the liver, and releases it as needed to help digest food — particularly fats — in the small intestine. Cholecystitis may be either acute (sudden and severe) or chronic (less severe attacks that occur from time to time).

Acute cholecystitis

Acute cholecystitis in about 90 percent of cases is caused when the outlet of the gallbladder or the duct leading from it is plugged by a gallstone (a stone formed in the gallbladder from cholesterol, a fatty substance, and sometimes from calcium or bile pigments). Unless the stone becomes dislodged, inflammation and pressure build up behind it. In severe cases, the swollen gallbladder may not receive enough blood, resulting in partial tissue death and gangrene. The gangrene may perforate the gallbladder, causing bile to spill into the abdominal cavity. An abscess (collection of pus within a cavity) usually forms around the area of gangrene, and bacteria may infect the gallbladder fluid. Occasionally, the re-

sulting leakage of infected bile produces a general infection (peritonitis) of the entire area around the abdominal organs. However, not all gallbladder attacks progress to this extreme; they may subside only to be repeated another time. Cholecystitis may also result from a blockage caused by enlarged blood veins in the common bile duct that the gallbladder shares with the liver. Rarely, infection may spread to the gallbladder from the nearby pancreas.

Acute cholecystitis often begins following a meal rich in fat (which requires more bile production), such as fried foods, chocolate, and cream. The individual may awaken in the middle of the night with indigestion, gas, and a sharp pain in the upper right quarter of the abdomen, which is often hard and tender to the touch. Pain may also appear in the middle of the abdomen and spread up to the tip of the right shoulder blade. The pain is steady and severe, gradually decreasing and finally disappearing in 12 to 18 hours unless there are complications. Vomiting is likely and provides some relief. There is little fever, unless the bile duct as well as the gallbladder is inflamed. If jaundice (yellowing of the skin, caused by bile pigment in the blood) is present, the symptoms are likely due to a gallstone blocking the common bile duct.

Radionuclide scanning confirms a diagnosis of cholecystitis (in this procedure, the patient takes in traces of radioactive material that travel to the affected area and radiate a picture onto the screen of a scanner). X rays and ultrasound, in which sound waves are bounced off internal structures to form an image of them, may also be used to locate gallstones.

Treatment of the acute attack consists of rest, intravenous feeding (from an IV bottle into the vein) but no food by mouth, pain-killing drugs, and antibiotics if needed. Because attacks are likely to recur, however, the real solution is surgical removal of the gallbladder. This is done immediately if complications develop. Preferably, however, it is performed a few days after the attack has subsided. If the patient has another illness, that is best brought under control before the operation is performed.

Chronic cholecystitis

Chronic cholecystitis is a continued inflammation of the gallbladder, with repeated attacks over time that are similar to but milder than those of acute cholecystitis. There are usually stones in the gallbladder; whether they develop before or after the emergence of the disease is unknown. The exact causes of chronic cholecystitis are not understood, although occasionally bacterial infection is the reason. Diet, heredity, and hormones appear to be involved, and the disease is more likely to affect women than men.

The pains of chronic cholecystitis commonly appear over the pit of the stomach and in the upper right quarter of the abdomen; they may be mild to unbearable. Pains usually come on suddenly and are normally steady, but may be sepa-rated by pain-free intervals of 15 minutes to an hour. The average attack lasts about an hour, although pains may disappear after 15 minutes or continue for several hours. Although the pains may appear together with nausea, gas, belching, and after eating fatty food, these indications may not be directly related to the disease.

Diagnosis of the disease is based on the symptoms and sometimes can be confirmed by X rays. The patient drinks a special chemical (designed to show on an X ray) that is absorbed by a normal gallbladder but not by an inflamed one. If the gallbladder does not show up in the X ray, the patient may have the disease. The doctor must make a careful investigation of other possible causes of the symptoms, including peptic ulcer (in the stomach or duodenum, the beginning of the small intestine), inflammation of the pancreas, and bowel disease.

The ideal way to treat chronic cholecystitis is to remove the gallbladder, together with any gallstones in the duct leading from the liver to the duodenum. If it is not clear that the symptoms are caused by gallbladder inflammation, or if the patient cannot withstand an operation, other methods are used. These include a low-fat diet (which lowers the need for bile) and weight reduction, plus antacids and other medications.

Cirrhosis

Cirrhosis is a disease in which the cells throughout the liver are progressively destroyed. They are replaced by nodules (swellings) containing normal new cells but also by much connective tissue that alters the structure of the organ. The flow of blood and lymph through the damaged liver is much less efficient, and eventually the liver fails.

Causes

Cirrhosis is the liver's attempt to rebuild itself and continue despite injury—from whatever cause. The injury may be a sudden and massive infection, as from hepatitis. It may occur in a less severe manner over months or years, as in chronic active hepatitis or in obstruction of the bile ducts within the liver. The latter process starts with inflammation, then scarring, then closure of the ducts. A similar condition is caused by obstruction of external bile ducts by a stone, scar, inborn defect, or tumor. The damage may be done over an even longer time, slowly and steadily, by alcohol abuse.

Alcoholism is by far the most common cause of cirrhosis. Once thought to be due to the poisonous effect of alcohol on the liver, its damage is now believed to result chiefly from malnutrition. Alcoholics get most of their calories from alcohol and so their diets are dangerously unbalanced. Lack of protein in the diet of an alcoholic, for example, causes scarring in a vital area of the liver. Other causes include:

- Some powerful medications—chemicals such as methotrexate, an anticancer drug; halothane, an anesthetic; and oxyphenisatin, a medicine used in enemas—may also cause liver damage
- Inborn errors in physical or chemical processes of the body
- Syphilis
- Passive liver congestion caused by a clot blocking the large (hepatic) vein carrying blood to the heart, or by an inefficient heart that cannot accept a normal flow of blood from the liver.

Symptoms

Frequently, cirrhosis is not suspected until it is well advanced, for it imitates many other diseases. Symptoms include a general weakness, a vague sick feeling, loss of appetite, loss of weight, and a loss of interest in sex. There may be a dull abdominal ache, nausea, constipation, or diarrhea. In a malnourished patient, the tongue may be inflamed. Many symptoms are the result of high blood pressure in the portal vein, which brings nutrient-bearing blood from the intestinal area to the liver where the blood is processed. In cirrhosis, the liver cannot handle a normal flow of blood, so the pressure in the portal vein rises. One result is that fluid from the blood is lost into the abdominal cavity. The fluid buildup may press against the diaphragm (the muscular wall separating the abdominal and chest cavities) and interfere with breathing. New blood vessels (collateral vessels) form to carry away the excess blood into the general circulation. There may be bleeding in the esophagus (food pipe) or stomach, when new collateral vessels burst under pressure. The patient may vomit blood. Serious, life-threatening hemorrhage may occur.

Other symptoms include an enlarged, firm liver and enlarged spleen; a mottled redness of the mound of the palm at the base of the thumb; "spider veins" on the skin of the upper body; loss of hair from chest and pubic area; diminishing testicles; and tingling sensations on the skin of the hands and feet.

Diagnosis

Proof of cirrhosis of the liver is furnished by liver biopsy. A hollow needle is inserted through the skin and into the liver itself to obtain a tissue sample for analysis. Tissue from a diseased liver reveals destruction of cells and scarring. Other diagnostic procedures include radionuclide scanning (in this procedure, the patient takes in traces of radioactive material that travels to the liver and illuminates a picture of the organ onto the screen of the scanner). X-ray pictures are taken of the gallbladder and of bile ducts inside the liver and leading from it. Blood and urine tests reveal important clues, including bile pigments in the blood, low red blood cell count, vitamin and mineral deficiencies, and protein in the urine.

Treatment

Treatment aims first to remove the cause of the original injury. Thus an alcoholic patient needs to stop drinking, is placed on a well-balanced moderate-to-high-protein diet, and is given larger than usual doses of multivitamins (supplemental vitamins include A, B complex, D, and K—which cannot be stored in the ill liver—and folic acid). If a stone is obstructing an external bile duct and thus causing liver damage, it can be removed. Fluids and salt are usually restricted, to prevent fluid buildup in the body.

Good care includes plenty of rest and frequent small meals, rather than fewer large ones, to reduce the work load on the liver, and avoiding any infection that might cause new stress on the liver.

Prevention

Many of the various causes of cirrhosis of the liver cannot be predicted and guarded against — but the major one can be. Drinking moderately or not at all is the best way to reduce the risk of developing this serious disease.

Colitis

Colitis is a general term meaning an inflammation of the colon (large intestine). It is usually a chronic (long-term) condition that is characterized by sudden attacks followed by periods of remission (relief). It should not be confused with irritable bowel syndrome (also called spastic or mucous colon), which is not an inflammation of the colon (although it can resemble colitis with symptoms such as diarrhea and abdominal pain) and which has been associated with emotional factors.

Frequently, the term colitis is used synonymously with an entity known as "inflammatory bowel disease." There are basically three diseases incorporated under this term: ulcerative colitis, granulomatous colitis (Crohn's disease), and ulcerative proctitis. Ulcerative colitis involves only the large intestine (except in rare instances). Granulomatous colitis may involve any portion of the food tract, including the mouth, and on occasion may not involve the colon. Ulcerative proctitis, the least serious of the group, involves only the rectum, but can closely resemble ulcerative colitis.

Causes

In some cases, the cause of colitis is unknown, although it can be a result of a bacterial infection or, in older people, lack of blood to the colon.

Symptoms

Colitis may begin slowly with abdominal discomfort, mild diarrhea or constipation, and a general feeling of being unwell. As the condition becomes more severe, symptoms such as abdominal pain or bleeding from the rectum may appear. If the disease appears suddenly, the patient may experience fever, bloody diarrhea, loss of appetite, and weight loss.

Diagnosis

The diagnosis of colitis is based on a direct inspection of intestinal walls with the aid of a sigmoidoscope (or proctoscope), a lighted tube inserted into the colon through the anus, the opening to the outside of the body. A tissue sample of the intestinal wall may be taken to be examined for signs of infection.

Treatment

Persons with a mild case of colitis can usually be treated at home and be permitted a normal diet. More seriously ill patients may be treated in the hospital with a special diet to allow the digestive tract to rest; replacement (often intravenously) of fluids and salts lost during episodes of diarrhea and/or bleeding; and medications, for example, antibiotics to treat an infection or cortisone (and other drugs) to treat inflammatory bowel disease. Those individuals with severe cases of colitis may require blood transfusions and perhaps even surgery.

Colostomy

Colostomy is the creation of an opening (stoma) in the wall of the abdomen to which an opening in the colon (ostomy) is attached. Thereafter, the contents of the colon are eliminated through the stoma instead of through the rectum and anus.

The operation may be permanent, as when some operations for cancer of the rectum eliminate the normal exit for the bowel, or it may be temporary, as in the surgical correction of Hirschsprung's disease.

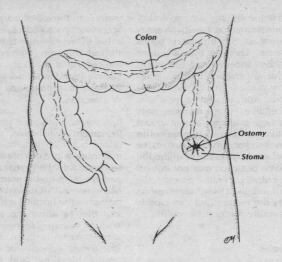

Colostomy is the creation of a stoma (opening) in the wall of the abdomen to which an opening in the colon (ostomy) is attached. The contents of the colon are then eliminated through the stoma rather than through the rectum and anus.

Correction of Hirschsprung's disease

In this inherited disorder of newborns, the last portion of the bowel lacks specialized nerves and cannot move normally. The healthy portion of the bowel above this segment is connected to the stoma and drains into a special waist-band diaper for several months until the baby is strong enough for the second step of the surgery. This involves removal of the defective bowel portion and connection of the healthy portion to the anus, permitting normal bowel movements and elimination of the stoma.

Permanent colostomy

A permanent colostomy does not prevent a person from leading a normal life. After the stoma has healed, or even before, the patient is taught how to empty the colon once a day by using irrigations (enemas) and a special collecting device. By manipulating the diet it becomes possible to time a bowel movement occasionally. At first, patients wear a pouch over the stoma to collect any leakage from the colon. An adhesive is used to form a tight seal around the pouch's opening and the stoma, and a deodorant in the pouch controls odor. However, after a while many individuals with so-called "dry colostomies" need only wear a stoma cap or small gauze patch over the stoma to protect it and absorb mucus secretions. Physical activities can be resumed, with or without a pouch, including swimming, other sports, and sexual relations. The only exceptions are heavy lifting, which could cause a hernia through the weakened abdominal muscles, or any activity that could injure the stoma or abdomen, such as hard contact sports.

To avoid infection of the stoma or irritation of the skin around it, the patient needs to wash the surrounding skin area with mild soap and water each day, then rinse and dry it. Special adhesive materials that protect and soothe the skin have become available. These are applied after cleaning the skin.

Support, encouragement, and practical advice from those who have undergone the operation are available through local chapters and the national headquarters of the United Ostomy Association.

Crohn's disease

Crohn's disease (also known as regional enteritis or ileitis) is characterized by an inflammation of a section or sections of any part of the digestive tract—most often of the ileum (the last one third of the small intestine). The disease may first appear as patches of tiny ulcers in the innermost lining of the intestine, with swelling of nearby tissue. Eventually the inflammation extends through all layers of the intestine, which becomes thickened, hard, and brittle. Deepening ulcers, scarring, and swelling may obstruct the intestinal tract.

Causes

The cause of Crohn's disease is unknown. However, research indicates that infection, immune disorders, or an inherited defect may play a part. There is some evidence of an increased incidence of Crohn's disease in Jews; blacks are least likely to develop the disease. The disease usually begins between age 15 and age 35, but can occur at any age.

Symptoms

Symptoms usually develop gradually, with spells of diarrhea (four to six stools a day, frequently bloody), low fever, weight loss, loss of appetite, general weakness, and steady or colicky pains in the abdomen, commonly on the right side. Milk, milk products, and coarse foods may make symptoms worse.

Occasionally an acute (sudden and severe) case resembles appendicitis, with sharp lower right abdomen pain, cramping, nausea, fever, and diarrhea. There may or may not be bloody stools. Also, an acute case can resemble infectious diarrhea.

Diagnosis

The chronic form of the disease can occasionally be mistaken for other problems, such as irritable bowel syndrome. However, a barium X ray of the small intestine may reveal the characteristic pattern of narrowed bowel sharply differentiated from healthy bowel. X rays of the large intestine may show characteristic "skipped areas" or areas of disease interspersed with normal bowel. Fistulas (see below) are also commonly seen on X rays. The doctor may also inspect the inner lining of the large intestine visually, with a lighted tube (inserted through the anus) known as a sigmoidoscope (proctoscope), looking for patchy areas of inflammation and taking a sample of tissue (biopsy) from the lining for inspection under a microscope. The examining doctor, probing the abdomen and pelvis, may detect a tender mass of thickened or matted loops of intestine.

Complications

Complications include abscesses (pus-filled cavities) and fistulas. Fistulas can be thought of as tunnels. They originate from an inflamed bowel and commonly burrow out into and around the anorectal area where upon examination they are seen as openings in the skin. These openings are often infected and discharging pus. Fistulas can also occur from bowel to bowel, bowel to bladder and/or vagina, and bowel to abdominal wall.

Perforation of the intestine can also occur, leading to peritonitis (infection and/or inflammation of the lining of the abdominal cavity). This is marked by severe abdominal pain with a rigid abdomen and is most often an acute surgical emergency. On occasion, a small perforation will be unnoticed; the immune system will then "wall off" the area creating an abscess.

Malnutrition is also a very common complication of Crohn's disease, as areas of inflamed intestine cannot properly absorb nutrients. The incidence of cancer of the colon and rectum is also increased in patients with Crohn's disease.

Treatment

An acute case of bloody diarrhea occurring in young people may be caused by infection and be unrelated to true Crohn's disease. If so, complete recovery is possible, with no further attacks. Chronic Crohn's disease, however, is another matter. At present there is no cure for it. At times surgery is necessary to remove entirely a section of diseased bowel, drain an abscess, or eliminate a fistula. This relieves the condition for a time, but symptoms almost always recur and another operation may be necessary. Treatment of the disease is directed at making the patient as comfortable and functional as possible by reducing the symptoms. Disability may be mild or severe.

A diet rich in calories and vitamins with adequate protein is desirable, to compensate for the patient's poor absorption of food from the intestine. Individuals with severely inflamed or obstructed bowels may be placed temporarily on intravenous feeding or a special no-residue diet. Patients with anemia need supplements (such as iron, folic acid, or Vitamin B$_{12}$) and sometimes blood transfusions, and those with severe diarrhea or dehydration (loss of body fluids) may need intravenous fluids.

Cramps and diarrhea are frequently controlled by various medications that relax the bowel wall, while preparations such as psyllium may help to firm stools.

Antibiotics are used short-term to treat abscesses and infected fistulas. Sulfa/salicylate combination drugs may be used continually to curb inflammation and prevent acute episodes, particularly in disease involving the large intestine. In addition, a cortisone drug known as prednisone, taken by mouth, is a mainstay in treating flare-ups of symptoms.

Diverticulitis

Diverticulitis is the inflammation and/or infection of little sacs or pouches (diverticula) that have ballooned out through the walls of the colon (large intestine). The pouches form when the inner lining of the colon is forced under pressure through weaker spots in the colon's muscular layer. The existence of the pouches (as a condition, not a disease) is referred to as diverticulosis.

Diverticulosis may be present in about one third of the people over 60 in the United States, and both its incidence and the frequency of complications increase with age.

Causes

One theory as to the cause of diverticulosis is that abnormal movement of the colon (possibly because of too little bulk in the diet) produces intense pressure that forces intestinal lining through the weak spots in the muscular layer. Most people with simple diverticulosis have no symptoms. Occasionally, however, a pouch next to a blood vessel may ulcerate, causing it to bleed. If the vessel is an artery, severe bleeding can result, seen as bleeding from the anus. Shock and possible death may result if the condition is not treated.

It has been estimated that about one fifth to one fourth of the people with diverticulosis may develop the symptoms of diverticulitis. Diverticulitis develops when a mass of hardened waste matter (called a fecalith) forms in a pouch and reduces the blood supply to the thin walls of the pouch (by means of pressure against the wall), making them more liable to infection by the bacteria of the colon. The inflammation that follows can lead to perforation, abscess (an enclosed sac of pus around the perforation), or infection of the lining of the abdominal cavity (peritonitis). Not infrequently, the inflamed section of bowel attaches to the urinary bladder or vagina, burrowing out from the colon to create a fistula (channel) that leaks infection into the other organ. Repeated inflammation can cause thickening of the wall of the colon, narrowing the colon and causing partial or sometimes total obstruction.

Symptoms

Symptoms include intermittent cramping pains and tenderness, usually in the lower left abdomen but sometimes in other areas of the lower abdomen in which case the pains may resemble those of appendicitis. Pain that worsens during urination may indicate that the inflamed colon is attached to the bladder. Stool (feces) and/or air in the urine may indicate a colon-to-bladder fistula. Constipation or constipation alternating with diarrhea is common. Fever is usually present with acute attacks.

Diagnosis

The diagnosis of diverticulitis usually is made if there is a history of pain in the left lower quadrant (quarter) of the abdomen accompanied by fever and a change in bowel habits. A physical examination may reveal a mass in the left lower quadrant along with extreme tenderness. After the acute episode has subsided, the examining doctor may insert a proctoscope (a lighted tube) through the anus and up the colon to see if there is any evidence of cancer that might be causing the symptoms. A barium (X-ray contrast fluid) enema and X ray is usually done to further rule out cancer of the colon and to locate diverticula, obstructions, and fistulas.

Treatment

Treatment of severe diverticulitis begins with bed rest in a hospital and intravenous (in the vein) feeding with nothing by mouth (to give the intestine a rest). Antibiotics are given if there is fever or other evidence of an infection. If peritonitis (inflammation and/or infection of the lining of the abdominal cavity) develops, it may be necessary to operate. The inflamed section of the colon may simply be cut out and the remaining sections joined, or, more often, a temporary colostomy (in which the colon empties through an opening in the abdominal wall to the outside) may be necessary. Later, after all inflammation and infection has subsided, this is reconnected to the remaining colon or rectum.

Prevention

A diet with plenty of bulk appears to be a way to avoid diverticulosis, the pouching that precedes diverticulitis. Those people who have developed diverticulosis should eat a relatively high-fiber diet. Supplements, such as psyllium, which increase bulk, may be recommended to move the stool through the colon at a normal rate.

Fistula

A fistula is any abnormal, tubelike passage or channel within a body tissue or tissues, usually between two internal organs, or leading from an internal organ to the body's surface. A fistula is sometimes created by surgery for diagnostic or therapeutic purposes. Others occur as the result of injury or congenital (present at birth) defects.

Types

A fistula may develop at virtually any body site. One very common type of fistula is the anal fistula that usually develops as the result of a break, or fissure, in the wall of the anal canal or the rectum (leading from the intestine to the outside of the body) or because of an abscess (an enclosed cavity of pus) in the area. Another common type of fistula is the vaginal fistula, which may follow a difficult labor and childbirth. This fistula is between the bladder and the vagina, causing urine to leak into the vagina. In another type of vaginal fistula, between the vagina and rectum, feces escape through the wall of the rectum into the vagina. Another fistula, the intestinal type, extends from the bladder to the intestine and allows urine to leak from the bladder into the intestines. Fistulas at other sites in the body can be caused by tuberculosis actinomycosis (a type of fungal infection), diverticulitis, or another disease.

Symptoms

Each type of fistula can produce its own peculiar set of symptoms, depending on its location, its size, and its depth. Typical symptoms are pain in the affected region and an abnormal discharge through the skin—particularly if the fistula affects the anus or vagina—which can be seen on examination of these areas. Often the fistula itself is a site of frequent infection and discomfort. The anal fistula usually has recurrent abscesses and constant watery discharge.

Treatment

In almost all cases, surgery is recommended as the only effective treatment. Vaginal fistulas are frequently corrected following childbirth, and the surgery is nearly always successful. In the case of anal fistulas, surgery is recommended unless severe diarrhea, active ulcerative colitis, or enterocolitis is present, in which case the healing of the surgical wound would present many problems and complications. Usually these infections are treated before surgery.

Prevention

Avoiding injury to body tissues is probably the only specific preventive measure against the occurrence of fistula. Prompt diagnosis and treatment will lessen the possibility of secondary infections and abscesses.

Gallstones

Gallstones are hardened masses that consist mainly of cholesterol,

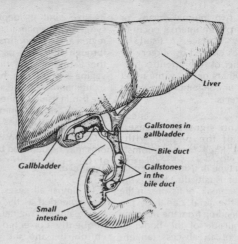

Liver

Gallstones in gallbladder

Bile duct

Gallbladder

Gallstones in the bile duct

Small intestine

Gallstones can form in the gallbladder or bile duct and cause inflammation of the gallbladder or even liver damage if they block the flow of bile from the gallbladder to the small intestine.

a substance regularly found in animal fats, blood, bile (fluid produced in the liver and stored in the gallbladder that is required for fat absorption in the small intestine), the liver, and other tissues. The stones form in the gallbladder or in the bile duct leading from the gallbladder into the small intestine, where food is digested and nutrients absorbed into the blood.

Causes

When bile contains excessive amounts of cholesterol in comparison to other ingredients, the unnecessary cholesterol separates from the solution and forms stone-like masses. Unfortunately,

these stones cannot be prevented by controlling cholesterol intake in the diet. Cholesterol from food passes into the blood, and there is no relationship between cholesterol levels in the blood and cholesterol levels in the bile.

In addition to concentrated bile and bile salts, several other factors contribute to the formation of gallstones. Eating too much fat, infection, liver disease, and forms of anemia — such as sickle-cell anemia—can lead to gallstones.

Pregnancy, obesity, or diabetes can also increase the risk of gallstones. Overweight people who frequently lose and gain large amounts of weight seem more susceptible to gallstones, as do women who have had two or more children. Although reasons are unclear, twice as many women as men over age 40 develop gallstones.

Symptoms

By themselves, gallstones often produce no signs of disease. About half the people with gallstones have no symptoms. Symptoms that do appear are usually chronic (long-term) in nature, causing discomfort and pain in the upper abdomen, indigestion, nausea, and intolerance of fatty foods. Sometimes stones pass through the bile duct into the intestines to be excreted naturally.

However, symptoms can occur if the stones lodge in the bile duct. In an acute gallbladder attack, a sharp pain often on the right side of the upper abdomen may travel to the back and under the right shoulder blade. Frequently, the pain develops suddenly after a meal and leads to fever, chills, vomiting, and possibly jaundice (yellowing of the skin and whites of the eyes caused by excess bile pigment). These symptoms occur after a stone that was previously free-floating in the gallbladder becomes trapped in the bile duct.

Complications

Serious complications of liver damage or jaundice may develop if stones block the flow of bile. Pressure from the stones may also cause inflammation and damage to nearby organs.

When gallstones remain in the gallbladder, the organ may become inflamed with a condition called cholecystitis, which causes severe pain 30 to 60 minutes after eating.

Diagnosis

Gallstones that show no symptoms may be detected by an X ray of the gallbladder called a cholecystogram. A cholecystogram is taken after the patient swallows a tablet containing dye which outlines the gallbladder and any stones that may be present. Some physicians use ultrasound rather than X ray; ultrasound is a procedure in which sound waves bounce off internal body organs and construct a visual image.

Treatment

For acute attacks of gallstones with severe and prolonged symptoms, doctors recommend a cholecystectomy (surgical removal of the gallbladder). This treatment is one of the most common forms of abdominal surgery, since the gallbladder is not necesssary to maintain life. Many doctors even suggest removing a gallbladder containing stones that is not causing symptoms to avoid future complications.

As an alternative to surgery, some researchers are investigating a drug to dissolve cholesterol gallstones. There is also some experimentation being conducted to see if gallstones can be dissolved with localized forms of high-intensity radiation.

Gastroenteritis

Gastroenteritis is an inflammation of the lining of the stomach and the intestine.

Causes

Gastroenteritis can be caused by bacteria or viruses; by allergic reactions to certain foods or to certain drinks; by infectious diseases, such as typhoid fever or influenza; by food poisoning; by overconsumption of alcohol; or by certain drugs.

Symptoms

Symptoms include headache, nausea, vomiting, diarrhea, and gas pains in the stomach and the intestine. Often, the individual will feel that gas is "caught" in certain portions of the intestine. On occasions, the intestines will seem to cramp, producing severe pain.

Diagnosis

The first task in treating gastroenteritis is to identify the cause or causes of the inflammation. Blood tests and cultures for viruses or bacteria may be done. If the problem is caused by an allergic reaction, the source of the reaction may be identified by allergy tests.

Treatment

Antibiotics can be administered for bacterial infections. A variety of medicines (many nonprescription) can ease the effects of stomach cramps and gas pains. Diarrhea may necessitate replacement of lost water. If the patient is a victim of heart disease, lost fluid (and resulting imbalances in the electrolyte and fluid balance) may cause irregular heartbeat.

Prevention

Maintaining a clean kitchen, eating in restaurants where the kitchens are kept clean, washing fresh foods thoroughly, and cooking foods carefully are all safeguards against bacterial and viral infections. Identification of allergy-causing foods and moderation in alcohol consumption also help prevent gastroenteritis if these are the causes of the problem.

Hemorrhoids

Hemorrhoids, often called piles, are enlarged veins inside or just outside the anal canal, which is the opening at the end of the large intestine. As veins swell, they cause severe inflammation and discomfort.

Causes

In most cases, hemorrhoids are the result of individual toilet habits whereby some people postpone normal bowel functioning. Habitual postponement of bowel movements can lead to loss of rectal function and undesirable straining during elimination. Straining irritates veins and slows the flow of blood, thereby contributing to swollen or inflamed veins. Postponing bowel movements may also cause stools retained in the bowels to lose moisture. When feces become dry and hard, the added strain of constipation encourages hemorrhoids.

Diet plays a major role in the development of hemorrhoids. A diet containing a high proportion of refined foods, such as white flour and sugar, rather than foods with natural roughage increases the likelihood of constipation and, therefore, the likelihood of hemorrhoids.

Another source of hemorrhoid irritation comes from pressure on the veins from diseases of the liver or heart or from a tumor. Pregnancy also contributes to the development of hemorrhoids because the enlarged uterus increases pressure on the veins. Moreover, prolonged pressure from pushing during labor and delivery can inflame the area. Although women appear to develop hemorrhoids during pregnancy, recent research suggests that they probably had the condition prior to pregnancy.

Hemorrhoids seem to be more prevalent in some families. However, this tendency has been attributed to similar dietary and personal habits.

Symptoms

Hemorrhoids may take years to develop and almost always result in irritating symptoms. The first signs of hemorrhoids include itching and some discomfort during and after bowel movements. Continued straining during elimination will eventually produce slight swelling of the lining of the anal canal. This swelling may not be noticed until hard stools scrape the anal lining and cause slight bleeding—an early clue that a hemorrhoid may have developed.

With prolonged straining, a portion of the anal canal may jut out of the anus during a bowel movement. At this stage, the elastic connective tissue is still strong enough to pull the hemorrhoid back into the anal canal unassisted, so the individual may not notice the growing problem. However, with persistent pressure, the protruding tissue may remain outside the anus after a bowel movement and need to be manually returned to the anal canal. Once outside the anal canal, the hemorrhoid creates a dull aching sensation.

A more involved problem develops when the hemorrhoid is difficult or impossible to return, and permanent swelling at the anal opening interferes with elimination. Then the patient may postpone bowel movements in an effort to avoid pain. Instead of helping, this intensifies the problem, because it leads to constipation.

Diagnosis

To diagnose a hemorrhoid, a physician inspects the anal canal, often with special instruments. An anoscope (short, lighted tube) inserted into the anus can reveal the condition of the rectal lining. A sigmoidoscope, which is a longer instrument, shows a view of the inner area of the colon.

Treatment

Painful hemorrhoids can be treated at home by applying cold water compresses directly to the anal area for five to ten minutes until pain is relieved. Some people reduce pain by taking hot baths. Over-the-counter preparations cannot cure hemorrhoids, but they can relieve itching and swelling. Should symptoms worsen after application of any remedy, its use should be suspended and a doctor consulted. Chemicals in these preparations may produce an allergic reaction. Nonirritating laxatives may also be occasionally useful in softening stools and easing bowel movements.

In the early stages of hemorrhoid development, adjustment of personal habits may prevent progression of the condition. A bowel movement should never be delayed, once the urge is felt. During bowel movements, straining should be avoided. A diet including plenty of roughage—natural grains, fresh fruits, and vegetables—also softens stools.

For severe cases of hemorrhoids, a doctor may recommend a surgical procedure called hemorrhoidectomy to remove dilated portions of the affected veins and tie off the remaining parts of the vein. A newer procedure called cryosurgery removes the hemorrhoid, but with less pain and fewer postoperative complications. With this technique, the hemorrhoid is frozen with an extremely cold probe. As the frozen tissue dies, the hemorrhoid falls off within several days. Physicians perform cryosurgery in their offices within a few minutes. The only postoperative symptom is a slight watery discharge for a few days.

Another technique used to eliminate internal hemorrhoids is rubber band ligation. Here, the doctor ties off the hemorrhoid's blood supply with a special instrument. This procedure causes the hemorrhoid to die and drop off within three to nine days. The physician performs the procedure in the office, but there is one drawback. The patient must return for several treatments, because only one hemorrhoid can be treated per visit. Once the hemorrhoid dies, brief spotting of blood and minor itching may occur.

Hepatitis

Hepatitis is a viral infection of the liver that is characterized by jaundice, a yellowing of the skin and whites of the eyes.

Causes and types

The disease is caused by several viruses, but the most common virus strains of hepatitis are hepatitis A, or infectious hepatitis, and hepatitis B, or serum hepatitis.

Both strains enter the body as

minute organisms and attack cells in the liver. Hepatitis A passes through the digestive tract and is transmitted from person to person by contaminated food or water or through the stools of an infected person. This form may occur as epidemics in places where sanitation is poor and sewage contaminated. Incubation, the time between exposure to the disease and the appearance of symptoms, is between 14 to 40 days. Sometimes, hepatitis A is so mild that symptoms never appear, but the infected person can still transmit the disease as a carrier of infection.

With hepatitis B, the virus enters the bloodstream, either from transfusion of contaminated blood or from contaminated needles, especially among drug users. Hepatitis B begins more gradually than does hepatitis A, so the disease may be present 40 to 180 days before the onset of symptoms. In addition, the virus can live in almost all body fluids, including saliva, semen, urine, and tears. This allows hepatitis B to be transmitted by sexual contact or by more casual contact such as sharing toothbrushes or razors.

Hepatitis may also result as a complication of the viral infection called infectious mononucleosis.

Symptoms

Early signs of hepatitis are general fatigue, joint and muscle pain, and loss of appetite. Nausea, vomiting, and diarrhea or constipation may follow with a low-grade fever of 102°F or less. As the disease develops, the liver enlarges and becomes tender. Chills, weight loss, and distaste for smoking appear along with the characteristic jaundice. Jaundice results from an accumulation of yellow bile pigment in the blood that turns the skin and whites of the eyes yellow.

In hepatitis A, the disappearance of jaundice generally signals the beginning of recovery. However, in hepatitis B, the virus may persist for years or the duration of a lifetime.

Any sudden rise in fever, extreme drowsiness, or severe prolonged pain requires immediate medical supervision to avoid permanent liver damage. Chronic, long-term hepatitis can lead to irreversible liver failure or cirrhosis. Cirrhosis is a condition in which normal cells of the liver are replaced by fibrous scar tissue that inhibits liver function.

Diagnosis

To determine the extent and severity of hepatitis, a physician analyzes blood and urine specimens from the suspected hepatitis patient. If the disease has progressed, the patient may have yellow skin and soreness in the upper abdomen over the liver.

More severe chronic hepatitis may require a liver biopsy, in which a needle is inserted into the liver to obtain a sample of liver tissue. In this procedure, local anesthetic is usually injected into the upper abdomen to eliminate discomfort from the test.

A new blood test is under investigation that will speed the diagnosis of hepatitis B and identify carriers of the virus.

Treatment

Because hepatitis is caused by a virus, there is no cure. Even treatment is limited, especially for acute hepatitis. Once the virus attacks, recovery is usually up to the body's regular defense system.

To encourage the healing process, physicians advise patients to avoid all strenuous activity. Strict bed rest is more important during the acute phases of hepatitis. More serious cases may require hospitalization to insure inactivity. Some of these patients may also need an exchange blood transfusion to aid recovery if the body cannot overcome contamination by itself. In addition, all hepatitis patients must avoid alcoholic beverages, because processing alcohol puts a tremendous strain on the liver.

Prevention

People exposed to hepatitis can prevent or minimize the disease by obtaining an injection of gamma globulin, a disease-fighting substance in the blood. Gamma globulin usually defends against virus A and offers a modest protection against virus B. In either case, if hepatitis develops following an injection, gamma globulin seems to reduce symptoms.

Scientists are also investigating a new vaccine against hepatitis. A vaccine is a preparation of the disease-causing agent that is introduced into the body to stimulate the body to produce antibodies whose job it is to fight the disease. For now, hepatitis vaccine is only recommended for people who are in direct contact with hepatitis carriers, but the vaccine will eventually become available for more widespread use.

Hernia

The term hernia refers to any abnormal protrusion of part of an organ or tissue(s) through the structures that normally contain it. In this condition, a weak spot or opening in a body wall allows part of the organ to bulge through. A hernia may develop in almost any part of the body; however, the most common sites are the abdominal and groin areas.

Although a hernia is often popularly called a "rupture," this is a misleading description. Nothing is actually "torn" or ruptured in a hernia. A hernia can be congenital (present at birth) or acquired; in the latter case, it is often the result of some stress or strain on the body wall involved.

Common types of hernias

Although there are literally as many types of hernias as there are sites or locations in the body, the following are some of the most common hernias:

- Umbilical hernia, protrusion of part of the intestine at the navel or umbilicus (seen mostly in infants)
- Inguinal hernia, a protrusion of a loop of intestine into the groin where the folds of abdominal flesh meet the thighs, often the result of increased pressure in the abdomen because of lifting, coughing, straining, or accidents (accounts for about 75 percent of all common hernias)
- Diaphragmatic hernia (also called hiatus hernia) occurs when a portion of the stomach protrudes above the diaphragm, the muscular wall separating the chest and abdominal cavities, into the chest. Normally, the esophagus (the passageway from the throat to the stomach) passes through a tight muscular collar that prevents the stomach from squeezing up into the chest cavity
- Scrotal hernia, an inguinal hernia that has passed into the scrotum, the bag of skin behind the penis that contains the testes
- Femoral hernia, a protrusion of a loop of intestine into the femoral canal, which is a tubular passageway that carries nerves and blood vessels from the abdomen into the thigh (this type of hernia is more common in women than in men)
- Incisional hernia, a hernia that occurs after an operation at the site of the surgical incision; often this type of hernia is due to excessive strain on the healing tissue (excessive muscular effort, lifting, coughing, or extreme obesity which puts pressure on a weakened area).

Conditions of hernias

Hernias can also be classified by their condition:
- Irreducible hernia, one that cannot be restored by manipulation
- Reducible hernia, one that can be returned to "normal" by manipulation
- Incarcerated hernia, a hernia that cannot be reduced through treatment, but is not obstructed or strangulated
- Strangulated hernia, one that is tightly constricted, cutting off the blood supply of the affected tissue.

Symptoms

Because of the many different types of hernias, the symptoms will vary slightly depending on the cause and the body part(s) involved.

Diagnosis

Diagnosis of a hernia can usually be made by thorough visual examination and by studying the patient's medical history and symptoms.

Treatment

For small, nonstrangulated or nonincarcerated hernias, various supports and trusses can sometimes offer temporary, symptomatic relief. However, the best treatment is surgical closure or repair of the muscle wall through which the hernia protrudes. Surgical repair of a hernia is called herniorrhaphy. When the weakened area is very large, some strong synthetic material may be sewn over the defect to reinforce the weak area. Postoperative care is simple and involves protecting the patient from respiratory infections that would cause him/her to cough and sneeze, thus placing strain on the suture line. Recovery is usually quick and complete.

Prevention

Avoiding strain or pressure on any body wall, especially those of the abdomen and groin area (in men), is the only real preventive measure against hernias.

Ileostomy

An ileostomy is the surgical opening (stoma) through the abdomen into the ileum, the lower part of the small intestine. An ileostomy is performed whenever the large intestine and rectum must be removed because of disease or abnormalities. The opening into the small intestine then becomes an artificial anus through which waste material is expelled, since waste matter can no longer travel through the normal anus.

The waste matter that is discharged through the stoma is collected in a bag that the patient wears continually. Because this waste matter does not pass through the large intestine where water is absorbed from the waste matter, the material excreted through the stoma is watery. Eventually, the waste matter becomes firmer, but it never becomes solid.

Patients learn to care for their ileostomies in the hospital after the operation. Equipped with this knowledge, a patient can lead a normal life with an ileostomy.

Irritable bowel syndrome

Irritable bowel syndrome, also called spastic colon or mucous colitis, is a collection of symptoms caused by irritability and irregularity in the movement of both small and large intestines. The syndrome is usually influenced by emotions. Feelings of nervousness, anxiety, guilt, depression, or anger may bring on this very common disorder. Coffee, raw fruits and vegetables, hormones, drugs, and overuse of laxatives can promote it, as can an inability of the body to digest the natural sugar in milk.

Symptoms

Not a disease, irritable bowel syndrome is a collection of symptoms that includes both constipation and diarrhea, often alternating and sometimes accompanied by straining and abdominal cramps. Stools may be loose or compacted and may include mucus, which has been manufactured as a lubricant by the irritated bowel lining. Gas, bloating, nausea, headache, or fatigue may accompany the other symptoms.

There are two main types of irritable bowel syndrome. The first is spastic colon, which often begins at mealtime and is marked by cramps or a dull aching pain in the abdomen, usually the lower part. The pain may disappear after a bowel movement. The second type of irritable bowel syndrome is painless diarrhea, which is characterized by an urgent need for a bowel movement upon awakening or during or right after a meal. Incontinence (involuntary loss of bowel control) can occur.

Diagnosis

For anyone who appears to have irritable bowel syndrome, the doctor will first want to rule out diseases with similar symptoms. The patient may be asked to bring in a stool specimen to be cultured and examined for traces of blood and parasites. The colon may be x-rayed, following a barium enema. The doctor may insert a sigmoidoscope (a lighted tube) into the colon through the anus, the opening at the end of the intestine, to check for serious disorders such as ulcers that can lead to ulcerative colitis.

Treatment

If no organic disease is found, the doctor will reassure the patient and discuss ways in which the symptoms can be relieved. There may be methods by which the patient can reduce the anxiety or depression that may be causing the syndrome. The doctor may prescribe a tranquilizer, sedative, mood elevator, or antispasm medicine — but only on a short-term basis, so that the individual does not become dependent on a drug. Long walks, bike rides, or other exercise may help to relax the person while promoting better bowel action. If constipation is a problem, the doctor will advise the patient to add bulk such as whole bran to the diet; to stop depending on laxatives; and to take pills that absorb water, add bulk, and help to stabilize the large bowel. If diarrhea is present, avoiding laxative foods, such as beans, may help. Patients bothered by gas will be warned against foods such as cabbage. Milk may even be barred from the diet. Most people, except many of northwest European origin, lose the ability to digest the natural sugar (lactose) in milk by the time they are 20 years old. A test for this is an oral dose of lactose. If it results in diarrhea and bloating, it is a tip-off that the symptoms could have been caused entirely or in part by drinking milk.

If irritable bowel syndrome continues despite the treatment, it is important to remember that it is not dangerous. However, to be on the safe side, a regular physical checkup should be scheduled with your doctor — every year — especially if you are over 40.

Jaundice

Jaundice is a yellowish discoloration of the skin, whites of the eyes, mucous membranes, and other tissues of the body, and is caused by the abnormal accumulation of bile pigment (or bilirubin) in the blood.

Bilirubin consists primarily of the hemoglobin of used red blood cells and is found in bile, a bitter, yellow-green fluid that aids in digestion by breaking down fat. Bile is secreted by the liver, stored in the gallbladder, and discharged into the intestine when it is needed for digestion.

Causes

In many cases, jaundice occurs when bile is prevented by obstruction from being discharged into the intestine. The obstruction may be caused by gallstones, by tumors or, uncommonly, by parasites in the bile ducts. Jaundice may also be an accompanying sign of hepatitis, a disorder in which the inflamed or damaged liver cannot process the bilirubin it receives. Occasionally, jaundice appears if too many red blood cells are too rapidly destroyed, sometimes as a result of an anemic condition, and the liver cannot accommodate the excess. In addition, jaundice is associated with, or symptomatic of, many other diseases in which the normal functioning of the liver is disrupted. These diseases include certain cancers and certain viral and parasitic infections. Over 50 percent of full-term and 80 percent of premature newborns show signs of jaundice by the second or third day after birth. In most of these cases, however, the condition is nothing to worry about and

disappears in a week or so.

Symptoms

When jaundice occurs, the liver usually has become enlarged and functions less effectively. Bowel movements may be clay-colored, and urine can vary in hue from light yellow to a brownish green. Jaundiced skin ranges in color from lemony yellow to dark olive green.

Diagnosis

Routine blood testing will determine the origin of most cases of jaundice, but occasionally it may be necessary to observe the bile ducts, by means of an X ray. Certain dyes injected into the blood will collect in the liver and bile ducts to show the point of obstruction on an X ray. Other alternatives include ultrasound, in which sound waves bounce off internal body structures and form an image of them, and a CAT scan, a special technique that provides a cross-sectional picture of the area.

Treatment

If a backup of bile is observed, surgery to eliminate the obstruction may be indicated. Otherwise, treatment will be determined by the nature of the cause of the jaundice.

Periodontal disease

Periodontal disease, or periodon-

Plaque buildup

Receding gum tissue

Bone deterioration

Pockets of bacteria

The left side shows what periodontal disease can do; the right side shows a healthy tooth, bones, and gums.

titis, is a progressive deterioration of the gums and bones around the teeth.

Causes

One theory is that the condition begins with an accumulation of bacteria and food particles that lodges within tissues surrounding the teeth. These bacteria emit toxins (poisons) that cause gum tissues to swell, bleed, and erode.

Stages of periodontitis

Gingivitis, inflammation of the gums, is the first stage of periodontitis. Pyorrhea (running of pus), the second stage of periodontitis, results when the soft tissues are separated from the bone and teeth leading to "pocket" formation.

Pockets of bacteria and pus accumulate around the teeth leading to weakening of the fibers holding the teeth in their sockets as well as to destruction of the bone supporting the teeth. As the disease advances, teeth become loose and fall out. They may also move out of alignment with one another and cause problems with chewing.

Symptoms

In the early stage of periodontal disease, gums become sore, red, and slightly swollen. They may be sensitive to the touch and bleed when brushed or flossed. Pus in the gums around the teeth signals the beginning of the second disease stage. If pus remains in the gum tissue without draining, pain and swelling can result.

Diagnosis

A dentist diagnoses the beginning of periodontal disease by examining the swollen gums and the deposits of bacteria and plaque around the teeth.

Treatment and prevention

Once detected, continued care of the mouth at home can help prevent extensive periodontal disease and reduce gum problems.

Oral hygiene to prevent gum disease is the same as treatment to prevent tooth decay. Ideally, the mouth needs to be cleaned after every meal. More realistically, a thorough cleansing before bed may minimize the chances of gum disease. Dentists suggest brushing teeth with a soft-bristled brush. Gentle movements within the crevices dislodge decay-causing material, while firm strokes over the teeth remove plaque.

Flossing is recommended to clear plaque from between teeth. After brushing and flossing, vigorously rinsing the mouth with mouthwash containing antimicrobials (substances that kill bacteria) can also help eliminate bacteria formation; but mouthwash alone cannot prevent plaque.

For self-checking, a dental mirror provides a view of the teeth and gums in the back of the mouth. Disclosing wafers, which when chewed discolor plaque, reveal any invisible film to be removed.

For advanced cases, a dentist may scrape the affected tissue pockets and apply antiseptics (germ-killers) every few months in an effort to kill the bacteria. Should this procedure fail to check the spread of the disease, surgery by a periodontist (gum specialist) may be needed to remove deep pockets in the gum. Once the bacteria are eliminated, good oral hygiene practices should control the disease.

Peritonitis

Peritonitis is a term used to describe an inflammation and/or infection of the thin double-layered membrane (peritoneum) covering the abdominal organs.

Causes

The condition occurs when the peritoneum is invaded by bacteria, toxins (poisons), bile (a substance produced by the liver and stored in the gallbladder), blood, or urine. Because the peritoneum is well-sealed, the only way it can be infiltrated is when one of the hollow organs of the abdomen ruptures; when a solid organ is somehow damaged, causing it to leak; or when there is a penetrating injury from the outside. For example, if the bladder is ruptured in an accident, sterile urine is discharged into the peritoneal cavity. Although germ-free, the urine is quite irritating, thereby causing a "chemical peritonitis." If, however, the colon is perforated, fecal contents, containing loads of bacteria and toxins, are discharged. This creates a bacterial peritonitis. Both of these conditions are extremely serious and must be immediately remedied.

Symptoms

A main symptom of peritonitis is severe pain that intensifies with any movement and often forces the person to lie very still with legs drawn up. The abdominal area is very tender and grows rigid; commonly there is vomiting, fever, and dehydration (loss of body fluids). When the peritoneum is inflamed, fluid begins to leak out of the blood vessels into the peritoneum. If not corrected, this may lead to shock (failure of the circulatory system because of loss of blood volume). After some time, the abdomen may swell. This is a danger sign that the intestines have become paralyzed and bloated with air.

Treatment

These symptoms and signs signify a need for immediate medical care, including intravenous (injected through the veins) antibiotics to fight infection. Intravenous fluids are also given to restore lost volume. In addition, usually a tube is inserted through the nose and into the stomach to relieve the bloating and remove pooled fluids. After the patient is stabilized with these procedures, surgery to remove or repair the cause of peritonitis is done. Chances for recovery are usually excellent.

Pyloric stenosis

Pyloric stenosis is a narrowing of the passage between the stomach and the small intestine. The stomach has two openings: at the top, where it joins with the esophagus, which is the food passage between the throat and the stomach, and at the bottom, where it joins with the small intestine. The lower opening is called the pylorus.

Causes

Pyloric stenosis (stenosis means narrowing or constriction) can be caused by many conditions including cancer, spasm, a nearby ulcer in the part of the intestine directly below the pyloric opening, gastritis (inflammation of the stomach), or enlargement of the pyloric sphincter muscle (the muscle that rings the pyloric opening and controls its movement).

Symptoms

In the case of congenital (present at birth) pyloric stenosis, ten days to three weeks after birth the infant will experience regurgitation (weak "spitting up" of part of the stomach's contents), projectile vomiting (vomiting with great force), weight loss, and dehydration (loss of body fluids) without appetite loss. Adults with pyloric stenosis experience discomfort in the upper and middle portion of the abdomen, pain, bloating of the abdominal area, nausea and vomiting, and weight loss.

Treatment

In mild cases of pyloric stenosis, the condition can be treated by taking small feedings or meals, restoring normal fluid levels, and administering anticholinergic drugs (drugs that block the strength of the nerve impulses that are making the pyloric muscle contract).

In severe cases, a pyloromyotomy (a lengthwise incision into the pyloric muscle) may be indicated. Also, a portion of the pyloric sphincter muscle may be removed.

Tooth decay

Tooth decay (or dental cavities or caries) is the gradual destruction and loss of minerals in the enamel (outer layer) and dentin (the bony second layer) of a portion of a tooth, which causes it to become soft, discolored, and porous.

Causes

A combination of factors causes tooth decay. The actual destruction is probably done by bacteria and by-products of their metabolism such as acid. These bacteria feed on sugars and starches that cling to the teeth. They live and multiply to become dental plaque. The plaque is made up of sugars, starches, bacteria, and proteins, and builds up on dental surfaces, especially near the gums and in other hard-to-clean areas. Here the production of acid is concentrated. The plaque prevents the saliva from performing its natural protective function.

Symptoms

When the cavity has progressed into the dentin or begins on the surface of an exposed root, the tooth becomes sensitive to touch and to rapid temperature changes. Sweet foods can cause pain as dissolved sugar enters the cavity. Bacteria may pass through tiny tubes in the dentin and inflame the pulp, which contains blood vessels and nervous tissue, producing toothache.

Diagnosis

The cavity reveals itself to the examining dentist as a darkened area or as a softness that "gives" when probed with a sharp instrument. It is also detected by X rays.

Treatment

Cavities are treated by drilling out the decayed material and replacing it with a filling. In front teeth, where appearance is important, the filling may be of porcelain cement or a plastic resin (which is also used to fill pits and tiny cracks in the enamel). In other teeth the filling is usually silver-colored or an alloy of gold, which is the most durable material. Where a tooth is badly damaged with involvement of the root canal, the dentist removes all decay, fills the cavity and/or root canal with cement, then grinds and tapers the outer surfaces and covers them with what is known as a gold crown. On teeth toward the front, the gold crown is overlaid with porcelain to provide a natural appearance.

Prevention

To prevent decay, teeth should be cleaned daily with a soft-bristled brush, preferably after each meal, to remove food particles and plaque. Equally important is the use of dental floss to remove debris between the teeth. Avoiding sweet, sticky foods, or at least rinsing or brushing shortly after eating them, may also help prevent decay. A child's teeth will be more resistant to decay if the child drinks water containing the proper amount of fluoride in the first 12 years while the teeth are developing. If the water supply is not fluoridated, a vitamin supplement containing fluoride can be taken daily. Adults and children alike can benefit by using a fluoride-containing toothpaste or mouthwash.

Ulcer

An ulcer is an open sore or erosion on the surface of an organ or tissue. The most common ulcers erupt in the digestive tract, in which case they are known as peptic ulcers. Peptic ulcers can appear in the lining of the esophagus (tube leading to the stomach), stomach, or duodenum (beginning of the small intestine).

Causes

Although the cause of a peptic ulcer is unconfirmed, scientists believe that the more common duodenal ulcers may result from excessive amounts of digestive juices produced by the stomach. The stomach may increase acidic secretions after coffee, alcohol, aspirin, and other painkillers are consumed, or after cigarettes are smoked. Therefore, these substances are thought to contribute to ulcers.

The less common stomach ulcers may be due to an inherent weakness in the wall of the stomach. However, this weakness may result from the same environmental conditions that aggravate duodenal ulcers.

Emotional stress may play a role in ulcer development. However, physicians distinguish between stress as a factor by itself and the way certain people deal with stress that would make them susceptible to ulcers.

Heredity plays an important role in contributing to ulcers since people who have a history of ulcers in their family seem to have a greater likelihood of acquiring the condition. Furthermore, for unknown reasons, people with Type O blood are more likely to develop ulcers. In addition, liver disease, rheumatoid arthritis (inflammation of connective tissue), and emphysema (overinflation of the lungs' air sacs) may increase vulnerability to ulcers.

Symptoms

Ulcers can produce mild symptoms resembling heartburn or indigestion, or severe pain radiating throughout the upper portion

The most common ulcers are those that affect the stomach or the duodenum, the beginning section of the small intestine.

of the body. The most common discomfort of ulcers is a burning in the abdomen above the navel that may feel like hunger pangs. Pain comes about 30 to 120 minutes after eating or in the middle of the night when the stomach is empty. At this time, the stomach's acidic juices are more apt to irritate the unprotected nerve endings in the exposed ulcer. Usually, pain subsides after eating or drinking something or taking an antacid to neutralize stomach acid.

Some people experience nausea, vomiting, and constipation. Blood in feces (discoloring it black), blood in vomit, extreme weakness, fainting, and excessive thirst are all signs of internal bleeding, and may appear with more advanced ulcers.

While ulcers are not life-threatening, they can cause serious damage if left untreated. Ulcers may corrode nearby blood vessels and cause internal seepage of blood or massive internal bleeding (hemorrhage). A perforated ulcer may penetrate an adjoining organ, causing infection. In addition, scar tissue growing around the ulcer may lead to an intestinal obstruction.

Diagnosis

Physicians diagnose peptic ulcers primarily by X ray. The patient swallows barium, a chalky substance, and stands in front of a fluorescent screen. As the X-ray tube moves down from the shoulder, the barium shows an opaque outline of the digestive tract that allows the doctor a view of any abnormalities.

When an X ray is inconclusive, the doctor inserts a gastroscope (long, flexible lighted tube) through the mouth and down the esophagus to see the ulcer. Stomach ulcers require a gastroscopic examination and a biopsy (removal of tissue sample for analysis) to confirm that the ulcer is not actually a cancer showing up as an ulcer on the X ray.

Treatment

Treatment for ulcers involves relieving the irritation so healing progresses naturally. Over-the-counter antacids counteract stomach acid and relieve symptoms, but they can cause complications. For example, sodium bicarbonate, a primary antacid ingredient, contains large amounts of sodium (salt) that can aggravate kidney disease or high blood pressure.

For more problematic ulcers, a physician may prescribe other preparations to promote healing. Anticholinergic drugs delay emptying of the stomach and keep the lining cushioned against acidity. Antispasmodic drugs relax digestive tract muscles and relieve tension if stress is a contributing factor to a particular ulcer case. Various new medications either form a protective coating against the acid in the stomach (sucralfate) or inhibit gastric acid secretion (cimetidine and ranitidine). With any drug, caution is suggested as side effects can outweigh their benefits.

Although recent studies have shown that a bland diet is unnecessary for ulcer management, a mild diet may be recommended until acute symptoms disappear. Thereafter, many doctors suggest avoiding only those foods known to cause stomach distress.

The effect of milk on ulcers is also questionable. Its neutralizing action on stomach acid is mild and temporary at best. Nevertheless, people who substitute milk for proven irritants, such as alcohol or caffeine, are less likely to stimulate their ulcers.

Most ulcers heal within two to six weeks after treatment begins. To prevent recurrence, patients should still refrain from cigarettes, caffeine, alcohol, or other known stimulants that would stimulate stomach acid production or irritate the digestive tract lining.

When drug therapy and diet cannot cure an ulcer, surgical removal may be necessary. Surgery follows repeated ulcers or ulcers that are life-threatening, such as perforated ulcers. Sometimes, surgeons remove a portion of the stomach and parts of the vagus nerve (which controls digestive secretions) to reduce stomach acid production.

Ulcerative colitis

Ulcerative colitis is a chronic, inflammatory disease of the colon (the latter section of the large intestine), characterized by bloody diarrhea. The lining of the colon becomes ulcerated — exhibiting open erosions.

Causes

Although there is a familial tendency to develop ulcerative colitis, the cause of the disorder is unknown. Any age group may be affected, but it tends to begin in persons between the ages of 15 and 40.

Among possible contributing factors are infection, immunological derangement (some breakdown in the patient's protective system), lack of protective elements in the bowel wall, either nervous or psychological disturbances, and alterations in the nature of the connective tissue in the colon. However, the best clue as to cause is the strikingly higher proportions of the disease in certain families.

Symptoms

The first sign of ulcerative colitis is usually a series of attacks of bloody diarrhea. The attacks can vary in intensity and duration and are usually interspersed with normal periods. The onset of the attacks may be severe, with sudden violent diarrhea, high fever, symptoms of abdominal inflammation, and bacterial invasions. Often, an attack will be preceded by mild lower abdominal cramps and the appearance of small amounts of blood or mucus in the feces.

If ulceration is confined to the rectum and terminal portion of the colon, the bowel movements may be normal or very hard and dry, with discharges of mucus full of red and white blood cells between stools. If the disorder extends to other portions of the colon, however, stools become looser and more frequent (perhaps 10 to 20 per day), and the patient suffers severe cramps, watery stools, fever, anemia, and loss of appetite.

Complications

If the condition persists in this severe form, hemorrhage (internal bleeding) is the most common complication. In toxic colitis, a serious complication, the colon loses muscular tone and dilates almost completely, resulting in perforations of the organ. The risk of colon cancer and cancer of the bile ducts is also increased in patients with ulcerative colitis.

Diagnosis

Ulcerative colitis is diagnosed through medical history, a stool examination, and sigmoidoscopy (in which a lighted, flexible tube is inserted into the colon for a visual examination of the interior). X ray studies with a barium enema are indicated except in cases where risk of perforation makes the barium enema procedure a potential danger for the patient.

Treatment

Mild cases of ulcerative colitis can be managed by adequate physical and mental relaxation, since the disease appears to be stress-related in some patients; a normal diet low in high-fiber fruits and vegetables and possibly milk; and antidiarrheal medication. More severe cases may respond to a drug known as sulfasalazine. In cases that do not respond to sulfasalazine therapy, hydrocortisone (artificial hormones) may be given by enema injection once or twice a day.

THE KIDNEYS
AND URINARY
SYSTEM

The urinary system includes those organs of the body that produce and eliminate urine, a combination of water and waste products passing out of the body as fluid. By controlling urine flow, the system maintains proper water balance throughout the body. Individual parts of the urinary system monitor concentration of salts and other necessary nutrients.

Functions of urinary system organs

The organs responsible for control of nutrients in the blood are the two kidneys. Kidneys are the bean-shaped structures located in the back of the abdomen. Their chief functions are to filter waste from the blood and insure reabsorption of essential nutrients back into the bloodstream. In the kidney, waste products combine with water to form urine.

Urine passes from each kidney into the bladder through tubes called ureters. The bladder stores the urine prior to elimination from the body. A muscle around the exit from the bladder prevents urine from escaping. When the bladder is about half full, the body feels an urge to empty the organ. At this time, the muscle relaxes to release the urine through the urethra.

The urethra is a tube that conveys urine from the bladder to the exterior of the body. The female urethra is about an inch and a half long and is enclosed within the body. The male urethra passes through the penis and is approximately eight inches long. For the male, the urethra serves the dual function of transporting urine and semen (fluid from male reproductive organs). Semen is ejaculated during sexual intercourse, during which urine is automatically blocked from leaving the bladder.

Disorders of the urinary system

Changes in urine and urinary habits that do not seem to have an obvious cause, such as drinking more liquids than usual, may be symptoms of disease.

Some symptoms requiring medical attention—if they last for more than a day or two—are changes in frequency, timing, control, quantity, and color, as well as accompanying pain.

A doctor should be contacted immediately if there is extreme pain while urinating; blood in the urine; a noticeable decrease in frequency (a symptom of kidney

This drawing shows the urinary system of a female. The blood is filtered through the kidneys, and the waste products, plus excess body water, are sent as urine through the system for excretion.

failure); or strong color changes or cloudiness, accompanied by pain or fever.

Changes in urine or urinary habits may be caused by a variety of disorders involving the kidneys, urinary tract, bladder, and prostate (a doughnut-shaped gland surrounding the male urethra), among others. The exact cause of a urinary problem is often related to the type of symptom displayed.

Increased frequency may be caused by inflammation of the kidneys, bladder, or urethra; diabetes (an imbalance in blood sugar level); or an enlarged prostate.

A change in timing of urination, usually in the form of very frequent nighttime awakenings accompanied by the urge to urinate (called nocturia), is often coupled with painful urination, a poor stream, or difficulty in starting. These may be symptoms of an inflammatory or infectious disease within the urinary tract, as well as tumors or other disorders that result in increased pressure on the bladder.

Difficulty in controlling, starting, and maintaining the flow may also be symptoms of an inflammation of the prostate gland. Inability to hold back urine is a common problem of elderly people as their control of the bladder muscle weakens. Also affected by this problem are women in the late stages of pregnancy. In this case, the weight of the uterus presses heavily on the bladder without letup.

Changes in the quantity of urine normally produced can also signal disease. Producing an excessive amount of urine (called polyuria) may be a symptom of kidney disease, diabetes, or glandular disorders.

Slight changes in the color and clarity of the urine day to day are normal, but strong color changes and extreme cloudiness may signal infection, tumors, kidney stones, prostate problems, or cysts along the urinary tract.

Pain while urinating, most commonly in the form of a burning sensation felt along the urethra, may be a sign of a lower urinary tract infection. Excruciating pain across the abdomen or the back may signal the presence of kidney stones.

Treatment of urinary problems usually involves treating the underlying cause of the sudden change, which can range from mild infections to very serious diseases. An accurate diagnosis by a physician is the first step to proper treatment of these disorders.

Cystitis

Cystitis is an inflammation of the urinary bladder; the term, however, is commonly used to mean bladder infection.

Causes

Occurring in women much more often than in men, it is usually caused by bacteria that have invaded the urethra, the tube that transports urine from the bladder to the outside of the body, and entered the urinary bladder. Women are more susceptible than men because their urethras are so short (approximately one inch versus seven to eight inches in men), thus presenting less distance for the bacteria to travel. In addition, in women the external openings of the urethra, vagina (birth canal), and anus (intestine) are so close together that bacteria can easily migrate from one to another. Almost always the bacteria responsible are of various types that normally live harmlessly in the human intestine, but which can contaminate or invade the area around the opening of the urethra and enter the bladder. Obstruction is also a common cause of urinary tract infection. When obstruction occurs, the bladder may not empty properly. The remaining urine in the bladder then creates a breeding ground for bacteria to multiply. Causes of obstruction can include tumors, stones, or an enlarged prostate gland (the male reproductive gland located at the base of the bladder surrounding the urethra).

Besides blockage, the urethral lining may have a defect which allows bacteria to enter the tract. For example, frequent intercourse

Prostate gland

Bladder

Urethra

Anus

Urethral opening

The male urethra is about seven or eight inches long.

Bladder

Uterus

Urethra

Vagina

Anus

The female urethra is about one inch long.

Cystitis is nearly ten times more common in women than in men because the urethra is much shorter in women than in men. Therefore, the infecting bacteria have less distance to travel in women.

may traumatize the urethra, disrupting its lining and making it more susceptible to infection.

Cystitis in men is uncommon. When it does occur, the usual cause is an infection that has spread from an inflamed prostate gland or that has developed in the bladder because of an enlarged prostate. Bladder infections in men, unless from an obvious cause, usually require detailed evaluation such as a kidney X ray and possibly cystoscopy, an examination by means of a flexible lighted tube (called a cystoscope) inserted through the urethra.

Urethritis, an infection or inflammation of the urethra only, is common in both men and women and is usually acquired through sexual intercourse with an infected individual. Gonorrhea and nongonorrheal urethritis (in which the infectious agent, although acquired through intercourse, is different from that of gonorrhea) are the two most common examples of this. There are, of course, nonvenereal causes of urethritis also.

Symptoms

The symptoms of cystitis include a painful sensation or burning upon urination, a frequent and often urgent need to urinate (even awakening one at night), and occasional low back pain. These symptoms, along with bloody urine, are known as "hemorrhagic cystitis" and occur quite commonly in women. Although quite frightening, this is most often a minor, easily treatable condition. In men, however, bloody urine is not usually attributable to hemorrhagic cystitis and demands immediate investigation. With the exception of visibly bloody urine, all of the above symptoms can be present in urethritis which is also commonly accompanied by a discharge. High fever, chills, upper (usually one-sided) back pain with or without any of the above symptoms usually indicate a kidney infection (pyelonephritis) and

demand the immediate attention of a doctor.

Diagnosis

Along with the above symptoms and signs, the diagnosis of urinary infection rests on the urinalysis and culture. The presence of moderate to large amounts of white blood cells, along with at least 100,000 colonies of any one bacterium in a culture, provides conclusive evidence of infection.

Not infrequently, it is difficult to determine which part of the urinary tract is infected, or if there is infection at all. In women, the opening of the urethra normally has some white blood cells and bacteria present. Therefore, in order to keep the urine specimen free from these contaminants, a midstream specimen is usually requested. The reason for this is that the first spurt of urine is thought to wash away the normal debris and the rest of the urine is now uncontaminated and provides a pure culture. For the vast majority of simple cystitis cases, this procedure is quite adequate; however, if a question exists as to the validity of the specimen or if for some reason the specimen must be absolutely free of contaminants, a catheter (thin, flexible tube) may be inserted into the bladder through the urethra. In women, this is an easy procedure and eliminates vaginal and/or anal (opening from the intestines) contaminants. If the catheterized specimen is free from pus and/or bacteria, the symptoms are of another condition — commonly vaginitis or urethritis. In a man, the procedure is somewhat more difficult and usually not necessary. If prostatitis is the suspected cause of the infection, the diagnosis is usually made by the physician inserting a gloved finger into the anus and directly feeling the gland. An infected prostate is usually quite tender and has a characteristic "boggy" feel. A specimen of prostatic fluid is usually obtained (by massaging the gland at the time of examination) through the urethra for culture.

Even with the above techniques, the differentiation between different sites of infection of the urinary tract is often not a simple matter and can have important implications as to treatment. The experience of the physician, the patient's history as to signs and symptoms (such as discharge, recent intercourse, back pain, or fever), along with still more sophisticated diagnostic techniques are all important in making the correct diagnosis.

In difficult chronic cases of cystitis in both men and women, in which the cause of recurring infection may be an obstruction or drainage problem, contrast fluid may be placed into the bladder by means of a catheter and X-ray pictures taken of the bladder and of the urethra during urination. The X rays may detect narrowed portions of the urethra, stones, and incomplete emptying of the bladder (which promotes cystitis). The bladder might also be examined by means of a cystoscope—a flexible lighted tube inserted through the urethra. Most often these procedures are preceded by an intravenous pyelogram in which contrast material injected through a vein is eliminated by the kidneys, providing an X-ray picture of the kidneys, ureters (tubes from the kidneys to the bladder), and the bladder.

Treatment

Treatment of first-time cystitis is by means of antibiotics by mouth for seven to ten days. Recently, large single doses of drugs have been found to work well in many cases. Recurrences may be treated in the same way if due to a different organism. If the same organism is causing the trouble, the condition may require larger doses of medication and/or treatment for up to four to six weeks. If the cystitis still persists, daily doses of medications may be necessary for up to six months. It is important that dosage instructions be followed exactly, because a person is vulnerable to a new infection or a reinfection of the same bacteria if the entire course of recommended drug therapy is not completed. Some individuals are prone to repeated episodes of cystitis or upper urinary tract infection. If an anatomic defect, such as a narrowed urethra, exists, dilatation (enlarging) may be needed. If stones are present, they may need to be removed surgically. If an infected prostate is the source of infection, antibiotics are usually tried first; surgery is a last resort. If no obvious reason for recurrent cystitis is found, the patient may be placed on low doses of antibiotics for long periods of time (this is called prophylactic — or preventive — therapy).

Prevention

Women may be able to guard against recurrent cystitis by front-to-back wiping with toilet tissue and soap and water cleansing after each bowel movement. They should also try to urinate immediately after sexual intercourse to wash away infecting bacteria that might enter the urethra. Loose, absorbent underclothes allow evaporation and absorption of body fluids and thus help prevent infection. Both men and women should drink plenty of fluids and urinate frequently, completely emptying the bladder each time.

Dialysis

Dialysis is the removal of wastes and other undesirable substances from the blood by means of a membrane that is selective in what it allows to cross. In the healthy body, this task is performed by the kidneys.

Hemodialysis

In a patient suffering from temporary or permanent kidney failure, however, this can be done with an artificial kidney machine and is known as hemodialysis. Two plastic tubes, one connected to an artery and one to a vein, are implanted in the patient's arm or leg. During dialysis, which can take three to five hours per treatment, blood from the artery tube enters the machine and comes into contact with a thin (commonly cellophane) membrane. Wastes from the blood pass through the membrane into circulating fluid on the other side. The blood cells themselves, along with other protein elements, are not allowed across the membrane. The cleaned blood is then piped back into the patient through the vein tube.

Peritoneal dialysis

Another method is called peritoneal dialysis. Here, the individual's own peritoneum (lining of the abdominal cavity) is used as the membrane. A sterile plastic catheter (tube) is passed into the abdominal cavity and a solution of glucose (a sugar) and mineral salts is periodically injected into and withdrawn from the cavity. The fluid comes into contact with delicate blood vessels in the peritoneum. Because of the difference in concentration of certain elements in the blood and the fluid, fluids and wastes from the blood are caused (by complex biologic principles) to pass through the peritoneal membrane wall into the dialysis liquid, which is withdrawn and replaced by a new liquid. The passage of material from one side of a membrane (the blood side) to the other (dialysis fluid side) is based on the same principles of the above mentioned hemodialysis.

Continuous ambulatory peritoneal dialysis

A new method called continuous ambulatory peritoneal dialysis has greatly lowered the cost of dialysis and made it more convenient. It can be done at home by the patient without the complex equipment and the skilled supervision that has made machine dialysis so expensive. A tube is surgically implanted in the patient, just below the navel. About every four to five hours and just before bedtime, the patient empties a bag of fresh dialysis fluid into the abdominal cavity through the tube and drains out the old fluid. This insures that fluid remains in the cavity, soaking up waste from the blood, while the patient sleeps or goes about usual daily activities. The procedure takes about 30 minutes each time but enables the patient to be independent and mobile.

Glomerulonephritis

Glomerulonephritis is an inflammation of the capillaries (tiny blood vessels) in the filtering units of the kidneys, called glomeruli, where wastes are drawn from the blood to form urine. The disease can be caused by an infection in the kidneys, but most often it is due to an allergic or immune response to infections in other parts of the body, particularly streptococcal infections such as strep throat, or to drugs or poisons in the bloodstream. The immune response occurs as an inflammation of the capillaries in the glomeruli. The capillaries become congested and surrounded by blood cells and pus. Fluid builds up in surrounding tissue, sometimes causing the kidney to enlarge. Protein, which should

remain in the blood, is discharged into the urine by the diseased glomeruli, and there is a general fluid buildup in body tissues. These two signs—fluid buildup (edema) and albumin (a form of protein) in the urine—are the two chief indicators of the disease first described in 1827 by English physician Richard Bright. (The disease used to be called Bright's disease, but doctors today are more likely to refer to it as glomerulonephritis from "glomeruli"; "nephro," referring to the kidney; and "itis," meaning inflammation.) If the disease continues to progress, the tiny arteries in the kidney become thickened and scarred so that some can no longer carry blood. The parts of the kidney they serve shrink and change. The eventual result of this process over many years may be total kidney failure. However, the great majority of patients with acute glomerulonephritis recover within one to two years. Only 5 to 20 percent develop chronic glomerulonephritis cases.

Causes

Although many different kinds of infections can lead to glomerulonephritis, including pneumonia, bacterial infection of the heart, secondary syphilis, malaria, hepatitis, and measles, by far the most common cause is streptococcal infection of the throat, tonsils, or skin.

Symptoms

Symptoms of glomerulonephritis begin one to six weeks after an initial infection such as strep

Glomerulonephritis is an inflammation of the tiny blood vessels of the glomeruli, the kidney's filtering units that draw wastes from the blood to form urine.

throat. The patient has headaches, a mild fever, a puffy face, pain in the area between the ribs and the hip, and decreased urine output. The urine may be bloody or coffee-colored. Shortness of breath may occur, together with increased heartbeat and a rise in blood pressure. A urine test for protein and red blood cells confirms the diagnosis. In extreme cases, the bloated condition of the body from accumulated fluids can cause the symptoms of heart failure, including rapid heartbeat, heart enlargement, and congestion of the lungs.

Treatment

Treatment consists of bed rest until one to two weeks after tests of blood, blood pressure, and of the urine reveal that the kidney is back to normal. Sodium (salt) and protein may be restricted or even forbidden for a time. Fluids are restricted until the output of urine returns to normal. Heart failure is treated with restriction of salt and water and with use of oxygen and the drug digitalis. Any infection is treated promptly with antibiotics.

If the disease is still present after one to two years, it may be considered chronic. Typically, the damage to the kidney continues to progress, but so slowly that the patient is without symptoms except for evidence in the urine including protein and red and white blood cells. A normal life may be possible for 20 or 30 years until the kidney can no longer function. At that time, replacement with a kidney transplant or periodic cleansing of the blood with a dialysis machine is necessary for life.

Guarding against infection, injury, and fatigue can help prevent flare-ups of the disease. Intake of protein may have to be limited, depending upon how the kidney is working. Plenty of fluids and normal activity are desirable, but strenuous exercise should be avoided, to prevent fatigue.

Incontinence

Incontinence is the loss of voluntary bladder or bowel control. It occurs frequently in children and in older persons.

Causes

Most often, incontinence is caused by some other underlying condition, such as a problem with the urinary tract—infection, inflammation, or pain—or with the muscles that control the bladder or bowel. It may also be caused by epileptic seizures, brain or spinal cord tumors or injuries, or a stroke. Successful treatment of the underlying cause clears up the problem of incontinence.

Stress incontinence is the involuntary leakage of urine on coughing, sneezing, straining, or laughing. This type of incontinence is common in women whose muscles have been weakened by childbirth.

Treatment

Although the first step in treating incontinence is to detect and correct any underlying problem, it is important to remember that many children have not established complete bladder and/or bowel control before they are four or five years old. Children of any age may have occasional accidents especially if they are ill or exhausted.

Persons who have problems with incontinence can help themselves by going to the bathroom often and regularly, by arranging sleeping and living quarters near bathrooms, and by wearing clothes that can be removed quickly and easily. It may also help to keep a bed pan or chamber pot next to the bed. If the problem is a urinary one, the incontinent person should drink only a small amount of water, if any, before going to bed. If the problem is bowel incontinence, the person should eat a lot of high fiber foods to establish regularity and should also keep in mind that bowels tend to move about one hour after a meal has been eaten.

While there are drugs available to aid in controlling urination, no drugs are yet available for controlling bowel movements.

Kidney failure

The kidneys are two bean-shaped organs located in the back of the upper abdomen. Their functions are to filter chemical wastes from the blood, excrete these wastes in the form of urine, and regulate body concentrations of water and nutrients. When kidney failure occurs, certain abnormalities within the kidneys prevent them from functioning normally, leading to chemical imbalances and the buildup of toxic (poisonous) substances and fluid within the body. This may eventually lead to organ damage and possibly death.

Forms of kidney failure

There are two forms of kidney failure. In the acute form, there is a sudden malfunction of the kidneys leading to a rapid buildup of toxins and fluid within the body, often within several hours. In the chronic form of kidney failure, there is a slow, progressive malfunction of the kidneys leading to a slow buildup of toxins and fluid, often occurring over several months to years.

Causes

Numerous conditions can cause kidney failure. Untreated high blood pressure, kidney stones or other urinary tract blockage, adverse reactions to chemicals or drugs, serious injury, infectious disease, shock following surgery, heart attack, blood transfusion with incompatible blood, severe dehydration (loss of body fluid), complications during pregnancy, immunologic disease, or congenital (existing from birth) kidney defects may all lead to kidney failure.

Symptoms

The most characteristic symptoms of kidney failure are a reduction in urine volume and edema, a condition in which fluid accumulates in the tissues. As a result, feet and hands and the area around the eyes may swell and become puffy. Urine color may change indicating kidney disease. In kidney failure, the urine may be bloody, wine-colored, or cloudy.

More generalized signs of kidney failure include drowsiness and fatigue, loss of appetite, diarrhea, nausea, dry skin, and difficulty in breathing. Delirium, coma, and death will eventually occur in untreated cases.

Diagnosis

Analysis of blood and urine samples is used to diagnose kidney failure. Urine tests may reveal substances such as white blood cells, sugars, or protein that have slipped through the normally efficient filtering system of the kidneys. Similarly, when the kidneys are not filtering waste materials from the blood, blood analysis identifies the waste products that remain in the blood. X rays or ultrasound scans of the kidneys may determine any structural abnormalities or blockage.

Treatment

In the case of acute kidney failure, treatment begins with diagnosing and correcting the cause of the kidney damage and restoring normal kidney function as rapidly as possible. For example, shock may be treated with blood transfusions or kidney stones may be surgically removed.

Complete bed rest is essential as the kidneys recover. In addition, limited fluid intake, except in cases of unusual fluid loss from diarrhea or vomiting, relieves the strain on the sensitive kidneys. Physicians often recommend a low-protein diet to reduce the extra strain that is required to process the waste products of protein metabolism in the kidneys.

Should these measures prove ineffective, the patient may be helped by dialysis. Dialysis is a process that cleans and filters toxic substances from the blood by an artificial kidney machine. Most dialysis patients receive treatment by traveling to the hospital three times a week. However, a newer portable technique allows more freedom for dialysis patients.

In the case of chronic kidney failure, destruction of the kidney has progressed to the point where treatment cannot bring kidney function back to normal. Treatment of these patients involves a diet low in salt and protein and dialysis at least three times a week. Dialysis will offer a chance to prolong life, but it is not a cure for the kidney failure. Only surgically replacing the damaged kidneys will cure the kidney failure. In recent years, methods of matching kidney donors with recipients have improved, thereby limiting transplant rejection and serious complications. Today, kidney transplants are a highly successful treatment for chronic kidney failure.

Kidney stones

Kidney stones are deposits of mineral or organic substances that form in the kidney. Their size may vary from that of tiny pebbles to walnut-like formations.

The formation of kidney stones depends upon what types and amounts of excess substances are found in the urine, the fluid mixture of water and waste products produced in the kidney and excreted from the body. When abnormally high levels of minerals, such as calcium, are in the urine, they may condense into hard masses, forming stones in the kidney.

Causes

Increased levels of calcium in urine may come from drinking large quantities of milk. Eating foods rich in Vitamin D, which helps the body absorb calcium, can also contribute to an overaccumulation of calcium. In addition, fractured bones can release extra calcium that may condense into stones in the kidney.

Certain disorders encourage building of mineral deposits in the kidney. Gout is a joint disease that results from high blood levels of uric acid (a waste product from breakdown of protein) that crystallizes into stones in the urine. Urinary infections that impede bladder function can also cause reten-

Kidney stones are formed in the kidney but may migrate to the ureter, creating an obstruction with swelling and damage above the blockage.

tion of urine that then harbors higher concentrations of elements that can solidify into stones. In addition, overactive parathyroids (endocrine glands that regulate calcium absorption) permit increased mineral absorption into the body, and this may lead to the development of kidney stones.

Middle-aged men and people with gout or chronic urinary tract infections are more susceptible to kidney stones. However, in many cases, no one can pinpoint the cause of the kidney stones.

Symptoms

Kidney stones may remain inactive for years and never produce any symptoms. On the other hand, some stones can cause problems as they pass out of the kidneys, including severe pain and tenderness over the affected kidney, frequent and painful urination, nausea, blood in the urine, fever, chills, and extreme exhaustion.

A more serious condition develops as the stone enters the ureter (the tube that carries urine from the kidney to the bladder) where it lodges and produces excruciating pain across the back, abdomen, and reproductive organs. If blockage occurs in the urethra, the tube that conveys urine from the bladder to the outside of the body, urine output decreases. The trapped urine may back up, distending and injuring the urinary tract. This situation requires immediate medical treatment to prevent loss of consciousness, shock, and possible kidney damage.

Kidney stones that are too small to be noticed may still cause damage to delicate tissues as they move through the urinary tract, scraping organ linings and leaving internal scars.

Diagnosis

To determine the type of kidney stone formation, a physician analyzes the blood and urine samples. X rays or an ultrasound scan, in which high-frequency sound waves bounce off internal body structures and outline their image, reveal the location and nature of the stones.

Treatment

The recurrence of kidney stones may often be controlled by diet. Reducing or eliminating intake of foods with high levels of stone-producing minerals can prevent worsening of the condition and the formation of new stones.

Since calcium contributes to kidney stones in most cases, the diet should be low in milk products and Vitamin D foods. Gout patients should decrease their protein intake, since uric acid is a by-product of protein digestion.

As yet, there are no drugs available to dissolve kidney stones. Doctors may prescribe painkillers if the pain from the movement of a stone is too great. Other medications inhibit absorption of calcium from the blood.

For kidney stones too large to pass, surgical removal may be necessary. However, a new less intrusive method of treating kidney stones is under investigation. It involves using tiny shock waves to disintegrate the stones so they can pass out of the system painlessly.

Prevention

To prevent recurrence of kidney stones, patients need to drink about three or four quarts of water a day to dilute their urine. Drinking large amounts of fluid, sometimes throughout the night, reduces urine concentration so stones cannot form. Surplus water can also flush the system of any small stones.

Proteinuria

Proteinuria is a symptom of kidney problems marked by an excess of proteins in the urine.

Causes

Proteinuria can be caused by, among other conditions, kidney malfunctions, heart disease, the consumption of certain foods, pregnancy and adolescent changes, and overexertion from certain sports such as jogging, marathon running, and boxing.

Symptoms

In most adult cases of proteinuria, the disorder is first diagnosed as an unexpected finding in a routine physical examination. Usually, the person will experience no symptoms and will be essentially healthy, with no evidence of kidney disease. The total protein excretion in the urine in these early-diagnosed cases is usually less than 1000 mg per day (the norm is less than 150 mg per day). Nevertheless, the majority of patients do not show any deterioration of kidney function.

In about half of the diagnosed cases, proteinuria ceases spontaneously within a year to several years. However, there are instances in which the patient continues to lose greater and greater amounts of protein in the urine. Eventually, high blood pressure and kidney failure may develop.

When proteinuria is constant, measures of protein excretion should be made on a regular basis. In these tests, the total protein excreted in the urine in a 24-hour period is measured.

Treatment

Treatment of proteinuria depends on its cause and its severity. As mentioned earlier, many cases disappear spontaneously. However, the patient should be carefully monitored and tested regularly in order to note any change in the condition. Any change in the protein level should be followed with other appropriate testing of kidney function.

Pyelonephritis

Pyelonephritis is a bacteria-caused inflammation of the kidney, affecting both the kidney tissue and the renal pelvis (the funnel-shaped expansion of the upper end of the ureter where it joins the kidney).

There are two types of pyelonephritis, *descending* and *ascending*. In the descending type, bacteria reach the kidney through the bloodstream, infecting first the kidney tissues themselves, and then "descending" or moving downward to infect the renal pelvis of the kidney. In the more common ascending type, the bladder is infected first, and the infection then spreads by moving upward to the kidney.

Causes

Causes of pyelonephritis may include scars from previous infections, urinary tract infections, abnormal growth of the prostate (a male gland secreting fluids), kidney stone and tumors, stagnation of urine due to backflow from the bladder, diabetes mellitus (a condition of excess sugar in the bloodstream), and pregnancy.

Symptoms

Symptoms of pyelonephritis are low back pain, difficulty in urinating, burning sensation upon urination, edema (swelling, including puffiness under the eyes), mental confusion, nausea, vomiting, and — in extreme cases — loss of consciousness. Although some cases of chronic (recurring) pyelonephritis can be traced to an acute onset or initial attack, with persistent, recurrent bacterial infections following, there are many cases in which there is no such acute phase. Often patients will have no real evidence of past or current infections.

Treatment

Acute pyelonephritis is treated with antibiotics given orally or intravenously (through the vein). Recurrent episodes should be treated with any of a number of appropriate antibiotics. Chronic pyelonephritis requires careful management and frequent reevaluation. Patients should be treated with an antibiotic even during periods when they feel no symptoms and receive long-term therapy after that.

THE ENDOCRINE SYSTEM

The endocrine system is a set of glands that release hormones into the bloodstream. Hormones are chemical substances that are secreted by organs or by cells of organs in one part of the body and are carried in the bloodstream to other organs or tissues where they control or regulate the structure or function of these distant organs.

Hormones can be considered chemical messengers: they are "targeted" at certain cells in the body, and their arrival in those cells causes certain activities to occur. In general, hormones have three major tasks. They regulate the activities of differing systems so that they can act together in a coordinated manner to achieve an end result. For example, the hormone adrenaline acts on the heart to increase its rate and force of contraction and on the blood vessels to increase blood flow to certain areas so that the body can cope with stress. Hormones also help control the type and rate of body growth and metabolism, and they help the body maintain a consistent internal environment.

Endocrine glands are so named because they secrete hormones internally into the bloodstream. No ducts transport the chemicals. In contrast, exocrine glands release their secretions through tubes or ducts (for example, sweat glands produce fluid that flows to the skin's surface through tubes or ducts).

Pituitary gland

Several glands with different functions comprise the endocrine system. However, all endocrine glands come under the control of the pituitary, or master, gland. The pituitary gland lies at the base of the brain. Its job is to receive messages about the need for a particular hormone and secrete either the hormone or substances that cause the manufacture and release of a hormone in response. For instance, if there is a need for more thyroid hormone, the pituitary is stimulated to secrete thyroid-stimulating hormone that causes the thyroid gland to increase production. By triggering responses throughout the endocrine system, the pituitary gland controls many body functions, including growth, response to stress, and energy regulation.

Thyroid gland

The gland directly responsible for body energy regulation is the thyroid gland. The thyroid is located in front of the throat above

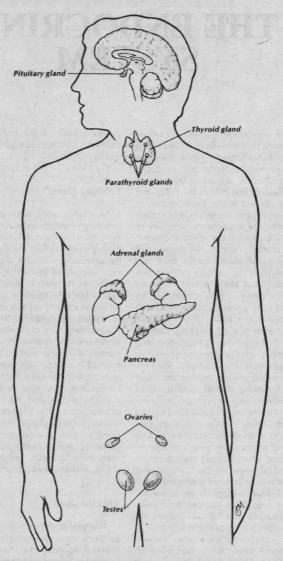

Pituitary gland

Thyroid gland

Parathyroid glands

Adrenal glands

Pancreas

Ovaries

Testes

The endocrine system is composed of glands that release vital hormones into the blood.

the top of the breastbone. It consists of two main sections or lobes on either side of the trachea that are connected by a narrow band of tissue called the "isthmus."

Parathyroid glands

Behind the thyroid glands are the parathyroid glands. Parathyroid glands control calcium levels in the blood by secreting parathyroid hormone.

Pancreas

The other glands in the endocrine system are located within the abdominal cavity. Specialized cells in the pancreas, produce two hormones needed to maintain stable blood sugar levels in the body. Insulin helps body cells utilize glucose for energy, thereby regulating the amount of sugar in the bloodstream. To balance this action, the hormone glucagon stimulates the liver to release its stored sugar into the blood, thus raising the blood sugar level.

The pancreas also functions in digestion of foods. Other cells in the pancreas produce special chemicals called enzymes that are secreted directly into the small intestine through ducts. These enzymes help break down food (particularly fats and starches) in the small intestine.

This varied activity of the organ means that the pancreas functions as both an exocrine and endocrine organ.

Adrenal glands

Other glands critical to normal body functions such as fluid balance, reaction to stress, and reproduction are the adrenal glands. Each of the two adrenal glands lies above a kidney. The adrenal glands have two distinct parts: the cortex (outer layer) that secretes steroid hormones and the medulla that secretes adrenaline and noradrenaline. Adrenaline and noradrenaline are responsible for the changes in heart rate, blood pressure, and level of usable glucose (sugar) that are necessary to cope with stress. In addition, adrenal glands in both men and women produce small amounts of the sex hormones known as androgens (male) and estrogens (female).

Sex glands

The primary responsibility for hormone production for the reproductive system is with the testes (male sex glands) and ovaries (female sex glands). Testes are two oval-shaped organs in the scrotum, the external pouch of skin behind and under the penis. They produce sperm and male sex hormones that provide male sex characteristics of penis development, body hair growth, voice changes, and increased muscle mass. Two ovaries in the female pelvis secrete the hormones estrogen and progesterone which govern the development of secondary female characteristics including ovulation (monthly release of egg from ovary), breast development, and body hair growth.

The endocrine system has a large influence on the way we feel and act. In turn, our energy and other needs in any given situation set the activity of the endocrine system. This feedback relationship is crucial in maintaining our general well-being.

ACTH

ACTH (adrenocorticotropic hormone), also known as corticotropin, is a hormone (a chemical "messenger" that acts upon a body process) produced by the pituitary, a pea-sized gland that is attached by a stalk to the base of the brain. ACTH is also manufactured synthetically or extracted from the pituitary glands of cattle and sheep and used as a drug.

Functions

ACTH travels through the bloodstream to affect the adrenal glands, two small but very important organs located over each kidney. It stimulates the cortex, the outer layer of the adrenal glands, to produce various hormones known as steroids. These include the corticosteroids (the most important of which is cortisol), androgens, which are male sex hormones (also produced in far smaller quantity by the adrenal gland in the female), and mineralocorticoids. The first of these, cortisol, has numerous functions. It is important in protein formation and breakdown, blood sugar control, reduction of inflammation, and is necessary for the body to mount an effective response against severe stress, be it a disease or multiple injuries with resultant shock. Androgens also have many functions, mainly the development and maintenance of male sex characteristics, reproductive capability, and musculature. They are also important in bone marrow function and protein biochemistry. Mineralocorticoids are steroid hormones involved in maintaining salt and water balance in the body.

Drug forms

The drug forms of ACTH and the corticosteroids are used to treat a disease in the same way the natural hormones would or as substitute or supplement hormones for people who have lost the ability to manufacture their own. The primary difference is that ACTH acts less directly and more generally. It stimulates the adrenal glands to enlarge and produce more steroids that then perform their various functions throughout the body. Corticosteroid drugs, on the other hand, can be administered to the part of the body that needs them most. Thus, a dab of hydrocortisone cream will eliminate a rash and a hydrocortisone injection will diminish the swelling of a painful knee joint virtually without affecting any other part of the body. Sometimes, however, corticosteroids are considered for generalized use throughout the body. In those instances, corticosteroids have an advantage over ACTH in that they can be taken by mouth and may be given in doses that far exceed what the body's adrenal glands can produce. ACTH must be injected because it would otherwise be destroyed by digestive enzymes, which do not affect the corticosteroids. Regardless of why or how they are used, all are powerful drugs that must be used with great care.

Addison's disease

Addison's disease is a gradually worsening condition occurring when the adrenal cortex, the outer layer of the adrenal glands, fails to produce enough hormones to meet the needs of the body. The adrenal glands, situated just above each kidney, produce many different hormones—chemicals which travel through the bloodstream and have specific effects on cells in another part of the body.

Causes

Formerly, the cause of this disease in 70 to 90 percent of the cases was tuberculosis or a fungal infection. However, in recent years, the disease is most commonly referred to as idiopathic, or "of unknown cause." The predominant theory is that most cases of Addison's disease are due to autoimmune destruction of the adrenal cortex; that is, the body produces antibodies against its own tissues, leading to their ultimate breakdown. Other known causes include partial destruction of the adrenal cortex by cancer, surgery, or degeneration of the tissue, or by deposits of amyloid, an abnormal body substance. A similar condition known as secondary adrenal insufficiency is caused by failure of the pituitary (a small gland attached to the base of the

brain) to produce enough of the hormone known as ACTH, which stimulates the adrenal cortex to produce its hormones.

Symptoms

Early symptoms of Addison's disease are weakness, fatigue, and a tendency to become faint when arising suddenly from a bed or chair. Increased pigmentation of the skin, producing a "tan" all over the body on exposed and unexposed areas alike with even darker pigmentation on creases and bony pressure points, occurs in most cases. (The increase in pigmentation is caused by overactivity of the pituitary gland as it tries to stimulate the failing adrenal cortex by producing more ACTH thereby also increasing production of a related substance that actually causes the pigmentation.) In certain places the tan may be broken by completely white patches, known as vitiligo. Black freckles appear on the forehead, face, shoulders, and neck. There may be skin discoloration around the nipples, and the mucous membranes of the mouth may have dark blue patches.

Later symptoms include weight loss, loss of fluid in body tissues, low blood pressure, and sometimes loss of appetite, nausea, vomiting, diarrhea, dizziness, and inability to keep warm.

The most alarming symptoms are those of an adrenal crisis, which requires immediate attention and hospitalization. Signs of this are extreme weakness; severe pains in the lower back, abdomen, or legs; collapse of the circulatory system; and a shutdown of the kidneys. Such a crisis may be brought on by severe stress such as infection, injury, surgery, or by a loss of salt through perspiration during hot weather.

Diagnosis

One laboratory sign of Addison's disease is a high level of ACTH but a low level of cortisol (an adrenal hormone) in the blood. This indicates that the pituitary gland is working overtime to stimulate the adrenal cortex with ACTH to produce cortisol, but the cortex is failing to produce.

Treatment

The basic treatment for Addison's disease is to provide steroid hormones, principally cortisone, to replace those not being produced by the adrenal cortex. An additional steroid drug may be added to the cortisone as part of the continuing treatment. It enables the body to retain salt, which helps the body retain water in tissues and blood. In doing so, it prevents the loss of salt and fluid that causes the low blood pressure of severe Addison's disease.

The outlook for patients on hormone treatment is excellent. Good medical supervision and intelligent patient cooperation can prevent emergencies caused by a sudden withdrawal or neglect of treatment or by an increased need for hormones because of infection, injury, surgery, pregnancy, or other stress on the body. It is important to avoid infection, to treat infection that develops as

soon as possible, and at all times to carry a card or wear a bracelet describing the condition and the need for cortisone. It is also critical to take the medication reliably and to be in touch with a physician who can increase or decrease the dosage as the need arises. With proper care, a person can lead a normal life.

Prevention

Prevention of Addison's disease, except by eliminating certain known causes such as tuberculosis, will probably have to wait until more is known about the mysterious failures of the adrenal cortex.

Corticosteroids

Corticosteroids are hormones produced in the outer layer (cortex) of the adrenal glands, two small organs that lie atop the kidneys. (Hormones are chemical "messengers" manufactured by body cells and carried by fluids to another location, where they control a body process.) There are more than 30 corticosteroids. Together, they regulate processes throughout the body and are essential to life. They are divided into three groups: mineralocorticoids, glucocorticoids, and sex steroids.

Functions

Mineralocorticoids exert control on the distribution of body fluids and the sodium and potassium mineral salts dissolved within them. Without the mineralocorticoids, the tissues and blood become depleted of salt and water. The blood decreases in volume, causing a drop in blood pressure that can result in collapse of the blood circulation system (shock).

Glucocorticoids help regulate the body's use and reserves of sugars and proteins, among other complex metabolic processes. They assist various chemical processes throughout the body, and also participate in the inflammation response. (Cortisol, one of these hormones, is known for this effect. For example, as medication — called cortisone — it reduces the swollen joints of arthritis and can eliminate skin rashes.) Finally, these hormones also participate in the body's reaction to stress.

The sex steroids include androgens (such as testosterone, also produced in the male testes) and estrogens (also produced in the female ovaries). Men and women have both male and female hormones in their systems. However, the abundance of androgens in men produces beard growth, enlarged muscle development, and other male characteristics. In women, an abundance of estrogen produces feminine characteristics such as breast development.

Production of corticosteroids is under control of ACTH (adrenocorticotropic hormone), which is released by the pituitary gland located near the base of the brain. ACTH travels in the bloodstream to the adrenal cortex and stimulates the cortex to produce corticosteroids. The pituitary gland is regulated by the hypothalamus, a part of the brain.

Cushing's syndrome

Cushing's syndrome is a group of abnormalities resulting from an excess level of the hormones produced by the outer layer (cortex) of the adrenal glands, small glands that lie atop the kidneys. (Hormones are chemical "messengers" manufactured by body cells and carried by fluids to another location in the body, where they control a body process.) The hormones produced in excess are chiefly cortisol, which has many complex functions; other hormones that regulate the body's use of sugars and proteins; sex hormones; and a hormone that controls the distribution of fluids and salts in the body.

Causes

In most cases, Cushing's syndrome is caused by excess production of ACTH (adrenocorticotropic hormone), which is normally manufactured by the pituitary gland to stimulate the adrenal glands to produce hormones. This excess of ACTH can be caused by an ACTH-producing tumor (growth) in another organ, such as a cancer in the lung or pancreas; by overmedication with ACTH or cortisone drugs; by tiny nonmalignant ACTH-producing tumors on the pituitary gland; or by a nonmalignant (or occasionally malignant) cortisone-producing tumor on the adrenal gland. The effect of too much

ACTH for whatever reason is an overgrowth of tissue in the adrenal cortex, resulting in overproduction of all its hormones. Since the hormones produced by the adrenal cortex regulate processes throughout the body and are essential to life, excess production causes widespread disorders.

Symptoms

Some of the most obvious signs of Cushing's syndrome are a "moon-shaped" face, caused by excess fluid in the tissues; a fat trunk but thin arms and legs; and fat pads over the shoulders and neck, producing a "buffalo hump." These abnormalities are all caused by excess deposits of fatty tissue in these locations. Purple stretch marks on the skin (usually of the abdomen); poor wound healing (caused by excess cortisone, which suppresses body defenses); easy bruising; hairiness, acne, and decreased or absent menstruation in women, because of increased male hormones; enlarged breasts in men, because of increased female hormones; muscle weakness; fractures in weakened bones; and emotional instability are also part of the syndrome. The development of diabetes and high blood pressure is also very common.

Diagnosis

Diagnosis of Cushing's syndrome requires measurement of adrenal cortex hormones in the blood and urine. One clue is that in normal persons cortisol levels in the blood are high upon awakening but decrease during the day; in the Cushing's syndrome patient cortisol levels are high all the time. Various tests can determine whether the cause of the syndrome is a malfunction of the pituitary gland (in which case the disorder is known as Cushing's disease) or is a tumor on the adrenal gland or elsewhere. Tumors on the adrenal glands are located by X rays, ultrasound, and CAT scan (a technique using X rays of multiple and progressively deeper sections, yielding a more three-dimensional picture). CAT scans and other special X rays of the head can often locate tumors on the pituitary gland, which is located at the base of the brain.

Treatment

Cushing's syndrome is treated by restoring a normal balance of hormones. This may involve surgery, X-ray treatments, or drugs. Tumors on the adrenal glands are removed by surgery. If there is a tumor on just one adrenal gland, the other gland usually shrinks and becomes hardly productive. Hormone supplements are usually given before surgery and must be taken for weeks or months after surgery until the second gland returns to normal function. In a rapidly worsening case of Cushing's syndrome, in which the adrenal cortex is greatly enlarged on both adrenal glands, one treatment is to remove both adrenal glands. This is usually a last resort. More commonly, however, other methods such as chemotherapy (drug treatments), X-ray treatments of the pituitary gland to weaken it and lower its output of adrenal-gland-stimulating ACTH, or removal of any adenomas (nonmalignant growths) on the pituitary gland may be tried first. If these measures fail, the adrenal glands are removed and the patient must take daily supplements of adrenal cortex hormones for the rest of his or her life.

If Cushing's syndrome is being caused by production of ACTH by a cancer in another part of the body, the cancer is located and removed, if possible. However, in most cases it is inoperable, in which case drugs to suppress production of the adrenal glands are given.

Cushing's syndrome is a very serious and possibly fatal disease unless it is detected and treated early. The outlook is best for those whose condition is caused by noncancerous growths and who receive early treatment.

Those who must take replacement hormones after treatment should carry a medical identification card and immediately tell their doctors about any infections, injuries, or stressful situations that might require an increase in hormone dosage. They should also report signs of underdosage, such as weakness, dizziness, or fatigue, and of overdosage, such as swollen tissues and rapid weight gain. Anyone whose adrenal glands have been removed must always take replacement hormones; stopping these replacements for any length of time is fatal.

Diabetes mellitus

Diabetes mellitus, often called sugar diabetes, is a condition in which the body is unable to process properly carbohydrates (sugars and starches), which are the body's major source of energy.

Normally, digestion causes these carbohydrates to release a form of sugar called glucose into the blood. As the blood glucose level rises, the pancreas gland located in the upper abdomen is stimulated to secrete the hormone insulin. Insulin acts to reduce the sugar content in the blood by transporting glucose from the blood to body cells where it is used for fuel or to the liver where it is stored until needed for fuel.

When the pancreas produces insufficient insulin or the body cannot use the insulin it manufactures, diabetes results. Sugar concentrations accumulate in the blood as glucose circulates throughout the body without being absorbed. Eventually, the kidney filters sugar from the blood, and urine (the fluid mixture of water and waste products) carries the excess blood sugar from the body.

Types

There are two major forms of diabetes. Type I, or insulin-dependent, diabetes results from a defect of unknown origin in the

The islets of Langerhans in the pancreas secretes insulin, the hormone that helps the body cells absorb sugar for fuel. One type of diabetes may result from a defect in the islets of Langerhans, causing decreased production of insulin.

islets of Langerhans, the part of the pancreas that produces insulin. This form of diabetes can develop in very young children.

With Type II, or insulin-independent, diabetes the pancreas functions adequately, but the body is unable to use insulin efficiently. Sometimes, a shortage of insulin-receptor cells (sites throughout the body where interaction of sugar and insulin occurs) allows the insulin to float in the bloodstream without working properly. Obesity often contributes to the problem as excess fat cells displace insulin-receptor cells.

Since Type II appears most often in adults over the age of 40,

this form may evolve from a gradual slowing of insulin production within the pancreas. In addition, other disorders of the endocrine system (glands that secrete hormones into the bloodstream) may cause hormonal imbalances that disturb insulin-sugar regulation.

Research shows that people who have Type II diabetes in their families have a greater tendency to acquire the condition. Women are more likely to be affected, but chances of developing Type II for all adults doubles with every decade past 40 years.

In some women, pregnancy triggers diabetes. The disease usually subsides after childbirth.

However, women who show signs of diabetes during pregnancy and deliver babies weighing over ten pounds have a greater risk of diabetes later in life.

Complications

Even though patients with diabetes can usually control the condition, untreated diabetes can lead to serious complications. Extremely high blood sugar levels place great strain on other organs. Diabetes may trigger atherosclerosis, hardening and narrowing of arteries that carry blood throughout the body. Insufficient blood supply contributes to heart attack; stroke; kidney disease; eye disorders, such as retinopathy; impotence; death of tissue due to inadequate blood circulation; gangrene; and even death.

Symptoms

Symptoms of Type I diabetes are excessive thirst and urination, fatigue, altered vision, fainting, irritability, and slow-healing cuts and bruises. Weight loss may occur despite constant hunger and voracious eating.

The same symptoms may signal Type II diabetes, or no symptoms may show at all. Physicians frequently detect this form when they perform routine examinations or tests for other problems.

Diagnosis

Should no symptoms be obvious, doctors can diagnose diabetes by analyzing blood and urine samples for elevated sugar concentrations. They may also test blood for extra insulin and urine for excess ketones. Ketones are the end products of breaking down fat for energy. Since people with diabetes do not use sugar normally, their bodies burn fat for fuel and eliminate the ketone end products in the urine.

Treatment

Both forms of diabetes mellitus require a treatment plan that maintains normal steady blood glucose levels. Once blood sugar levels are under control with insulin injections, diet, or medication, a person with diabetes can usually lead a normal life.

Type I, or insulin-dependent, diabetes requires injections of insulin to regulate blood sugar levels evenly all day. If blood glucose concentrations rise, the body may signal an imbalance by displaying symptoms of weakness, fatigue, and thirst. These symptoms mean that increased insulin is needed. However, if blood sugar levels become too low, an insulin reaction sets in, causing dizziness, hunger, fatigue, headache, sweating, trembling, and — in severe cases—unconsciousness. A quick remedy for this problem is to eat simple sugar, such as candy.

Ideally, a doctor can prevent these fluctuations of sugar levels by coordinating the type and timing of insulin injections with meal content and energy output. A special diet is important to balance daily insulin injections. Young children with diabetes, in particular, need sufficient calories to grow and develop normally. Insulin requirements for persons with

Type I diabetes differ widely among individuals. Some patients may maintain balanced blood sugar levels with one insulin injection taken before breakfast. Other patients may require several insulin injections per day. Furthermore, insulin requirements may change as the patient grows older, undergoes surgery, becomes pregnant, or develops another unrelated illness.

Most people with Type II, or insulin-independent, diabetes can regulate their condition by proper diet. Sometimes, oral antidiabetic drugs, which work by stimulating the pancreas to produce more insulin, may be prescribed. However, there is some evidence that these drugs may be no more effective in controlling diabetes than diet alone. In addition, some investigators feel that these drugs may increase the incidence of death caused by cardiovascular diseases; however, this has not been fully proved.

A controlled diet is critical for diabetes control. Overweight individuals need to lose weight. Thereafter, emphasis is on eating balanced meals that will sustain recommended weight. Fats need to be limited to reduce chances of atherosclerosis, and the diet should be low in simple sugars. The diet should include plenty of fibrous roughage, such as is contained in fruits, vegetables, and whole grains; fiber in the diet has been shown to reduce or slow sugar absorption in the digestive tract. Your doctor can provide a medically approved diet plan with food exchanges that allow flexibility with regular family meals and dietary needs.

With either type of diabetes, follow-up is important to plan diet, determine changes in insulin dosage, and retest blood and urine for blood sugar levels. Careful control of blood sugar levels can enable a person with diabetes to lead a normal life.

Goiter

Goiter is an enlargement of the thyroid gland, characterized by a swelling at the front of the neck.

Causes

Goiter may be caused by a lack of dietary iodine which is necessary for the production of thyroid hormone. In this case, the thyroid gland enlarges in an attempt to produce more hormone. When this happens, the cells in the gland enlarge, but do not increase in number. If iodine deficiency is minor, the condition is usually confined to young women. Men and school-age children are affected if the iodine deficiency is severe.

Goiter was at one time common in areas where there is a lack of iodine in the soil and water. Since the ocean is the basic source of iodine, inland areas were the most deficient (in the United States, the Great Lakes region was such an area; in Europe, mountainous inland regions in the Alps often had inhabitants with iodine defi-

Goiter is a swelling in the neck caused by an enlarged thyroid whose cells have enlarged to produce more thyroid hormone.

ciency). In recent times, however, iodized table salt has solved this problem.

Some forms of goiter are associated with an overactive thyroid gland, that is, the diseased thyroid produces more hormone than the body needs.

Symptoms

In the case of an overactive thyroid, the symptoms accompanying the swelling in the neck include nervousness, weight loss, bulging eyes, rapid heartbeat, and occasionally high blood pressure. Sometimes a person with goiter shows signs of an underactive thyroid, such as sluggishness, weight gain, dry skin and hair, and fatigue. Often, however, the only symptom of goiter is the swelling in the neck.

Treatment

The chief objective of goiter treatment is reduction of the swelling. The first step is usually to suppress the thyroid gland's over-functioning. If the goiter is caused by simple iodine deficiency, small doses of iodine can be given. Sometimes, administering synthetic thyroid hormone, in an attempt to halt the gland's increased efforts to produce the natural hormone, will reduce the enlargement. If treatment is started early enough, surgery to remove enlarged portions of the gland can be avoided. On the other hand, surgery is sometimes necessary in cases in which the size of the goiter interferes with normal breathing.

Hirsutism

Hirsutism is excessive hair growth in areas that are not usually hairy in women—usually the face, breasts and chest, and abdomen.

Causes

Some degree of hirsutism is present in about 30 percent of women, and it may accompany some primary disorder as a secondary symptom. Family and racial tendencies, however, account for a good percentage of hirsute women. While some hirsutism stems from a primary disorder, many cases have no known cause. It is thought, though, that hirsute women all have hair follicles that are hypersensitive to normal female androgen levels. (Androgen is a male sex hormone, but certain levels of it are normally present in women.)

In some cases, hirsutism is only one sign of virilization (or masculinization) characterized by acne, balding, and increased muscle mass, as well as by hirsutism. This condition can be caused by overactive adrenal glands (which secrete some sex hormones), ovarian tumors, adrenal tumors, steroid medications, and other causes. However, the majority of hirsute women are not masculinized. A more common cause of hirsutism is polycystic ovaries, a condition marked by numerous cysts on the ovaries (female sex glands) that leads to infrequent menstruation or absence of menstruation, absence of ovulation, obesity, and enlarged ovaries.

Hirsutism is also seen in Cushing's syndrome, a condition that in women is characterized by excessive fat tissue in the face, neck, and trunk; absence of menstruation; convex curvature of the spine; high blood pressure; and muscular weakness. Mild hirsutism also appears in a young girl with an underactive thyroid. Absence of, or damage to, the pituitary gland, anorexia nervosa (self-inflicted starvation or excessive dieting), and some drugs such as the corticosteroids and certain birth control pills can also cause hirsutism.

Symptoms

The only symptom of hirsutism itself is excessive growth of hair in normally hairless areas in women: face, neck, breasts and chest, and abdomen. The hair may be soft and fine or coarser, depending on many factors.

Diagnosis

Diagnosis is usually confirmed through visual examination and medical history.

Treatment

The treatment of hirsutism is directed at removing the cause, if it is identified. For example, adrenal hyperplasia (an abnormal increase in the number of cells in the adrenal gland) can be suppressed by corticosteroid drugs. Patients with polycystic ovaries can be treated with low-dose estrogen birth control pills or with other drugs.

In some cases, however, removing the cause does not diminish the hair growth. In these cases, hair removal is recommended for cosmetic reasons. The only safe, permanent local treatment is electrolysis, destroying the individual hair follicles by an electric current. Temporary measures, such as plucking, shaving, waxing, using a depilatory wax or chemical, will temporarily mask the problem but electrolysis is the only permanent solution to hirsutism.

Prevention

Other than prompt diagnosis and treatment of the primary cause or disorder (provided there is one), there are no known preventive measures for hirsutism.

Hyperthyroidism

Hyperthyroidism is a condition that results when an overactive thyroid gland produces too much thyroid hormone. The thyroid gland is a small butterfly-shaped gland located in front of the windpipe above the top of the breastbone. It affects every tissue in the body by secreting thyroid hormone which helps maintain body temperature, convert food to energy, and regulate growth and fertility. The pituitary gland, which is the control center for all endocrine glands, regulates the production of thyroid hormone by secreting thyroid stimulating hormone (TSH) when a need for thyroid hormone is present. In addition, adequate iodine is necessary for the production of thyroid hormone. Iodine in the blood is obtained either from substances taken into the body, such as food, or from the breakdown of thyroid hormone itself.

In hyperthyroidism, the thyroid gland somehow malfunctions. The pituitary gland will sense the increased levels of thyroid hormone and shut off the stimulation. However, the abnormal gland is no longer sensitive to this mechanism.

Graves' disease

Hyperthyroidism is a descriptive term that encompasses different disorders. Graves' disease, a common form of hyperthyroidism, is probably due to the presence of an abnormal chemical stimulator of thyroid hormone production. This disease occurs most often in the young, particularly those in their 30s and 40s. It is also more common in females than in males. The occurrence of bulging eye(s) and distinctive skin problems is also a part of Graves' disease. The thyroid gland itself is frequently enlarged, smooth, and soft. Along with these unique features, patients with Graves' disease exhibit the symptoms and signs common to all forms of hyperthyroidism, including rapid heartbeat, weight loss despite increased appetite and food intake, generalized hyperactivity, tremors, increased sweating, severe nervousness and emotional instability, alterations of menstruation and fertility, and weakness.

Toxic multinodular goiter

Toxic multinodular goiter, another common form of hyperthyroidism, is a condition in which nodules (lump-like clusters of thyroid tissue) somehow form and secrete abnormally large amounts of thyroid hormone. These nodules function independent of normal regulatory mechanisms. In contrast to Graves' disease, this condition is common in the middle-aged and elderly. Bulging of the eyes rarely occurs, and the gland is not uniformly enlarged, but lumpy. There has been no chemical mediator defined in this illness. Toxic multinodular goiter, of course, also produces the aforementioned symptoms and signs common to the hyperthyroid state.

Diagnosis

The diagnosis of hyperthyroidism is made by the history and physical examination and confirmed with laboratory data. Naturally, the level of thyroid hormone in the blood must be significantly elevated, and this can be determined by a simple blood test. Further documentation

and quantitation is obtained through the use of nuclear medicine scans utilizing radiolabeled iodine. Since iodine is necessary for the production of thyroid hormone, the injected, labeled iodine will gravitate to the thyroid yielding not only a picture of the gland, but a precise estimate of the degree of hyperactivity.

Treatment

Treatment of hyperthyroidism depends on which condition is present. However, treatment of the hyperthyroid state in general has several common elements. The drug propranolol, a beta blocker, is commonly used to block the adrenaline overstimulation seen in hyperthyroidism which greatly contributes to the tremors, increased heart rate, and sweating. This drug, although it diminishes symptoms, does not get at the root of the problem: too much thyroid hormone. To decrease the amount of thyroid hormone being produced, antithyroid drugs such as propylthiouracil are used. These drugs actually interfere with the production of thyroid hormone. However, this is again usually only a temporary solution, since when the drug is stopped, the excess production may resume. The definitive therapy of hyperthyroidism is the actual destruction or removal of most or all of the gland by the use of radioactive iodine or surgery.

Graves' disease is usually first treated by blocking the adrenaline overstimulation with propranolol. Simultaneously, an antithyroid drug is started. Usually this drug is maintained for a period of one to two years and then tapered off. With this approach, relapse (recurrence) is not at all uncommon. If relapse occurs or if the level of thyroid hormone is normalized, the choice then is how to reduce the amount of thyroid tissue. Whether surgery or radioactive iodine is used depends upon many complex factors and is a very controversial subject in medicine. One would be best advised to seek the opinion of a physician well-versed and experienced in the treatment of this disease before choosing. It is to be noted that both of these treatments frequently result in too little thyroid hormone in the blood, but this problem is easily remedied by supplementation with synthetic thyroid hormone.

The treatment of toxic multinodular goiter is somewhat less controversial. After blocking with a beta blocker and, frequently, normalizing hormone levels with an antithyroid drug, destruction of the gland with radioactive iodine is the therapy of choice.

Hypoglycemia

Hypoglycemia is the body's inability to maintain enough glucose in the blood. Glucose is a sugar released into the blood from digestion of carbohydrates.

During normal digestion, increased glucose levels trigger the secretion of the hormone insulin from the pancreas located in the upper abdomen. Insulin acts to reduce the sugar level in the blood by helping certain body cells absorb the sugar for fuel.

Reactive hypoglycemia

If the pancreas continues to produce insulin longer than necessary or produces too much insulin relative to the level of glucose in the blood, abnormally low blood sugar levels result. This condition is called reactive hypoglycemia. Reactive hypoglycemia is a condition caused by an oversecretion of insulin and consequent rapid lowering of blood glucose levels producing symptoms of hypoglycemia in response to a glucose load. Reactive hypoglycemia is also known as postprandial (after meals) hypoglycemia as it occurs only in response to food.

The specific causes of reactive hypoglycemia are unknown in most cases. However, certain conditions (for example, rapid emptying of the stomach with consequent absorption of a large glucose load that occurs in those patients who have had part or most of the stomach removed) commonly are associated with reactive hypoglycemia.

Fasting hypoglycemia

Another type of hypoglycemia, fasting hypoglycemia, has several known causes. Basically, fasting hypoglycemia is caused by either an insufficient production of glucose or an overutilization of the glucose present in the blood. Often, these two factors are combined to create a low fasting blood glucose level. In addition, the presence of an insulin-producing tumor on the pancreas may contribute to fasting hypoglycemia. Because alcohol disturbs the regular sugar storage and release mechanisms within the liver, heavy drinkers are at greater risk of developing the disorder. Fasting hypoglycemia can also occur in anyone who has not eaten for an unusually long interval, but this is a temporary situation. Chronic hypoglycemia is uncommon.

Symptoms

Hypoglycemia symptoms include fatigue, nervousness, perspiration, dizziness, headache, hunger pangs, visual impairment, and accelerated heartbeat. The condition may also bring anxiety, concentration problems, confusion, and blackouts. If sugar deprivation continues unchecked, severe hypoglycemia can produce convulsions (short-term loss of consciousness involving the nervous system and producing jerking muscle movements) and possibly deep coma (prolonged loss of consciousness).

Diagnosis

To diagnose hypoglycemia, a doctor analyzes a blood sample to detect abnormally low sugar levels. Blood drawn during an attack of the condition provides the most accurate assessment, since symptoms can then be correlated with actual blood glucose levels.

Treatment

Treatment for hypoglycemia often is aimed at the underlying cause of the disease. For example, a pancreatic tumor may require surgery to remove the growth, and a hypoglycemic reaction to insulin overdose by diabetics may necessitate adjustment of insulin dosage until the body balances sugar and insulin.

With most cases of reactive hypoglycemia, however, there is no known cure for the pancreas' tendency to overproduce insulin when it is not needed. The most effective treatment involves avoiding all foods that generate attacks.

A good diet is one that is low enough in sugar and starches to moderate the body's overreaction to sugar intake and rich enough in protein to help maintain gradual elevations of blood sugar. By eating smaller meals more frequently, levels of sugar concentrated in the blood may remain more stable.

It is important to note that true hypoglycemia is an uncommon condition. Since many of the symptoms of anxiety and hypoglycemia are alike, the two diagnoses are sometimes easily confused.

Hypothyroidism

Hypothyroidism is a disorder in which an underactive thyroid gland produces too little thyroid hormone. The thyroid gland lies in front of the windpipe above the top of the breastbone. Its job is to secrete thyroid hormone that influences every tissue in the body by participating in maintenance of body temperature, conversion of food to energy, and regulation of growth and fertility. The pituitary gland, which controls all endocrine glands, regulates the amount of thyroid hormone that is produced by raising or lowering the amount of thyroid-stimulating hormone (TSH).

Causes

The exact cause of hypothyroidism is unknown. However, the disorder may result from chronic (long-term) thyroid inflammation or deficiency of pituitary hormone. Autoimmune (destruction of the body's own tissue by its immune system) diseases of the thyroid are also a common cause of hypothyroidism. In addition, heredity may play a role in the development of thyroid imbalance. Also, women seem more prone to thyroid disorders, but the exact reason is unconfirmed. For some women, pregnancy triggers the hormone imbalance.

Hypothyroidism can also develop after suppression or partial removal of the thyroid gland as treatment for hyperthyroidism, a condition resulting from an overactive thyroid that produces too much thyroid hormone.

Symptoms

People with hypothyroidism may be overweight, easily exhausted, and subject to recurrent infection. They may also experience menstrual disorders, intolerance of cold, dry skin and hair, puffiness of hands and face, and mental illness.

Prolonged hypothyroidism may cause signs of reduced general body functioning. Anemia, a deficiency of red blood cells, may result from diminished function of the bone marrow, where red blood cells are formed. Heart rate may decrease, and reflexes become sluggish. In addition, an electroencephalogram, which measures brain waves, may reveal irregular patterns.

Diagnosis

To diagnose hypothyroidism, a series of tests may be given. First, a blood test measures the amount of thyroid hormone in the blood. Pituitary thyroid-stimulating hormone is also measured. If thyroid production is too low, the level of TSH should be greatly increased (to push the thyroid to produce). If this is not the case, there may be a pituitary abnormality at the root of the problem.

Treatment

Since hypothyroidism develops from a shortage of thyroid hormone, the most effective treatment is thyroid hormone supplements. Supplements are either natural hormones extracted from the thyroid glands of animals or synthetic hormones. Both types control the problem, but the natural form is usually less costly. Although treatment provides the necessary hormone control, hypothyroidism often continues throughout life. Thus, the individual may require lifelong follow-up to monitor treatment.

Ketosis

Ketosis, also known as keto-acidosis, is an abnormal condition that occurs when the body burns fat instead of glucose (a sugar that is the body's chief source of energy) and, as it does so, emits more poisonous by-products (called ketones) than the body can tolerate. Under normal circumstances, ketones are broken down into carbon dioxide and water by the liver and other organs.

Causes

Ketosis occurs most often in those people with insulin-dependent diabetes mellitus, a disorder in which the pancreas produces little or no insulin, a hormone secreted into the bloodstream to regulate glucose levels. This imbalance, in turn, prevents the body from absorbing enough glucose and forces it to obtain its energy by burning fat. Ketosis is also a consequence of starvation, another condition in which the body must rely excessively on stores of fat for energy.

Symptoms

The most common symptoms are a vinegar-like breath odor,

increased thirst and urination, weakness, abdominal pains and generalized aches, nausea, and vomiting. If allowed to continue unchecked, ketosis can lead to breathlessness and possible coma.

Diagnosis

Ketosis is diagnosed by testing the glucose and ketone levels of blood or urine, although the urine test is a less accurate reading.

Treatment

An injection of insulin ends diabetic ketosis. Diabetics are especially susceptible to ketosis before their condition is diagnosed, while they are fighting an infection, or when they neglect their diet or medication. Treatment of ketosis caused by starvation consists of feeding the individual sugar-containing substances by mouth or administering glucose solution intravenously (into the vein).

Pancreatitis

Pancreatitis is an inflammation of the pancreas, an organ located behind the stomach, close to the liver and gallbladder.

The pancreas has many functions. The exocrine pancreas secretes digestive enzymes (proteins that help chemical reactions along), for example, amylase, which aids in the breakdown of starches, and lipase for the breakdown of fats. The endocrine pancreas secretes hormones directly into the bloodstream, such as the hormones insulin and glucagon, which are critical to the body's processing of glucose (sugar).

The existence and degree of inflammation in the pancreas may be hard to determine not only because of the gland's hidden position and dual purpose, but also because symptoms are easily confused with other abdominal disorders.

Causes

Pancreatitis commonly results from an obstruction of the pancreatic ducts. Why these blockages occur is often hard to determine. It has been observed that the majority of pancreatitis cases are related to gallbladder disease or alcoholism. Acute attacks are frequently associated with gallstones or alcoholic binges. If hereditary factors are involved, the disease may begin in childhood, as early as eight or ten years of age. Direct blows to the abdomen or injury during an operation may also lead to pancreatitis, sometimes a year or more after the event. Mumps and other viral infections; drugs including steroids (cortisone), diuretics, and oral contraceptives; and tumors have all been connected with pancreatitis.

Symptoms

The disease is characterized by the sudden onset of steady, severe, boring upper abdominal pain (frequently radiating to the mid-back) accompanied by nausea and persistent vomiting. Eating, or even the sight of food, may seem to bring on the pain or to make it worse. Vomiting provides no relief, a feature which can distinguish it from some stomach or intestinal disorders. Fever, shock, jaundice (yellowish discoloration of the skin), dehydration, bleeding, and infection may occur in severe attacks. After an acute episode of pancreatitis, tissue debris, blood, and pancreatic enzymes may form a "pseudocyst," that is, an organized collection of material without its own true sac. Rupture or enlargement of a pseudocyst can be a very serious or even fatal event. If a pseudocyst is formed and is not resolving on its own, surgery is necessary to drain it.

Diagnosis

Blood and urine tests as well as microscopic tissue examination may be inconclusive, but can at least be helpful in excluding other abdominal disorders. A newer test, endoscopic retrograde cholangiopancreatography, enables visual inspection of the pancreatic ducts through an X ray. The technique is performed by inserting a gastroscope (a lighted tube) through the mouth and stomach into the duodenum (beginning of the small intestine). In the duodenum is the opening to the common bile and main pancreatic ducts. A special device is inserted through this opening and X-ray contrast material is injected. From the films taken, obstructions, tumors, or characteristic ductal patterns associated with chronic pancreatitis can be seen. This test is usually not performed within several weeks of an attack of pancreatitis.

Treatment

The patient is usually hospitalized from three to 14 days for a mild to severe acute attack. Correction of an underlying problem, such as removal of stones, improves the chances for complete recovery.

Initial treatment is aimed at relieving the pain and reducing stomach secretions which can stimulate the pancreas. Pancreatic function is diminished by eliminating eating and drinking and by suctioning out stomach acids to allow the pancreas to rest. Large pseudocysts which do not dissolve on their own may require surgical drainage to prevent rupture. During convalescence, a low-fat, high-protein diet should be followed and antacids may be prescribed. If the disease is chronic, it may be necessary to use pancreatic extracts to supplement insufficient volume of enzymes secreted by the diseased pancreas. This helps to normalize digestion thereby maintaining reasonable nutritional status.

Chronic pancreatitis is an indication of continued degenerating tissue damage which may impair pancreatic function. In some cases of recurrence, surgical exploration might be considered to locate a previously unidentified blockage or to remove diseased tissue; however, surgery is unlikely to help the patient who continues to drink alcohol to excess.

Pituitary gland

The pituitary (also called the *hypophysis cerebri*) is a small gland located just beneath the base of the brain, between its two frontal lobes, and directly above a cavity called the sphenoid sinus.

Functions

The pituitary gland has two lobes or parts, each with its own function. The front, or anterior, lobe secretes the following hormones: *somatotropin* (also known as growth hormone that affects the body's general growth); *thyrotropic hormone* (also known as thyroid stimulating hormone that acts on the thyroid gland to stimulate production of thyroid hormone); *adrenocorticotrophic hormone* (ACTH—which stimulates the adrenal cortex); two gonadotropic hormones (follicle-stimulating hormone and luteinizing hormone that are concerned with maturation and release of egg and sperm cells); and *prolactin* (which acts on the mammary glands to promote the secretion of milk).

The posterior lobe of the pituitary secretes the following hormones: *oxytocin* (which stimulates smooth muscle tissue to contract and is critical in labor of childbirth); and *vasopressin* (which regulates the kidney's function of taking or releasing water in the system).

Disorders of the pituitary gland

Despite its relatively small size, the pituitary gland is so important

THE ENDOCRINE SYSTEM 385

Back *Front*

Posterior pituitary *Anterior pituitary*

The small pituitary gland is one of the most important glands in the body.

to bodily functions that it is sometimes called the "master gland." Disorders of this gland, often the result of tumors, can result in disastrous abnormalities in growth and body maintenance. Excessive secretions of growth hormone by the anterior lobe produces giants, while deficient secretion produces dwarfs (if disorders in secretions occur during the years in which the skeleton would be growing naturally). If oversecretion occurs after a person has become an adult, a condition called *acromegaly* results, in which the victim's hands, feet, jaws, and facial bones grow disproportionately large.

A condition known as diabetes insipidus (which is unrelated to the more common diabetes mellitus, or high blood sugar levels) is one of the malfunctions of the posterior lobe. With this disorder, there is a deficiency of vasopressin, resulting in abnormally high urinary output of water. Control can be regained with the use of synthetic vasopressin to inhibit excessive water release.

Prostaglandins

Prostaglandins are fatty acid substances, similar in chemical structure to hormones, that occur naturally in the human body. Like hormones, prostaglandins appear to regulate or trigger activity in various tissues and organs. The first prostaglandin was isolated in the human prostate gland, which is how the substances got their name. More than 16 prostaglandins in six groups have now been identified.

Functions

Prostaglandins stimulate smooth muscle, affect heart rate, influence blood pressure, and contract the uterus. Prostaglandins affect the cardiovascular (heart and blood vessel) system, the central nervous system, the gastrointestinal (digestive) system, the endocrine (hormonal) system, and the urinary tract. In the endocrine system, for example, a prostaglandin triggers the release of the vital growth hormone by the pituitary gland (which is located at the base of the brain and controls a number of body functions).

Drug forms

Medical researchers have been experimenting with various preparations of synthetic prostaglandins as drugs, for both diagnosis and treatment of disease. One prostaglandin stimulates contractions of the uterus in childbirth, so a prostaglandin preparation can help speed up some cases of difficult labor. Another prostaglandin has been used to reduce blood pressure in research subjects, but is not yet available as a prescription drug. Prostaglandins are also being studied in the treatment of asthma, emphysema (a serious respiratory disease), shock (a sudden, dangerous slowing down of blood circulation), and even the common cold. Researchers have successfully used a prostaglandin to halt the growth of leukemia and melanoma, two types of cancer, in cells in the laboratory.

THE MALE REPRODUCTIVE SYSTEM

The male reproductive system consists of those structures in the male body designed to create life. The system includes the two testes, a network of ducts, a set of glands, and the penis.

Testes are two oval-shaped glands located in the scrotum, a pouch of skin hanging behind the penis. Their job is to produce male sex hormones (called androgens and testosterone) and sperm (sex) cells. Sex hormones control secondary male sex characteristics from puberty on, including penis growth, body hair growth, voice change, and increased muscle mass.

Testes discharge sperm cells into the epididymis, the first structure in the duct system. Other passageways include the two vasa deferentia (the plural of vas deferens), the ejaculatory duct, and the urethra. The entire duct system transports sperm from the testes to the outside of the body.

The epididymis runs along the top and side of each testis. Inside the epididymis are several ducts which direct sperm from the testis into the vas deferens. The vas deferens, or continuation of the epididymis, loops up into the body before descending into a duct in the seminal vesicle gland.

This duct from the seminal vesicle joins the ejaculatory duct. From here, the duct stretches through the prostate gland and enters the upper segment of the urethra, the tube that connects the bladder to the outside of the body. At different times the urethra functions as an exit tube for urine as well as for sperm.

As sperm travel through the duct system, they combine with fluids from the male glands. The two main types of male glands are the seminal vesicles and the prostate gland. Seminal vesicles each lie near the underside of the bladder (storage depot for urine before elimination from the body). They discharge a sticky, thick fluid that unites with the sperm cells emerging from the testes.

The prostate gland is a small doughnut-shaped organ positioned so that it completely surrounds the urethra. The prostate gland secretes an alkaline (basic) substance that makes up the major portion of seminal fluid, which carries sperm outside the body.

The sperm, or male reproductive cells, are protected from acid (present both in the male urethra and in the vagina) by this alkalinity of the prostate's secretions.

A front view of the male reproductive organs.

Sperm are also capable of the greatest mobility (ability to move) when in a slightly alkaline medium. Proper prostate secretion is thus essential to proper sperm action.

Sperm mixed with glandular fluids is called semen. Semen forms in the urethra and travels out of the penis during sexual excitement, or ejaculation.

The penis is the external organ that propels sperm into the female during sexual intercourse. When sexually excited, the large internal spaces, or corpora cavernosa, within the penis fill with blood. As the penis engorges, it becomes rigid enough to enter the female vagina, or entryway to the female reproductive system.

Gynecomastia

Gynecomastia is the development of breasts in a male. Breast enlargement is a normal, short-term development in some newborn boys whose breasts enlarge in response to female hormones they received from their mother during pregnancy. The condition may also appear at puberty when the boy's body is undergoing normal hormonal changes.

A side view of the male reproductive organs.

Causes

In most cases, gynecomastia is a result of too much estrogen, a female sex hormone, in the male's body. Breast enlargement at birth and at puberty usually occurs because the estrogen level has not yet adjusted to normal (both females and males normally have estrogen in their bodies). Abnormal gynecomastia occurs when conditions or diseases, such as tumors of the testes (the male sex glands that secrete sex hormones) or an estrogen-secreting tumor on the adrenal glands, result in abnormally high levels of estrogen in the male's system.

Symptoms

Other than the obvious en- largement of the breasts, symptoms may also include tenderness in the breast and, in extreme cases, the secretion of milk. Teenaged boys with normal temporary gynecomastia may also show signs of embarrassment and even fear that they are abnormal.

Treatment

Gynecomastia should always be brought to the attention of a doctor. Most cases are temporary and normal. However, these individuals should be reassured that it is a normal and temporary condition. It is especially important that tumors of the adrenal glands or testes be ruled out or treated. If such tumors exist, they are usually removed surgically. In severe or prolonged cases, the excess breast tissue can also be removed by plastic surgery with no visible scarring.

Hydrocele

A hydrocele is a soft swelling around a testis and is noticeable as a soft mass in the scrotum, the bag of skin containing the testes. The term *hydrocele* means literally a sac of water.

There is a normal double-layered covering around each testis. Within these two layers there is usually just enough fluid for sufficient lubrication. Occasionally, however, the amount of fluid may increase, leading to the swelling around the testis. As a rule, most hydroceles in and of themselves are harmless and common, especially in older men.

Causes

Although a hydrocele may be caused by an injury or inflammation in the scrotum among other problems (this is called secondary hydrocele), quite often there is no apparent cause (this is known as primary hydrocele).

Symptoms

Although hydroceles are usually painless, symptoms may include pain and, of course, an obvious swelling.

Treatment

A small, painless hydrocele often requires no treatment. However, if the hydrocele becomes very large or painful, treatment may be indicated. Bed rest, ice bags, and painkillers such as aspirin may afford temporary relief. Usually, however, the physician will draw off the excess fluid with a needle, a procedure done under local anesthetic. While this may bring relief, it is not always a permanent solution, since excess fluid may build up again in the area. A more permanent resolution of the problem is surgical correction.

Impotence

Impotence is the inability to achieve and maintain an erection of the penis, which is necessary to penetrate the female vagina during sexual intercourse. Internal spaces in the penis (called corpora cavernosa) normally fill with blood during sexual excitement and cause the penis to become rigid and erect. Impotence is a partial or total impairment of this function.

Types

There are two types of impotence: primary impotence, in which a man is never able to have an erection adequate for sexual intercourse; and secondary impotence, in which a man quite often fails to complete intercourse to the satisfaction of both partners. Secondary impotence is the more common type.

Many men experience temporary impotence at some point in

their lives, but chronic (recurring) impotence can lower a man's self-esteem and put a strain on his marriage or social relationships.

Causes

Impotence can be caused by either physical or psychological problems. It may be brought on by job-related stress, fear of causing pregnancy, unresolved conflicts about sexuality, or fear of sex after a heart attack or major surgery. Emotional problems such as these, along with drug and alcohol abuse, are some of the leading causes of impotence.

Until recently, psychological problems were thought to be the only cause of impotence; but several physical disorders are now known to trigger the problem: an imbalance in the hormonal system, which may cause a decrease in production of testosterone, the male hormone necessary for an erection; certain drugs used to treat high blood pressure, although the reason for their causing impotence is not known; diseases of the nervous system, such as multiple sclerosis; structural abnormalities of or injury to the penis; and malfunctioning of the circulatory system, which can interfere with the blood flow to the penis necessary for an erection.

Symptoms

The major symptom of impotence is a repeatedly limp penis that is unable to penetrate the vagina during sexual intercourse.

This may be accompanied by a lack of interest in sex, but not necessarily infertility (the inability to father a child).

Diagnosis

Several tests can help to diagnose the cause of a case of impotence. A blood test will show whether adequate levels of testosterone are present. A blood pressure cuff specially designed to wrap around the penis, coupled with ultrasound (the use of sound waves to create an image of internal structures), detects blood pressure and blood vessel problems in the penis. Another test registers the size of erections that naturally occur during sleep; if these amount to at least a 20 percent enlargement of the penis, it can usually be concluded that no physical problem is causing the impotence.

Treatment

Impotence is treated with testosterone injections, surgery, penile implants, and psychological counseling. Testosterone injections may be used to relieve hormone problems, while surgery may be necessary to repair the veins and arteries that deliver blood to the penis. These procedures, however, are not always effective and therefore not recommended for everyone.

Penile implants represent a successful new treatment for impotence, with several varieties now in use. One is a silicone rod implanted in the corpora cavernosa, resulting in a penis that is semi-erect at all times. Another is a flexible silver wire surrounded by silicone, which, when implanted, allows the penis to be manipulated to an erect angle for intercourse. A third model consists of balloon-like cylinders implanted in the corpora cavernosa and attached to a container of fluid, which, when activated by a hand pump, fills them the way blood normally fills the penis during an erection.

Counseling by psychologists or trained sex therapists may be recommended for men whose impotence seems to be stemming from emotional problems; in addition, counseling may also help those with physical disorders in learning to deal with their impotence.

Prevention

Avoiding the abuse of alcohol and drugs, as well as eliminating or coping with stress, should help to prevent at least some episodes of secondary impotence.

Prostatitis

Prostatitis is an infection or inflammation of the male gland called the prostate. It predominantly affects older men, usually in the form of chronic (recurring) flare-ups. Though not a serious disorder, prostatitis can be irritating and uncomfortable because it disrupts normal urination; in advanced stages, it can cause bladder or kidney damage.

Located just below the bladder, the prostate is a small, doughnut-shaped gland that surrounds both the neck of the bladder and the urethra (the narrow tube which carries urine, from the bladder through the penis, to be expelled). As men get older, they sometimes develop an enlarged prostate, which may constrict the urethra and eventually trigger a condition called prostatism, which is a disruption of normal urination marked by prolonged effort or repeated attempts to start the flow, decreased force, and dribbling toward the end of the flow. Some urine is almost always left in the bladder, forming a fertile breeding ground for bacteria and subsequent infection common in prostatitis. Advanced cases of prostatism may cause a sudden, total blockage of urine flow, requiring emergency treatment because the backup of urine can lead to kidney and bladder damage.

Causes

An isolated bout of prostatitis can result from a sexually transmitted disease or a urinary tract infection when the bacteria from these disorders also infect the prostate gland. However, chronic prostatitis, the more common form, seldom results from an infection; in fact, its cause is unknown. It has been theorized that too much or not enough sexual activity may cause a chronic disorder, because the prostate secretes a substance during ejaculation which helps to transport sperm cells.

Symptoms

The most common symptoms

An enlarged prostate, caused by inflammation of the prostate gland, may constrict the urethra passing through and interfere with urination.

to look for, if prostatitis is suspected, are trouble in starting the urine flow, reduced force, and dribbling as it ends; increased frequency of urination; and increased feelings of urgency, even during sleep. An infected prostate may be marked by discomfort in the lower back and genital area, a burning sensation while urinating, fever, and chills.

Diagnosis

Prostatitis is diagnosed by an examination of the prostate to check its size, shape, and firmness. An infected prostate will be tender to the touch and, when it is massaged by the doctor, pus cells will be forced out and will then appear in the urine. A culture of the urine specimen will be examined for bacteria, although very often no bacteria are identified in a case of chronic prostatitis. However, a urinalysis may show some evidence of infection, and if a trace of blood is present, the urine will be additionally tested for the presence of malignant cells.

An enlarged prostate is diagnosed by means of a procedure called intravenous pyelogram (IVP), in which dye is injected into a vein in the arm and allowed to travel through the bloodstream to the kidneys, urinary bladder, and out through the penis. The dye will show any enlargement or obstruction in the ureters. Then the patient will be required to urinate; if the IVP shows a large quantity of urine left in the bladder, a partial obstruction caused by an enlarged prostate generally can be diagnosed.

Treatment

Most prostate infections can be treated quite successfully with antibiotics. Chronic nonbacterial prostatitis, however, is not treated with antibiotics. Instead, drinking large quantities of water and nonalcoholic fluids, as well as taking hot baths, is often recommended.

An enlarged prostate that causes symptoms is normally treated by surgical removal of the excess tissue through one of two procedures: transurethral surgery (performed through the urethra), in which the center of the prostate gland is scraped out by an instrument that has been inserted into the penis; or prostatectomy, a more complicated procedure requiring an incision in the lower abdomen or between the legs. There is little danger of impotency resulting from either of these surgical procedures, but they may lead to retrograde ejaculation, a harmless condition in which semen is passed back into the bladder to be expelled with the urine, rather than through the penis to be ejaculated during intercourse.

THE FEMALE REPRODUCTIVE SYSTEM

The female reproductive system consists of those structures within the female body designed to create and nourish new life. The system includes the ovaries, fallopian tubes, uterus, cervix, and vagina. Some doctors include breasts as reproductive parts, because they may nourish the new life after birth.

Although breasts, or mammary glands, are often considered organs of reproduction, they are actually a type of sweat gland. However, their development is regulated by the reproductive system. For example, hormones manufactured by the ovaries control breast growth during puberty (the time of life around 11 or 12 years when sex organs begin to mature) and milk production after childbirth.

The reproductive process begins in the ovaries. Ovaries are small, egg-shaped glands located in the lower abdomen. These glands monitor the cyclic functions of the reproductive system based on ovulation. Ovulation is the monthly production and release of a mature egg (occasionally two or more eggs). This action and other reproductive functions result from stimulation of hormones — estrogen and proges-

terone—secreted by the ovaries. Estrogen regulates the secondary sex traits of body hair growth, breast development, ovulation, and menstruation. Progesterone contributes to reproduction, as well as to enlargement of the breasts during pregnancy and milk production after childbirth. The two hormones coordinate to control the menstrual cycle.

Once an egg is released, it travels through the fallopian tubes. There are two fallopian tubes and they extend from each ovary into the uterus. Their reproductive function is to contain the egg until fertilization (union between the egg and sperm, or male sex cell) takes place. Fallopian tubes direct the sperm to the egg and then propel the fertilized egg into the uterus.

The uterus is a pear-shaped hollow organ normally about the size of a lemon. Its muscular walls are lined with rich, soft tissue called the endometrium. Each month the lining adds layers in anticipation of receiving and nourishing a fertilized egg. Should conception (union of sperm and egg) occur, the lining nourishes the fertilized egg in the uterus until birth. However, if the egg remains unfertilized, the uterus sheds the

A side view of the female reproductive organs.

A front view of the female reproductive organs.

endometrium and the unfertilized egg, which leave the body as menstrual discharge.

The cervix is a narrow opening to an inch-long canal. The canal connects the lower end of the uterus to the upper portion of the vagina. This canal transports sperm on their way to fertilize an egg and is the passageway for menstrual discharge and babies leaving the uterus.

The vagina, or birth canal, is a passageway leading from the uterus to the outside of the body. In the average adult woman, it measures four to five inches in length. Although vaginal walls are normally close together, they separate to accommodate a descending baby during childbirth and the erect male penis during sexual intercourse.

The vagina produces natural secretions that provide continual lubrication and cleansing of the organ. The amount of secretion may vary with the menstrual cycle and emotional state.

Amenorrhea

Amenorrhea is defined as the absence of menstruation. There are two categories of this disorder. Primary amenorrhea is the failure to begin menstruating by the age of 16; secondary amenorrhea, the more common of the two conditions, is the absence of three or more periods in a row in a woman who has been menstruating for some time. Primary amenorrhea is specifically defined at the age of 16 and can go on indefinitely; secondary amenorrhea is usually a temporary condition, since the

periods generally resume when the underlying cause for the interruption has been corrected.

Causes

Primary amenorrhea may be caused by endocrine gland disorders (such as hyper- or hypothyroidism); genetic abnormalities; damaged or missing ovaries, uterus, or vagina; or an excessively thick hymen (the membrane that covers the vaginal opening in young girls), which prevents the menstrual blood from flowing out.

Secondary amenorrhea is caused, most commonly, by pregnancy. It can also be triggered by strenuous sports training; poor nutrition; drastic weight gain; jet lag; certain medications, including birth control pills; serious surgery or disease; emotional shock; or the loss of a certain percentage of body fat.

Symptoms

The symptoms that commonly accompany primary amenorrhea indicate abnormal or inhibited physical development; the young girl may fail to develop breasts or body hair, indicating that a genetic disorder may be present that is preventing her from attaining sexual maturity. These girls are also usually short.

Secondary amenorrhea has no symptoms other than the absence of menstrual periods.

Diagnosis

Diagnosis of both categories will probably include a pregnancy test to rule out that possibility as the cause, as well as tests to determine genetic or hormonal disorders and X rays to check the reproductive organs.

Treatment

Primary amenorrhea may be treated with an extensive hormone therapy program to stimulate physical development or, if the cause is a thick hymen, with surgery to open the hymen. Some cases of primary amenorrhea, however, are untreatable.

Secondary amenorrhea may be treated with a hormone that will trigger ovulation and reestablish the menstrual cycle. However, quite often this condition will reverse itself without treatment, especially if the cause is merely an interruption in the patient's normal routine, an emotional upset, or, of course, pregnancy.

Prevention

Maintaining good nutrition habits and a normal weight and avoiding overexerting sports can probably be beneficial in preventing secondary amenorrhea; no specific precautions can be taken, however, to prevent primary amenorrhea.

Cystocele

A cystocele is a protruding into the vagina of a portion of the urinary bladder. This is often a result of damage during childbirth of the wall of fibrous tissue that normally separates the vagina and the bladder. This may happen during the birth of a baby of any size. However, women who have never delivered a baby may also develop a cystocele. A cystocele may not appear until menopause, when the damaged or weak area weakens further, permitting the rear and base of the bladder to protrude into the vagina. At the same time, or separately, there may also be a bulging into the vagina of a portion of the rectum (final part of large bowel) or small intestine or urethra (the tube through which urine leaves the body). There may also be a prolapse of the uterus (in which the uterus drops through the vagina and in very severe cases protrudes from the vagina opening).

The bladder's protrusion into the vagina creates a pool of stale urine in the bladder which cannot be easily emptied and which becomes a breeding ground for bacteria. Cystitis (inflammation/infection of the bladder) with its symptoms of painful and difficult urination often results.

Symptoms

A woman with cystocele may feel a fullness in the vagina and may find it difficult to empty her bladder completely (she may be able to do this by urinating a second time). However, many women with cystocele have no symptoms at all.

Diagnosis

Diagnosis is made by examining the inside of the vagina where a bulge can be seen in front of the cervix (the neck of the womb that protrudes into the vagina). Also, if a catheter inserted into the bladder after urination can draw out more than two ounces of left-over urine, a cystocele is definitely suspected. A special X ray in which dye is inserted into the bladder will reveal the bulged-out section of bladder.

Treatment

The preferred treatment for cystocele is surgery to repair the damaged wall and put the protruding section of bladder back in its original place. A pessary (a device inserted into the vagina to support the vagina and reduce the cystocele) may be used in women who refuse or cannot withstand surgery. A cystocele does not always require treatment. However, if frequent bouts of cystitis occur, some form of treatment will be necessary.

DES

DES (diethylstilbestrol) is an artificial (man-made) estrogen (female sex hormone) used to treat a variety of disorders.

The drug was popularly prescribed to prevent miscarriage from the early 1940s until it was found to be ineffective and was banned for this use by the Food and Drug Administration in 1971. It is now linked to an increased incidence of adenocarcinoma—a rare cancer of the glandular cells of the reproductive organs — in daughters of the several million women who took DES to prevent miscarriage and other pregnancy complications. Recently, testicular cancer in male offspring was also associated with maternal DES use.

Although experience has shown that the chance of developing a malignancy is small, children exposed to DES before birth run a higher than average risk for benign (noncancerous or precancerous) growths and for structural changes involving the reproductive organs (vagina, cervix, and uterus in women; penis, testicles, and urinary tract in men), as well as for infertility problems. These abnormalities usually appear after puberty, generally in the late teens to early 30s, years after the exposure.

Because of these potential problems, DES should not be taken by a woman who is pregnant or suspects that she is pregnant. DES may be used safely in nonpregnant women to treat a variety of disorders including certain vaginal conditions and estrogen deficiency that may occur at menopause or after the surgical removal of the ovaries. DES may also be used as a post-coital contraceptive (the so-called "morning-after pill"). Since DES is a hormone that may produce a variety of effects on the body, its use must always be supervised by a physician.

Recently, DES has been shown to be effective in some patients in reducing the growth of advanced prostate cancer in men and certain forms of breast cancer in both sexes.

Although the incidence of serious complications is small, physicians strongly advise that individuals who were exposed to DES because it was taken by their mother should be routinely examined to detect any developing abnormalities.

Dilatation and curettage

Dilatation and curettage, also called a D and C, is the surgical scraping of the lining of the uterus after the cervix (neck of the uterus) has been dilated (expanded). This minor procedure is often done to diagnose disease of the uterus (such as cancer) or to correct extreme or prolonged bleeding. It is also used to perform an abortion and may be employed after a miscarriage (an involuntary expulsion of an unborn baby — before it is able to live on its own— from the uterus) to remove any remains of tissue, thus lowering the risk of hemorrhage and infection. Dilatation alone may be performed to enlarge the passageway out of the uterus. This might be done in the case of a severely narrowed cervix to eliminate painful menstruation caused by restricted flow of menstrual fluid. For treatment of this problem, multiple dilatations may be necessary since the cervix will often again become narrow after several months.

The lining to be scraped, known as the endometrium, consists of a mucous membrane richly supplied with blood vessels. It grows anew each month to provide a potential nesting place for a fertilized egg and forms an attachment to the placenta that nourishes the baby-to-be. If no fertilization occurs, the endome-

trium is shed during menstruation and a new one begins to grow.

The procedure

A D and C is performed in an operating room under sterile conditions. Anesthesia may be general (the patient is put to sleep) or local. The lower bowel and urinary bladder must be empty; an enema (to empty the bowel) may be required before the operation.

The patient rests on her back with her feet up in stirrups. The surgeon inserts metal dilators of progressively larger sizes into the opening of the cervix, the cervical canal, until it is open enough to permit the insertion of the surgical instruments. An alternate method of cervical dilatation employs a small tube of dried seaweed that is left in the cervical canal for eight to 12 hours. As the seaweed absorbs moisture from the cervical canal, it expands and enlarges the canal.

A curette, a scraping instrument designed for this purpose, is used to remove endometrial tissue. Special forceps may also be used to remove tissue.

The principal risks of a D and C are hemorrhage, infection, and perforation (puncture) of the uterus. The latter is more possible during pregnancy because the uterus is especially soft and thin at that time.

When the operation is finished, an absorbent pad is placed over the entrance to the vagina. Following the operation, the pad is checked every 15 minutes for two hours, and excessive bleeding

Dilatation and curettage (D and C) is the surgical scraping of the lining (endometrium) of the uterus after the cervix has been dilated (enlarged). The procedure is done with a curette, a special scraping instrument.

reported to the physician.

Mild painkillers should be enough to control discomfort from the operation. If there is pain in the abdomen that cannot be relieved in this way, or that is continuous or sharp, it should be reported immediately. Some difficulty in urinating may be expected immediately after the procedure.

In most cases, the patient stays in bed for one to two hours following surgery but then may resume normal activities. Most women return home several hours after the operation or the next day. Many daily activities can be resumed immediately, and in a week all normal physical activities may be resumed. Sexual intercourse should not be attempted, however, until after the next visit to the doctor, when the doctor can determine if and when sexual relations can be resumed.

Dysmenorrhea

Dysmenorrhea is the term for painful menstruation. It occurs most commonly in teenagers and in women who have never been pregnant.

There are two types of dysmenorrhea. Primary dysmenorrhea is a recurring condition usually beginning shortly after the onset of menstruation in a young girl. Secondary dysmenorrhea develops later in life after a woman has been menstruating for some time.

Causes

The cause of primary dysmenorrhea is thought to be the release of prostaglandins (substances which stimulate uterine contractions) from the lining of the uterus shortly before a menstrual period begins. The resulting contractions will constrict blood vessels in the uterus, causing pain in the same way that a decrease in blood supply to the heart results in chest pain. The reason for this excessive production of prostaglandins is not known. Dysmenorrhea is usually secondary to—that is, a result of—other reproductive problems, such as fibroid tumors, a narrow cervix, or endometriosis (the displacement of tissue from the lining of the uterus to areas elsewhere in the body).

Symptoms

The major symptoms of both types of dysmenorrhea are cramps or pain in the lower abdomen, possibly extending around to the back. Nausea, vomiting, diarrhea, headache, fatigue, and nervousness are mainly associated with primary dysmenorrhea. These symptoms usually appear at the beginning of or slightly before the menstrual period, and may last several hours or several days.

Dysmenorrhea is not a serious condition, but it can be annoying, uncomfortable, and even incapacitating. Since secondary dysmenorrhea usually indicates that another affliction is present, treatment should always be sought for this condition.

Diagnosis

Diagnosis will include a complete physical exam as well as medical and menstrual histories. If the symptoms are present from the onset of menstruation at puberty, primary dysmenorrhea is usually the diagnosis. If symptoms have appeared suddenly in a woman who has menstruated for some years, secondary dysmenorrhea can be assumed and further diagnostic evaluation of the reproductive organs may be necessary to determine the disorder that is causing the dysmenorrhea. Ultrasound examinations, in which sound waves bounce off internal structures forming a visual image of them, or X rays may help in determining the underlying disorder.

Treatment

Recently, primary dysmenorrhea has been treated successfully with nonsteroidal antiinflammatory drugs (including ibuprofen, naproxen sodium, meclofenamate sodium, diflunisal, and mefenamic acid) which, when taken just before a period is to begin, act to suppress the release of prostaglandins and thereby reduce the contractions that are causing pain.

Secondary dysmenorrhea is treated by correcting the problem that is causing it; for instance, endometriosis can be treated with hormone therapy or surgery, thus relieving the source of the dysmenorrhea.

Home remedies often help to ease menstrual pain and relieve pressure. These include a hot water bottle or heating pad placed on the abdomen; hot baths; and lying on the back with the knees bent. Also, interestingly, childbirth may relieve dysmenorrhea problems, possibly because of the enlargement of the cervix (mouth of the uterus) or destruction of some nerve fibers in the uterus.

Dyspareunia

Dyspareunia is difficulty or pain for a woman during sexual intercourse.

Causes

Dyspareunia may be caused by a resistant hymen (the membrane that partially or completely covers the opening to the vagina); or inflammation or injury of the vagina, urethra (the urinary tube), vulva (the lips and other structures around the opening to the vagina), or the anus (the opening of the large intestine). It can be the result of scar tissue forming around an episiotomy (a surgical cut to enlarge the opening of the vagina before childbirth) or surgery to repair the vagina. Other organic causes include tight muscles in the area around the vagina, an "hourglass" contraction of the vagina, a divided vagina, inflammation of the cervix (the neck of the uterus), prolapsed (fallen) uterus, infected fallopian tubes (which lead from the ovaries to the uterus), and endometriosis (in which bits of tissue from the lining of the uterus grow outside the uterus on various organs in the pelvic cavity, including the ovaries and fallopian tubes).

Inadequate lubrication of the vagina is a common cause of dyspareunia, as is an unconscious tightening of the vaginal mus-

cles—perhaps the result of fear, unreadiness, or unwillingness to perform the sex act, or other psychological reasons. Improperly fitted or improperly lubricated birth control devices (condoms or diaphragms) and an allergy to contraceptive spermicides are other causes.

Treatment

Treatment for dyspareunia is correction of any underlying disease, injury, or structural defect if such a problem exists. For some couples, psychological or psychiatric counseling is helpful in removing psychological barriers to sexual intercourse that may result in dyspareunia.

Water-soluble lubricating jelly (not petroleum jelly), obtainable in any drugstore, provides a good vaginal lubricant. Estrogen creams can be used along with water-soluble jelly to restore lubrication to a dry vagina after menopause. Soothing anesthetic creams and temporary avoidance of intercourse can relieve the soreness of dyspareunia.

Endometriosis

Endometriosis is a condition in which tissue from the lining of the uterus detaches itself and grows elsewhere in the abdominal cavity outside the uterus. It occurs only in women during the childbearing years, especially in women between the ages of 30 and 40.

Endometriosis develops when the tissue that normally lines the uterus (called endometrial tissue or the endometrium) displaces itself and grows on the outside of the uterus, on the ovaries, the intestine, or anywhere else in the abdomen. The endometrium normally thickens and swells during each menstrual cycle in preparation for possible pregnancy, then breaks down and flows out of the body during menstruation if no pregnancy occurs. When endometriosis develops, the displaced endometrial tissue continues to swell and bleed each month, but it has nowhere to flow. The body responds to the presence of this accumulated blood by building scar tissue around it that builds up month after month, finally leading to the formation of blood-filled pockets or cysts (often called "chocolate cysts") on the affected organs.

Causes

The exact cause of endometriosis is not known, but several conditions are thought to lead to its development: menstrual blood may flow backwards through the fallopian tubes and into the abdominal cavity, but the reason for this is not known; the cervix or vagina may be blocked so that the menstrual blood cannot flow out normally; or surgery or another condition may lead to the displacement of some tissue from the uterus.

Symptoms

The symptoms of endometriosis are pain during, immedi-

ately before, or immediately after the menstrual period; pain during intercourse; discomfort in the lower urinary tract or intestine; irregular or excessively heavy menstrual flow; bleeding from the rectum; blood in the urine; and infertility. These symptoms may vary from person to person. Some women may experience all of these symptoms, while others may experience only one or two.

Diagnosis

Endometriosis is diagnosed with a complete medical and menstrual history. Two pelvic examinations may be performed, one during menstruation and one between periods, to determine the changes in the reproductive area during the cycle. The doctor may also perform a laparoscopy, in which a small, lighted tube is inserted into the lower abdomen through a tiny incision; any displaced tissues can usually be seen through the tube.

Treatment

Treatment of this disorder involves halting the condition, reducing the pain, and restoring normal menstruation and fertility. The best way to halt endometriosis is to modify the body's natural hormone secretions with drugs in order to stop menstruation and ovulation for some time, thus allowing the endometrial tissue to shrink. Naturally, the patient will be unable to become pregnant during this type of drug therapy, but since endometriosis often causes infertility, many patients are already unable to conceive. Two types of drugs are usually used in this treatment. Birth control pills as well as several other medications that modify female hormone secretions are sometimes prescribed in high enough doses to stop menstruation and ovulation. However, an excessive dosage often brings with it undesirable side effects such as nausea, fluid retention, and the possibility of blood clotting.

A new synthetic hormone called danazol creates a condition similar to menopause, causing menstruation and ovulation to stop and the endometrial tissue to shrink almost immediately, but without some of the side effects associated with hormonal drugs. However, danazol can be expensive and in some cases is not effective.

If drug therapy is unsuccessful, surgery may be necessary, involving either the removal of scar tissue and endometrial tissue or, in advanced cases, the removal of the uterus and ovaries, rendering the patient sterile.

Prevention

There are no specific measures that will prevent the development of endometriosis, but pregnancy and breast-feeding often have a beneficial effect on this condition because, in interrupting the menstrual cycle, they prevent the buildup of tissue. Childbirth enlarges the cervix, which may be beneficial in the prevention of endometriosis. The disease is seen more often in women who have postponed childbearing until their late 20s or 30s, so becoming pregnant earlier in life may help to reduce the risk of developing endometriosis in later years.

Fibrocystic disease of the breast

Fibrocystic disease is a condition in which benign (noncancerous) lumps form in the breast, either temporarily or for the duration of the childbearing years.

This condition is not dangerous in itself, but it has been found that women with certain forms of fibrocystic disease are two to four times more likely to develop breast cancer than other women. To complicate matters, the presence of these benign lumps makes it difficult to detect any new, possibly dangerous growths.

Cause

The exact cause of fibrocystic disease is not known. However, the tendency to develop it may be inherited. Also, it is seen more often in women who have never breast-fed a child, but the reason for this is not known.

Symptoms

The most noticeable symptoms of this disorder, obviously, are the lumps, which may take the form of either solid masses or fluid-filled sacs called cysts. Large cystic lumps near the surface may be moved about freely, unlike can-

There is some fibrous tissue in the normal breast to support the milk glands.

Rib

Fat

Mammary (milk) glands

Fibrous tissue

Extra fibrous tissue

Cysts

In the fibrocystic breast, there is extra fibrous tissue and solid or fluid-filled lumps (cysts).

cerous lumps that are usually firmly attached to surrounding tissue. Changes in the body's hormone secretions during the menstrual period tend to increase slightly the size of the lumps and cause additional pain, but the cysts reduce in size following the period. Other symptoms may include a slight discharge from the nipple as well as persistently

heavy and tender breasts, not only before and during menstruation, as is commonly seen in healthy breasts, but all the time.

Diagnosis

Diagnosis will include a physical exam and, possibly, one of two additional procedures: mammography (breast X ray) or diaphanography, an examination of the breast tissue by shining a light through the translucent tissue. Either of these procedures will determine whether the lumps are fluid-filled cysts or solid masses. If they are found to be solid, a biopsy (the removal of a small piece of tissue for analysis) may need to be performed in order to detect the possibility of cancerous cells.

Treatment

Fibrocystic disease often requires no treatment. In some cases lumps may disappear in a few months. However, cysts which are unusually large or particularly bothersome may be drained of their fluid by the insertion of a hollow needle in a procedure called aspiration. If there are many small lumps or continuous development of new ones, other forms of treatment may be necessary to prevent the formation of cysts. Birth control pills may be prescribed, as they act to equalize the amount of hormones present in the body during the monthly cycle; however, birth control pills have also been found to cause cysts in some women. Large doses of Vitamin E have also been effective in treating this disorder.

Prevention

Relieving or preventing fibrocystic disease may be promoted by discontinuing or drastically limiting the intake of nicotine and a chemical called methylxanthine, found most commonly in coffee, tea, cola, chocolate, and some cold medications. It is thought that both nicotine and methylxanthine may promote the growth of fibrocystic tissue.

Because of the greater risk of breast cancer with certain forms of this disorder, women with fibrocystic disease should have a physical exam at least twice a year, report any new growths or enlargements of existing lumps, and perform a self-examination of their breasts each month following the menstrual period.

Fibroid tumors

Fibroid tumors are solid, noncancerous growths composed of smooth muscle fibers and connective tissue that appear in and on the uterus. They are thought to be the most common abdominal tumor, found in about 25 percent of all women over the age of 30 and more often in black women. Cancer rarely develops in fibroid tumors.

These tumors vary in size and shape, usually grow slowly, and cause few problems. They may grow in the walls of the uterus or out from the uterus; only rarely, they may appear on the cervix; and occasionally they fill the entire uterus, push through the cervix, and appear in the vagina.

Complications

Sometimes fibroid tumors do cause complications. If they become very large, they may press on surrounding organs (for instance, on the intestine or bladder, which may result in constipation or frequent urination). If they extend into the uterus, heavy and prolonged menstrual periods may result. If pregnancy occurs, the tumors tend to enlarge and may cause complications as the unborn baby grows.

Causes

The cause of fibroid tumors is not known, but their growth seems to be related to estrogen, a female hormone, since these tumors rarely appear before puberty and tend to recede by the menopause years. They most commonly appear in the middle to late reproductive years, when the estrogen level is at its peak.

Fibroid tumors may occur along with other disorders, such as endometriosis (the displacement of tissue from the lining of the uterus to outside the uterus) or pelvic inflammatory disease (an infection of the fallopian tubes).

Symptoms

The symptoms of fibroid tumors are dysmenorrhea (pain during menstruation); a gushing or flooding of menstrual flow; occasionally, abdominal pain (although pain is not usually a symptom unless a complication develops, such as a twisting of the tumor, cutting off its blood supply and causing severe pain); and, if the tumor is advanced, a noticeably enlarged abdomen. Sometimes these tumors display no symptoms and are simply discovered during a routine physical exam.

Diagnosis

Diagnosis begins with a physical examination and may include curettage (scraping the uterus walls) or endometrial biopsy (removal of some tissue from the lining of the uterus) to test for cancer. X rays as well as ultrasound (a technique that uses sound waves to outline internal structures) may also be used to view the location and nature of the tumor.

Treatment

Fibroid tumors may require no treatment at all, other than regular checkups with the doctor. Those that are causing complications may require one of two types of surgery: the removal of the tumor (called a myomectomy), recommended for women in their early reproductive years whose symptoms are somewhat mild and who desire a future pregnancy; or the removal of the uterus (called a hysterectomy), usually recommended for older women or for those who do not want to become pregnant, as this operation makes pregnancy impossible.

Hysterectomy

Hysterectomy is the surgical removal of the uterus and its cervix. Removal of the uterus may be done through an abdominal cut or incision or through the vagina (the top of the vagina is stitched together after the uterus is removed). The latter procedure requires no external incision and, therefore, leaves no external scar.

Hysterectomies may be either

total or partial. The total hysterectomy involves the removal of the entire uterus. A partial hysterectomy means removal of only the body of the uterus and not the cervix.

When hysterectomy is performed, the ovaries and fallopian tubes may also be removed. However, there are pros and cons to removing healthy ovaries, particularly in women who have not yet reached their natural menopause. While the removal of the uterus itself causes the termination of menstruation and the inability to bear children, the removal of the ovaries (oophorectomy) causes the patient to prematurely experience the other bodily changes of menopause, which are brought on by the loss of the female hormones produced by the ovaries. For this reason, physicians remove the ovaries only with strong reasons.

Reasons for hysterectomy

Hysterectomies are performed for a number of reasons. They are most commonly performed when the uterus is diseased. Symptomatic fibroid tumors, uterine prolapse, and cancer of the uterus are common reasons for a hysterectomy. Cysts and tumors of the ovaries or fallopian tubes may also require a hysterectomy.

Contrary to common belief, a hysterectomy, in and of itself, does not interfere with, or diminish the pleasure of, sexual intercourse, nor does it cause weight gain.

Leukorrhea

Leukorrhea is an abnormal discharge from the vagina. All women will have some normal discharge, and this results from a secretion of mucus by the cervix (neck of the uterus) and the vagina. This normal discharge helps to lubricate the vagina and, to some extent, prevent infection. At the time of ovulation, when an egg is released from the ovary, this discharge is most noticeable, but it is generally present during the entire menstrual cycle.

Symptoms

An abnormal vaginal discharge usually has the following characteristics: it may be heavy, it may be associated with itching of the genital organs and anal area, and it may have a disagreeable odor.

Causes

Abnormal discharge is usually caused by an infection of the vagina, but it may also be caused by an infection of the cervix, a tumor or other abnormal growths, the presence of foreign matter in the vagina such as a tampon, or, less commonly, an inflammation of the vagina caused by chemicals in douches or contraceptive creams or jellies.

Vaginal infections are usually caused by one of three different organisms: a fungus, a parasite, or by a variety of bacteria.

Diagnosis

To diagnose the cause of the discharge, the doctor will perform a pelvic examination and will often take a sample of the discharge and look at it under the microscope. Sometimes a culture of the discharge may also be taken so that the organism causing the problem can be grown in the laboratory and identified.

Treatment

Once the cause of the abnormal discharge has been identified, specific steps will be taken to treat it. If the discharge is caused by bacteria, oral antibiotics or antibiotic vaginal creams may be prescribed. Specific oral drugs or vaginal creams will be prescribed if the discharge is caused by either yeast or trichomonad. In some cases, a biopsy of the cervix or vagina may be required if the doctor suspects that a tumor may be causing the discharge.

Douching with vinegar and water or other solutions available at the drugstore generally will not cure the discharge even though symptoms may improve for a few days. A woman with an abnormal vaginal discharge should consult her doctor before attempting to treat herself.

Mastectomy

Mastectomy is the surgical removal of a breast or part of a breast, usually as a treatment for cancer.

Types

There are several types of mastectomy, each characterized by the muscles, glands, tissues, or skin removed.

- Lumpectomy—removal of the tumor along with some of the surrounding breast tissue
- Partial mastectomy—removal of the tumor along with approximately one half of the breast
- Simple mastectomy—removal of the entire breast and possibly some of the lymph nodes in the armpit
- Modified radical mastectomy—removal of the entire breast plus more of the armpit lymph nodes than in the simple mastectomy
- Radical mastectomy—removal of the entire breast, all the lymph nodes in the armpit, and the chest muscles
- Extended radical—removal of breast plus additional tissue in the chest as well as the armpit lymph nodes and chest muscles
- Super radical mastectomy—removal of the same tissues and muscles as in the extended radical but in addition tissues and lymph nodes up into the neck.

Determination of type

The type of mastectomy is determined by whether the cancer is still localized in the original site or whether the cancer has spread into neighboring lymph nodes. The lymph nodes in the armpit will have a biopsy done on them—a biopsy is the removal of a small tissue sample to examine it for malignant cells. In addition, other tests may be done to determine if the cancer has spread to other areas of the body.

There is some question about how extensive the surgery needs to be. Some studies have shown

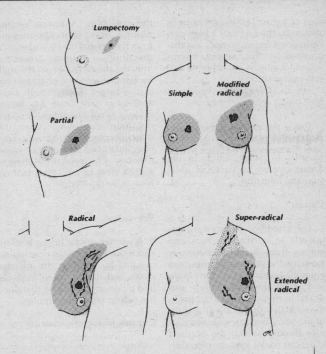

The shaded portions show the area affected by each type of mastectomy.

that the survival rate for a specified period of time is the same regardless of the type of operation. Therefore, it would seem that the simplest procedure is indicated. However, there are differences of opinion in medical circles, and a woman facing a mastectomy should thoroughly discuss all of the procedures and available options with her doctor.

Treatment

The operation is performed while the patient is under general anesthesia. Afterward the patient remains hospitalized for about a week and may begin radiation therapy or chemotherapy. Periodic checkups are advised every six to 12 months.

Prevention

One of the best preventive measures a woman can take is establishing the habit of a monthly breast self-examination. This simple routine can detect a cancerous lump before it spreads beyond the breast. The effectiveness of breast self-examination is shown by the fact that a high percentage of breast tumors are discovered by the patients themselves during a monthly breast self-examination.

See also Cancer for instructions for a breast self-examination.

Mastitis

Mastitis is inflammation of the breast caused by bacterial invasion and infection.

Causes

This condition occurs most frequently in nursing mothers and comes from bacteria, normally found on the skin and nipples, that enter the breast through the nipple and infect the milk glands and ducts. In many cases, it occurs in the third to fifth day after the birth of the baby, because cracked nipples through which the bacteria enter the breast may develop during the first week of breast-feeding.

Symptoms

Symptoms of mastitis include pain, swelling, redness, high fever, and a tender lump in the breast. Sometimes the lymph glands in the armpit next to the affected breast may be tender and swollen. In cases of severe infection there may be pus in the breast.

Treatment

The treatment for mastitis is antibiotic medication to combat the infection. A breast-feeding mother may continue nursing from the normal breast and should discontinue nursing from the infected breast but expel the milk by hand to prevent engorgement of the breast. Even though most antibiotics will enter the breast milk in small quantities, this will not harm the baby. When the infection clears up, nursing from the infected breast can be resumed. Occasionally, if there is a great deal of pus, the pus may have to be drained.

Prevention

A woman who is breast-feeding can reduce the risk of developing mastitis by keeping the nipples clean and dry between feedings and by wearing clothing that does not rub or irritate the nipples.

Chronic fibrocystic mastitis

Another more common form of mastitis is not infectious and is called chronic fibrocystic mastitis. In this condition breasts contain small cysts and nodules and are usually very painful. This condition is readily treated by a physician, who will check to be sure that the cysts and nodules are not cancerous.

Menopause

Menopause is the normal, natural stage in a woman's life when her menstruation and ovulation cycles stop, ending her reproductive years. Also called climacteric or the change of life, it occurs around age 50 but can start anywhere between the ages of 40 to 60. During the years immediately preceding its onset, menstrual periods may become scant and irregular.

Cause

Scientists do not fully understand what causes menopause but they believe that it is triggered when the female sex glands, the ovaries, stop responding to the gonadotropic (sex gland) hormones that are secreted by the pituitary gland to control normal function of the ovaries. The ovaries' subsequent decline in the production of the female hormone estrogen sets off the bodily changes.

Symptoms

Physical symptoms may include hot flashes (a warm and flushed feeling that comes over the face, neck, and chest and lasts a few minutes at a time but recurs throughout the day), excessive perspiring, dryness in the vagina (which can lead to painful or difficult intercourse), pounding heartbeat, joint pains, headaches, itching skin, increased facial hair, and decreased armpit and pubic hair.

Nonphysical symptoms are depression, anxiety, irritability, apprehension, decreased ability to concentrate, lack of confidence, and insomnia.

Symptoms may last from a few weeks to more than five years. Not every woman experiences the same changes, other than an end

to menstruation; about 25 percent notice no other changes, 50 percent discern some physical and/or psychological symptoms, and the other 25 percent note very uncomfortable or distressing symptoms.

During this time, it can also be difficult for a woman to face the aging process and its physical ramifications, the end of the childbearing years, and a sense of uselessness because of a possible decrease in family responsibilities.

It is important not to attribute all physical changes to menopause to the point of overlooking the symptoms of disease. This is a good time to schedule an examination and discuss the bodily changes with a doctor. A woman should see a doctor immediately if she starts to bleed in between menstrual periods, bleeds excessively, or has another period six months or more after they had apparently stopped.

Effect on fertility

Fertility and the need to practice birth control at this stage depend upon a woman's age at the time of her last period. Under age 50, a woman can still conceive for up to 24 months after the date of her last period; over 50, conception is possible for up to one year.

Treatment

Treatment for the physical symptoms of menopause includes replacement of the female sex hormones, commonly estrogen or a combination of estrogen and progesterone in tablet or vaginal cream. The lowest effective dose is administered (because of possible side effects) for the first few months and then tapered off (unless symptoms reappear) until the changes in the ovaries are completed.

Artificial estrogen can help a woman's psyche, bones, joints, and skin but it does harbor potential side effects, including coronary or cerebral thrombosis and cancer of the uterus. Estrogen is not given to women with circulatory or liver disorders and is carefully controlled when prescribed to those with diabetes, epilepsy, and heart or kidney disease. Progesterone is not prescribed for women with liver disease and is carefully controlled in those with asthma, epilepsy, and heart or kidney disease. The benefits and hazards can be discussed with a doctor; other medication is available to treat certain menopausal symptoms in women who cannot take hormones.

Treatment for the psychological or emotional symptoms may include tranquilizers, antidepressants, sleeping pills, or psychotherapy.

It is important to remember that any treatment merely lessens the discomfort of menopause; it cannot stop or slow down menopause.

After menopause, a woman may be more prone to osteoporosis (a disease that makes bones porous and brittle) and high blood pressure. Both of these conditions can be controlled under medical supervision.

Menorrhagia

Menorrhagia is a term referring to an abnormally long—more than seven days—or heavy menstrual flow, frequently accompanied by the passing of large blood clots.

Causes

It is a common problem, one that is often caused by a disturbance in the hormones controlling the menstrual cycle. It can also be caused by fibroid tumors in the uterus, inflammation of the pelvis, and hypothyroidism (underactive thyroid gland).

The condition, which is especially common in women nearing the late 30s and 40s, seldom indicates the existence of a serious disorder. However, it may result in iron deficiency anemia because of excessive blood loss.

Diagnosis

If this abnormal menstrual flow continues over a long period of time, a physician should be consulted. The physician may perform a number of tests to determine whether there is a serious underlying cause, as well as do a Pap test, a cervical biopsy (tissue sample from the cervix), or a biopsy of the uterine lining to check for cancer. The physician may also do a blood test to check for iron deficiency anemia.

Treatment

It is suggested that persons having this disorder reduce the level of their activities during menstruation and be sure to get enough iron so that they will not become anemic.

Menstruation

Menstruation is the monthly breakdown and discharge of the endometrial tissue that lines the uterus. The endometrial tissue thickens during each menstrual cycle to prepare the uterus for possible pregnancy. Approximately midway through the cycle, ovulation occurs. Ovulation is the pro-

cess in which an ovary—one of two glands near the top of the uterus that secrete female sex hormones—releases an egg. Extending from either side of the uterus are the fallopian tubes, which are four to five inches long with finger-like projections at their ends. When the ovary releases an egg, the projections on the nearby tube sweep the egg into the tube where it slowly inches toward the uterus.

If during that time, the egg is fertilized by a sperm, the male reproductive cell, it moves to the uterus and implants itself into the rich uterine lining where it grows

Stages of menstrual cycle

Fallopian tube

Egg   Ovary

Endometrium

Uterus

In the first stage while the egg is still inside the ovary, the endometrium (lining of the uterus) is fairly thin.

When the egg is released and begins to move into the fallopian tube, the endometrium begins to thicken in preparation for a possible pregnancy.

The egg moves through the tube toward the uterus. This is the point at which conception may occur. The egg is met by the male sperm cell in the fallopian tube, and the fertilized egg moves on to the uterus. During this time the endometrium continues to grow.

If conception does not occur, the endometrium ceases to grow and thicken. At this stage, the endometrium breaks down and is discharged, along with the unfertilized egg, from the uterus. This is menstruation. (In this drawing, the egg has been enlarged for the sake of illustration; normally the egg is only visible under a microscope.)

for the next nine months. If the egg does not become fertilized, the uterine lining breaks down and passes, along with the unfertilized egg, out of the cervix (neck of the uterus) on through the vagina and out of the body. This discharge is known as menstruation, and this monthly cycle is controlled by the female hormones, estrogen and progesterone, secreted by the ovaries.

Young women start menstruating and ovulating at puberty, which occurs between the ages of nine and 14, and normally do so every month (except while pregnant) until they reach menopause around age 50 or so.

Menstrual disorders

Menstruation may be accompanied by complications of varying degrees of seriousness in many women at some point in their reproductive lives. The most common problems are dysmenorrhea, painful menstruation; amenorrhea, the absence entirely of a menstrual period or the missing of several periods; and premenstrual tension (PMT), distinct feelings of irritability and discomfort in the days before the period begins.

For many years the symptoms of these disorders have been attributed to emotional factors.

Research, however, has shown that most are caused by very real physical changes, and many new methods of treatment have been developed.

Although the disorders themselves are generally not dangerous, they can be physically and emotionally incapacitating. Furthermore, they may be symptoms of a disease in the reproductive organs. Therefore, medical treatment for annoying symptoms accompanying menstruation should always be sought to be on the safe side.

Oophorectomy

Oophorectomy is surgical removal of an ovary, either one of the two female sex glands situated above and on either side of the uterus. The ovaries are almond-shaped organs, about 1½ inches long, that produce an egg for fertilization each month and also secrete the female sex hormones. An oophorectomy is a major operation, usually performed through either a vertical or horizontal incision in the abdominal area but occasionally through an incision in the vagina.

Removal of one ovary (unilateral oophorectomy) may include a salpingectomy — removal of all or part of the nearby fallopian tube that transports eggs to the uterus. Removal of both ovaries is a bilateral oophorectomy. A bilateral salpingo-oophorectomy—removal of both ovaries and both fallopian tubes — ends a woman's ability to conceive children. A hysterectomy (removal of the uterus) is generally performed in conjunction with a bilateral oophorectomy because the uterus has no purpose without either ovary and, if left, can harbor tumors later on.

Reasons for oophorectomy

Oophorectomies correct a number of conditions in which the ovaries are the site of the trouble, including an ectopic pregnancy, in which the embryo is lodged in the ovary, and benign (noncancerous) and malignant (cancerous) ovarian cysts and tumors. In women with recurrent cancer or endometriosis (a condition in which parts of the uterine lining are displaced outside the uterus), physicians do oophorectomies intentionally to stop hormone production, which tends to aggravate the problem. Breast cancer, as well, may be dependent on hormones to grow; about one third of the women with breast cancer show a decrease in breast cancer growth after removal of their ovaries.

For a woman in her childbearing years, doctors make every effort to save any healthy ovarian tissue. Because the ovaries are fed by an excellent blood supply, they heal quickly and even a small bit of preserved ovarian tissue will function, secrete hormones, and discharge eggs. The woman remains fertile and avoids an early menopause.

Oophorectomy with hysterectomy

Some physicians recommend a bilateral oophorectomy when the

uterus must be taken out. There are pros and cons to removing healthy ovaries. Arguments for their removal are: it eliminates the possibility of ovarian cancer, since the hysterectomy may interfere with blood supply to the ovaries; a small number of women will develop cystic ovaries and pain, requiring a second operation anyway; and, if a woman is in her 40s, the ovaries will naturally stop functioning within a few years. Arguments against a routine oophorectomy are: it causes the onset of premature menopause, which brings with it greater risks of high blood pressure and osteoporosis (loss of bone mass); the abrupt loss of hormone production is less natural than the gradual tapering off of a natural menopause, provoking severe menopausal symptoms, such as hot flashes and vaginal shrinkage; and estrogen, the hormone usually prescribed after a bilateral oophorectomy, may increase the risk of breast cancer.

In women past menopause, for whom fertility is no longer an issue and in whom the ovaries are no longer producing estrogen anyway, both ovaries and uterus are commonly removed even if only one ovary is abnormal.

Ovarian cysts

Ovarian cysts are abnormal swellings or sac-like growths on an ovary, either one of the two female sex glands that produce eggs and female sex hormones. Ovarian cysts may be liquid-filled or semi-fluid.

Most cysts are small but can vary in size from less than an inch in diameter to as big as 15 to 20 inches in diameter and, depending on their size, type, and location, can be symptom-free or can cause severe pain and complications. They are common among women between the ages of 20 and 50 and can grow alone or in groups, on one ovary or both. Approximately 85 percent are benign (noncancerous).

Causes

The origin of most ovarian cysts is unknown. In some instances, they develop from an abnormal egg. Others originate as eggs that stay in the ovary instead of leaving after they ripen. Still others are related to abnormalities in the ovary.

Types

Polycystic ovaries (the Stein-Leventhal syndrome) are ovaries in which the eggs are never released after they mature. Multiple small cysts within both ovaries are seen in this condition. Excessive and abnormal body hair growth and the development of acne may result from hormonal imbalances caused by polycystic ovaries. Women with endometriosis (uterine tissue that grows outside the uterus) tend to develop growths on the ovaries. Dermoid cysts are commonly found in women under the age of 30; they arise from the ovarian cells that produce the eggs, and the cysts may contain fragments of hair, teeth, bone, and sweat and oil glands.

Symptoms

Symptoms of ovarian cysts vary with the type of growth. Some bear no symptoms and are only discovered during a routine pelvic examination. Others cause firm, painless swelling in the lower abdomen; pain during sexual intercourse; frequent urination (if they press against the bladder); irregular vaginal bleeding; an increase in body hair (if they affect the hormone-producing capabilities of the ovaries); or pain, nausea, and fever (if the cysts rupture or grow on stalks that get twisted).

Cysts can rupture during sexual intercourse, a fall, childbirth, surgery, or for no apparent reason. The resulting effect depends upon how irritating the cystic fluid is to the surrounding tissues, which immediately emit a fibrous material, or adhesions, to defend themselves against the contents of the cyst. The situation can be dangerous if the fluid is infected, cancerous, or extremely irritating.

Diagnosis

Ovarian cysts are diagnosed by pelvic, or vaginal, examination or laparoscopy (a surgical procedure in which a telescopic-like instrument is inserted through the abdominal wall to view the pelvic organs). Sometimes they are difficult to diagnose accurately because symptoms can resemble acute appendicitis or other abdominal problems. In addition, it can be hard to determine if a cyst is malignant or not and if it is actually on the ovary or some other pelvic organ. Ovarian cysts that develop during pregnancy are also difficult to diagnose.

Treatment

Some cysts require no treatment if they are small, not creating any problems, or are likely to disappear on their own. If treatment is necessary, cysts may be drained with a laparoscope, but most are removed surgically. Removal involves either taking out the entire ovary (oophorectomy) or taking out only the cyst (cystectomy).

If the ovarian cyst proves to be cancerous, it is necessary to remove both ovaries, both fallopian tubes, and the uterus since the cancer may have spread from the ovarian cyst to these other structures. If an ovarian cyst is found in a woman after menopause, it must always be removed since these cysts often prove to be cancerous. Removal of both ovaries, both tubes, and the uterus is also performed in this case.

Ovulation

Ovulation is the process in which an ovary—one of two glands near the top of the uterus that secrete female sex hormones—releases an egg. The egg develops in a small

During ovulation the ovary releases the ripe egg, which moves up the fallopian tube toward the uterus.

fluid-filled sac called a follicle. When ovulation occurs, this sac ruptures, releasing an egg from the ovary.

Extending from either side of the uterus are the fallopian tubes, which are four to five inches long with finger-like projections at their ends. When the ovary releases an egg, the projections on the nearby tube sweep the egg into the tube where it slowly inches toward the uterus.

If during that time, the egg is fertilized by a sperm, the male reproductive cell, it moves to the uterus and implants itself into the rich uterine lining where it grows for the next nine months. If the egg does not become fertilized, the uterine lining breaks down and passes, along with the unfertilized egg, out of the cervix (neck of the uterus) on through the vagina and out of the body. This discharge is known as menstruation.

Ovulation is regulated by a complex system of hormonal and chemical secretions from the ovaries, the hypothalamus (part of the brain), and the adjacent pituitary gland (the master gland controlling most hormone secretions).

Young women start ovulating — and menstruating — during puberty, which occurs between the ages of nine and 14, and normally do so every month (except while pregnant) until they reach menopause around age 50 or so. Some women feel cramps in the lower abdomen during ovulation. The only other ways to recognize when ovulation is happening are to take body temperature before rising in the morning with a special thermometer or to count 14 days from the first day of the last menstruation in an average 28-day cycle. However, the length of the menstrual cycle can vary. Sperm that has been ejaculated inside a woman's vagina as long as two to three days before the release of the ripe egg can still fertilize it. Therefore, there is an almost seven- to ten-day period during which a woman can become pregnant during each cycle.

Pelvic inflammatory disease

Pelvic inflammatory disease (PID), or salpingitis, is an infection of a woman's fallopian tubes, two four- to five-inch long ducts that conduct egg cells from the ovaries to the uterus. Although the term is widely used to refer to infections of all the parts of the pelvic cavity above the vagina, PID is properly restricted to the fallopian tubes.

Causes

The causes of PID are not always fully known, but it is usually caused by certain bacteria transmitted during sexual intercourse, an intrauterine device (IUD) that has become infected, or certain vaginal infections. One of the commonest agents causing PID is gonorrhea, a widespread sexually transmitted disease.

It is suspected that a woman is more vulnerable to PID if her cervical canal (the opening from the vagina into the uterus) has been dilated at some point by either recent surgery or recent childbirth or miscarriage. Under normal circumstances, the cervix prevents bacteria from the vagina from entering the uterus.

Symptoms

PID symptoms include severe pain and tenderness in the lower abdomen, fever, a foul-smelling vaginal discharge, early menstrual bleeding, pain during sexual intercourse, nausea, vomiting, fatigue, and pain during urination or defecation.

Complications

If it is not diagnosed early, the infection can cause abscesses (pus-filled cavities) to form in the fallopian tubes or around the ovaries (the female sex glands, which secrete female sex hormones and discharge eggs). PID can also damage and irreversibly scar pelvic tissue and, if the tubes are blocked, PID can prevent conception. The infection can also result in bacteria entering the bloodstream and spreading to other parts of the body and in peritonitis (inflammation of the membrane lining the pelvic and abdominal cavities).

Diagnosis

It is important to seek medical attention as soon as symptoms occur so the infection can be treated before it worsens and spreads. The physician will take a sample of fluid from the cervix to identify the infecting organism.

Treatment

The doctor will prescribe antibiotics to fight the infection and aspirin or other painkillers for pain relief. The woman may be advised to rest in bed, abstain from sexual intercourse, and apply heat to the lower abdominal area. These measures generally succeed in curing the infection; if not, the woman may have to enter the hospital to receive antibiotics intravenously (in the vein). In some cases, a laparoscopy (a view of the internal organs through a special tube) or possibly surgery to drain blocked tubes or abscessed tissue may be required. Sometimes, the damage is too extensive and the fallopian tubes, the uterus, and the ovaries may have to be removed. This will cure the infection; however, conception will then be impossible.

Prevention

A woman can minimize her chances of contracting PID by taking precautions any time her cervix is dilated; for example, by avoiding tampons, sexual intercourse, douches, and tub baths for at least several weeks after childbirth, an abortion, D and C (dilatation and curettage, surgical scraping of the interior lining of the uterus), or miscarriage. She should check with her doctor regarding when these activities may be resumed. Also, if a woman suspects she may have gonorrhea, she should have this treated before PID develops.

Premenstrual tension

Menstruation is the process in which the endometrium, or inner lining of the uterus, sloughs off the buildup of tissues triggered each month by hormonal releases to prepare the womb for the fertilized egg cell. If the egg is not fertilized, menstruation, in the form of a slow, bloody discharge over four or five days, ensues. Premenstrual tension is the nervousness, irritability, and bloating experienced by some women during the week before their menstrual period begins. In the past, this and other menstrual problems were thought to be caused by emotional instability or hysteria, but modern research has shown that there are physical reasons for menstrual disorders.

Cause

Premenstrual tension is thought to be caused by fluctuations in the production of female hormones in the course of the menstrual cycle. These hormonal changes apparently increase the amounts of salt and fluid retained in the body (called edema) during the week before the period begins. Neither the exact cause for this fluid and salt retention nor the reason for its effect on certain women is fully understood.

Symptoms

The symptoms of premenstrual tension appear during the week preceding menstruation and usually disappear as soon as the menstrual flow begins. In addition to nervousness and irritability, this disorder is characterized by a bloated or puffy feeling that results from fluid retention. Other symptoms include depression, headache, fatigue, tenderness in the breasts, and acne.

Treatment

Premenstrual tension is often treated by reducing salt intake or taking medications (called diuretics) which help to eliminate excess fluid from the tissues. Tranquilizers as well as psychological counseling may be recommended for cases in which emotional problems are an underlying cause. A balanced diet, moderate exercise, and adequate rest may also be beneficial in treating the condition.

Prevention

A reduction of salt intake in general may also help to prevent the initial edema that may often accompany premenstrual tension.

Prolapse

Prolapse involves the collapse, falling, or change in position of tissue or an organ so that it turns outward, falls down, or reverses its position in reference to surrounding tissue. Prolapse is caused by injury, disease (with internal swelling), parasitic infestation (such as worms), or other inflammation.

Prolapse of the uterus may be one of three types, depending on severity: (1) first degree prolapse, in which the uterus sags downward to cause the cervix (the womb's opening) to fall to a point where it is flush with the entrance to the vagina; (2) second degree prolapse, in which the cervix is outside the vagina; and (3) third degree prolapse, in which the entire uterus is outside the vagina.

Treatment

If the prolapse is the result of injury or stress, a surgical repair may be indicated, in which the prolapsed organ is returned to its proper place and sewn or stapled into position. If the prolapse is the result of disease or swelling, the cause of the prolapse must first be controlled and then eliminated. Afterward, the organ or tissue is returned to its original position and secured there. A prolapsed uterus can make future childbirth difficult and may damage other organs.

Rectocele

Rectocele is a condition in which a portion of the rectum, the tubular-shaped organ at the end of the intestinal tract, protrudes into the vagina.

In this second degree prolapse of the uterus, the organ has fallen to a point where the cervix is outside the vagina.

Cause

The usual cause of this condition is a weakening of the back wall of the vagina due to the stretching caused by childbirth.

Symptoms

A minimal protrusion may produce no symptoms or a mild pressure sensation during bowel movements. More severe protrusion of the rectum may lead to chronic constipation and painful bowel movements.

Diagnosis

A rectocele is easily diagnosed by the doctor during a pelvic examination. After straining or coughing, the rectum may be seen bulging into the vagina.

Treatment

Rectocele is not a dangerous condition and generally requires no treatment. If severe constipation or painful bowel movements develop, surgical repair is often curative. Mild symptoms may be relieved by avoiding straining and heavy lifting and by drugs and diet that will ensure a soft bowel movement.

Toxic shock syndrome

Toxic shock syndrome (TSS) is a rare, sometimes fatal disease that develops very suddenly and progresses rapidly when the *Staphylococcus aureus* bacterium enters the bloodstream. TSS was first defined in 1975, when its link to the use of tampons was suspected. Since then, almost 90 percent of all reported cases have occurred in menstruating women under the age of 30 who use tampons. About three in 100,000 menstruating women have contracted toxic shock syndrome. Five to 15 percent of these cases have been fatal.

Toxic shock syndrome occurs when the bacterium enters the bloodstream and produces a toxin (poison) that causes leaks in cell walls allowing blood to seep into the tissues. This results in a sudden, very dangerous drop in blood pressure, shock, and sometimes death.

In serious cases, the low blood pressure and the weakened cell walls (which allow foreign bodies to enter) can leave the victim susceptible to further complications, such as heart and liver damage. Often the body does not produce enough antibodies (protective substances) to fight off this invasion, so TSS can easily reoccur.

Causes

This disorder is caused by a toxin which is produced by a bacterium, but the identity of this toxin and why it is produced in certain cases remain a mystery. Moreover, the bacterium can be present in the body without producing the toxin.

The exact link between toxic shock syndrome and the use of tampons also remains somewhat vague. Although their use is considered to be a definite risk factor, tampons do not actually cause the disease, but they may promote the growth of bacteria that leads to it.

Researchers now theorize that the new "superabsorbent" tampons as well as tampon applicators may be responsible for triggering TSS. The superabsorbent tampons may swell so much that they entirely fill the vagina, totally blocking the elimination of blood and creating a breeding ground for infection; also, these tampons tend to be left in the vagina hours longer than the less absorbent varieties, again increasing the chances for infection. Tampon applicators, moreover, may accidentally scratch the walls of the vagina, allowing bacteria to enter.

However, since 10 percent of all cases occur in men and nonmenstruating women, the bacteria can apparently enter the body in ways other than through the vagina. Toxic shock in these cases often occurs when the body has been weakened by major surgery, severe burns, or cases of boils or abscesses. Also, women who have recently given birth are at a higher risk of developing TSS because the vagina (or birth canal) is more susceptible to the invasion of bacteria at this time.

Symptoms

The symptoms of toxic shock syndrome are high fever, vomiting, diarrhea, a rash that looks like sunburn, peeling of skin on the soles and palms, blurred vision, and disorientation.

Treatment

Immediate emergency medical treatment should be sought by anyone noticing the symptoms of TSS. This will almost certainly mean hospitalization, during which the patient will be given therapy similar to that administered to poison victims. Fluids or whole blood transfusions are given to raise blood pressure, an ice blanket is used to reduce fever, and antibiotics are administered to fight the infection.

Precaution

The best precaution that can be taken to prevent toxic shock syndrome is probably to discontinue or limit the use of tampons, especially the superabsorbent variety. Tampons can still be safely worn, but they should be changed every three to four hours and alternated with sanitary napkins as often as possible, especially before going to bed, as they tend to remain

inserted for much longer periods of time during sleep.

Vaginitis

Vaginitis is any one of a number of bacterial or fungal infections and inflammations of the vagina (the female passageway from the uterus to the outside of the body), usually marked by burning and itching of the external genital organs. A discharge may or may not be present.

An untreated infection can become chronic (recurring) or can lead to a urinary tract infection. Pregnant women, as well as those who have diabetes or gonorrhea (a sexually transmitted disease), are at a higher risk of developing vaginitis.

Vaginal infections can be transmitted to male sexual partners, but usually with no serious results. However, vaginitis is not considered a sexually transmitted disease, since it is not contracted or transmitted only by direct sexual contact.

Causes

Vaginitis is caused by an imbalance of the microorganisms normally present in the vagina, resulting when some outside factor causes one of the strains to reproduce more quickly than the others. Possible causes include birth control pills, which, because of their high estrogen (a female hormone) content, cause the vaginal lining to change in such a way that it is more likely to nourish microorganisms that cause infection; certain antibiotics, which may kill bacteria that normally help to maintain the microorganism balance in the vagina; a warm, moist, environment, often caused by tight pants or pantyhose, nylon underwear, or a wet bathing suit, which creates a breeding ground for infection; and the chemical irritation arising from the excessive use of douches, feminine hygiene sprays, bubble baths, talcum powder, and scented or colored toilet paper.

Vaginitis tends to occur more often in the summer, because excessive heat and moisture are known to trigger the disease.

One variety of the disease, called nonspecific, noninfectious vaginitis, is not caused by this overproduction of microorganisms, but rather by an irritation from some outside source. However, vaginitis is most commonly caused by one of three microorganisms: *Candida albicans*, or monilia (a fungus); *Hemophilus vaginalis* (a bacterium); or *Trichomonas vaginalis* (a protozoan, or one-celled organism). Each type displays a slightly different set of symptoms and requires a specific method of treatment.

Symptoms

The fungus *Candida albicans*, or monilia, results in severe itching of the external genital organs and pain during intercourse. A thick, white discharge from the vagina, resembling cottage cheese in texture and having a "yeasty" odor, is the reason why this condition is more commonly known as a yeast infection. This is the variety of vaginitis most frequently contracted by diabetic and pregnant women.

The bacterium *Hemophilus vaginalis* causes a creamy white or grayish, foul-smelling discharge. The presence of *Trichomonas vaginalis,* also accompanied by itching and burning as well as a greenish-white discharge and foul odor, is more likely to appear during or immediately following menstruation.

Noninfectious, nonspecific vaginitis is characterized only by irritation and dryness, usually with no discharge.

Men can be infected by the bacterium or protozoan varieties during sexual contact, but they usually display no symptoms.

Diagnosis

Vaginitis is diagnosed by determining which of the three microorganisms is causing the infection by examining a smear of vaginal discharge under a microscope.

Treatment

Treatment will vary somewhat according to the type of microorganism that has been causing the problem. Those infections caused by a fungus are treated with antifungal cream which is applied directly to the vagina.

Bacterial infections are treated with sulfa drugs or antibiotics, administered either orally or as vaginal suppositories (cones of medicine that are inserted into the vagina). Both partners are usually treated with oral antibiotics because bacterial infections can be transferred between the sexes.

An oral antibiotic called metronidazole is administered to women with protozoan infections and to their partners, as well; however, some studies have linked this drug to cancer and genetic damage in lab animals, so it should not be taken during the first half of pregnancy.

Nonspecific, noninfectious vaginitis is usually treated simply by removing or avoiding the irritants causing it, such as tight clothing, perfumed soaps, chemical sprays, or scented tissues.

Prevention

Some types of vaginitis can probably be prevented by using only nonscented, white toilet paper; wearing cotton underwear and loose-fitting pants; and avoiding the overuse of douches and feminine hygiene sprays.

PROBLEMS OF COUPLES

Certain disorders affect only a male or a female. Nevertheless, a couple can encounter health problems in three areas: birth control or contraception, infertility, and sexually transmitted or venereal diseases. Decisions or problems in all three areas affect both partners.

Although sex is a topic that arouses much curiosity and interest, it unfortunately is also surrounded by many myths and misconceptions that can lead to needless anxiety. But societal attitudes have been changing, and there is now more free and open discussion about subjects that used to be considered taboo.

The best approach to solving any difficulties takes two ingredients: an understanding by both persons involved in a relationship of how the male and female sexual and reproductive systems work, and a willingness to communicate openly and honestly.

Responsibility for these areas of health should not be shouldered by either the man or the woman alone. Both partners need to work together to weigh consequences, consider alternatives, and provide mutual support.

Birth control

Couples who want to delay or prevent pregnancy can choose from several different kinds of contraceptives: physical devices (intrauterine devices); barrier methods (condoms, diaphragms); chemical methods (spermicides, pills); a combination of physical and chemical methods (diaphragm with a spermicide); permanent birth control (vasectomy for males or blocking fallopian tubes for females); or abstinence during the woman's fertile period.

Some birth control methods require a doctor's prescription; others can be purchased over the counter. Methods vary in effectiveness, convenience, and safety. It's a good idea for a couple to discuss with a doctor the advantages and disadvantages of the various methods of birth control, especially side effects, ease of use, and reliability. Choose the birth control method that suits you best as a couple; what works well for one couple may not appeal to another.

Infertility

On the other hand, about one out of every five couples who want to conceive a child finds they are unsuccessful at doing so. If pregnancy does not occur after a year of regular sexual intercourse without contraceptives, the man and woman may want to consult with an obstetrician/gynecologist or a urologist who specializes in infertility.

During the last ten years or so, medical science has made tremendous inroads into diagnosing and treating causes of infertility and has thus given new hope to childless couples. Improved testing procedures, new drugs that stimulate ovulation, and surgical techniques that can correct female or male structural problems or sometimes successfully reverse sterilization procedures have enabled many couples to become parents.

Sexually transmitted diseases

One of the risks of intimate sexual contact, especially for men and women who have more than one partner, is infection with a sexually transmitted disease (STD), also called venereal disease (VD). These diseases are caused by organisms that thrive in the warm moist environment within the reproductive systems and are transmitted by sexual contact.

Despite improved diagnosis and treatment for these diseases, their incidence has increased, probably because of the sexual freedom of the last twenty years that has resulted from more reliable birth control. Factors that directly affect the increase include: declining contraceptive use of condoms, which offer some physical protection from infection; the likelihood of people having more than one sexual partner and infecting others before they themselves develop symptoms; and increased sexual activity among teens, who are less apt to recognize symptoms or who fear admitting the fact to a medical authority.

Gonorrhea is the most prevalent of the STDs, but herpes, syphilis, and nonspecific urethritis are common enough to be of concern to sexually active people. Although with the exception of herpes, these diseases can be cured, the consequences of delaying treatment of these diseases are too important to ignore. Permanent sterility can result.

STDs are serious matters for pregnant women. The diseases can be transmitted to a baby as he or she passes through the birth canal and can critically affect the child.

A person who does become infected with any of these diseases must abstain from further sexual contact until the problem is checked. Any sexual partner(s) must also be informed of the possibility of infection and seek treatment, whether or not they develop symptoms.

Each of these problems encountered and shared by couples are discussed in more detail in the following sections.

Birth control

Birth control, also called contraception, is the voluntary prevention of pregnancy. A variety of methods are available for preventing pregnancy. Couples who use no contraceptive have a 90 percent chance of achieving pregnancy over a 12-month period.

Natural family planning

Natural family planning is based on calculating when a women ovulates—that is, releases the egg from the ovary each month —and is most fertile. The couple then abstains from intercourse during the fertile period.

The male's sperm can live in the female's body for about two days before fertilizing an egg. The egg can live for about 24 hours after ovulation. A day or two is added to this fertile period for safety's sake because it is so difficult to determine just when ovulation occurs. All told, a couple needs to abstain from intercourse seven to ten days a month in order to prevent pregnancy.

There are three methods a woman can use to determine when she ovulates. The temperature method is one of the most reliable. Each morning upon awakening and before getting out of bed, you take your temperature with a special basal temperature thermometer (which only measures temperatures between 96 and 100 degrees Fahrenheit) and record it on graph paper. At the end of a menstrual cycle, you will note that your temperature dropped suddenly on one day followed by a rapid climb for the next three days. The sudden drop in temperature indicates that you are about to ovulate. After ovulation your temperature rises quickly for three days and does not return to pre-ovulation levels until the beginning of the menstrual period. The safe days to have intercourse are from four days after the sudden drop in temperature until three or four days

No mucus several days after period

Thick, sticky mucus for several days

Slippery, stringy mucus indicating ovulation is occurring

Thick, sticky mucus or no mucus after ovulation

Mucus from the cervix (neck of uterus) undergoes changes as hormone levels vary during the menstrual cycle. Testing the mucus between thumb and forefinger indicates the changes shown here.

after the end of your period. It is important to become familiar with your cycle by recording your temperature levels for several months before relying on this method of birth control.

The mucus method may also help determine when you ovulate. Each morning you examine the mucus from the vagina and cervix. Cervical mucus undergoes changes as hormone levels vary during the course of the cycle. To determine these changes, you can blot the vaginal area each morning with a facial tissue and then test the mucus between your thumb and forefinger. You are watching for the following changes. After your period you will have several days with no mucus. This is followed by several days of a yellow or white thick, sticky discharge. There will then be one or two days when the mucus becomes transparent and very *slippery* with the consistency of raw egg whites. The mucus will form a string between the thumb and forefinger. This is when ovulation occurs. After ovulation the mucus again becomes thick and sticky or there may be no mucus at all. The fertile period begins with the yellow/white thick, sticky discharge and continues until about three days after the phase when the mucus is slippery with the consistency of egg whites. You should avoid intercourse during this time. In other words, the safe period is from three days after the slippery mucus stage to about three days after the end of the menstrual period.

The calendar method is also an option. You keep a record of your menstrual cycles for one year or more. You and your doctor then use the record to work out the probable day of ovulation, based on the fact that the average woman menstruates 14 days after she ovulates. However, any individual woman may vary from that average, so the calendar method is not precise.

Natural family planning is entirely natural and does not require the use of mechanical aids or drugs. The effectiveness rate for this kind of birth control is up to about 75 to 80 percent, depending on the care with which the techniques are followed. However, even in women with regular cycles, illness, fatigue, stress, or even a vacation can delay ovulation and throw off all careful calculations.

Spermicides

The spermicide is a chemical foam, cream, suppository, or jelly applied to the woman's vagina to kill sperm. Used alone, a spermicide is about 75 to 85 percent effective when used correctly. Some disadvantages of a spermicide are that it must be applied before each separate act of intercourse, it has chemical odors, and it may irritate the vagina. A chief advantage is that spermicides are readily available at every drugstore without a prescription.

Diaphragm

The diaphragm is a molded rubber cap that the woman places inside the vagina to cover the cervix, the opening of the lower end of the uterus that projects into the vagina. The cap blocks the sperm, preventing them from entering the uterus. Diaphragms come in different sizes and must be fitted by a physician. Used alone, the dia-

The diaphragm is a molded rubber cap that a woman places inside the vagina to cover the cervix, the opening of the lower end of the uterus. The diaphragm blocks the sperm, preventing them from entering the uterus.

phragm may occasionally fail, because it may not be inserted correctly or may shift slightly during intercourse. Used with spermicides, however, diaphragms are quite effective, with only about a 3 to 5 percent chance of pregnancy.

Condom

The condom, or "rubber," is a thin rubber or synthetic sheath that the man fits over his penis just before intercourse. A condom used alone is about 70 to 90 percent effective, depending on the care with which it is used. Several problems may occur with the use of the condom. For example, tiny holes or tears may develop in the sheath causing leakage of sperm.

Also, when the penis withdraws from the vagina as intercourse is completed, the condom sometimes breaks or unrolls partially inside the vagina — releasing its contents. However, a condom used regularly with a spermicide is approximately 95 percent effective in preventing pregnancy. Condoms have the great advantage of being readily available in any drugstore without a prescription. They also have the theoretical advantage of preventing the spread of venereal disease.

IUD

The intrauterine device (IUD) is a small plastic device inserted into the woman's uterus by a

The IUD, available in several shapes, is a small plastic device inserted into a woman's uterus by a doctor. It is thought that the IUD prevents pregnancy by causing changes in the lining of the uterus that disrupt the normal environment of the egg.

physician. It is available in a variety of shapes. The IUD has a string attached to it that hangs into the cervix, so the woman or her partner can check to be sure the IUD is still in place. The IUD apparently prevents pregnancy by causing changes in the uterine lining that disrupt the normal environment of an egg. For the woman who can use an IUD, the advantages are great, as she does not have to worry about contraception each day. The effectiveness rate is high, with only about a 5 percent chance of pregnancy.

However, severe menstrual cramps and increased menstrual bleeding may follow the insertion of an IUD. Sometimes these side effects lessen after a month or two. In other cases, severe cramps and prolonged bleeding continue, and the physician may advise removal

of the IUD. The IUD is also thought to increase the probability of pelvic infections and ectopic (outside the uterus) pregnancies.

Oral contraceptives

Oral contraceptives, or birth control pills, are the most effective reversible method of contraception. A woman taking the pill has less than a 1 percent chance of getting pregnant.

The pill — which is available by prescription only — uses synthetic female hormones, estrogen and progestin, to override the natural hormonal regulation that results in the release of an egg. The pill signals the pituitary gland, which directs hormonal activity in the body, not to release the hormones that would normally stimulate the ovary to release an egg.

Each day you take one pill, at about the same time of day, removing it from a container that has the required number of pills for one cycle — usually 21. From one to three days after you take the last pill for that cycle, your menstrual period begins. Menstrual periods may be lighter in flow, and cramps are reduced or absent.

If you forget to take one pill or more, menstrual bleeding may begin. In that case, you should continue taking the pills daily, but you should also use an additional contraceptive method, such as a condom, until after your next regular period.

Birth control pills are not recommended for women with a history of high blood pressure, of blood-clotting problems, of hepatitis, or of any cancer of the uterus or breast. A woman over age 35 who smokes heavily is advised to stop smoking if she wants to take the pill. Birth control pills should not be taken by a woman who suspects she may be pregnant. In addition, women with diabetes, epilepsy, heart disease, and thyroid disease may be advised not to take the birth control pill, depending on the nature and severity of the disease.

It is important for a woman on the birth control pill to report to her doctor if any of the following symptoms occur: severe headache, blurred vision, severe chest pain, sudden shortness of breath, and pain and swelling of the legs.

Contraceptive sponge

The contraceptive sponge is a disposable sponge-like device saturated with spermicide. A woman inserts the sponge into the vagina up against the cervix where the device works by continuously releasing spermicide for up to 24 hours. Additional applications of spermicide are not necessary, even for multiple acts of intercourse. There are other advantages as well: the sponge is available as an over-the-counter contraceptive that does not need a prescription; unlike a diaphragm, the sponge does not have to be fitted; and the sponge can be inserted ahead of time, which allows greater spontaneity in sex. The sponge has been found to be about 85 percent effective.

Because the contraceptive sponge is a relatively new product, some doctors think that more needs to be known about side effects. So far there have been a few cases of a local irritation or an allergic reaction; however, these have been mild and infrequent. There is also concern that the sponge could become a breeding ground for infection, especially if used improperly. You should consult your doctor about the sponge and its proper use before trying this method of birth control.

Sterilization

A woman may be sterilized by an operation that blocks the fallopian tubes that carry eggs from the ovaries to the uterus. A man may be sterilized by a procedure called a vasectomy, in which each vas deferens, the duct that carries the sperm from the testis, is cut. These procedures may be reversed, but

Vasectomy is a method of male sterilization in which each vas deferens, the duct that conducts the sperm from the testis, is cut.

only by complicated surgery that is not always successful. Therefore, physicians recommend sterilization only when the couple has decided without reservation that no further pregnancies are desired.

Genital warts

Genital warts (condylomata acuminata) is considered to be a sexually transmitted disease (a venereal disease—a highly contagious illness that is spread primarily through direct sexual contact). These growths are caused by a virus and appear on the external genital organs.

If left untreated, genital warts can grow quite large, causing discomfort during sexual intercourse, urination, and bowel movements. They are seen more frequently in uncircumcised men than in those who have been circumcised.

In women, pregnancy may make genital warts grow faster, but they usually shrink after the baby is born. They may even become large enough during pregnancy to block the birth canal, making a cesarean delivery necessary. The wart virus can also be transmitted from a mother to her child during birth, but there is no evidence that it causes any serious complications in infants, as do some other sexually transmitted diseases.

Cause

Genital warts are caused by direct sexual contact with an infected person. About 60 percent of all those exposed to them will develop the disease. However, the warts will not appear until six weeks to eight months after the initial exposure.

Symptoms

The only symptom of genital warts are the warts themselves, appearing most frequently on the penis, vagina, anus (opening from the rectum to the outside), and, less commonly, in the mouth or on the cervix (neck of the uterus). They are soft, moist, and pink, appearing alone or in clusters; cluster formations tend to resemble cauliflower in their uneven, puffy appearance. They are seldom painful, but they can be irritated by sexual intercourse; in fact, they often grow on parts of the sex organs that receive the most friction during sexual intercourse.

Diagnosis

Genital warts can usually be diagnosed by a simple physical examination because their appearance is so distinct. If there is any doubt, a sample of tissue from the wart can be tested to rule out other disorders such as cancerous growths or the swelling that often accompanies syphilis, another sexually transmitted disease.

Treatment

Genital warts are treated with a drug called podophyllin, applied directly to the warts, then washed off several hours later. More than one application may be necessary. Podophyllin is toxic in large quantities, however, so very large or troublesome warts are often removed by cryotherapy (a process in which liquid nitrogen freezes the growths off) or by heat treatments which dry out and destroy the warts.

A person who has developed genital warts or any other sexually transmitted disease should abstain from sexual activity until all tests have indicated that the disease is no longer present. A case of genital warts, as well as all sexually transmitted diseases, requires that every sexual partner of the infected person also be examined and treated, if necessary.

Prevention

Genital warts can be prevented, obviously, by avoiding sexual contact with someone who has the disease. However, since this cannot always be possible, it should be remembered that the chances of contracting these diseases increase with the number of different sexual partners a person has; therefore, limiting the number of partners can be beneficial in decreasing the chances of developing this disease.

Infertility

Infertility is defined as a couple's

Blockage in vas deferens
which carries sperm
from testis to penis

Penis

Testis
where sperm
is produced

Male infertility can be caused by a blockage anywhere in the tubes that convey sperm from the testes to the penis.

failure to conceive a child after one year of regular sexual intercourse without birth control. In about 40 percent of all cases of infertility, the problem lies with the male; in 60 percent it lies with the female or with both partners.

Infertility is not sterility. The term infertility implies that the condition can be treated and reversed, that it may be a temporary problem; the term sterility is applied to a permanent, irreversible inability to have children.

Recent research has shown that a woman's fertility drops off significantly between the ages of 31 and 35 and continues to decline thereafter until menopause, when it ceases. A man's fertility also declines after the age of 40,

although men can remain fertile until old age.

Causes of male infertility

One of the major causes of male infertility is a low sperm count. It is measured by the number of active sperm present in a milliliter (less than one-half teaspoon) of semen (the fluid ejected from the penis during intercourse). An average "sperm count" is 90 million sperm per milliliter; a count of 40 to 60 million is thought to be necessary for conception; when the count is less than 20 million, it is highly unlikely that the man can father a child, although since only one sperm is needed to fertilize the female egg, it is still possible.

A low sperm count can be caused by low levels of testosterone, the male sex hormone; by exposure to chemicals, pesticides, and radiation; by very frequent sexual intercourse, which depletes the sperm supply too quickly; and by heat (which slows sperm production) generated by wearing tight underwear or pants, sitting for long periods in hot cars or trucks, or working near ovens and kilns.

Infertility can also result if sperm cannot propel themselves through the female reproductive tract to reach the egg, or if sperm are irregularly shaped (only sperm with oval-shaped heads can fertilize an egg).

In addition to problems with the sperm themselves, male infertility can be caused by any obstruction in the tubes that convey the sperm from the testes to the penis. Infertility may also be caused by varicose veins in the scrotum (the pouch containing the testes), perhaps because the increased blood flow in these swollen veins brings extra heat to the area; or by a local infection or injury, although the infertility problem will probably reverse itself when the condition is corrected. In addition, surgical removal of part of the prostate gland, as well as the use of certain drugs for high blood pressure, can lead to retrograde ejaculation (a disorder in which the semen is passed backwards into the bladder, to exit with the urine, rather than out through the penis during ejaculation).

Causes of female infertility

A woman may be infertile because of a variety of conditions. It may be that she is not ovulating (releasing an egg each month); this is true in about 25 percent of all infertility cases. The fallopian tubes (through which the egg travels on its way from the ovary to the uterus) may be obstructed, often as a result of pelvic inflammatory disease (PID), which inflames the tubes and causes scar tissue to form. PID, in turn, can develop as a reaction to an IUD (intrauterine device used for birth control), a sexually transmitted disease, a ruptured appendix, or an infection of the lower reproductive tract. Endometriosis (the displacement of tissue from the lining of the uterus to outside the uterus) may also cause scar tissue to form that blocks the fallopian tubes. In addition, an imbalance of the female hormones estrogen and progesterone or of other hormones secreted from the pituitary or thyroid glands can interfere with the reproductive cycle. A weakness in the cervix (the neck of the uterus), sometimes resulting from a previous abortion or surgery, may render it unfit to hold the weight of a pregnancy; or a "hostile" cervix, one which creates an environment that in some way prevents sperm from surviving, may be the cause of the infertility.

Symptoms

The major "symptom" of infertility is the failure to conceive a

Female infertility can be caused by an obstruction in the fallopian tube through which the egg passes from the ovary to the uterus and in which the sperm and egg are united at conception.

child after regular sexual intercourse for a year. Other "symptoms" would depend on the cause of the infertility.

Diagnosis

Diagnosis of the reason for the infertility problem will usually begin with physical exams and complete medical and sexual (and, in the woman's case, menstrual) histories of both partners.

A fresh sample of the male's sperm will be examined under a microscope to determine the quantity and quality of the sperm. This will provide a sperm count and will also determine whether the sperm are adequately mobile which are necessary for conception.

To determine whether ovula-

tion is taking place in the female, the basal body temperature (the body temperature upon awakening, before eating or drinking) will be taken every morning for several months. If the temperature rises by 6/10 to 1 degree for a few days in the middle of the menstrual cycle, ovulation is probably taking place. An endometrial biopsy, a sample of the lining of the uterus, can also indicate whether or not ovulation is occurring.

Obstruction of the fallopian tubes can be diagnosed by injecting a dye into the reproductive tract and then taking an X ray. Another test consists of injecting carbon dioxide gas into the fallopian tubes and waiting for the patient to feel pain in the upper part of the body, indicating that the gas is passing through the fallopian tubes and that there are no obstructions.

A weakness in the cervix can be diagnosed through a physical exam and X rays; a hostile cervix can be identified by a microscopic examination of the mucus in the cervix shortly after sexual intercourse to determine the rate of sperm survival. Endometriosis is diagnosed by inserting a small, lighted instrument into the abdomen (called a laparoscope) through which the doctor can actually see the uterus, fallopian tubes, ovaries, and any displaced endometrial tissue that may be causing the infertility. Hormone imbalances in both men and women are diagnosed with blood tests.

Treatment

Treatment for a low sperm count caused by a testosterone deficiency usually consists of hormone therapy to increase testosterone levels. If the low sperm count is due to chemicals, radiation, or excess heat, these conditions need to be corrected or avoided. If the sperm count is low for some unknown reason, there is often little more that can be done.

If male infertility is caused by varicose veins, surgery may be necessary; if an obstruction exists somewhere in the tubes leading to and through the penis, microsurgery to open the blockage may correct this problem.

In females, failure to ovulate is often treated with a fertility drug called clomiphene to stimulate hormone production that regulates ovulation. About 60 percent of these patients become pregnant, and the chances of multiple births are very low. A stronger drug, which is a combination of certain pituitary gland hormones, may also be prescribed, but it carries with it a greater risk of multiple births.

Obstructed fallopian tubes may require microsurgery to open the blockage, or a new procedure in which an egg is removed and replaced beyond the point of the obstruction, where it waits to be fertilized normally. A hostile cervix can be treated with the female hormone estrogen, which stimulates the production of increased mucus necessary to transport the sperm. Sometimes sperm can be placed directly into the uterus, bypassing the cervix completely. Endometriosis can be treated with the surgical removal of displaced tissue and the scar tissue that has formed around it. Hormone imbalances can be corrected with hormone drug therapy.

Test-tube, or in vitro, fertilization is a new technique in which an egg is removed from the woman's ovary and is then placed in a test tube or special sterile dish containing the husband's sperm. Once the egg has been fertilized, it is then placed into the woman's uterus where it will continue to grow. This technique is primarily used in women whose blocked fallopian tubes cannot be opened by surgery.

Although recent advances in treating infertility have led to greater and greater success, about 15 percent of all female infertility problems and about 10 percent of all male problems remain undiagnosed and therefore untreatable.

Nongonococcal urethritis

Nongonococcal urethritis (NGU), also known as nonspecific urethritis, is a sexually transmitted disease that causes an inflammation of the urethra. A sexually transmitted disease, also known as venereal disease, is a highly contagious illness spread primarily through direct sexual contact.

Complications

NGU, left untreated, can lead to arthritis, prostatitis (inflammation of the prostate), and epididymitis (inflammation of the ducts leading from the testes) in men, and pelvic inflammatory disease (an inflammation of the fallopian tubes) in women. It can be transmitted from a mother to her baby during childbirth, resulting in ear infections and pneumonia; it has also been linked to an increased risk of stillbirths and sudden infant death syndrome.

Cause

NGU is transmitted by direct sexual contact with an infected person. It displays symptoms similar to gonorrhea, although it is not caused by the gonorrhea bacterium but by several others.

Symptoms

Sometimes no symptoms are evident when NGU is present; in other cases there is a discharge from the penis or vagina, painful and burning urination, and other symptoms similar to those of gonorrhea. In fact, NGU can occur at the same time that gonorrhea is present.

Diagnosis

Diagnosis of NGU is often difficult because there is no one simple test for it; a sample of secretions from the penis or vagina may be taken to determine if chlamydia is present, but many labs do not do this test and those that do may charge a very high fee. Therefore, NGU is often diagnosed by ruling out other disorders that may display similar symptoms.

Treatment

Penicillin has no effect on NGU, so this disease is treated with other antibiotics, such as tetracycline. This is the reason that treatment for gonorrhea, usually penicillin, will not affect NGU.

A person who has NGU or any other sexually transmitted disease should abstain from sexual activity until all tests have indicated that the disease is no longer present. It is necessary that every sexual partner of the infected person be examined and treated.

Prevention

NGU can be prevented by avoiding sexual contact with someone who has the disease. Since this is not always possible, it should be remembered that the chances of contracting NGU or any other sexually transmitted disease increase with the number of different sexual partners a person has.

PREGNANCY AND CHILDBIRTH

Pregnancy

Pregnancy is a condition in a female between the time one of her eggs is fertilized by a sperm (a male reproductive cell) and the time her child is born.

Conception

After the egg has been ejected from the surface of one of the ovaries (the organs in which eggs are formed), fertilization, also called conception, can occur in the fallopian tubes (two tubes linking the ovaries to the uterus, or womb). The fertilized egg (also called a zygote) travels down a fallopian tube into the uterus, where it attaches itself to the uterine wall. It remains there to grow and develop (it is called an embryo at an early stage; a fetus at a later stage of development) until birth (in most cases, nine months later).

Symptoms

Usually the first symptom noticed by a pregnant woman is a missed menstrual period. Nausea and vomiting ("morning sickness") are also common symptoms of pregnancy. During normal pregnancy, many changes take place in the mother's body. The abdomen stretches and the breasts enlarge, grow sensitive, and prepare to produce milk for the baby. Blood volume increases up to 30 percent; and breathing stems more from the chest and less from the abdomen, and the bladder pulls up higher into the abdomen (because of the increased abdominal space taken up by the growing fetus). The amount of blood flowing through the kidneys increases 25 to 40 percent (to eliminate wastes from both the mother and fetus). There is a slight increase in the acidity of the saliva (this may be one of the causes of the nausea and vomiting). In some cases, the skin may develop brown spots or splotches. A hormone called "relaxin" causes the bones of the pelvic area to widen during the tenth or twelfth week of pregnancy. Many of the mother's glands expand in size.

The nine months of pregnancy are usually thought of medically as three three-month periods or trimesters. During the first trimester, the woman may experience nausea and vomiting, her breasts and nipples will become enlarged, and her waistline may enlarge. In the second trimester, the uterus grows, abdominal

One month   Three months

enlargement becomes more apparent, and the woman can feel the fetus move. Many women feel their best during this trimester. During the last three months, the pregnancy tends to become a more cumbersome condition, and the woman may need more rest. The fetus often "drops" lower in the uterus in the last month.

Prenatal care

Most women wait until they have missed a second period before consulting their doctor. Once the doctor confirms the pregnancy, he or she will begin a program of prenatal (before birth) care. Prenatal care consists chiefly of making sure that nothing is wrong, in other words, that there are no complications. Good nutrition is important. The body's requirements for calcium and phosphorus, two essential minerals in food, almost doubles, and there is an increase in the demand for iron and many other elements. Gradual caloric increases are not only allowed but advisable, provided the additional food does not come from empty calories such as excess starches and sugars. Generally, if the woman was consuming 2,000 calories before pregnancy—with no weight gain—she

Six months   *Nine months*

should raise her intake to 2,200 or 2,400 calories in the early pregnancy period and she may be advised to increase that figure to 2,600 calories by the later stages. If the baby's weight is included, most women should gain approximately 23 to 26 extra pounds by the ninth month. This additional weight puts more stress on the back and on the legs, sometimes resulting in problems such as swayback or varicose veins (swollen veins close to the skin surface in the legs). These conditions can be eased by proper rest, exercise, and, for varicose veins, special hoisery.

Once the initial nausea and vomiting period is over (usually after two or three months), many women increase their calorie intake too much, sometimes in a mistaken attempt to "make up for what the baby is taking." As a consequence, they show drastic gains in weight, with all of the complications, such as swollen ankles, that such gains bring. At the other extreme are those mothers who cannot eat normally because the nausea symptoms persist throughout pregnancy. In each of these cases, both the mother and the fetus may suffer. If any sudden weight gain or loss is experienced, the physician should be informed.

Either through rapid weight

gain or inadequate kidney function, some women tend to swell significantly in the ankles and lower legs and, to a lesser extent, in the hands and fingers. Under no circumstances should non-prescription diuretics (drugs causing increased urinary output) be taken for this condition. The doctor should be consulted.

Proper rest and exercise are important throughout the pregnancy. In general, a woman can participate in most, if not all, of the activities and sports she was taking part in before her pregnancy. Her doctor can help advise her about any limitations.

Precautions

One of the most important aspects of prenatal care is safety in the use of medications. A pregnant woman, or one who even suspects she is pregnant, should never take a medication without her doctor's recommendation or approval. This caution includes over-the-counter preparations — even aspirin — as well as prescription drugs. In addition, a woman should not smoke during pregnancy, and she should limit, if not eliminate, alcoholic beverages. Smoking has been linked to miscarriage (the expulsion of the fetus before it is capable of surviving on its own), low birth weights, and prematurity. Alcohol, too, has been linked to miscarriage, and studies have shown that alcohol can affect the brain of the fetus. Products containing caffeine should also be limited. The best guideline to remember is that

no drug or substance can be assumed to be harmless during pregnancy.

It is important to remember that the womb may not protect the fetus as well as it was once thought. Many substances and organisms have been found to affect the development and survival of the developing fetus. It is estimated that 20 percent of all birth defects are directly related to environmental factors such as drugs, viruses, and vitamin deficiencies. Another 60 percent are caused by the interaction of an environmental factor and an inherited predisposition. So it is important for every woman who is contemplating pregnancy or is already pregnant to beware of the possible hazards to which her baby may be vulnerable.

The fetus is also susceptible to infections that affect the mother-to-be, especially rubella (German measles) and certain sexually transmitted diseases such as herpes. In addition, a pregnant woman should avoid immunizations with live viruses and postpone travel to foreign countries where infectious diseases are prevalent. Toxoplasmosis, an infection spread by eating or preparing uncooked meat or handling a cat's litterbox, presents another risk. The parasite that causes toxoplasmosis is harbored in the bodies of some food animals (pigs, sheep, and cattle) and in the intestinal tract of cats. You need not forgo meat nor get rid of your cat. You simply must be certain to cook meat thoroughly and to avoid emptying or cleaning your cat's litterbox. A woman's doctor may also advise against unnecessary X rays during pregnancy.

As the medical profession has learned more about inherited diseases, it has been able to offer genetic counseling to couples concerned about the possibility of having a child born with an inherited disease or abnormality. A genetic counselor or specialist in genetic diseases can calculate the chances of a couple's offspring being afflicted with a problem due to a family history or to the age of the parents. For some genetic diseases, tests can determine if one or both parents are carriers. However, genetic counseling cannot guarantee the health of a child. It can only supply facts and offer advice.

Childbirth

A normal pregnancy that runs its full time span is called a "full term pregnancy." Here, the baby is born after a full gestation (or developmental) period of 40 weeks or thereabouts. Sometimes the baby will come earlier, an event known as prematurity.

There are three stages to normal vaginal labor and childbirth. During the first, contractions of the uterus open the cervix (the mouth of the uterus). The plug of mucus that has been sealing the uterus off from the vagina for nine months is expelled. This is often followed by either a slow trickle or sudden gush of amniotic fluid as the amniotic sac in which the baby has been growing breaks. At this point, the woman should notify her physician and head for the hospital.

The second stage begins when the cervix is completely dilated. The contractions become much stronger, accompanied by an urge to bear down and push the baby along the birth canal. A doctor or midwife will instruct the woman to push down only during a contraction so that she conserves her energy and strength. After the baby emerges, the umbilical cord, which connects the baby to the placenta, is tied and cut. Today, in one out of six pregnancies, the delivery is performed by cesarean section.

The baby, who usually gasps and cries on delivery, is immediately checked by the obstetrician or pediatrician. After being cleaned off, the baby is handed to the new mother to hold.

Five or ten minutes later, the placenta, or afterbirth, is delivered or pushed out by more contractions of the uterus. After the physician is certain this third stage is completed, he or she will stitch any tears or incisions that were made in the vagina and give the woman medication to stop excess bleeding.

The entire birthing process can last anywhere from five to 24 hours; the average is about 12 hours. Childbirth usually takes longer if it is the woman's first delivery.

More and more expectant fathers are taking active roles in their wives' pregnancies by attending prenatal classes. And most hospitals now welcome fathers into the delivery rooms so they can participate in the miracle of childbirth and comfort and support the mother while she goes through labor.

Anesthesia

Anesthesia used during childbirth includes pudendal block, paracervical, spinal, epidural, and caudal anesthesia.

In pudendal block, local anesthetic is injected through the wall of the vagina or through the skin of the buttock to reach the pudendal nerve. Blocking off this nerve eliminates pain and feeling from the lower part of the vagina, the rear portion of the vulva (the external genitals), and the surrounding outside skin. It is often used when delivery is going well and the mother wants to push. Sometimes this type of anesthesia is used following a paracervical block, in which a local anesthetic is injected around the mouth of the womb.

Various types of spinal anesthesia are used in childbirth. In one popular method, with the patient sitting up, a heavy solution containing local anesthetic is injected between the fourth and fifth vertebrae of the lower back into the fluid-filled sac surrounding the spinal cord. The heavy solution mixes with the spinal fluid and settles downward, blocking off pain messages from below the waist for about an hour.

Epidural anesthetic has a similar effect and is injected at the same place, but instead of being introduced into the spinal fluid in a single shot, it can be fed for hours through a fine plastic tube that rests its tip against the tough dural membrane covering the spinal cord (hence the term epidural; "epi" means "upon"). The nerves are blocked where they enter the spinal cord to produce a numbing effect. An advantage of this is the fact that the dural membrane is not punctured, thus reducing the chances of complications, such as headache and infection.

Caudal anesthesia is the same as epidural except that the tube is introduced at the very tip of the spine, the "caudal" or "tail" area.

Because both the epidural and the caudal anesthesia can slow labor if given too soon, they are not given until the woman is in active labor.

Breast-feeding

After delivery, milk production and breast-feeding will begin in earnest and will continue for several months until the baby is capable of taking other nourishment, unless, of course, the mother prefers to start the baby on artificial formula. In this case, she will be treated with medication and icepacks to curtail milk production. Most doctors advise that breast-feeding is best for the baby's growth and future health.

After breast-feeding ends, the breasts will return to normal size.

On the following pages, you can read in more detail about certain subjects pertaining to pregnancy and childbirth.

Artificial insemination

Artificial insemination is the introduction of a man's semen (the

PREGNANCY AND CHILDBIRTH   449

fluid containing the sperm) into a woman's vagina or uterus by artificial means, usually by a special syringe, in the hope of accomplishing a pregnancy. The semen may be from the woman's husband or from an unknown donor.

Artificial insemination from the husband is sometimes done when the husband has a low sperm count—that is, when there are not enough sperm per unit of fluid to cause pregnancy. To obtain enough sperm, several collections may be made over days or weeks, frozen, and used in one insertion. Artificial insemination may also be used when one or the other partner cannot perform the sexual act in a normal manner, for example because of a physical condition or an emotional problem.

Donor

Artificial insemination from a donor can also be an alternative to adoption when the husband cannot father a child, whether because of low sperm count, absence of sperm, poor quality and lack of motion in sperm, or because of inability to perform sexual intercourse. It may also be considered when the husband carries an inborn defect that he does not want to pass on to his child. The woman's physician arranges for the sperm to be obtained from an unknown donor and inserts it at or before the time of her ovulation. This procedure should never be done without the husband's permission; in fact, in most states it is illegal without a legal agreement signed by both husband and wife.

Cesarean section

Cesarean section is the delivery of a baby by cutting through the abdomen and uterus and removing the baby through these incisions.

Types

Two types of cesarean section are performed:
- In the classic cesarean, a vertical cut is made directly down the center of the uterus in its thick upper section. The incision on the skin of the abdomen is also made vertically and extends from the navel down to the pubic bone. This operation is generally used only if the baby is lying in an abnormal position or if the placenta (afterbirth) is located in an abnormally low position in the cavity of the uterus. With this type of cesarean, there is more bleeding than with the second method, it is more difficult to repair the incision, and the uterus is more likely to rupture during a future pregnancy. For these reasons, the classic cesarean is seldom used today unless there are specific reasons for its use.
- The lower-segment cesarean is the more commonly performed operation. Here, the incision in the uterus is made in the lower, thinner section. This incision may be either a vertical cut or a curved, smile-shaped cut. For this operation, the incision on the skin may be either vertical down the middle or smile-shaped near the lower part of the abdomen.

Classic cesarean incision

Lower-segment cesarean incision

Bladder

A cesarean section is the delivery of a baby by cutting through the abdomen and uterus and removing the baby through these incisions. The two types of cesareans are the classic and the lower-segment; the incisions for each are shown here.

About 10 to 20 percent of births in the United States are cesarean. They should be performed only by a skilled obstetrician, accompanied by an anesthesiologist to administer anesthesia to the mother and a pediatrician (specialist in care of children) to check the baby at birth. Cesarean section is performed when delivery of the baby is necessary and when a natural vaginal delivery would cause injury to either the mother or the baby. Antibiotics, better anesthesia, and blood transfusions have made cesareans much safer than in the past.

Reasons

Some of the reasons for a cesarean section include:

- To save the baby's life when the umbilical cord (the unborn baby's supply line of oxygen and nutrients from the mother) is being pinched off during the birth process, or any other time the baby is not getting enough blood and oxygen to survive; this may be detected by abnormal heart rate patterns on the fetal monitor

- To prevent infection of the baby by dangerous bacteria in the surrounding (amniotic) fluid, or by a dangerous vaginal infection such as herpes

- To prevent injury to the baby during a breech birth, when the baby would emerge through the vagina buttocks or feet first rather than head first; many obstetricians believe that all breech births in first-time mothers and all premature breech births should be done by cesarean delivery

- To ease the birth or prevent injury when the baby is too large or the mother's pelvis too small for a vaginal delivery
- To deliver the baby if the mother fails to deliver after long labor
- To save the baby's life if problems with the placenta are cutting off blood supply to the baby
- To treat disease of the mother or baby that can be treated better if birth occurs rapidly
- To be safe if the mother has had a previous cesarean birth (the rule had been that any woman who has one cesarean must have cesarean sections on all following births; however, in recent years many vaginal deliveries have been performed successfully on women who had previous lower-segment cesarean sections).

Risk factors

Risks of a cesarean section include possible infection, bleeding, and dangerous blood clots that may get into the blood circulation. There is a small chance that the uterus will rupture during another pregnancy, before or during birth. The cesarean may be inconvenient for the mother, requiring her to stay in the hospital for five to seven days instead of going home with her baby in three days. She may not be able to see the baby for a number of hours after delivery if she has undergone general anesthesia. Breast-feeding may be difficult if the mother is being given strong medications to relieve pain, which keep her asleep for long periods of time. There is pain from the operation incision, and the mother's activity is restricted once she arrives home. It takes up to six weeks for complete healing of the incision. In addition, the extra expense for her and her baby is considerable. However, all of these costs are small if they save the baby from lifelong brain damage or save the life of infant or mother.

Conception

Conception is the union of a sperm cell from the father with an egg from the mother to form a new life.

Ovulation

During the course of her life, the average woman produces about 350 to 400 eggs, or ova, one for each menstrual cycle. The two organs in which the eggs mature, known as ovaries, are located near the top and on either side of the uterus (womb), and are connected with it by ducts known as fallopian tubes. In the midpoint of the 28-day menstrual cycle of the average woman, an egg matures in one or the other ovary, is expelled from the ovary during a process called ovulation, and starts to travel down its fallopian tube toward the uterus, propelled by the waving action of tiny hairs, known as cilia, that line the tube. If the egg meets sperm cells en route, conception may occur.

Conception is the union of a sperm cell from the father with an egg from the mother to form a new life. Once a month the woman's ovary releases an egg that travels through the nearby fallopian tube toward the uterus. If the egg meets sperm cells en route, conception may occur. Only one sperm can penetrate an egg.

Fertilization

Sperm cells — which look like tadpoles under a microscope — originate in the man's two testes, which are contained in a fleshy bag (the scrotum) that hangs beneath the penis. At the climax of sexual intercourse, an average of 300 million to 500 million sperm cells, floating in a teaspoonful of thick white fluid, spurt from the tip of the man's penis deep into the woman's vagina.

Immediately the sperm start swimming forward, propelled by their long waving tails and aided by contractions of the muscles of the woman's vagina and uterus. The goal of the sperm is to swim through the cervix, into the uterus, and up one of the fallopian tubes to fertilize a new egg just released from the ovary that produced it. Even if all goes well, however, only one of the millions of sperm will succeed. Millions of sperm are killed by acid secretions of the vagina or cervix or become trapped by mucus in the vagina (however, during the middle of the woman's menstrual cycle, when the egg is coming down a fallopian tube to be fertilized, the fluids are thinner, less acid, and less of a barrier; also there are alkaline chemicals in the fluid accompanying the sperm, which act to neutralize the woman's acids). Most of the remaining sperm fail to pass through the uterus and up one of the two fallopian tubes. During most of the woman's menstrual cycle, both tubes are empty and the sperm find nothing to fertilize. Only during a few days is an egg present in one of the tubes, and then it may be reached only by a few of the millions of sperm cells that began the journey. The sperm completely surround the egg, their thin long tails waving furiously in an attempt to force their pointed heads into the female cell. Finally one succeeds. The tail detaches, and the head moves toward the center of the egg. In seconds, a chemical change comes about in the egg that prevents the entry of any other sperm. Conception has occurred.

The fertilized egg

Unlike all other cells in the body, the sperm and the egg each contain only 23 chromosomes (chromosomes are the chemical "blueprints" that together determine all of the inherited characteristics of the baby to come). All of the other cells contain twice that number, 46. But in the first 12 hours of conception, the 23 chromosomes from the mother and the 23 chromosomes from the father join to form a new nucleus of 46 chromosomes. This is the basic unit from which the new individual will come.

During the next four or five days, as the fertilized human egg drifts down the fallopian tube and into the uterus, the original cell divides and subdivides into anywhere from 16 to 48 cells. In another two or three days the cluster of cells grows into many more and implants itself into the nourishing blood-rich lining of the mother's uterus, which soon forms the beginning of a placenta around the baby-to-be, called an embryo at this stage. Within about 17 days after conception, the placenta begins blood circulation to the embryo, in which various cells are specializing to form different parts of the baby's body. By the end of the seventh week of pregnancy, all of the basic structures of the body have been formed, and the embryo now is called the fetus until birth.

Ectopic pregnancy

Ectopic pregnancy is a pregnancy in which the fertilized egg develops outside the uterus. Usually it occurs in either of the two fallopian tubes which each extend some 4½ inches from the ovaries (egg-producing organs) to the uterus and through which the egg travels from the ovary to the uterus. In that case it is also known as a *tubal pregnancy*. However, on rare occasions the pregnancy starts to develop in the ovary, on the cervix (neck) of the uterus, or attached to the outside of a nearby organ in the abdominal cavity. (The ovary is not directly connected to the fallopian tube. There is a slight gap between them, which sometimes permits an egg to escape into the abdominal cavity.)

Causes

The usual cause of an ectopic (out of place) pregnancy is an obstruction or narrowing of the fallopian tube that prevents the egg from passing downward through the tube to the uterus. The obstruction or narrowing is usually the result of inflammation or scarring from an infection, such as gonorrhea, but it may also develop after abdominal surgery or because of a growth such as a pelvic tumor. Tubal infections caused by numerous other bacteria can occur after miscarriage or childbirth or during the use of an IUD (intrauterine device). If these infections are severe, blockage of the tube may result.

Complications

An ectopic pregnancy may be fatal unless it is promptly treated. The danger is that it will not be detected until it has ruptured (broken) the tube enclosing it, causing massive bleeding. Pregnancies located in other areas such as the ovary and cervix can invade large nearby blood vessels and cause massive bleeding.

Symptoms

Symptoms of ectopic pregnancy usually begin from two to four weeks after a woman misses her menstrual period. She may be bothered by sharp, continuous pains on one side of her pelvis (lower abdomen) and by slight bleeding from her vagina. With rapid bleeding, which usually does not occur until after the sixth week of the pregnancy, the patient may suffer from sudden sharp pains in the lower abdomen, from backache, low blood pressure, fainting, and even shock (collapse of circulation to the outer parts of the body).

Diagnosis

The examining doctor may discover a tender swelling on one side of the pelvis. Movement of the uterus (during a pelvic examination) may cause pain. When ectopic pregnancy is suspected, the patient is hospitalized immediately. Ultrasound pictures may reveal the outline of the expanding mass. In most cases, there is slow bleeding from the end of the fallopian tube into the abdominal cavity, which may be detected by inserting a hollow needle through the wall of the vagina beneath the cervix and drawing off blood. The diagnosis is confirmed by inserting a laparoscope (a lighted tube) through a small cut into the abdominal cavity to detect the ectopic pregnancy visually.

Treatment

Treatment for ectopic pregnancy is surgical removal of the pregnancy. When the pregnancy is in a fallopian tube, the entire tube and sometimes the ovary must be removed. However, it is sometimes possible to remove the pregnancy and reconstruct the tube.

A woman who has had one ectopic pregnancy has a 15 percent chance of having a second one. This does not mean that she should not try to become pregnant again—but that when she does try, she should be especially watchful for symptoms of ectopic pregnancy, and she should see her physician immediately so that the location of this pregnancy may be determined.

Episiotomy

An episiotomy is a surgical incision into the tissues surrounding the opening of the vagina during childbirth in order to make the delivery easier and to avoid extensive tearing of the tissues. The advantage of the procedure is that it substitutes a controlled surgical incision for excessive stretching and tearing of all the tissues. The incision itself is easier to repair later than a tear or break in the tissues would be.

Episiotomy is often performed for women who are having their first baby. With subsequent pregnancies, episiotomy may not be necessary, since the tissues surrounding the vagina have often been stretched sufficiently by the first delivery to allow an easy second delivery.

Types

The most common type of episiotomy is a midline incision made with surgical scissors from the midpoint of the vaginal opening directly downward toward the rectum. This type of incision carries one important risk: during the birth it might extend into the anal sphincter (the ring of muscle surrounding the opening from the intestine) or the rectum itself; however, it can be repaired easily and will eventually heal itself. To avoid the risks of entering the rectum, some physicians prefer the mediolateral episiotomy in which the incision is made at an angle, thus avoiding the rectum and anal sphincter.

Hyperemesis gravidarum

Hyperemesis gravidarum is a term that refers to excessive or abnormal vomiting during pregnancy. This type of vomiting is more severe than that caused by normal morning sickness, which usually clears up on its own within a few months. In hyperemesis gravidarum, the vomiting leads to starvation, loss of water in the body, and an imbalance in body fluids.

Symptoms of hyperemesis

gravidarum include loss of weight and dehydration. The condition is most often treated in the hospital through the use of anti-vomiting drugs and of intravenous feeding to correct the possible malnutrition, dehydration, and imbalance of body fluids. A pregnant woman should not attempt to treat herself with drugs for her vomiting without consulting her doctor.

Miscarriage

A miscarriage, in medical terms a spontaneous abortion, is the end of a pregnancy, brought on by the premature delivery of the fetus before the beginning of the twentieth week of pregnancy. At that point, the fetus is not developed enough to survive outside the uterus on its own. (After the twentieth week of pregnancy, a spontaneous abortion is considered a premature delivery or, if the baby is born dead, a stillbirth. A pregnancy that is ended artificially is commonly known as an abortion, although the medical term is termination of pregnancy.) Most miscarriages occur within the first 14 weeks of pregnancy.

It is impossible to know the number of miscarriages that happen during the first month of pregnancy before a woman realizes she is pregnant; the only indication is a slightly late menstrual period with a heavier than normal flow. However, about 10 to 15 percent of the known pregnancies end in miscarriage.

Types

There are different categories of miscarriages. A "threatened" miscarriage is experienced by about one out of every five pregnant women when they bleed vaginally during the first three months; although it may indicate a spontaneous abortion, with proper care it is rarely more than a threat and the pregnancy will continue normally. An "inevitable" miscarriage refers to a situation in which bleeding occurs and the cervix begins to dilate (open). A "missed" miscarriage occurs when the fetus dies in the uterus but is not naturally expelled, and the woman has no bleeding or pain to signify that the pregnancy is not progressing; the physician usually notices when the uterus stops growing.

Causes

The reason that a miscarriage occurs is not always understood, but it is believed that a fetus usually aborts because it is not developing normally. Several factors can contribute to a miscarriage including abnormalities in the father's sperm; disease in the mother, most notably an acute infection, glandular disorder, high blood pressure, kidney or heart disease, diabetes, or thyroid problems; abnormalities in the uterus; the mother's poor nutrition and use of cigarettes, alcohol, or drugs; environmental pollutants; or the mother's involvement in a severe accident or trauma.

The expulsion of the fetus

because of an abnormality is thought to be a chance event, not due to a problem or defect in either parent. Of women who miscarry once, most (80 percent) have a successful subsequent pregnancy. Women who miscarry two or three times, whether or not they deliver successfully in between, are known as "habitual aborters."

Symptoms

The symptoms of miscarriage are vaginal bleeding (from a few drops to a heavy flow) and cramps (either dull and constant or sharp and intermittent) in the lower abdomen or back. The bleeding can start suddenly or follow a brownish discharge. A solid clot of material or tissue may pass from the vagina. If possible, this should be saved for the doctor who may be able to examine it and determine a reason for the expulsion. A miscarriage can be complete—the uterus expels all the tissue — or incomplete—tissue remains inside the uterus.

A pregnant woman who starts bleeding or experiences pain should contact her physician immediately.

Treatment

There is no medical treatment to stop or avert an inevitable miscarriage. (The drug diethylstilbestrol, DES, was prescribed to deter miscarriages until it was discovered that it had little effect and could cause abnormalities in babies.) The physician generally directs the woman with symptoms to rest in bed and abstain from sexual intercourse.

After an inevitable, incomplete, or missed miscarriage, any remaining fetus or placenta must be removed by a surgical procedure known as dilatation and curettage (D and C) in which the physician expands the cervix and gently scrapes residual material from inside the uterus. Without this precaution a woman is more likely to be susceptible to infections caused by the retained tissue.

It is normal for a woman to feel depressed by the loss of the expected child, but it is usually safe for her to attempt to conceive soon afterward—six to eight weeks later—on the advice of her physician.

Prevention

More and more information is becoming available about the use of drugs and about the nutritional and environmental factors that can affect a pregnancy. It is advisable for a woman, at the beginning of her pregnancy, to seek counseling or educate herself so she is aware of the most up-to-date information on the substances and practices that may contribute to a miscarriage.

Placenta previa

Placenta previa is an abnormal condition after conception in which the fertilized egg, or zygote, travels to the lower portion of the uterus, to attach itself to a part of the uterine wall near or even over the uterine os (opening). In these cases, the placenta (a temporary organ in the uterus, which develops during pregnancy to conduct nourishment and oxygen from mother to unborn child) forms in such a way as to cover all or part of the uterine opening and thus interfere with normal delivery. There are three types of placenta previa: (1) partial, in which only a portion of the cervix (or uterine mouth) is covered; (2) complete, in which the cervix is completely covered; and (3) low-lying (or marginal), in which the placenta does not cover the cervix, but is close enough to it possibly to interfere with normal delivery. There is one placenta previa in every 100 to 500 pregnancies. They are more prevalent among women who have had two or more children than among those for whom it is the first pregnancy.

Cause

Placenta previa is not necessarily the result of a disease or of inadequate precautions on the part of the mother. The cause of this condition is unknown. Some authorities feel that a placenta will never implant on the same part of the uterine wall twice. If a woman has several pregnancies, only the lower part of the uterus may be left on which the placenta can implant.

Symptoms

The major symptom of placenta previa is painless vaginal bleeding. Profuse bleeding may begin as early as the 24th to 26th week of pregnancy, with no apparent cause. The blood will be bright red, indicating that it is fresh blood. Bleeding occurs as the placenta separates from the wall of the uterus near the uterine opening. This bleeding occurs without any injury (from a fall, for example). In some cases, the blood flow is light (spotting).

Diagnosis

Any vaginal bleeding during pregnancy is abnormal and should be reported to the doctor immediately. An ultrasound scan of the mother's abdomen will then be performed. If a placenta previa is present, this will be seen with the ultrasound scan.

Treatment

There are two types of treatment: delayed and active. The purpose of delayed treatment is to give the fetus time to mature so that it can survive a cesarean delivery (through an incision in the abdomen) and be mature enough to survive a premature birth. In the case of active treatment, the fetus is delivered by cesarean section as soon as possible.

The degree of vaginal bleeding will usually dictate the type of treatment. If vaginal bleeding is slight, delayed treatment is chosen. If vaginal bleeding is heavy, a cesarean section will be performed immediately.

Bleeding from placenta previa may be extremely heavy, leading to severe blood loss from the mother. This bleeding stops only after the fetus and placenta are delivered. Unless treatment is rapid, death of both the mother and the fetus may occur.

Toxemia of pregnancy

Toxemia of pregnancy is a severe condition which sometimes occurs in the latter stages of pregnancy and is characterized by high blood pressure; swelling of the feet, hands, and other extremities; and an excessive amount of protein in the urine. If allowed to worsen, convulsions and coma may set in. Toxemia of pregnancy is actually a misnomer from the days when it was thought that the condition was caused by toxic (poisonous) substances in the blood. The illness is more accurately called preeclampsia before the convulsive stage and eclampsia afterward.

Causes

The causes of toxemia in pregnancy are not clearly understood. It tends to develop more often among mothers from lower socioeconomic levels. One theory is that dietary deficiencies may

be at the roots of some cases. Also, there is the possibility that some types of toxemia are the result of deficiency of blood flow in the uterus, or womb.

Symptoms

Toxemia is divided into three stages, each progressively more serious and leading, ultimately, to death if not treated.
- *Mild preeclampsia symptoms:* swelling, high blood pressure, and protein in the urine;
- *Severe preeclampsia symptoms:* headache, dizziness, fever, drowsiness, tachycardia (interruption of natural heart rhythm), tinnitus (noise in the ears), double vision, nausea, vomiting, and abnormal urine production;
- *Eclampsia:* convulsions, coma, death.

Treatment

Toxemia in pregnancy cannot be completely cured until the pregnancy is over. Until that time, treatment includes stimulation of kidney functions, control of high blood pressure, control of convulsions, and, in severe cases, early delivery of the infant to insure the survival of the mother.

Prevention

There is no known preventive for toxemia of pregnancy. The first line of defense is the monitoring of all bodily functions in order to spot any preeclampsia symptoms as they first begin to appear.

CARING FOR YOUR CHILD

As a parent, you know better than anyone else when your child is not acting or feeling right. Sometimes there are visible signs of illness, like diarrhea or a fever; at other times, a change in your child's behavior alerts you to a problem, even though there are no physical symptoms. How can you better equip yourself to make the best decisions about your children's health?

First, educate yourself. Read thoroughly this chapter on childhood illnesses. Know what symptoms to watch for and what to do about them. Second, trust your instincts. If you feel there is a problem or an emergency situation, act on it. Third, ask questions. Don't be shy in dealing with doctors or other medical professionals; if you don't understand their answers, ask them to repeat the explanation.

When to call a doctor

Here are some rules of thumb about about when to call the doctor for common ailments:

- Fever: higher than 101°F for more than 24 hours; the child looks and acts extremely ill, is difficult to arouse, or is incoherent.

- Common cold: lasts more than ten days; accompanied by a fever higher than 101°F, a sore throat or pus-like nasal discharge for longer than two days, or a persistent cough or wheezing.
- Sore throat: pain present in throat for more than three days; accompanied by a fever higher than 101°F.
- Earache: pain lasts more than one hour; child looks very ill; child's temperature is higher than 101°F.
- Cough: accompanied by wheezing or difficulty in breathing; fever of more than 101°F; cough is persistent or is short, dry, and sharp; accompanying cold has lasted more than ten days.
- Headache: frequent headaches; child appears ill.
- Stomachache: pain is constant in the lower stomach for more than two hours; child has bloody stools; child vomits green or yellow matter more than twice.
- Vomiting: accompanied by fever; child is very ill—difficult to arouse; child vomits green or yellow matter more than twice; vomiting lasts more than twelve hours.
- Diarrhea: child does not urinate for eight hours; accompanied by vomiting; blood in the stools;

diarrhea lasts more than one day; fever of more than 101°F.

Illness in babies may be a little harder to detect. Call the doctor when an infant:

• Refuses to nurse or take liquids;
• Urinates very little;
• Vomits repeatedly;
• Becomes extremely fretful or lethargic;
• Becomes hoarse, has difficulty breathing, or has a crowing cry, especially if there is a fever and the baby appears sickly;
• Becomes fretful and pulls on ear;
• Has a marked increase in bowel movements; blood or mucus in the stool;
• Displays noticeable protrusion of the soft spot on the head.

Call your doctor if an existing condition is not improving or if you do not know what to do about certain symptoms. Although parents need to use common sense in calling the doctor, it is always better to err on the side of being overcautious. A doctor can often give directions and reassure you over the telephone.

Respiratory disorders account for almost half of all childhood illnesses. Fortunately, they are easy to diagnose, and the availability of antibiotics makes many respiratory infections fairly simple to cure.

Although children are needy in the sense that they cannot provide for themselves, they are remarkably tough when it comes to recovering from illness and overcoming physical disorders. This resilience sees them through a time of life when their undeveloped bodies make them the most vulnerable to mishaps, accidents, and germs.

Amblyopia

Amblyopia is the name for diminished vision in one or both eyes, usually without any obvious defect. (Amblyopia is not the same as nearsightedness, farsightedness, or astigmatism which can be corrected with eyeglasses or contact lenses.)

There are two main types of amblyopia, depending upon the cause: "lazy eye" amblyopia and toxic amblyopia.

"Lazy eye" amblyopia

"Lazy eye" amblyopia occurs frequently in young children whose eyes, because they are not parallel, do not line up images correctly (a condition known as strabismus). In order to prevent double vision (in which you see two images of everything instead of one), the brain suppresses the sight of one eye; the other eye does all the work. Thus the popular term "lazy eye" is used for the eye that is not working. The eye, like any other organ, will not develop properly if not used; therefore, the structures of the suppressed eye may atrophy (waste away) or fail to develop.

Unfortunately, there are usually no obvious symptoms of "lazy eye." By the time the condition is recognized, the eye may be permanently damaged. The child usually appears to see as well as the next boy or girl. On the other hand, sometimes the condition that causes the amblyopia may be very noticeable. The eyes may turn either inward or outward or one may be looking up while the other is looking down.

To fully restore sight in the lazy eye, treatment must begin before the child is four to six years of age. If the eyes are out of focus because some of the muscles of the eye are weaker than others, the condition may be corrected by special glasses or contact lenses, by eye exercises, by eyedrops in or a patch on the normal eye that diminishes the ability of the normal eye to focus thereby forcing the lazy eye to work, or occasionally by surgery. Follow-up by the doctor is needed until the child is at least ten years of age.

Prevention of "lazy eye" amblyopia can begin soon after birth. If the eyes of a baby in the first weeks of life are continually out of alignment or still out of alignment from time to time at six months of age, the condition should be investigated. Otherwise, there may be a possibility of amblyopia. A simple eye test given in the doctor's office or even at home or nursery school should be able to show that one eye is not working and that treatment is needed. It should not be delayed. The child will not "grow out" of either strabismus or amblyopia.

Toxic amblyopia

Toxic amblyopia, usually occurring in both eyes, can result from excessive drinking of alcoholic beverages over a long period of time (and may be due mainly to the poor nutrition of heavy drinkers, who get most of their calories from alcohol and so do not eat enough nourishing food). It is also found, rarely, in heavy cigarette smokers and in people exposed to various chemicals, including lead, methanol (wood alcohol), digitalis, chloramphenicol, and arsenic. The toxic substance causes swelling and irritation of the optic nerve around the site where it enters the eyeball, and if the irritation continues, it can cause lasting damage to the nerve and even total blindness.

Symptoms include pain on moving the eyeball and an increasing area of poor eyesight in or near the center of one's field of vision.

Treatment is to stop exposure to the poison, if it can be discovered. In lead poisoning, the patient is given medicine that combines with the lead and draws it out of body tissues. The treatment is known as chelation therapy.

If the cause is removed at once, vision may improve—unless there is permanent damage to the optic nerve.

Apgar score

The Apgar score is a general evaluation of a baby's condition, made one and five minutes after birth, to determine immediately if the newborn needs emergency care. The score was devised by the late Virginia Apgar, M.D. and is based on the letters of her last name.

Procedure

One minute and five minutes after birth, a delivery room nurse, anesthesiologist, or pediatrician rates the baby on five indicators, using a scale of 0 to 2:

A (Appearance): the baby gets a top score of 2 if the skin is completely pink; 1 if it is pink but hands and feet are bluish; and 0 if the entire body is blue (indicating lack of oxygen).

P (Pulse): a score of 2 is given for a pulse, or heart rate, above 100; 1 for less than 100; 0 for no pulse.

G (Grimace, or reflex irritability): to score a 2, the baby must cry vigorously when slapped lightly on the soles of the feet; a grimace or slight cry scores as a 1; no response gets a 0.

A (Activity): active motions score a 2; some movement of arms and legs is a 1; but a limp and motionless infant scores 0.

R (Respiration, breathing): strong efforts to breathe, together with vigorous crying, score a 2; slow, irregular breathing, 1; no breathing, 0.

Scores

Most babies score between 7 and 10 when tested one minute after birth. They are breathing well, crying, pinkish in color, active, and need no emergency measures.

Those babies who score from 4 to 6 usually need help immediately. The throat is suctioned to remove thick mucus, small blood clots, or bits of swallowed membrane (from the amniotic sac that enclosed the baby before birth). Oxygen is sometimes given to assist breathing and restore color.

The baby with the Apgar score below 4 is limp, pale or bluish, perhaps without heartbeat, and is in grave danger. The throat is suctioned and the baby is placed on a mechanical respirator which pumps air in and out of the lungs until the baby can breathe on his or her own.

A second Apgar score is taken five minutes after birth and recorded on the baby's chart beside the first score. The second score is a good measure of the baby's adaptation to the world outside the womb.

Autism

Autism is a form of mental illness (psychosis) in children. The word autism comes from "auto," the Greek word for "self," and literally means "self-ism." The autistic child is wrapped up in his or her own unrealistic inner thoughts, unable to communicate or relate to other people.

Causes

Although the cause of autism remains a mystery, several reasons for the disorder have been suggested. In some cases, an inborn mental defect may play a part, since many of these children from birth do not smile and do not accept affectionate cuddling. In other instances, severe mental or physical trauma during childhood may contribute to the disorder. The sex of the child may also be a factor; males are four times as likely as females to be autistic.

Symptoms

Autism is a collection of symptoms, of unknown cause, beginning in the first 30 months of life. The autistic child is very withdrawn, unaffectionate, and uninterested in people including parents, brothers, and sisters. The child seems to behave as if he or she is alone in the world. Accompanying this attitude is a speech and language disorder: the child may learn to speak late or not at all, and if speech develops it is odd and limited. One common practice is echolalia (repeating or "echoing" the last phrase or word of everything the other person says). Other marks of autism are a total resistance to change (even something so minor as rearrangement of furniture) and the repetition of meaningless acts such as rocking, arm-flapping, or head-banging. Finally, mental development is often uneven. Usually the child does best in non-language subjects and may learn best with methods that emphasize memorization and drill. There are no particular signs of nervous system defects, although half of all autistic children experience seizures before reaching their teens.

Diagnosis

In diagnosing autism, the doctor must distinguish it from childhood schizophrenia, a mental illness that usually strikes later than does autism but that may also cause a child to be silent and withdrawn. The doctor must also make certain that deafness or severely impaired hearing is not present. The child is given intelligence tests, to help determine the potential for training and education, and tests of the nervous system. A tranquilizer drug may be prescribed if needed for emergency use to quiet screaming or violent outbursts.

Treatment

An autistic child may have to be cared for in an institution or a specialized school. But day care programs for autistic children are available in some cities, and the trend is to train parents to care for their children at home (information about available programs may be obtained from The National Society for Autistic Children).

The method of treatment used by professionals today, and taught to parents, is known as behavior therapy. The main goals are to limit self-destructive or meaningless actions, to promote language development, and to make the child more social. In behavior therapy, the professional—or parent — works hard to develop a close relationship with the child, so that the child will want to imitate the adult. The adult also uses direct action such as rewards and praise to promote speech, playing with other children, self-care skills (such as dressing and washing), and helpfulness. With such methods, some autistic children of average or near-average intelligence are able to develop into normal adults.

Prevention

Unfortunately, because the cause is unknown, there is no recognized method of prevention.

Battered child syndrome

The battered child syndrome is a group of symptoms indicating that a child has been injured, usually repeatedly, by a parent, guardian, or other family member. The injury may be either physical, emotional, or sexual and is known as *child abuse*. Closely related is *child neglect*, in which the parent or guardian fails to provide for the nutritional, emotional, physical, or health needs of the child—even though resources such as food, shelter, clothing, and health care are available.

Causes

The principal cause of child abuse is a failure of self-control by the parent or guardian. There are four main reasons for this:

Inadequate parent. Many parents who abuse their children did not receive much love from their own parents and may themselves have been abused. They did not learn how to give affection and thus find it hard to develop a good relationship with their own children. They do not have a very high opinion of themselves. Easily frustrated, they lose their tempers and resort to harsh punishment methods that they learned as children. In addition, some abusing parents are simply mentally disturbed.

"Difficult" or "different" child. Some children are so overactive, irritable, or demanding that they drive a parent to unacceptable behavior. The parent strikes out and injures the child. Another reason may be that the child may not be able to perform as well as brothers or sisters, or as well as the parent expected, in school or elsewhere. The parent may lash out to punish the child for this "failure" or "defiance," either with blows or hurtful words.

"Lonely family." Some parents without close friends or relatives nearby, to help out and talk to, become overburdened with the constant demands of rearing children — especially small children. They lose their tempers and hurt their children, without meaning to do so.

Emergency. Some unexpected event, such as when a child breaks something or defies the parent, may cause the parent to strike out in a blind rage.

Symptoms

Physical symptoms of abuse include old and new bruises; scars from cuts and burns; serious damage to the eyes, mouth, or internal organs; and evidence in X-ray pictures of bone fractures in different stages of healing. The test of child abuse comes when parents cannot give reasonable explanations for the child's injuries.

Signs of emotional abuse are more difficult to spot. In babies, it may be failure to put on weight even though no illness is present. Children who are "too good," too anxious to please adults, but who do not get along well with other children and are mistrustful may be victims of emotional abuse. At school, they have trouble with teachers as well as with other children. Threats, ridicule, and unreasonable punishment by nonphysical means are some of the ways parents abuse their children emotionally.

Sexual abuse is fairly common, often by a parent or an older brother or sister. Of all kinds of abuse, it may be the hardest to detect. There are usually no physical symptoms, although venereal disease in a child is grounds for suspicion. The child may willingly consent to sexual activity or may be too embarrassed to reveal the facts to anyone outside the family. The most typical sexual abuse occurs when a father establishes a sexual relationship with his daughter often with the knowledge of the mother. The mother may be afraid to complain or may simply accept the situation. As in other forms of child abuse, sexually abused children often grow up to abuse their children just as they were abused.

Child neglect can be as harmful as child abuse. An extreme example is when a live newborn baby is found in a garbage can. Parents who did not want a child in the first place may not give it the love and attention it needs to do well. Babies who have been neglected emotionally may appear uninterested in people and even retarded.

Parents who neglect their children may be incompetent because of drug or alcohol abuse or medical problems, because of a depressed state of mind, or because of a whole set of problems they just cannot seem to handle.

Those most likely to abuse their children are young parents with their first child, unmarried adolescent mothers rebelling against their parents, parents who were abused as children, and parents of ill or premature babies who are separated from them shortly after birth. Such parents need special attention and support in order to get their families off to a good start.

Outside intervention

When physicians suspect child abuse, they are required by law in most states to report it to a government social service agency or welfare department. However, punishment of the parents is not the goal of the law. Jailing a parent might injure the child even more than the original abuse, if the parent is capable of being a good father or mother in the future. Removing the child from the family may be necessary to protect the youngster from future injury, but in most cases this is not done or the removal is only temporary. The child may simply stay in the hospital a few days while the case is studied and parents are interviewed. In many communities, a team made up of a social worker, pediatrician, psychiatrist, and other specialists talk to the child and parents and develop a long-term treatment plan. This often involves periodic visits by a social worker to the home and psychological help for one or both parents. Practical help such as day care for small children and household help by a trained homemaker can ease the burdens on an overworked mother. Trained nonprofessional "parent aides" can provide good support as can "Parents Anonymous" chapters — made up of parents who formerly abused their children.

Prevention

Even before the first child is born, planning is useful. The father should realize the need for his encouragement of the mother and help with the baby and chores. Perhaps relatives and friends or others can be lined up to help with emergencies or babysitting. If the baby is born ill or prematurely and must stay in the hospital intensive care unit after the mother comes home, parents should visit the baby at least every day and stay as close as possible so that the baby will not be a stranger when he or she comes home. Many mothers of young children find it helpful to get together once a week or so while their children play to share ideas and support each other.

Parents who are afraid they may abuse their children should talk to other parents about how they handle their problems with children and to their family doctor who may be able to provide the name of a specialist in family problems.

Cerebral palsy

Cerebral palsy (CP) is a general term to describe various disorders of muscle control, caused by brain or nerve damage usually before or around the time of birth. The damage may result when brain tissue becomes starved for oxygen for whatever reason. It may result from separation and bleeding of the placenta (the organ that unites the unborn baby to the wall of the uterus and provides nourishment to the baby) in late pregnancy or from disorders caused by diabetes of the mother.

Symptoms

Symptoms of CP range from simple clumsiness or slight incoordination of muscles to multiple handicaps that prevent normal life and movement. Frequently, the brain damage that causes CP also causes mental retardation, epilepsy, hearing problems, visual defects, and learning and behavior disorders. However, some CP children are normal except for disordered muscle control.

Types

There are four general types of cerebral palsy: spastic, athetoid or dyskinetic, ataxic, and mixed. Some 70 percent of people with CP are of the spastic type. They move stiffly and with great difficulty because their affected "spastic" muscles are constantly tense and tight. One arm and one leg may be affected, or both arms or both legs. Affected arms and legs appear thin and wasted, are weak, and are likely to twist and jerk. Walking on the toes, or with a "scissors" movement, is typical. When all four limbs are affected, the mouth, tongue, and palate may also be affected, interfering with speech, eating, and drinking and causing a constant drool.

Athetoid or dyskinetic CP accounts for about 20 percent of cases. Athetoid CP is characterized by continual slow, twisting movements of the fingers and hands during waking hours. Similar movements of the upper arm or legs and trunk may also occur. There may be sudden jerky movements as well. All of these symptoms are caused by damage to the basal ganglia, a mass of nerve-cell bodies at the base of the brain.

Ataxic CP results from damage to the cerebellum (lower brain) or nerves leading from it. Symptoms are weakness, lack of balance and coordination, tremor, difficulty with fine or quick movements, and a clumsy way of walking with feet wide apart.

Mixed CP occurs frequently. Often, spastic and athetoid types are combined. Ataxic and athetoid types are mixed less often.

In addition to the above disorders, about 25 percent of CP patients have convulsions—which usually can be controlled by anticonvulsant medicines.

Diagnosis

Early diagnosis and treatment of cerebral palsy are vital if a child is to develop as fully as possible. Any baby who may have suffered brain damage around the time of birth should be watched carefully for signs of CP (such a baby may have been born nearly lifeless, or very small and premature, or undergone severe infection after birth). Possible signs of CP in a baby include twitching, convulsions, back-arching muscle spasms, partial paralysis of the face, and very late development of the ability to lift the head, sit, crawl, speak, stand, and walk. Although it is difficult to diagnose any particular form of CP in the first two years of life, parents should report any suspicion promptly to their doctor.

An important part of the doctor's investigation into possible CP is to discover if there is any other reason for the symptoms. Some of the same symptoms are caused by other conditions requiring surgery or other specific treatment. Still other conditions result from diseases, such as progressive cerebellar degenerative disease, which continue to worsen. (Although CP never disappears, at least it does not get worse.)

Treatment

Treatment of a CP child requires many different elements. Ideally, it involves a physician working with a team of specialists in a special clinic, hospital, or other setting where their efforts can be coordinated. Someone with CP may need a series of medical diagnostic studies, psychological testing, speech therapy, physical therapy, special dental care, specially designed clothes, braces, corrective glasses, surgery, a hearing aid, special furniture, special schooling, and perhaps special institutional care. Occupational therapy can help the patient in self-care, including dressing and eating.

Because CP is a life-long condition, parents need to learn as much as possible about caring for a CP child. A good therapist will teach the parent how to continue the therapy at home. Every reasonable effort must be made to help the child become self-reliant. Parents can often get valuable advice and support from other CP parents and from professionals at the local chapter of the United Cerebral Palsy Association. Therapy for CP children and adults is

provided at rehabilitation centers sponsored by the National Easter Seal Society for Crippled Children and Adults and by various other agencies.

Prevention

Expectant mothers can guard against cerebral palsy in their unborn children by good prenatal care including an ample, well-balanced diet, rest, exercise, frequent checkups, and avoidance of drugs and infections. During labor and birth, the doctor can keep track of the baby's heartbeat by use of a fetal monitor and if necessary operate quickly to save the baby from brain damage caused by oxygen starvation. Expectant mothers with difficult pregnancies should try to deliver their babies at a hospital with a newborn intensive care unit, directed by a certified M.D. specialist known as a neonatologist. Here, premature and ill babies can be watched closely and cared for by specially trained nurses and doctors using the latest methods.

Circumcision

Circumcision is the surgical removal of the foreskin, the retractable sleeve of skin covering the glans (the head of the penis). Among some religious groups, the operation is performed as a religious ritual on the eighth day following birth. In hospitals, it is usually done on the last day before a baby boy goes home. In any event, if it is to be done for non-medical reasons it should be done in infancy and not later—when it is a more serious operation and might harm the child psychologically.

During the five-minute operation, which is done without anesthesia, the foreskin is carefully cut away. Dressing for the cut is petroleum jelly-soaked gauze applied to the incision. The incision heals rapidly, forming a dry scab that drops off after a few days. Although the incision should be kept as clean as possible, no other special care is necessary. Other than a few drops of blood that might be produced if the diaper rubs against the cut, there is no bleeding in a normal baby.

Reasons for and against circumcision

The decision for or against circumcision should be made by the parents before the baby's birth. There are two sides to the question. The operation became standard in American hospitals in recent decades as a cleanliness measure. In a young boy, the foreskin completely covers the head of the penis and cannot be pulled back very far. If the penis is not kept clean, urine and other substances can cause irritation of the glans and perhaps lead to infection between the foreskin and the glans. However, with normal care in cleanliness, this is not a problem. Even though the foreskin at first cannot be pulled

back very far because of bands of tissue that bind it to the glans, it is necessary to wash only the part of the glans that can be uncovered comfortably at any one stage. Gradually the bands of tissue dissolve by later childhood when the foreskin can be pulled back completely.

It has been argued that circumcision prevents cancer of the penis and cancer of the cervix (neck of the uterus) in the sexual partner of the circumcised man and may help prevent venereal disease. However, there is no solid evidence to support these statements.

The strongest argument in favor of circumcision today, apart from religious circumcision, is to prevent a boy from feeling "different" from his father, brothers, friends, or schoolmates who are circumcised. In addition, it is a little more convenient to wash a circumcised penis.

Very seldom is there a medical reason to perform a circumcision. It should never be done in the first day of life, or if the baby is ill or premature. Furthermore, it should be delayed indefinitely if there is any abnormality of the glans or penis, so that the foreskin can be used later as graft tissue to repair the defect. It should not be done if the mother was taking during pregnancy or is taking while breast-feeding any medication that promotes bleeding, such as anticoagulants or aspirin, or if there is any family history of hemophilia or other bleeding disorders.

Risks of circumcision include

local infection that may lead to significant hemorrhage and mutilation. Many medical authorities feel that there is no absolute medical reason for routine circumcision of the newborn. Adequate cleanliness and hygiene offer the same advantages of routine circumcision without the risks of the operation.

Parents, therefore, should consider all factors—cultural, religious, and physical—before making a decision about circumcision.

Cleft lip/cleft palate

Cleft lip and cleft palate, a defect in one of every 700 or 800 newborns, is characterized by a split running through all or part of the upper structure of the mouth. A cleft lip (or harelip) may be only a small notch near the center of the upper lip, or it may extend into the nostril. A cleft palate can be as minor as a split in the uvula, the little "finger" of tissue hanging down in the back of the throat. On the other hand, a cleft in the palate may divide the entire soft palate, the muscular tissue that roofs the rear of the mouth. In its most severe form, a cleft splits not only the soft palate but the entire hard palate (the bony roof of the mouth) and upper jaw, joining with a cleft lip. The cleft may even divide the palate into three parts, resulting in a split on either side of the nose, leaving a middle section of upper jaw and gum dangling.

Cleft lip happens in earliest pregnancy, soon after the fourth week when the baby's face starts to form. Bulges of tissue on either side of the face grow toward the midline to form the nostrils and lips. At about the seventh week they meet and join; if they do not, a cleft lip is the result.

A failure of development in the eighth week of pregnancy causes cleft palate. The palate is formed from two plates of tissue, which originally are on either side of the developing tongue. As the head and neck grow, the tongue moves downward and the tissue plates move into position and fuse into one—unless there is a mistake or weakness, which results in cleft palate.

Causes

The basic causes of cleft lip and cleft palate are not fully understood. There is obviously an inherited tendency toward the defects. More than one fourth of children with cleft lip also have a relative with a cleft. If parents without cleft defects have one child with a cleft, they have a 5 percent risk of having a second child with a cleft; if they have two children with clefts, there is a 12 percent risk of a cleft in future children. Perhaps some difference in the uterus, such as poor blood supply to the infant, combines with an inherited weakness to produce the error of development. Certain chemicals or medications, too many vitamins or not enough, and viruses have been suggested as possible causes of cleft defects.

Often cleft lip and cleft palate are associated with other birth defects. About one child in six who has a cleft lip, with or without cleft palate, has one or more other birth defects. A child who has only a cleft palate has up to a 50 percent chance of having another defect, such as joined fingers or toes, malformed ears, spina bifida, heart disease, or clubfoot.

Treatment

Treatment of a patient with a cleft lip and/or a cleft palate requires the services of a specialized team. Such a group includes a pediatrician, orthodontist, speech therapist, plastic surgeon, psychologist, audiologist, and otolaryngologist. Treatment may take place at a specialized clinic or hospital center or may be coordinated by a pediatrician who brings in different experts as needed.

Before any treatment can begin, however, steps must be taken to permit the child to eat. A cleft lip prevents normal sucking, while a cleft palate causes milk to run out of the nose, and may cause choking and vomiting. Special feeding devices are used, such as a nipple with an enlarged flange to cover the cleft or a regular nipple with enlarged holes. A small syringe with a short rubber tube, like one used to baste a turkey, may be used to feed a child with a cleft lip, although sometimes such a

child can breast-feed. In a few days after birth, an orthodontist skilled in cleft palate repair may be able to fashion an appliance that provides a temporary roof for the mouth, enabling regular feeding. At the same time, the appliance prevents the mouth from being distorted before the palate can be closed.

Surgery to correct a cleft lip is done in the first few days of life by some surgeons, because it will make the baby more acceptable to parents and make it easier to feed the baby by bottle. However, other surgeons delay the operation from two to eight months, so that surgery will not interfere with the growing bonds of affection between mother and baby (for one thing, the baby cannot breast-feed for six weeks after the operation) and to rule out other birth defects that might interfere with recovery.

Plastic surgery to correct cleft palate usually takes place in the second year of life. Some surgeons repair the soft palate first, when the child is between six and 18 months of age, and the hard palate much later — sometimes not until age five years. While early surgery helps the child's emotional and speech development, some surgeons wait because they are concerned that early surgery may cause distortion of growth in the middle third of the face. While waiting, the child wears an appliance that roofs over the mouth.

The problems created by cleft palate and cleft lip cannot be solved only by surgery. An orthodontist is needed for youngsters with cleft palate, not only to make appliances but to straighten teeth that are poorly positioned. A speech therapist aids the child in developing speech, which is altered because of missing or inadequate soft palate or artificial palate. A psychologist helps to treat emotional and social problems sometimes caused by being "different" in speech or appearance. An otolaryngologist is consulted to treat the middle ear infections that are common in young children with cleft palate and to inspect the child monthly for such problems. Finally, an audiologist is needed for those children who develop hearing loss because of middle ear infections. With proper care and encouragement and with modern plastic surgery, the average child with a cleft can make a good recovery.

Clubfoot

Clubfoot (*talipes*) is a common birth defect in which one and often both feet are fixed in an awkward, twisted position. The foot resists efforts to stretch or turn it back. In *talipes equinovarus,* the most frequent form, the foot points down and turns in while the front of the foot curls toward the heel. If not corrected, the condition worsens and interferes with walking. The person seems to walk on the ankle and the outside or inside edge of the foot.

Causes

The cause of clubfoot is unknown. However, it seems to involve heredity and something that happens in the womb to arrest development around the ninth week of pregnancy, when the baby's feet are being formed. Clubfoot may begin as a muscle abnormality. The Achilles (heel) tendon is shortened, the ankle and its muscles are deformed, and the heel bone is shortened and flattened to some extent.

Treatment

Correction of clubfoot should begin as early as the first week of life, while the bones, muscles, ligaments, and tendons are soft and pliable. Usually the correction is done in separate stages, not all at once. In the talipes equinovarus form, the first stage is to uncurl the front of the foot away from the heel. The next is to turn the foot so that the sole faces outward. The third stage is to put the foot in a cast with the toes pointing up. This may require surgery to lengthen the Achilles tendon and to free the ankle joint.

Correction takes place in a series of small, painless, gradual adjustments. Typically, the therapist flexes and stretches the foot by hand and then fixes it in a cast in a partially corrected position. After a week or so the cast is removed, the foot is manipulated again, placed in a still better position, and a new cast applied. Sometimes, instead of making a new cast each time, wedges are placed inside the existing cast to adjust the foot. The entire casting process may take three months.

Once the correction is made, it must be followed up with exercises, devices which hold the feet in place at night while the baby is sleeping, and orthopedic shoes. A "night splint" often used consists of corrective shoes with soles joined by a flat metal bar that keeps the feet in exactly the right position.

Because clubfoot sometimes recurs, periodic checkups are necessary until the child becomes an adult. However, in most cases, the correction is completely successful and the individual can walk and run normally.

If early treatment has not succeeded, or if a child is not treated until age nine or ten, more extensive surgery is required. This is followed by several weeks with the foot in a cast. Usually this has satisfactory results. The foot is rather stiff, but this does not prevent the individual from engaging in the most active sports.

Somewhat separate from but related to true clubfoot is *metatarsus varus,* in which the front of the foot turns inward. Known as "apparent clubfoot," or "pigeon toe," this is a milder deformity that may not be diagnosed in the first several weeks. Unlike a true clubfoot, the apparent clubfoot can be moved easily into a correct position. Usually it can be corrected by manipulation, without the need for casts or surgery.

Congenital hypothyroidism

Congenital hypothyroidism is a condition present at birth that leads to defective physical and mental development because of a deficiency of thyroid hormone. If untreated, a person born with congenital hypothyroidism grows to a maximum height of three or four feet, with a large, flat, broad head; short forehead; puffy wide-set eyes; broad, short, upturned nose; thick lips; large tongue protruding from a drooling mouth; narrow chest; potbelly; swayback; rough skin; dry hair; and severe mental retardation. In former times, these individuals were often found in inland areas where foods contain little iodine, which is necessary for the body to produce thyroid hormone. The ocean is the basic source of iodine, so people living away from the ocean and its iodine-rich seafood are more likely to develop hypothyroidism.

Causes

Congenital hypothyroidism can result from a defect in development of a child before birth. The thyroid gland in the newborn child may be missing or underdeveloped, which may have been caused by a severe deficiency of iodine in the mother's diet during pregnancy. Rarely, congenital hypothyroidism is caused by an inherited absence of a body chemical needed to produce thyroid hormone. When hypothyroidism first occurs in children over age two, it is usually due to an inflammation of the thyroid gland resulting from an immune disorder. It can also be caused by disease of the pituitary gland or hypothalamus.

Symptoms

Hypothyroidism need never develop in an infant. Many states now require that the blood of every newborn be tested for thyroid hormone level.

If a baby is not treated, the first symptoms of congenital hypothyroidism begin between age three and six months, or whenever the mother stops breast-feeding (breast milk contains tiny quantities of thyroid hormone). The baby is "too good," in the sense that he or she seldom cries (when the baby does cry, it is a strange hoarse cry), sleeps more than normal, is inactive, and thus is easy to care for. This behavior is a result of the baby's lack of thyroid hormone, which regulates the rate of body processes, and increasing mental retardation. The baby's movements are slow and awkward, and the child has feeding difficulties, is constipated, and develops jaundice. The stomach protrudes, and a hernia may develop at the navel.

At this time the characteristic facial features of a child with hypothyroidism start to show: the thick tongue, which interferes with breathing; the wide-set eyes; the turned-up nose; and also a dull expression indicating mental deficiency. The baby's heart beats slowly, resulting in poor circulation and cold skin. The hair is dry and dull. Teeth come in late and decay easily.

The child who develops hypothyroidism after age two is typically short and fat, with short legs and arms and a head that appears too large. Sexual development in an older child may be delayed.

Diagnosis

Diagnosis of congenital hypothyroidism may include not only a blood test for thyroid hormone levels, but also administration of radioactive iodine, which normally would concentrate in the thyroid gland and reveal itself on the screen of a radiation scanner. Of course, if a child has no thyroid gland, that does not happen. X rays may also be used to detect delayed development of the skeleton, and an electrocardiogram may be ordered to reveal heartbeat patterns.

Treatment

Treatment for congenital hypothyroidism is lifelong replacement of thyroid hormone with a synthetic substitute, ideally starting at birth. Those who receive the supplemental drug starting before the age of three months usually seem to grow and develop normally. Children born without a thyroid gland are even more at risk than those whose thyroid gland works poorly and if not treated by three months of age are retarded for life even though their growth is corrected.

Prevention

Mothers-to-be can help prevent congenital hypothyroidism in their offspring by eating a well-balanced diet that includes iodine-rich foods like fish and by using iodized salt or an iodine supplement. At birth, the child's blood should be tested for thyroid hormone level.

Croup

Croup is a hoarse, barking cough that sometimes follows a cold or fever in very young children, most commonly those under the age of two years. A croup attack may occur only once for a short period and never reoccur, or it may linger or reappear when it seems to be gone.

Causes

Croup is caused by a viral infection of the larynx (voice box). The characteristic barking cough is produced when air forces its way through the child's swollen larynx. The air passageways in a child's throat are very narrow; therefore, when an infection causes swelling, there is little room for air to pass through, and breathing can

be severely hampered. Also, the windpipe and the bronchi (the main breathing tubes that connect the windpipe and the lungs) may become blocked with mucus, further impairing breathing.

Symptoms

The identifying symptoms of croup are a deep, barking cough and breathing difficulties, especially when breathing in. Sometimes a fever and hoarseness are also present. The child may gag while coughing, causing vomiting that usually relieves the cough. The coughing attack often occurs in the evening and usually lasts less than an hour.

Symptoms that indicate a worsening condition include blue skin and lips, drooling, and extreme exhaustion. When the croaking sound continues while the child is inhaling, a condition called stridor has developed. If any of these symptoms occur or if there are severe breathing difficulties, medical help should be obtained *immediately*.

Treatment

Croup can be treated at home by first, and most importantly, calming the child. The barking cough, especially when accompanied by difficult breathing, can frighten anyone, especially a child, and this fear can only aggravate the symptoms. To calm the child, he or she can be asked to visualize what is happening in the throat; the child can picture the tubes to the lungs opening wide, allowing air to pass freely. Sometimes the child can be told to imagine a relaxing scene or to listen to a calming bedtime story. A relaxed child will respond much better to home remedies.

The goal is to relieve the cough by reducing the inflammation and swelling in the larynx. This can be accomplished by breathing in moist air from a humidifier or vaporizer, by leaning over a pan of hot water with a towel draped over the head, or by sitting in a steamy bathroom with a hot shower running. Moist air reduces the swelling and makes breathing easier. Of course, precautions should be taken to protect a young child from being scalded while taking part in these treatments, and the child should never be left alone.

Drinking extra fluids (not milk or orange juice) at room temperature is also recommended. Cough medicine will not help, and may even harm, a child with croup, nor any other object into the mouth in an attempt to aid the breathing. In a severe case, drugs can be administered to control the inflammation in the throat; also, antibiotics can sometimes control the infections connected with croup.

Prevention

It is not known why some children develop croup after a cold or fever and others do not; therefore, there is really no way to prevent croup.

Fontanelles

Fontanelles are the gaps between the bony plates of an infant's skull. The largest and most noticeable of these gaps is the "soft spot" on top of the head and toward the front, which lies between four bone plates. There is also a groove that runs like a center part toward the back of the head, where a much smaller soft spot is located. The fontanelles serve two purposes. During birth, they permit the head to adapt without injury to being squeezed as it passes through the birth canal. After birth, they permit the brain to grow. During the first two or three years of a child's life, the skull plates grow toward each other until they meet, covering the soft spots. However, the plates do not fully knit together until shortly before adolescence, when the brain stops growing.

The baby's soft spot is supported by tough membrane and does not have to be treated more delicately than any other part of the head. It is normal for it to be slightly depressed, to tense up when the baby cries, and to pulsate in rhythm with the heartbeat. (Contrary to what many believe, the pulsation is not that of an artery directly beneath the soft spot. Instead, it is caused by changes in the pressure of cerebrospinal fluid, which surrounds and protects the brain and spinal cord.)

Fontanelles are the gaps between the bony plates of an infant's skull. Fontanelles permit the head to adapt without injury to being squeezed during birth, and after birth they allow room for the brain to grow. Eventually, the bones meet and knit together.

Gilles de la Tourette's syndrome

Gilles de la Tourette's syndrome is a childhood disorder marked by intense tics (twitchy, repetitive movements of certain muscles) which may be either single or multiple. It begins, generally in boys, around the age of seven or eight years. At first the tics are simple: facial twisting, blinking, grimacing, shoulder shrugging, or twitching. Later the tics progress to vocal tics accompanied by psychological involvement.

Causes

The causes of Gilles de la Tourette's syndrome are unknown. It is still disputed whether the disorder is of physical or of psychological origin.

Symptoms

The symptoms of Gilles de la Tourette's syndrome are at first limited to the muscles in the face, head, neck, and shoulders. At first, and often as the first symptom, there are incomprehensible gasping or breathing noises from the larynx (voice box) as if the patient were barking, wheezing, or gasping for air. As the tics spread to the shoulders and arms, there are shoulder shrugs and twitches, and twistings of the neck and arm.

Next, vocal tics, such as grunting, sniffling, snuffing, shouting, and "barking" sounds, begin to develop. As the vocal symptoms worsen, the patient begins to exclaim in a loud voice words or phrases with obscene meanings or common "swear words." Echolalia (repetition by the patient of all that is said to him or her, almost automatically) is often seen. The patient will seem to "fixate" on a word or phrase and repeat it over and over with increasing speed. Often, too, the individual will spasmodically and automatically repeat or mimic the actions of those around him or her.

The symptoms of Gilles de la Tourette's syndrome tend to come and go, especially as the patient approaches puberty and adulthood. Tics that are very violent during waking hours often stop during sleep. Some tics are intensified by emotional upheavals. Unlike most movement disorders, Tourette tics are often suppressed in school or social settings and expressed more often when the patient is alone or with family members. In some cases, the tics are capable of being suppressed by voluntary control. The excessive swearing, however, unlike many of the other Tourette symptoms, only appears in the presence of others. Some patients attempt to cover it up by coughing, thus developing another tic. Often symptoms decrease in adult life and disappear, only to return during a period of stress. Mental activity remains normal.

Diagnosis

Diagnosing Tourette's syndrome is often difficult, since the early stages often resemble common childhood tics seen in many young school-age children. Also, early and middle-stage symptoms are difficult to distinguish from certain brain conditions, which can produce similar symptoms. However, Gilles de la Tourette's syndrome can often be diagnosed with some assurance as the course of the illness unfolds.

Treatment

Tourette's syndrome can be treated with medications starting with small doses and increasing the dosage until the tics are controlled. Often a combination of drugs is used, depending on the individual case. Group psychotherapy can be helpful in some cases, although it seems to be of limited use in most. In extreme cases, leukotomy, or surgical interruption of white nerve fibers of the frontal lobe of the brain, is considered.

Prevention

At present there are no known preventive measures for Tourette's syndrome.

Hyaline membrane disease

Hyaline membrane disease (HMD) is a respiratory distress syndrome, occurring in premature infants in which the newborn does not have fully functioning lungs. It is the leading cause of illness and death in premature infants.

Cause

The cause of HMD is the birth of the infant before the structures that manufacture *pulmonary surfactant* are developed. In order to begin inhaling and expanding normally, the newborn's lungs require the presence of a substance (pulmonary surfactant) that reduces the surface tension of the alveoli, the tiny air sacs at the end of bronchial tubes where oxygen and carbon dioxide waste are exchanged. Without this reduction in surface tension, the air sacs tend to collapse when the infant breathes out. This, in turn, pro-

duces incomplete expansion of the lungs. The end result is that the blood that is passing through the lungs is not fully oxygenated, at least not sufficiently to sustain life.

The symptoms of hyaline membrane disease are easily observable. There is a blue tint to the skin, from lack of oxygenation of the blood; symptoms of oxygen deprivation; irregular heartbeat; rapid, labored, and shallow breathing; flaring of the nostrils; grunting when breathing out; and swelling of tissues.

Treatment

Treatment for HMD is aimed at maintaining necessary oxygen levels. The problem is lack of the ability of the lungs to oxygenate blood—until the lungs develop that ability, oxygen must be provided in such a way as to prevent damage to the infant.

Fluids, serum glucose (sugar), and electrolytes are provided by intravenous (into the vein) feedings. An oxygen face mask is used to provide warmed, moisturized oxygen with a continuous positive pressure. In more severe cases, a ventilator is necessary to breathe for the infant.

The condition will either clear up on its own as the lungs develop and begin to produce surfactant in about three to five days, or the infant will not survive.

Prevention

The best preventive measure is to guard against premature labor.

The mother should be carefully monitored during the last weeks of her pregnancy for any signs of premature labor. In the case of diabetic mothers, the lungs and its structures may not yet be fully formed until the fortieth week of pregnancy, so this disease is possible at full term in these cases.

Hydrocephalus

Hydrocephalus is an abnormal accumulation of cerebrospinal fluid within the cavities or hollow spaces of the brain. Normally, cerebrospinal fluid is secreted in the cavities of the brain and absorbed by a membrane that surrounds the cavities. If the membrane does not absorb the fluid or if the fluid is blocked, the fluid builds up in the cavities. The fluid buildup causes the head to become enlarged and the brain to become compressed or reduced in size. This condition has sometimes been referred to as "water on the brain" when, in reality, it is water *in* the brain.

Hydrocephalus in infants

When hydrocephalus occurs in an infant, the loosely connected bony skull plates pull apart to accommodate the swelling. As a result, the head becomes greatly enlarged. In addition to having an oversized head, the child with hydrocephalus may have an abnormally enlarged forehead and swollen or enlarged blood vessels in the scalp. This condition

can lead to paralysis, blindness, mental retardation, inability to speak, and convulsions.

Hydrocephalus is usually the result of a brain infection or malformation in the unborn baby prior to birth. While the baby's head may not appear abnormally large at birth, it expands rapidly from month to month, and if untreated the child usually dies by the end of the second year. If the blockage is only partial, the individual may live for a number of years, or may even live a full life.

Hydrocephalus in children and adults

Although hydrocephalus is usually a congenital (present at birth) condition, appearing in infants, it can occur later in childhood as a result of an infection or tumor. It can also occur in adults as a result of these same causes.

Diagnosis and treatment

Early diagnosis, which is accomplished through the use of X rays and CAT scans, is vital to a possible cure or recovery. Surgery can make it possible, in some cases, to bypass the blockage or obstruction, causing the fluid buildup to escape through other exits. Often a small tube is shunted from a brain cavity into the abdomen or into a major blood vessel, and fluid drains from the brain into the abdomen or blood vessel. As the child grows, the tube may become blocked, again allowing pressure to build in the brain. If this happens, the tube will be replaced or the blockage removed. When surgery is successful, the probability of mental retardation is greatly reduced, and the prospects of normal development are increased.

Hyperkinesis

Hyperkinesis is a nervous disorder that affects mostly children. The condition is characterized by very high levels of physical activity, consistently impulsive and immature behavior, and extremely short attention span. It is four to five times more commonly seen in boys than in girls.

Also known as minimal brain dysfunction, attention deficit disorder, and, most commonly, hyperactivity, this condition is thought to be the result of a deficiency or malfunctioning of chemicals in the brain called neurotransmitters, whose job it is to transmit impulses between the nerves.

Although hyperkinesis does no physical damage to the body, it can trigger long-lasting social, emotional, and educational problems. For example, hyperkinetic children cannot sit still and concentrate for long periods, so they may have trouble with reading, writing, and arithmetic. They often appear to be immature, uncoordinated, and boisterous and may have trouble getting along with classmates, teachers, and parents; consequently, they

often suffer from a poor self-image.

Causes

The cause of hyperkinesis is not known, but several theories have surfaced in recent years. One states that the additives, preservatives, and colorings found in processed foods have a toxic or allergic effect on some children, resulting in hyperkinesis. Another theory states that a genetic defect or damage to a fetus during pregnancy causes this disorder. A third theory holds that, when deciding upon taking action, the brain has two systems—one which inspires immediate action and one which encourages hesitation and consideration—and that the neurotransmitters which control the "hesitation" response are malfunctioning in the hyperkinetic child. None of these theories has been proven or disproven.

There are no specific risk factors associated with this disorder, but it is thought that parents who were hyperkinetic tend to have children who also suffer from it.

Symptoms

A variety of symptoms point to a case of hyperkinesis. The hyperkinetic child is overly active, fidgety, restless, overly talkative or boisterous, impulsive, and seemingly uncoordinated. In school, this child has a very short attention span and seems to forget facts quickly, disrupts the classroom, does school work hastily and incorrectly, skips or adds words when reading, laughs too loud and hard, and prefers to play with younger children.

Diagnosis

There are no specific tests to help diagnose hyperkinesis. These symptoms seem to be present in all children to some degree, and since hyperkinesis is rather vaguely defined, the symptoms displayed by an individual child suspected to be hyperkinetic need to be carefully observed. The quantity, intensity, and duration of these symptoms may single out hyperkinetic children from others who are merely bored with school or who are having other behavior problems.

Treatment

Drug therapy has proved to be the most successful (and controversial) treatment for hyperkinesis. Several stimulant drugs appear to have a calming effect on hyperkinetic children because they affect the neurotransmitters' "contemplative" response (the one which encourages hesitation before action). However, these drugs have been shown to have unpleasant side effects such as stomach cramps, colds, nervous mannerisms, and even stunted growth. Therefore, many children on this therapy are required by their doctors to take "drug holidays" to give their bodies a break

from the side effects of the medication.

Special diets which attempt to eliminate all food additives have been prescribed in keeping with the theory that additives cause hyperkinesis. Studies on this treatment have been either inconclusive or contradictory. However, many parents report dramatic changes in behavior after this treatment, although part of the change may be due to the extra attention paid to the child whose meals have to be specially prepared.

Parents can help to influence the child's actions, in addition, by praising or rewarding good behavior and ignoring or punishing bad behavior.

Immunization

Immunization is the means of producing immunity, or resistance by the body to a specific disease. Doctors employ two types of immunization: *active* and *passive*.

Active immunization

Active immunization is accomplished by injecting weakened or killed viruses or bacteria into the body. This stimulates the body's natural defense system. Certain specialized white blood cells—which are manufactured in the bone marrow, are circulated in the blood, and are stored in lymph nodes and elsewhere—produce substances known as antibodies, carried in the bloodstream, that are tailor-made to fight the invading organisms. They remain in the body for years, sometimes a lifetime, to protect it against that particular disease.

Passive immunization

Passive immunization involves injecting ready-made antibodies—usually extracted from the blood of animals that have been immunized solely for the purpose of producing antibodies to be used in passive immunization. Passive immunization is borrowed immunity and is only temporary but serves to protect a person who may already be infected until the body has time to create its own antibodies.

Immunization can provide protection against measles, mumps, rubella (German measles), polio, whooping cough, diphtheria, and tetanus, all of which can cripple or kill.

Children's immunizations

To be completely protected against diphtheria, tetanus, and whooping cough (pertussis), a child needs a shot of the combination diphtheria-tetanus-pertussis (DTP) vaccine at two, four, six, and eighteen months and a booster shot upon entering school around age five years. When the child gets the DTP shots, he or she should also receive by mouth a drop of the oral polio vaccine (although since there are usually only four doses of polio vaccine, the child

does not receive it at six months of age). At 15 months a child should have a combined shot for measles, rubella, and mumps. He or she should be tested for tuberculosis at the end of the first year and receive a tetanus-diphtheria booster shot between 14 and 16 years of age.

Parents who do not have a family physician can call their local public health department. It usually has supplies of vaccine and may give shots free.

Nephrotic syndrome

Nephrotic syndrome is a disorder most commonly affecting children in which the glomeruli, tiny clumps of blood vessels in the kidneys that filter urine, do not work properly. The defective glomeruli allow proteins, most notably albumin, to escape from the bloodstream and seep into the urine while letting fluid that should be eliminated as waste accumulate under the skin.

Causes

Nephrotic syndrome is caused by other diseases that affect the kidneys and although it is a relatively rare disorder, it is a serious one that requires careful treatment for children who are afflicted by it. The syndrome causes a vulnerability to other infections, including peritonitis (inflammation of the lining of the abdominal cavity), and the risk that the condition may persist and develop into chronic glomerulonephritis and eventually kidney failure.

Symptoms

As a result of fluid accumulation, the child's body gradually swells up (edema), becoming especially bloated around the face, abdomen, and ankles. In addition, the child urinates very little, about one fifth the normal amount. The syndrome usually affects children between the ages of one and six years, more often boys than girls.

To prevent complications, a doctor should be consulted as soon as a child either urinates less often or has unusual swelling in the face, abdomen, or ankles.

Diagnosis

If initial blood and urine tests point to nephrotic syndrome, the doctor will order more tests and possibly a kidney biopsy (tissue sample) to confirm the diagnosis.

Treatment

With proper medical care, usually in a hospital where medication (diuretics to eliminate excess fluid and steroids to control inflammation) and diet (high in protein and low in salt) can be carefully supervised, the condition can be controlled. Symptoms are likely to clear up after a few weeks and the child can finish recuperating at home, sometimes with no aftereffects, other times with a relapse after several weeks or months.

Osteomyelitis

Osteomyelitis is inflammation of the bone and bone marrow due to a pus-producing bacterial infection. It is considered a childhood disease, occurring most often in boys between the ages of five and 14, but it also occurs among adults. Since the introduction of antibiotics, osteomyelitis is rare in the United States, but it is still common in countries lacking good medical care and proper nutrition.

Causes

Although bone is fed essential oxygen and nutrients by blood vessels, blood may also carry bacteria, which tend to settle in the capillaries of the long (arm and leg) bones. Germs can also reach the bones directly from adjacent infected tissue or through an open wound or fracture. Usually osteomyelitis affects only one area of the bone or bone marrow, but can attack more than one bone at a time.

Symptoms

Symptoms include: pain and excruciating tenderness near a joint or at the affected area; fever in the 102° to 104°F range; redness; and swelling. Although a physician can often diagnose osteomyelitis from the visible symptoms, X rays and blood tests confirm its presence.

Treatment

The child with the condition is often hospitalized and given antibiotics in liquid, tablet, or intravenous (into the vein) form. Doctors may drain the pus and clean the area in a minor surgical procedure and then immobilize the limb in a splint. The child is released from the hospital once the healing begins, but may have to take antibiotics for six more weeks.

Complications

Complications may prolong treatment. Possible complications are blood poisoning (septicemia); destruction of the bone; spread of the infection to a nearby joint, possibly resulting in a permanent deformity or stiffness; transference of the infection to the surface of the skin where it erupts as an abscess; damage to the bone cartilage (elastic connective tissue) that retards bone growth; and suppurative (infectious) arthritis.

Chronic (long-term) osteomyelitis is a possible delayed complication of acute (sudden) osteomyelitis, especially if it results from a fracture or the presence of a foreign body in the wound such as a bullet or metal surgical piece. The major signs of chronic osteomyelitis are a flare-up or reopening of an abscessed wound, with a fluctuating discharge of pus and pain, and bone that feels thickened and is covered over by scars. X rays show irregular bone and pieces of dead bone. Chronic osteomyelitis can be prevented by immediate antibiotic treatment of the acute variety.

Treatment for chronic osteomyelitis may be extensive. It may take several successive operations to remove all the dead bone and tissue, completely drain the abscess, and repair bone when possible. Large doses of antibiotics may be required.

Prevention

To prevent osteomyelitis, clean and disinfect all wounds thoroughly and, especially in children, apply a bandage to keep the area clean until it has healed.

Patent ductus arteriosus

Patent ductus arteriosus is a congenital (present at birth) heart disorder in which the ductus arteriosus, an extra blood vessel present in the fetus (unborn child) which allows the blood to pass from the pulmonary artery to the aorta (two of the main blood vessels leading directly from the heart), fails to close after birth. It is most common in premature babies.

If the ductus arteriosus fails to close after birth, incorrect flow of blood will put a strain on the baby's heart.

During the gestation period (the nine months of fetal growth and development in the uterus), the fetus is immersed in amniotic fluid and, thus, the lungs are not used. Therefore, the blood bypasses the lungs through this extra vessel, and the fetus receives oxygen from the placenta (which nourishes the unborn child).

If the ductus arteriosus remains open after birth, blood continues to flow through it. Since blood continues to bypass the lungs, it carries less oxygen than is required to supply body tissues.

Cause

In most babies, the duct begins to close before birth and is completely closed by age three months. The reasons for this normal closure, or for failure to close, are poorly understood.

Symptoms

Although obvious symptoms are rare, the affected infant may display shortness of breath or develop congestive heart failure.

Treatment

Patent ductus arteriosus can be treated with medication if diagnosed early (various prenatal—before birth—tests have become available in recent years for diagnosis if the condition is suspected) or can be eliminated by tying off the duct in a simple surgical procedure.

Phimosis

Phimosis is a constriction of the foreskin (skin fold over the head of the penis) that prevents the foreskin from being drawn back over the head (glans).

Causes

The cause of phimosis is either congenital (present at birth) or acquired. The acquired form is usually due to an infection involving the penis that leaves adhesions — growths of tissue that adhere both to the inner aspect of the foreskin and to the glans itself. Phimosis also prevents debris (common dirt, dead cells, and normal fluid secretions) from escaping, thereby causing the debris to stagnate between the foreskin and glans providing an excellent place for bacteria to grow. Once infection is established, ulceration of the glans and swelling of the lymph nodes in the groin can occur.

Treatment

The definitive treatment for this condition is circumcision — the surgical removal of the foreskin. If, for some reason, this must be delayed, there must be careful attention to keeping the area clean and dry and free from infection until the situation is corrected.

Pinworms

Pinworms is a term that refers to a condition in which the gastrointestinal tract and occasionally other sites such as the female reproductive tract are infested by any of a variety of worms, called *oxyurids*. These worms are tiny (about 3 to 10 millimeters in length).

Cause

The usual cause of the infestation is the ingestion (consumption) of the worm's fertilized eggs by eating food contaminated with the eggs. Contamination results from contact with fingers that have been in contact with feces. Eggs can also survive on bedclothing and linens for two or three weeks.

Symptoms

Many children who have pinworms do not have obvious symptoms. Such symptoms that may occur are itching around the anus (the opening from the large intestine to outside the body), accompanied by inflammation of the anal tissues. After being ingested, the eggs hatch and release their larvae into the upper portion of the small intestine. The larvae mature as they pass up through the first part of the large intestine. After mating, the adult male worms die and the females migrate on down the large intestine to the anal region, where they lay their eggs around the anus. The eggs are transferred from the anus to the mouth on the child's hands, and the cycle continues. Pinworms can be transmitted to other children and adults in the same manner. Also, the hatched larvae can migrate back through the anus and into the bowel.

Worms can also cause irritation, inflammation, and obstruction in the appendix. In addition, pinworms can work their way into a female's vagina and urethra (the passageway from the bladder to the outside) and cause inflammation and/or infection in the vagina, the reproductive system, and the bladder.

Diagnosis

Aside from noting the symptom of itching, the diagnosis is made by identifying the eggs or worms under a microscope. An easy and inexpensive way to accomplish this is to wrap a piece of cellophane tape—sticky side out — around a tongue depressor. This swab is then placed against the anal area. The contents from the swab are then transferred to a slide for microscopic examination. This procedure should be done in the morning before bathing and on several consecutive days.

Treatment

Treatment of pinworms is not difficult. Usually one dose of the drug pyrantel pamoate is sufficient. Other medications are also available. In addition, in group infestations, all members should be treated simultaneously, and their bedclothes, linens, and underwear laundered at the same time. Also, the eggs around the anus should be removed by cleaning the anal area thoroughly at the time of treatment. Reinfestation is common, and when symptoms develop, another course of treatment is necessary.

Prevention

It is important to teach children clean eating habits, to encourage them to wash their hands frequently, and to keep an eye open for other children who may be infected (as evidenced by scratching around the anus).

Reye's syndrome

Reye's syndrome is a type of encephalitis (inflammation of the brain) that also affects the liver. It is a somewhat rare, noncontagious disease that strikes children under the age of 18, often after they are recovering from a viral infection such as influenza or chicken pox. It is most commonly seen in children between the ages of five and 11 years and most often between December and March.

Reye's syndrome is a serious disease that requires immediate treatment. It is fatal in 25 percent of all cases.

This disorder is different from other types of encephalitis because it not only causes the brain to swell but also causes fatty deposits to collect in the liver, thereby resulting in malfunctions in both organs. Brain damage, coma, or death can result if it is not diagnosed and treated quickly.

Cause

The exact cause of Reye's syndrome is not known, but since it almost always follows a viral infection, it has been theorized that the virus combines with another unknown substance in the body and produces a damaging poison.

Symptoms

The symptoms of Reye's syndrome are sudden vomiting, abnormal sleepiness or hyperactivity, and confusion. Convulsions and coma may occur as the disease progresses.

Diagnosis

Early diagnosis is crucial. Reye's syndrome is diagnosed by careful observation of the symptoms; testing of a sample of cerebrospinal fluid (the clear fluid of the central nervous system, produced in the brain) but only if there is no suspicion that there is increased pressure in the brain; blood tests to determine the presence of liver damage; and tests of the blood sugar level because it is often low in young children who develop this disease.

Treatment

There is no known cure for Reye's syndrome. Treatment usually consists of helping the child to weather the first few days of the illness, maintaining normal blood sugar levels and reducing pressure on the swollen brain. Usually, if the child survives for three or four days, the symptoms will subside and recovery will follow.

If blood sugar is low, normal levels should be restored with the injection of glucose, a form of sugar, into the veins. Increased pressure on the brain from the swelling is also reduced with medication.

Prevention

There are no specific steps to prevent Reye's syndrome. How-

Severe scoliosis can be seen when viewing a child from the back, and even mild scoliosis can be noticed when the child bends at the waist. Bending forward rotates the chest making one side of the back more prominent.

ever, although it has not been proven that aspirin causes or promotes Reye's syndrome, it is recommended that aspirin not be given to children with a viral infection, especially chicken pox and influenza.

Scoliosis

Scoliosis is sideways curvature of the spine. There is usually a main curve in one direction and an upper and/or lower curve to compensate for it in the opposite direction.

Causes

Scoliosis can result from unequal leg lengths, or it may be due to defective development of the vertebrae (backbones) while an unborn baby is growing in the uterus. Paralysis of trunk muscles on one side of the body caused by polio, cerebral palsy, or muscular dystrophy; tilting of the pelvis in hip disease; or deformities of the spine caused by rickets or rheumatism can also lead to scoliosis.

There is no known cause, however, for the most common kind of scoliosis, known as idiopathic (cause unknown) scoliosis. It occurs during childhood and results in the curvature of a previously straight spine. Before the age of three years, mostly boys are affected, with an upper curve to the left and a lower curve to the right. Between the ages of four and ten years, both boys and girls are affected in equal numbers, and the curves are varied. Most prevalent is the adolescent form, usually affecting girls between age ten and the time their skeletons mature. Most often, the upper spinal area (behind the chest) curves to the right, with compensating curves to the left in the lower neck area and in the small of the back. If untreated, scoliosis can produce diminished lung capacity, back pain, spinal arthritis, and disk disease.

Symptoms

Parents should be alert for the signs of scoliosis, which may be noticed first as an apparently uneven hemline, unequal pant legs, or one hip higher than the other. To inspect your child, ask the child to stand up straight with shirt off while you observe from the rear. Notice if one shoulder is higher than the other or if one shoulder blade sticks out. With the arms hanging loosely at the sides, notice if one arm hangs away from the body farther than does the other. See if one hip appears higher or more prominent than the other. See if the child seems to tilt to one side. Finally, ask your child to bend forward, arms hanging in front and palms together at the level of the knees. A hump on the back at the ribs or near the waist may be a sign of scoliosis, as may be any "one-sidedness" noticed in the tests above.

Diagnosis

If you have any suspicions, report them to your child's doctor, who will give the child a similar checkup and if necessary take X rays or call in an orthopedic surgeon to confirm the diagnosis.

Treatment

Treatment of scoliosis may involve only exercises if the curvature is mild. Sit-ups, exercises to stretch the spine, and breathing exercises may strengthen the muscles of the trunk enough so that they will correct the situation. Frequent X rays and physical examinations are needed to determine if the exercises are working.

More severe scoliosis may require a special brace, which is constructed of a leather or plastic pelvic girdle holding one vertical brace in front and two in back, connected to a ring around the neck. This often must be worn 24 hours a day, except when the patient is bathing or exercising, until the child's skeleton has matured. It is adjustable for growth.

The most severe scoliosis requires spinal-fusion surgery, in which certain vertebrae (backbones) are fused together, with stabilization provided by metal rods, cable, and/or staples. Before the operation, the patient needs to be placed either in a body cast for

Spina bifida is a defect of development in which there is defective closure of the bony encasement of the spinal cord causing the meninges (membranes surrounding the brain and spinal cord) to protrude as a sac from the opening.

three to six months or in dynamic traction (with weights and pulleys) for seven to ten days. Frequent checkups are needed after surgery to make sure that the correction is being maintained.

Spina bifida

Spina bifida is a congenital (present at birth) defect of development in newborn infants, marked by a defective closure of the bony encasement of the spinal cord, through which the meninges (membranes covering the brain and spinal cord) may or may not protrude as a sac. If they do protrude, the condition is known as spina bifida cystica; if not, it is spina bifida occulta. This defect can range all the way from a form with few visible symptoms to a completely open spine. The cause is unknown.

Description

Spina bifida commonly affects the chest and lower back regions of the spine and extends for three to six vertebral (backbone) segments. The sac, if there is one, may collapse while the child is still in the uterus, but fills with cerebrospinal fluid soon after birth. If the sac is not covered with skin, it can rupture and perhaps lead to meningitis (inflammation of the meninges).

Spina bifida can be accompanied by varying degrees of paralysis, depending on involvement of the spinal cord and/or its nerve roots. Since the paralysis is usually present in the fetus, it can lead to problems such as clubfoot or dislocated hip. In addition, the paralysis may affect the sphincters (closure muscles) of the bladder and rectum, resulting in genitourinary disorders and damaged kidneys. An abnormal convex shape to the curve of the spine may occur and can hinder surgical closure. Hydrocephalus (accumulation of cerebrospinal fluid within the skull) also accompanies many cases of spina bifida.

Diagnosis

The laboratory analysis of the condition begins with X rays of the spine, skull, hips, and lower extremities, if malformed. Urine tests are also necessary. Further tests depend on the extent of the defect but may include a CAT scan and an evaluation of the cerebrospinal fluid.

Treatment

Treatment requires an extensive evaluation of the child's condition by neurosurgeons, urologists, orthopedists, pediatricians, and in some cases, social service workers and psychiatrists who work with the parents. Closure of the defect assures a better outcome. Long-term survival and lifestyle depend on the type and extent of the defect to the spine, other defects present, the infant's general health, and treatment resources. It should be remembered that in addition to surgical closure of the spine, the infant may need other more extensive surgery to repair accompanying problems. The most common complications are loss of kidney function, clubfoot, dislocation of the hip joints, scoliosis (curvature of the spine), pressure sores, muscle weakness, and spasm.

Prevention

There is at this stage no known "prevention" for spina bifida; however, diagnosis through amniocentesis is growing progressively more accurate.

Strabismus

Strabismus is commonly referred to as "squint-eye" or "cross-eye." Technically, the term refers to a deviation of one eye from parallelism with the other.

Causes

Amblyopia, or reduced visual sharpness, results from suppressing the image from the deviating eye to avoid confusion. Disuse of one eye, as in cases of severe injury or impaired vision due to disease, may result in this form of strabismus.

Strabismus is usually present at birth (unless, as in the case of amblyopia, it results from later injury to one eye or impaired vision because of disease). The exact cause of congenital strabismus is unknown.

Symptoms

Symptoms include obviously crossed, wandering, or "squinting" eyes, except in some cases in which the lack of parallelism of the eyes is so subtle it cannot be seen.

Diagnosis and treatment

Complete evaluation of the eyes is essential to determine if there is involvement of a serious ocular (eye) or neurological (nerve) disorder in strabismus. If muscle imbalance alone is responsible, the strabismus can be treated easily with corrective glasses or contact lenses. Surgical restoration of the muscle balance can be done in more extreme cases. Eye exercises are effective in many less severe cases. Permanent visual loss can result if strabismus is not treated before the child is four to six years old.

Sudden infant death syndrome

Sudden infant death syndrome (also called SIDS and crib death) is the unexplained and sudden death of a baby who apparently is perfectly well when put to bed but dies silently in its sleep, often without any signs of a struggle. SIDS is the second leading cause (after accidents) of death in infants from two weeks to one year of age, with 8,000 to 10,000 deaths per year in the United States. Most frequently, deaths occur in the third or fourth month of life, with a higher death rate among boys, children of teenage mothers, infants from poor families, and babies who were premature. There are more deaths in the winter than in the summer. SIDS is a worldwide phenomenon.

Search for the cause

SIDS, before it was known by that name, used to be blamed on smothering in the bedding, but this diagnosis is inaccurate. It is also not attributable to vomited food clogging the airways, to bottle feeding, nor to any known cause that parents could prevent. Parents who have lost one child to SIDS are not known to be at higher risk of losing another in the same way.

Some investigators believe a combination of conditions is necessary to trigger SIDS, including a narrowed and inflamed airway, temporary airway obstruction, chronic oxygen deficiency, and irregular breathing, leading to a spasm of the trachea (windpipe) and death. Research is continuing.

Counseling for parents

Parents who lose a child to SIDS are totally unprepared for the death and usually have overwhelming guilt feelings — that something they did or did not do caused the death of their child. SIDS, however, is not the parents' fault. An autopsy will prove this fact. Doctors and nurses who take the time to discuss the death fully with the parents can be very helpful. So can another parent who has lost a child to SIDS. There are now many local chapters of the National Foundation for Sudden Infant Death Syndrome or the International Guild for Infant Survival, both of which can be valuable counseling and information sources.

Undescended testes

Undescended testes is a condition in which one or both of the testes (male gonadal or sex glands) do not descend into the scrotum (a small sac located between the legs), but remain in the abdomen, where they have developed before birth. This condition is also called cryptorchidism or cryptorchism and is not uncommon.

If the testes do not descend, they often degenerate or atrophy (shrink), and thus do not secrete into the system the male sex hormones that they would have ordinarily supplied. This, in turn, can cause the elimination or suppression of the development during puberty of secondary male sex characteristics such as body hair, heavier musculature, deepening voice, and so forth. Damaged sperm, or insufficient production of them, can also result from undescended testes, especially if the situation is still present in adolescence or adulthood. If one testis is damaged but the other testis is descended and normal, sexual development and reproduction function are normal.

Causes

The causes of this condition are not clearly understood. It is conjectured that perhaps a membrane in the abdomen gets in the way. If only one testis is undescended, the problem is most likely mechanical in nature; if both are involved, the underlying cause may well be hormonal.

Treatment

Treatment for this condition is controversial. In deciding upon treatment, three important considerations must be kept in mind: the potential lack of fertility of the testes, if they do not descend; the probability (or lack of probability) that they will descend without intervention; and the chances of the undescended testes becoming malignant (cancerous). Hormone therapy is sometimes effective, but in many cases where it is successfully applied, it is thought by some doctors that the testes would

Kidney

2nd month
of pregnancy

3rd month

6th month

8th month

9th month

The male sex glands, the testes, develop in the abdomen and gradually descend downward into the scrotum before birth. Occasionally this progression does not occur, and the child is born with undescended testes.

probably have descended by themselves anyway. Surgery to bring the testes into the scrotum is usually a successful treatment if done before the age of five years.

Sometimes, the testes can be made to descend by manipulation of the tissues around them.

There is no known preventive for undescended testes.

EMOTIONAL HEALTH AND MENTAL ILLNESS

Emotional and mental problems vary greatly in degree. Today, many mentally healthy people turn to therapy for help in coping with an emotional crisis—such as the loss of a loved one, a divorce, or the inability to initiate or sustain a relationship. On the other end of the scale are people who are so disturbed that they cannot function well enough to take care of their basic needs.

All of us experience emotional ups and downs throughout our lives and are prone to feelings of anxiety, fear, guilt, or depression. It is when these feelings seriously interfere with a person's ability to carry on with work or to deal with home or social life that a problem exists.

Warning signs

The borderline between "normal" and distorted actions and feelings is not scientifically exact. However, there are general warning signs of emotional or mental difficulties that warrant professional help:
• Severe anxiety that is not attributable to reality;
• Unreasonable fears of people, places, or events;
• Prolonged depression or the inability to recover from a major crisis or loss;
• Difficulty in getting along with other people or in holding a job;
• Self-destructive behavior such as compulsive drinking, gambling, or drug use;
• Sexual dysfunctions, such as impotence, frigidity, promiscuity, or perversion;
• Sleeping difficulties, insomnia, recurring nightmares;
• Feelings of hopelessness or confusion, suicidal thoughts;
• Inability to make simple decisions, moodiness, feeling out of control;
• In children, failure at school, disruptive behavior at school and home, senseless destruction, delinquency, frequent physical complaints.

Since some medical disorders (for example, low blood sugar, overactive thyroid) can produce physical symptoms that resemble an emotional problem (anxiety, shakiness), the first step in seeking treatment is to arrange to have a thorough physical examination. In addition to ruling out a physical problem, the person can also ask the doctor for a referral to a competent therapist or mental health agency.

Types of professional help

There are several different kinds of professional therapists qualified to treat emotional and mental difficulties:

• Psychiatrists are doctors with a medical degree plus three or more years of training in psychiatry. Psychiatrists are the only therapists qualified to prescribe drugs. They are licensed by state and certified by their specialty board.

• Clinical or psychiatric social workers are professionals with a master's degree and/or a doctorate in mental health plus two years of internship in a clinical setting. They are certified by state and listed in the *National Registry of Health Care Providers in Clinical Social Work*.

• Clinical psychologists are therapists with a doctorate in psychology and one year of supervised clinical training. Psychologists are licensed by state or certified by their specialty board or listed in the *National Register of Health Service Providers in Psychology*.

• Psychiatric nurses are nurses with master's degrees in psychiatry or mental health, accredited by the American Nurses' Association Division on Psychiatric and Mental Health Nursing Practice.

• Psychoanalysts are psychiatrists or clinical psychologists with special psychoanalytic training. However, a person with little or no training can use the title of psychoanalyst — be careful to check the person's credentials. At present, psychoanalysts are licensed only in California but others may be listed in *The National Registry of Psychoanalysts*.

• Pastoral counselors are members of the clergy with training and/or degrees in psychology or social work. They are certified by the American Association of Pastoral Counselors.

Finding help

One of the biggest keys to success in therapy is finding and selecting a qualified professional with whom the person seeking treatment feels comfortable. Before making an initial appointment, ask the therapist about his or her credentials. During the first appointment, ask for an explanation of the methods or forms of therapy the therapist uses; for an estimate of how long treatment may last and how much it will cost; and for an opinion on the results that can be expected.

The patient seeking treatment should ask himself or herself these questions: Do I feel comfortable talking to this person? Do I trust him or her? Do the proposed method of treatment and the expected results sound plausible? It may take more than one appointment or session with the therapist to answer these questions. If you have doubts, it is perfectly permissible to shop around for another therapist. It is also possible that, after meeting with you, the therapist may feel unqualified to work successfully with you; he or she may refer you to another professional.

Types of therapies

There are many kinds of therapy, but the most common are:
• Psychoanalysis: intensive psychotherapy (four or five times a week for several years) that aims to change long-standing personality problems;
• Individual psychotherapy: one-on-one discussion between therapist and patient about problems, worries, emotional attitudes, and ways of coping with life;
• Group therapy: shared experiences in a group of peers who may offer criticism and praise;
• Family therapy: therapy to solve problem interactions between or among family members;
• Behavior modification: a therapy method that involves breaking old habits that cause problems and relearning new ways of dealing with people;
• Drug therapy: treatment with medication, mostly used for people with severe problems, often in conjunction with another form of "talk" therapy;
• Relaxation training or biofeedback: behavior modification often applied to eliminate physical symptoms such as tension headaches.

There is a lot of misinformation about the subject of emotional and mental illness that is left over from the days when little was known about the workings of the mind and body. Some people still attach a stigma of "crazy, unpredictable, and dangerous" to those who have sought and received treatment for mental or emotional disorders. Such labels are not only unfair but usually inaccurate; the number of persons with problems who pose any threat at all to others is very small.

Fortunately for all of us, emotional and mental illness is gradually becoming better understood and accepted as a disease that can be treated and cured. Even more importantly, emotional health is being recognized as a goal that should and can be attained.

Anorexia nervosa

Anorexia nervosa is an eating disorder that strikes mostly young women who suppress the urge to eat and continue to lose weight to the point of malnutrition and starvation. It can be fatal, because an anorexic can literally starve herself to death while she continues to think of herself as fat.

Anorexics continue to starve themselves because they mistakenly believe that they are fat and need to diet. The result is not only an unattractively skinny appearance, but also an end to menstrual periods (which very frequently cease when a certain percentage of body fat is lost), and, most importantly, the destruction of healthy muscle and organ tissue, which, when starved, the body uses as energy sources.

Those at risk

Ninety-five percent of all anorexics are female; most are teenagers from upper or upper-middle class homes. About one in 200 women of this age and social class is estimated to have anorexia nervosa.

Anorexia seems to be a psychological disorder as well, as it often develops in young women with deep-seated problems, although the classic anorexic may not seem to be a "troubled" teenager. The young girl who has always been "perfect," obedient, and who has tried to fulfill all the wishes of her parents, teachers, and friends may become anorexic due to a subconscious need to have total control over at least one area of her life.

Impending adulthood and all that it entails may scare the anorexic into dieting away all that reminds her of her developing maturity: her larger breasts, curved hips, and fuller thighs. The lack of menstrual periods, too, is a reminder of the happier days of childhood.

Our culture's obsession with thinness as the ideal in beauty can also trigger the desire in an adolescent girl to diet down to her "perfect" weight; often a casual remark that a girl is slightly overweight has led to a case of anorexia in a susceptible person.

In addition, people with jobs or hobbies that require strict weight control, such as athletes, ballerinas, and fashion models, may find that simply watching their weight has become an obsession with dieting. In fact, the few males who develop this disorder often do so in an attempt to qualify for an athletic team.

Symptoms

The major symptom of anorexia nervosa is drastic weight loss to the point of extreme underweight, which can be accompanied by overly vigorous exercise that burns off the few calories that are consumed. Anorexics cannot be convinced to eat with threats or reasoning; they have a distorted body image that tells them they are fat even as they view their extremely thin bodies in a mirror.

Despite the refusal to eat more than tiny amounts of particular foods, the anorexic may be obsessed with the idea of food. She may prepare elaborate meals for others or go on eating binges followed by vomiting, which can be self-induced (bulimia), and may use laxatives excessively. Menstrual periods stop completely, and a growth of fine, downy hair appears all over the body.

Diagnosis

Positive diagnosis of anorexia nervosa will require the doctor

A person with anorexia nervosa has a distorted body image that makes her think she is fat even as she views her extremely thin body in a mirror.

first to rule out that the extreme weight loss has been caused by a serious illness such as cancer, infectious disease, disorders of the digestive organs, or inadequate absorption of vitamins and minerals. Anorexia can usually be positively diagnosed when the patient displays the classic symptoms before the age of 25 and has lost 25 percent of her original body weight.

Treatment

Anorexia is sometimes treated with hospitalization and forced feeding; but usually, anorexics can be treated on an out-patient basis by a doctor, psychiatrist, or specialist in eating disorders, whose job is to convince the anorexic that she must eat and gain weight, but that she will not be allowed to become fat. Her distorted body image as well as her eating habits must be changed in order for her to conquer this disorder. Most importantly, the underlying psychological problems must be exposed and resolved. Often, this means psychological therapy for both the anorexic and her family.

Bulimia

Bulimia is abnormal and excessive eating, usually caused by emotional factors. Victims of the disorder overeat far beyond the needs of their bodies. In extreme cases, they resemble alcoholics, employing food instead of drink as an escape from the problems of life. When distressed, they may even go on food binges and eat themselves into a stupor. Sometimes they may feel guilty after overeating and induce themselves to vomit.

Causes

To a bulimia victim, food provides a way to relieve stress. Some think that excessive eating is an unconscious attempt to recapture the feelings of security experienced in childhood when food was received from the mother. Psychiatrists have speculated that overeating may also represent a hunger for affection that was denied in early childhood when the child's attention was focused on the mouth and eating. It may be a substitute for affection, attention, or sexual relations that the

person is not now receiving. It may be an outlet for hostile feelings, since food is being destroyed by the acts of biting and chewing. Finally, the person may unconsciously seek to become more important and safer by becoming larger—through weight gain.

Bulimia is sometimes found among mental patients, especially those who have regressed to babyish behavior. Excessive eating may also result from hyperthyroidism (overactivity of the thyroid gland), whose victims burn up great quantities of calories without adding weight. In a very small percentage of cases, bulimia may be caused by damage to the appetite control center of the brain.

Treatment

Attempts to cure bulimia have not been very successful and have frequently caused the patient to become even more distressed. However, it is generally agreed that a logical first step is to help the patient discover the emotional causes of his or her disorder. This may require individual or family counseling by a psychiatrist or clinical psychologist, who also tries to help the patient gain confidence, become more sociable and self-reliant. New satisfactions are sought to replace those formerly found in overeating. A diet and exercise program may follow.

Delirium

Delirium is a confused mental

state marked by disorganized or incoherent speech and hallucinations (imagined perceptions believed to be real). Often the person is unaware of time or place; is fearful, excited, and restless; and suffers from delusions. The heartbeat is rapid, the pupils of the eyes are dilated (enlarged), and sweating is common.

Causes

The condition can occur because of fever, disease, injury, poisons in the system, or mental disease. It may result from the sudden withdrawal of alcohol or another drug upon which the individual has become dependent; from liver, kidney, or heart failure; or from deficiencies in certain B vitamins or thyroid hormone. It can also be caused by pressure on brain tissue — as in meningitis, brain cancer, or an abscess—or a bruising or bleeding of brain tissue.

Symptoms

Delirium often develops rapidly and fluctuates in severity. The patient usually cannot remember what has happened during the delirious period and does not recall past events well. Depending on its cause, delirium may last from hours to weeks. Partial or complete recovery depends on the nature, severity, and treatability of the underlying cause.

Treatment

Treating the underlying disease or condition is the first step in treating delirium. In the meantime, the patient should be cared for patiently and sympathetically in a quiet, relaxed, simple environment. Every effort should be made to answer questions, remove fears, and keep the patient in touch with reality.

Depression

Depression is a psychological condition characterized by prolonged sadness, combined with other negative mood symptoms, such as loss of interest in others, in work, and in recreation; indecisiveness and inability to concentrate; anxiety; apathy; loneliness; lowered self-esteem; and self-blame.

Temporary depression

Deep sadness or depression is a normal reaction of an emotionally healthy person to discouraging life events such as loss, separation, death of a family member, and disappointment. It is probably a protective reaction, enabling you to withdraw from everyday concerns long enough to sort out your feelings and prepare yourself for a new approach to life.

Temporary depression can also occur because of normal chemical changes in the body. Two examples are premenstrual depression and postpartum (after childbirth) depression, both thought to be linked to female hormone activity. In addition, certain drugs, including oral contraceptives, reserpine (used to lower high blood pressure), alcohol, and some sedatives, may cause a side effect of depression in some people. Certain infections including influenza, viral hepatitis, infectious mononucleosis, and tuberculosis can depress one's mood, as can a deficiency of Vitamin B_{12}, an over- or under-production of hormones by the outer layer of the adrenal gland, or various diseases of the nervous system.

Normal depression, which is a reaction to a specific disappointment or loss, is temporary. It can be helped by the support of family and friends or simply by the passage of time and by steps the person takes to change his or her life situation. Medication is not usually necessary, nor is any other treatment. However, a visit to a physician can provide valuable assurance that the depression is not abnormal.

Severe depression

Severe depression is another matter. Unlike normal depression, which is sometimes called *reactive* depression because it is a reaction to a specific circumstance, this disorder does not have an obvious cause. Also, the reaction is out of proportion to the seeming cause, and it may continue for weeks or months.

The causes of severe depression are unclear. Loss of a parent at an early age or growing up in a cold, critical, unstable, or unfriendly family setting may make it hard for a person to deal with life's losses and disappointments. A certain type of deepest depression, melancholia, may be caused by a chemical deficiency and is sometimes treated with the medication lithium carbonate. Finally, a small percentage of severe depression is linked to mental disease.

Symptoms

The symptoms of severe depression include crying spells, slow speech, agitation, hopelessness, helplessness, withdrawal from usual activities, recurring thoughts of death and suicide, and irritability. (Some of these symptoms also occur in moderate depression, to a lesser degree.) Early awakening, insomnia, fatigue, loss of appetite, weight loss or gain, loss of sexual desire, and imagined pains are also common. Depressed patients with certain mental diseases may hear voices accusing them of unpardonable sins, see visions of coffins or dead relatives, believe that others are watching or persecuting them, and suffer delusions that they are terribly worthless, sinful, or incurably ill.

Sometimes periods of deep depression alternate with periods of elation, high hopes, grandiose ideas, and overactivity. This is known as a manic-depressive condition. When in the manic state, the person is overwhelmingly confident and inexhaustible, racing from thought to thought. Eventually, however, the mood changes to blackest despair.

Diagnosis

Diagnosis of severe depression can be complicated. Some depression is "masked." The person is "smiling on the outside, crying on the inside" and may not even realize his or her depressed mental condition. Instead, the depression is expressed in physical symptoms, such as headaches or backaches that have no physical cause. In addition, the person may seem to have lost all emotion, including the ability to take pleasure in anything.

The examining physician needs to rule out any possible physical causes of the depression, such as that induced by disease, deficiencies, or medication. Drug abuse and alcoholism may be involved—but perhaps as results rather than causes of the depression. Schizophrenia and other mental disorders must be considered.

Treatment

Treatment for depression does not usually require hospitalization. Exceptions are those cases in which the patient is suicidal, in a stupor, agitated and out of touch with reality, or physically deteriorated as a result of the depression. Hospital treatment for the first three types of cases may involve treatment with drugs known as antidepressants or may include four to eight treatments of electroconvulsive therapy (ECT). In ECT, the patient is put to sleep with a general anesthetic and electric current is passed through the brain. This results in a seizure like that of epilepsy. After a brief period of drowsiness, the patient is often alert and in a clearer state of mind than before the treatment.

Most severe depression, however, can be handled out of the doctor's office with drugs, psychotherapy (counseling by a psychiatrist or psychologist, or preferably a combination of the two), with office visits once or twice a week at the beginning of treatment and fewer later if improvement occurs. It is extremely important to find professionals who are not only knowledgeable, but also reassuring and encouraging, as well as trusted by the patient. Elaborate psychotherapy over a long period of time is often not called for unless there is a serious personality disorder. If the depression is a secondary result of a serious physical illness, individual reassurance and support groups may provide the best help.

Lithium carbonate is used to treat manic-depressive illness both in its extreme form and its more moderate form, known as cyclothymia. In the latter type, the person alternates between brief periods (usually days) of gloom and elation.

Suicide is a major risk in depression and should especially be guarded against when the person seems to be recovering from the depression but is still feeling "low," when anniversaries of landmarks in the person's life occur, and in the days preceding menstruation.

Depression is the most common form of emotional disorder. It should not be disregarded and often can be reduced or eliminated with proper support and treatment.

Electroconvulsive therapy

Electroconvulsive therapy (ECT) is a treatment procedure in which an electric current is passed through the brain to create a convulsion of the central nervous system. Based on the belief that electric shock breaks down disturbed mental patterns, ECT is used chiefly in severe depression and manic-depressive illness (alternating periods of depression and elation). Occasionally, it is employed to arouse a schizophrenic patient from catatonia (an unresponsive state).

Procedures

Prior to treatment, the patient is examined, given appropriate laboratory tests, and may undergo an electroencephalogram (brain wave test) to detect any brain injury that might be related to the condition. Such an injury would rule out the use of ECT. Usually ECT is given early in the morning,

because the patient must not have had anything to eat or drink for eight hours before treatment. The patient is put to sleep briefly by an anesthetic given intravenously (into a vein). Electrodes are placed on one or both sides of the head and electric current administered. The seizure that results lasts from five to 20 seconds. Recovery is rapid; after half an hour or an hour of drowsiness the patient is usually alert and willing to talk. Some temporary memory loss is common, and headaches sometimes occur. However, the use of general anesthesia has prevented spinal injuries and the anxiety that used to precede shock treatments. It is said that serious complications of ECT arise in less than 1/10 of 1 percent of all cases.

A usual course of ECT treatments is two or three times a week for three to four weeks. A faster method, in which the patient's heart rate is monitored with an electrocardiograph, employs repeated surges of electric current in one to three sessions.

Hyperventilation

Hyperventilation is abnormally rapid and deep breathing, which serves to draw large quantities of air in along with expelling too much carbon dioxide.

Causes

Although hyperventilation can result from physical disease that interferes with the oxygen/carbon dioxide exchange in the lungs, most often hyperventilation is a physical response to stress, anxiety, and emotional upset. It begins slowly and builds up to a point at which symptoms appear and the person panics. The breathing then becomes even more rapid and difficult.

Symptoms

The diminished blood level of carbon dioxide can lead to buzzing in the ears; a tingling feeling in the fingers, toes, and lips; and light-headedness. It may also be marked by tightness in the chest and a feeling of suffocation—that is, the inability to breathe. Hyperventilation attacks may last up to half an hour or longer and may recur several times in a 24-hour period.

Symptoms of hyperventilation may be strikingly similar to those of heart disease and other serious illnesses. The individual experiencing these symptoms should, therefore, see a doctor to rule out the possibility of any of these more serious conditions.

Treatment

The symptoms of hyperventilation can often be relieved by having the person breathe into a paper bag. In this fashion, he or she immediately inhales back into the body the needed carbon dioxide he or she has just breathed out into the bag. In this way, the normal level of carbon dioxide in the blood can be restored.

Hypochondria

Hypochondria is the persistent and exaggerated worry — usually based on self-diagnosis — an individual has about his or her health, even though the person is not actually ill nor likely to become ill. It is sometimes referred to as *hypochondriasis,* which was originally thought to be the region of the stomach that was the center of melancholy or sadness.

Description

Hypochondria reflects an often morbid concern over any unusual physical or mental sensation or feeling. For example, to the hypochondriac, a headache indicates a brain tumor; a cough has to mean tuberculosis; and a mole is sure to be cancerous. Despite test results and reassurances, this person is convinced that he or she either has a serious illness or will have one very soon.

Symptoms

Frequently, the hypochondriac complains of pain or discomfort in the stomach, chest, head, or neck. Symptoms common among hypochondriacs include nausea, loss of appetite, vomiting, and belching. These symptoms become worse after the person has received expressions of sympathy and concern from family members or friends. In addition, the hypochondriac often makes repeated visits to doctors and uses numerous nonprescription drug items.

Treatment

Hypochondria is very difficult to treat. It has been estimated that only a small percentage of persons afflicted with this disorder recover completely. Psychotherapy is sometimes useful in such situations; however, it is often of more help if the individual can be encouraged to divert the energy spent on worrying about his or her health to more productive interests and activities.

Mania

Mania is a term that refers to an abnormal elevation of mood, characterized by wild excitement, overactivity, and lack of concentration. It is also characterized by excessive irritability, hostility, and sometimes violence.

Mania is the opposite of depression in the manic-depressive disorder, in which periods of elevation alternate with periods of depression, with periods of normalcy in between.

Symptoms

Persons in the manic stage are likely to go on spending sprees; start, but not finish, new projects; become sexually promiscuous; exhibit restlessness and distractibility; and chatter rapidly and often incoherently. In addition, their judgment is often impaired. Because persons in the manic state think they are functioning at their very best, manic individuals overestimate personal capacity for activity. As a result, many overextend themselves, becoming involved in many activities without considering the consequences.

Treatment

Mania and manic-depressive disorder are usually treated with medication and/or psychotherapy. The medication most commonly used is lithium carbonate. Lithium is most useful in preventing manic episodes. However, it may require several weeks for lithium to be effective and blood tests to monitor blood levels are essential since excessive lithium levels can cause serious side effects. It is not known exactly how lithium works to combat mania, although it has been shown that lithium affects chemical transmitters in the central nervous system.

Paranoia

Paranoia is a mental disorder or personality disorder characterized by delusions of grandeur and suspicion of persecution.

Symptoms

Paranoid personalities display unreasonable distrust and constant unfounded suspicion that others are out to do them harm; interpret innocent comments as personal attacks; develop grandiose or exaggerated estimations of their own worth, yet feel that others do not recognize their value; believe they are the center of attention because everyone else openly criticizes them; and strenuously defend their fears with reason and logic.

Occasionally, paranoia shows itself as unwarranted and extreme sexual jealousy.

An internal conflict between the need for recognition and the compulsion to guard certain aspects of emotional life may be the root of paranoia. Often, unconscious sexual conflicts play a role in the development of paranoia.

Paranoia differs from paranoid schizophrenia, a much more serious problem in which the individual not only has delusions of grandeur and a persecution complex, but also demonstrates deranged thought processes, hallucinations, and other signs of disturbed personality.

Treatment

True paranoia can generally be helped with psychotherapy and medication, if necessary.

It is important to remember that almost everyone exhibits some harmless, short-lived paranoia from time to time, usually from excess worry over an embarrassment or from disappointment.

Phobia

Phobia is a psychological disorder characterized by persistent, abnormal, and unfounded dread and fear of something that is not inherently dangerous or threatening to most people. It is also a suffix or word ending, which denotes unreasonable fear or abhorrence of a specific element as in claustrophobia, an intense fear of being closed in.

A phobia resembles acute or chronic anxiety but, unlike "free-floating" anxiety, it is linked to specific environmental stimuli: heights, open places, the state of being alone, travel, even blushing. True phobia affects fewer than 1 percent of the total population.

Causes

Phobia, like anxiety, seems to occur more often in some families. The anxiety itself is a fearful reaction to the emergence of forbidden or unconscious drives. In most cases, a set of psychological mechanisms called *projection* and *displacement* focuses the anxiety on specific external objects, persons, or situations that then come to stand for or represent the original cause of the anxiety. In shifting attention to the secondary symbol, the patient learns to use avoidance of the object or situation (spiders, heights, open places, and so on) to prevent rearousal of the painful anxiety. The "choice" of the phobic object is often at random; it may be the first object, location, or situation at hand when the original anxiety first appears.

Symptoms

Often, the very thought or mention of the phobic object induces anxiety in the patient. The closer he or she comes to the reality of the situation, the more the anxiety mounts towards panic. As a result, the patient spends more time avoiding the phobic stimulus and this very avoidance often begins to restrict his or her daily activities. Examples include the man or woman who cannot travel because of fear of flying or the victim of agoraphobia who avoids all open places in order to remain secluded at home where he or she feels "safe."

Common phobias

The symptoms of the phobias depend, of course, on the phobic object. *Agoraphobia* (a fear of open, public places, such as stores, malls, parks, theatres, or stadiums, or of crowds and crowded situations) is the most common phobia, accounting for about 60 percent of all such cases. This abnormal fear of being in open places greatly restricts the life of the person with agoraphobia, who in extreme cases will not leave home — except perhaps if accompanied by a close friend or relative. The first sign of the condition may be a panic attack when out in public, with feelings of anxiety, restlessness, breathlessness, rapid or irregular heartbeat, and approaching doom. Thereafter, the person may stay at home to prevent another panic attack. Often, the agoraphobic person experiences the phobia selectively — he or she can face the phobic situation fairly well in the company of someone close or trusted.

Another common phobia, *claustrophobia*, is an intense and unrealistic fear of being confined in an enclosed space, such as an elevator or small room. Commonly, the claustrophobic person becomes anxious even at the thought of being "trapped" in a small room or passageway. If the person unexpectedly has to face the phobia, as when caught in a stuck elevator, real panic may result.

Unlike some phobias such as a fear of mice, snakes, or spiders, which the average person seldom sees, claustrophobia can cripple one's vocational and social life since enclosed spaces are part of the everyday environment.

Other phobias, called simple phobias, involve objects. Some are childhood phobias, such as fear of the dark or of animals, and disappear with age. But adults, too, experience phobias of specific objects or situations: spiders, heights *(acrophobia),* or being alone *(monophobia).* If the objects are easily avoided, as with spiders or snakes, there is usually no great problem. However, fear of flying may cause great inconvenience for a person whose work or social life involves constant air travel, and monophobia may handicap a worker whose job requires long periods of isolation to complete a project.

The phobias of function, or social phobias, are those in which the presence of others causes the anxiety. Among the most common are *erythrophobia* (a fear of blushing) or the fear of eating, which makes the patient incapable of eating in the presence of others or in a public place such as a restaurant or cafeteria.

Phobias usually begin in early adulthood and follow a long course of alternate improvement and worsening of symptoms. Agoraphobia, the severest of the phobias as well as the most common, is the least likely to show significant improvement. The longer the patient has phobic symptoms (any time period over a year), the less likely he or she is to achieve a complete recovery.

Treatment

A type of psychotherapy called insight therapy may be helpful in less severe cases; patients learn to recognize the real, underlying object of anxiety and come to see the phobic object as merely symbolic of the "real" fear. More extreme cases often respond better to behavioral therapy in which the patient is deconditioned to the phobic stimulus by being required to confront the stimulus. At the same time, the patient is encouraged to try various relaxation techniques to combat anxiety. In the most severe cases, a technique called flooding is used in which

the patient is forced to experience prolonged phobic anxiety with a constant exposure to the dreaded object or situation.

Although drug therapy alone generally is less effective than when it is combined with psychotherapy, minor tranquilizers and antidepressants often can help delay or dull the onset of panic attacks.

Psychosomatic illness

Psychosomatic (or psychophysiological) illnesses are a broad, loosely-defined group of disorders in which physical symptoms are of mental, emotional, or psychological origin. They are not specific "diseases" or "disorders," as these terms are commonly used, but, instead, symptoms that are at least partly psychological in origin.

There are many ways in which psychosomatic illness can be fully defined. In some cases, psychological factors can contribute directly or indirectly to the cause of some physical disorders, as with heart disease and Type A (heart attack-prone) personalities, who show aggressiveness, competitive drive, preoccupation with deadlines, a chronic sense of impatience, and a feeling of time urgency. On the one hand, a Type A patient's heart attack is not psychosomatic in that the illness itself is of physical and not psychological origins, but on the other hand, the personality type can be linked rather definitively with this set of physical symptoms.

There are other cases in which psychiatric symptoms are direct expressions or symptoms of disease, as in disorders involving the nervous system or endocrine (hormone-producing) organs. In other cases, psychological symptoms occur as reactions to the physical illness, especially if the illness is recurring or chronically disabling.

Thus, the term "psychosomatic symptoms" or "psychosomatic illness" covers all these cases, but common usage confines the term "psychosomatic" to conditions in which psychological factors appear actually to cause the illness.

Causes

Current thinking on psychosomatic illness suggests that social stress may appear disguised in somatic form—that is, in the form of physical symptoms. Often the patient overlooks or denies the underlying emotional disturbance. Subsequent testing fails to reveal the source of the problem in many cases and diagnosis is vague.

Psychosomatic symptoms

Almost any type of symptom that can be imagined by a patient can be psychosomatic in origin. In fact, it is estimated that one third of all patient complaints to a doctor may be at least partially psychosomatic in cause. Sometimes, the patient may have previously experienced the symptom as a real condition, and at a time of social stress the symptom "reappears." Or the patient has a real illness or injury, is treated and cured, but still insists the symptoms are persisting. Occasionally, the patient may "borrow" the symptoms from another person (for example, he or she complains of chest pains while caring for a relative with a heart attack).

While almost any sort of symptom may be psychosomatic, the most typical complaint is pain—facial pain, headaches, generalized abdominal pain, backache, painful menstrual cycles in women, and so on.

Munchausen's syndrome

There is also a psychological disorder called Munchausen's syndrome, which is the technical name for pathological malingering or chronic fictitious illness. This syndrome involves repeated fabrications of illness, usually acute, dramatic, and generally convincing, by a patient who goes from doctor to doctor, hospital to hospital, clinic to clinic, for treatment. Many of the "patients" have studied medical textbooks closely and have learned to mimic the symptoms of unusual or dramatic diseases. Sometimes they even practice self-mutilation and give themselves abscesses, scars, rashes, even infestations of pinworms and other organisms. In some bizarre variations, a child or other relative is used as a surrogate patient and the parent or other relative will falsify medical history, injure the other person with drugs, add blood or bacteria to urine and blood samples, all in order to simulate a disease of his or her choice.

Diagnosis

Diagnosis of psychosomatic disorders is often difficult since the patient may be quite skilled at manipulation and deception or may be unaware of his or her own motivations.

Treatment

For patients with true psychosomatic disorders, such as those with Munchausen's syndrome, successful treatment is rare. Often, complying with the patient's wishes for treatment or testing relieves the symptoms temporarily, but usually the demands grow, and if the doctor refuses additional or more dramatic treatment methods, the patient often becomes angry and moves on to another doctor, clinic, or hospital. Psychiatric treatment is often refused or circumvented. Therefore, treatment is usually limited to early recognition of the true nature of the disorder, avoidance of risky or expensive procedures and testing, and refusal to administer unwarranted medication. If the patient can accept any kind of counseling or psychiatric help, that will, of course, become the treatment of preference.

Schizophrenia

Schizophrenia is not a single mental disorder, but rather a group of mental disorders that impair functioning and that are characterized by psychotic symptoms involving disturbances of thinking, feeling, and behaving. Among the characteristics common to most types of schizophrenia are withdrawal from reality, delusions, hallucinations, ambivalence, inappropriate emotional responses, and bizarre behavior.

Causes

Most cases of schizophrenia are considered to be "caused" by a complex interaction between inherited and environmental factors. Approximately 10 percent of close relatives of schizophrenics are diagnosed as schizophrenic themselves sometime in their lives. A genetic susceptibility appears to be an important factor in schizophrenia, but it should be stressed that schizophrenia is not "inherited." Even if the susceptibility is there, the obvious signs of the illness are connected to stressful life events and the individual's ways of coping with them.

Schizophrenia is not confined to any single age, race, sex, socioeconomic, or racial/ethnic group. It has a worldwide distribution, affects persons of all ages (although it commonly starts in later adolescence or early adult life), and seems to be a bit more prevalent in lower socioeconomic groups (however, some authorities guess that this is misleading; the diagnosed schizophrenic's inability to focus on career, profession, education, and related matters allows him/her to drift farther and farther down the socioeconomic scale. One interesting side note: most of those who develop schizophrenia in later life are widowed, unmarried, or handicapped.

There is no specific personality type that can be singled out as "pre-schizophrenic." Many schizophrenics do show such traits as extreme sensitivity, shyness, lack of emotion, anti-social behavior, and paranoid attitudes early in life, but an equal number of people with the same symptoms lead normal lives.

Symptoms

The onset of schizophrenia may be sudden or gradual. However, even in cases with an acute or abrupt onset, there will be definite stages: a prodromal period of increasing withdrawal and disintegration of previous levels of functioning; then a residual phase, with the onset of persistent delusional beliefs and emotional withdrawal. In the full-fledged schizophrenic state that follows, some or all of these symptoms may occur:

- **Thought disorders.** Clear, goal-directed thinking becomes increasingly difficult and thought/speech grow more diffuse. Sudden, incomprehensible changes of subject, fringe associations, a private symbolism, and obvious flaws in reasoning occur. Some patients report a thought block while others claim their thoughts are broadcast and shared.
- **Emotional changes.** Lack of emotion and inappropriate emotion are the most common symptoms, but mood disturbances (depression, excitement, anxiety, elation, perplexity) are also common.
- **Perceptual disorders.** "Hearing voices" is the most common, but all the other senses may be affected as well. The "voices" often are giving a running commentary on the patient's behavior or seem to be talking about him or her.
- **Delusions.** Delusions may involve persecution, illness (hypochondria), religious ideas, jealousy, sexual problems, grandeur, thought blockage or broadcasting, telepathy, or special significance (such as the belief that one is the Messiah or is the victim of a conspiracy).
- **Catatonic symptoms.** These can range from hyperactivity and excitement to stupor and immobility. Assuming odd positions for long periods of time can occur, and affected mannerisms (exaggerated gait, grimacing) are common.
- **Violent behavior.** Self-mutilation and petty crimes, as well as suicide, are common

especially when committed at the command of the "voices." Violent schizophrenics often commit a crime in the quest for recognition or acclaim and may seek out someone in an authoritative position, such as a parent or teacher, or a popular "authority figure," such as a movie star or political figure.

- **Nonspecific symptoms.** These include withdrawal from reality, abnormal activity (rocking, pacing), eccentric dress or grooming or dishevelment, perplexity, ritualistic behavior and "magical" thinking, depression, anxiety, anger, and hypochondria.

Diagnosis

The *diagnosis* of schizophrenia normally requires that the patient and his/her illness meet at least these specific criteria: (1) presence of certain psychotic symptoms, delusions, hallucinations, and formal thought disorders; (2) deterioration from an earlier level of functioning; (3) continuous symptoms for a period of at least six months; (4) onset before age 45; (5) symptoms not traceable to other emotional disorders; and (6) symptoms not due to organic mental disorders or mental retardation. Diagnosis must also rule out "mimicking" conditions, such as drug dependence, infectious disorders, and other mental disorders such as simple paranoia or manic-depressive syndrome.

The diagnosis of schizoaffective disorder is often made when the physician cannot draw a clear line between true schizophrenia and other emotional disorders. It often covers cases of an isolated incident (or incidents) of schizophrenic behavior with no recurrence.

Treatment

The chief treatment measures for schizophrenia include drug therapy, psychotherapy, counseling including social support, and gradual rehabilitation and retraining. For a first illness or acute relapse, hospitalization is usually indicated in order to stabilize the patient's condition. However, hospitalization for more than a few months may be inadvisable; if the patient is able to function outside of an institution, leading some semblance of a normal life may actually be therapeutic.

The drugs usually prescribed are antipsychotic medications. When patients refuse to continue oral doses of antipsychotic drugs, long-acting injections are often preferable to reduce the risk of relapse. Patients who display remission of symptoms should be given a "drug holiday" at intervals to test functioning without drugs, but careful observation and monitoring of symptoms should continue. Antidepressants may be substituted in some cases.

Electroconvulsive therapy is used only for catatonic patients or for those with the severest, most immobilizing depressions.

The cornerstone of most treatment programs is psychotherapy. Occupational therapy and gradual social involvement should also be arranged, as should a structured rehabilitation program. Careful control of environmental pressures is important. Both over-stimulation and understimulation should be avoided.

It should be remembered that schizophrenia is not necessarily a chronic disorder. About 30 percent of patients recover completely and most of the remaining ones show marked improvement, although impaired emotional response and lowered drive usually persist. With treatment, even active cases can be controlled within four to eight weeks.

No specific preventive measures are known at this time.

Senility

Senility is the term applied to the mental and physical deterioration associated with old age. While the term covers both physical and mental problems, most people think of mental deterioration when they hear the word.

Causes

The causes of senility are many: arteriosclerosis (hardening of the arteries); heart disease (with an accompanying loss of oxygen to the brain and other body tissues); lung disease (with a decrease in the lungs' ability to oxygenate blood); blood vessel diseases; and diseases of the liver, the kidneys, and other organs. Senility is not linked to a single disease, nor is it thought to be inevitable (some people are mentally alert at ages past 100). However, the years take their toll, and chronic disorders hasten senility. Life-long harmful habits are also a cause of early senility; alcohol, tobacco, and drug use are among the worst offenders.

Symptoms

Gradual loss of physical and mental vigor is the most common symptom of oncoming senility. A lack of interest in the surroundings or in activities once enjoyed is another symptom. Victims experience a loss of complex skills, such as the ability to do puzzles, math problems, logic problems, or even their personal checkbook balances. If the onset of senility is sudden, as it is with a condition called Alzheimer's disease, the victim will often be in a panic, as he or she feels mental powers deteriorating more and more each day. Short-term memory is one of the first faculties to go, and many victims are completely aware of the fact that their minds are deteriorating.

Physical senility is gradual, unless a chronic illness accelerates the process. The skin becomes dry and loses its resilience, the muscles lose their tone and become weak, the bones lose their strength and become brittle, and the organs gradually fail in their functions.

Prevention

While there is no way to stop the clock, there are many ways that one can continue leading a vigorous, active life all the way into the 60s, 70s, and 80s. Regular exercise; balanced diets; avoidance of toxic substances such as tobacco, alcohol, drugs, carbon monoxide, and other pollutants; and proper amounts of vitamins and minerals seem to have a positive effect on people at any age. Protection from debilitating disease and avoidance of injury (falls, broken bones) can also add years of activity to the lives of the elderly.

Much of mental senility could be avoided by simply not "turning off" the mind upon retirement. To stay mentally active takes an act of will. The mind begins to deteriorate quickly if it is not used—in some ways similar to the shrinking that unused muscles experience.

HEREDITY AND INHERITED DISEASES

In order to consider heredity and the hereditary aspects of diseases, it is important to understand the basis of heredity—the gene.

Genes

A gene is the basic unit of hereditary characteristics in the cell. A gene is a component of DNA which, in turn, is a component of chromosomes. Chromosomes are threadlike coils within every living cell that contain the "blueprint" or "genetic code" for the cell. This code is contained in strands of DNA, which is the basic building block of chromosomes and which is composed of genes. Each gene is an instruction for a particular characteristic. (It has been estimated that each cell contains about five feet of coiled DNA strands and each strand carries about 100,000 genes.)

When a cell, in the process of growth, divides itself, the DNA ladder splits apart down the middle; each side of the ladder then forms a duplicate of itself on the other side to create a complete new ladder.

It is the genes, then, as part of the structure of the DNA, that determine both what a cell is and how it works. It is as if a computer program not only told the computer what to do but helped to form the machine itself.

Consequently, cells that are coded to develop into tissue for the human liver, for example, do so because that is what their genetic coding tells them to do. Cells that give rise to bone tissue do so because that is what their genes tell them to do. The same goes for blue eyes, long fingers, brown hair, and all the other characteristics that an individual human body exhibits.

Sex cells

Each cell in the human body contains 46 chromosomes, made up of genes. The only exception to this rule are the sex cells—the ovum and sperm—each of which contain only 23 chromosomes. When these sex cells unite, as in the fertilization of the ovum by a sperm, the result is the full complement of chromosomes with genes that are donated by both parents. Since each parent

Chromosomes

Detail of
chromosome structure

DNA molecule

Protein-coated
DNA strand

Genes are contained within the chromosomes of every cell in the body. Chromosomes are threadlike coils that contain the genetic code for the cell. Chromosomes are composed of DNA, which has a spiraled, ladderlike structure. The composition and arrangement of the DNA determines the genetic code of the cell.

donates only 23 chromosomes (half of the genetic coding that makes each parent a unique individual), the resulting offspring is a blending of a portion of each parent's genetic material.

Dominant or recessive

The traits that genes give rise to are called *dominant* or *recessive*. A recessive gene usually carries a trait that does not appear because it is overridden by a dominant gene. Eye color provides an example. Usually, when one parent has brown eyes and the other parent has blue eyes, the offspring will have brown eyes. This means that for this particular union of genetic material, brown eyes are a dominant genetic characteristic, while blue eyes are recessive. Of course, it does not always work this way, and sometimes a child will have green or hazel eyes from a union of brown-eyed and blue-eyed parents. Furthermore, the brown-eyed child may have inherited the recessive blue-eyed trait. If, in the future, the brown-eyed person's recessive blue-eyed trait combines with another recessive blue-eyed trait in creating a new individual, the two recessive traits may override the brown-eyed trait, and the new individual will be blue-eyed.

Mutation

Genes sometimes mutate. This means that for some reason (a malformed gene, effects of toxic substances or disease, radiation, or even—as some have speculated—a chance collision between a gene and a radioactive particle) the offspring exhibits physical or mental characteristics that are not evident in either parent. The same is true in the case of recessive genes: sometimes, a gene that is normally recessive shows up in offspring when least expected. It can be as simple a phenomenon as, for example, a deformed ear that is shared by a great uncle or a grandparent but by no other member of the family.

The discovery of the structure of the DNA molecule has opened a new era in biological research, the most recent branch of which is called genetic engineering. In this field, through complex procedures and high technology, researchers hope to be able to eliminate diseases such as cancer by altering the genetic coding of the human body and its immune system.

Celiac disease

Celiac disease, or celiac sprue, is a chronic disorder of the small intestine caused by sensitivity to gluten, a protein found in wheat and rye and to a lesser extent in oats and barley. The disorder causes poor absorption by the intestine of fat, protein, carbohydrates, iron, water, and Vitamins A, D, E, and K. Removal of gluten from the diet normally brings improvement.

Causes

The basic cause is probably an inherited defect found mostly in people of northwestern European ancestry. For example, it affects one person in 300 in west Ireland, approximately one in 5,000 in the United States, and twice as many women as men. One theory about celiac disease has it that the body reacts to gluten and the related gliadin as if they were a virus or bacterium. When food containing gluten reaches the upper loop (jejunum) of the small intestine, antibodies in the intestinal wall are stimulated. In the process, for some unknown reason, the intestinal villi, which are hairlike projections through which food from the intestine is absorbed into the bloodstream, are destroyed. Destruction of the villi is almost total in the upper loop, less so in the rest of the small intestine. Poor absorption of food and water is the result. Another theory states that gluten/gliadin acts as a direct toxin or poison to the intestinal wall. One or both of these theories may be true.

Symptoms

Symptoms of celiac disease may begin in infancy when the child starts eating wheat cereal or other foods containing gluten. The child does not thrive, suffers painful bloating in the abdomen, and passes pale, foul-smelling, bulky stools. Failure to absorb enough iron produces anemia, a deficiency of oxygen-carrying red blood cells. Poor absorption of protein may cause edema (swelling of body tissues). There is little fat on the body. Growth may be stunted, signs of vitamin deficiency appear, and softening of bones may produce bone deformities and fractures. Sometimes the symptoms disappear in adolescence and reappear in adulthood.

Adults with celiac disease have many of the same symptoms, including bulky, foul-smelling stools, weight loss, vitamin deficiencies, swelling of body tissues, anemia, and bone pain. The disease may begin as late as age 60. It can also cause strange sensations in hands and feet, dry skin, eczema, acne, cessation of menstruation, mood changes, and irritability.

Diagnosis

The most definite test for celiac disease is an examination under the microscope of a piece of tissue taken from the wall of the small intestine. (The sample is taken with the aid of a flexible tube with a cutting instrument at the tip that is inserted through the mouth into the intestine.) Several samples may be taken. The specimen from a celiac patient has almost no villi and appears as an alternating flat and bumpy surface with a disorganized network of blood vessels. Various blood tests, taken after the patient has eaten specific substances, reveal how well the intestine has absorbed these substances. In addition, blood tests may reveal low levels of protein, calcium, potassium, and sodium. Tests of stools reveal excess fat in the waste.

Treatment

The primary treatment of celiac disease is to remove all gluten from the diet, which is easier said than done. Hot dogs, ice creams, commercial soups and sauces, candy bars, and all kinds of baked goods can be sources of gluten (even small amounts of gluten must be avoided). Many doctors refer the patient to a dietitian for detailed lists of foods to avoid and for advice in following a healthful diet, which should be high in calories and protein and low in fat. Vitamin and mineral supplements are given as needed. In stubborn cases, a cortisone drug may be given which will often result in improvement.

Recovery is most dramatic in children. For most patients, the outlook is good. In severe cases, complete return to normal bowel function and normal absorption may take months or may never occur. For that reason, and to rule out other diseases of deficiency or poor absorption, it is best to see a doctor as soon as symptoms appear. This is one ailment that is almost completely treatable.

Cystic fibrosis

Cystic fibrosis is a serious hereditary disease characterized by abnormal secretions that affect many parts of the body, primarily the lungs, pancreas, and digestive tract.

Description

When cystic fibrosis is present, the exocrine glands release abnormal mucus, sweat, or other secretions into the body. (The exocrine glands are those glands through various ducts and across membranes in order to transport vital chemicals throughout the body and to keep the membrane linings moist.) The most serious effects of cystic fibrosis occur when faulty mucous glands release an overly thickened, gummy mucus rather than the normal clear, free-flowing fluid. This thick mucus accumulates in the glands, causing swelling, forming cysts, and, more importantly, blocking various ducts throughout the body. This abnormal mucus secretion can affect many areas of the body. One of its most serious complications occurs when mucus in the lungs, which is normally present to sweep the lungs clean of bacteria and foreign particles, becomes thick and sticky, accumulating in the airways and creating a breeding ground for infection rather than preventing it. Consequent infections produce still more mucus, and the airways, already narrowed from the swelling, become even more clogged. Recurrent infections can lead to long-term breathing difficulties, and the condition becomes seri-

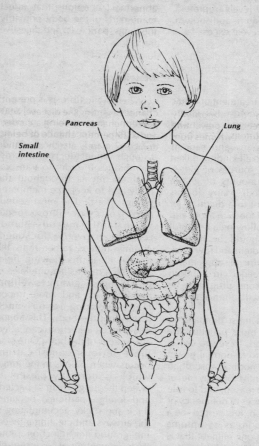

Cystic fibrosis is a disease characterized by abnormal secretions that affect many body parts, particularly the lungs, the pancreas, and the intestinal tract. In the lungs, thick mucus hampers breathing and promotes infection. Thickened secretions can obstruct the ducts in the pancreas and block the passage of pancreatic digestive enzymes into the small intestine.

ous. Most patients die from respiratory failure caused by obstruction of the airways and by persistent infections.

Also affected by this disorder is the pancreas, the long, thin organ that secretes digestive juices through a series of ducts into the small intestine. These ducts can be blocked by the abnormally thickened secretions, preventing important digestive enzymes from being transported to the small intestine where they are needed to digest fats. Similarly, the reproductive system may show these effects of cystic fibrosis. Reproductive tract secretions are also thickened, so that mucus may block the pathway of the ovum (egg) and make it difficult for female patients to become pregnant. Likewise, about 98 percent of male patients are sterile because a duct through which the sperm normally travels is blocked by thickened mucus.

Heat exhaustion is another problem related to this disease, because of the large salt loss through excessive sweating.

Cause

Cystic fibrosis is caused when a gene (a unit in a cell that determines an inherited characteristic in the body) is defective and adversely affects the exocrine glands so that their secretions become abnormal. This defective gene is recessive, meaning that it must be inherited from both parents for the child to suffer from the disease. If the gene is received from only one parent, the child is a carrier but will not get the disease. About 5 percent of the white population in the United States are carriers, with much lower incidence in black and Oriental populations. Approximately one in every 400 marriages takes place between two carriers. A child of two carriers has a 25 percent chance of getting the disease, a 50 percent chance of being a carrier, and a 25 percent chance of being completely free of the defective gene.

Symptoms

The symptoms of cystic fibrosis may show up at birth or may not appear until adolescence. About 10 percent of babies are born with a plug in their intestinal tract which requires surgery, but this condition is not exclusive to cystic fibrosis.

Typically, children afflicted with the disease eat well but gain weight slowly and show signs of malnutrition because the fat in their foods is excreted from the body without being used; the pancreas has been prevented from releasing the enzymes necessary to digest fat, so digestive problems are common and stools are large and foul-smelling. In addition the patient usually has excessively salty sweat, a chronic cough accompanied by mucus discharge, rapid and difficult breathing, and fatigue and muscle cramps from salt loss. Sinusitis (inflammation of the air-filled cavities in the facial bones), nasal polyps (growths in the nose), and a barrel-shaped chest from over-inflated lungs may also develop in some patients.

Many symptoms are indications of other, less serious, disorders, so unfortunately, cystic fibrosis cases often remain undiagnosed or undetected for some time while the disease progresses.

Diagnosis

Diagnosis usually includes a physical exam, medical history, chest X ray, and sweat test to determine the patient's salt level. Most cystic fibrosis patients have excessively salty sweat, although salt level doesn't indicate the severity of the condition. Tests of the stool and digestive juices can show how well the pancreas is functioning.

Treatment

Although cystic fibrosis cannot be cured, its symptoms can be relieved to some extent. Patients are advised to monitor their diet and health habits carefully: to reduce the fats in their diets; to eat very nutritious foods with high amounts of essential minerals and vitamins; to take salt tablets; to take pancreas enzyme tablets to aid digestion of fats; to take antibiotics, use aerosol mists, or receive vaccinations in order to fight specific respiratory diseases; to use mist tents; to exercise regularly; and to practice postural drainage (lowering the head below the chest) in order to help drain mucus from the clogged lungs.

Prevention

There is no means of preventing cystic fibrosis today. Researchers continue to look for a reason why the defective gene causes mucus to become abnormal, as well as for a way to identify carriers of the gene. One new test may break some ground; it measures certain chemicals present in the amniotic fluid (the liquid that surrounds a fetus in the womb) so that an unborn baby with the gene can be identified. Meanwhile, scientific advances in this area have at least helped those afflicted to live more comfortably with the disease. Until the 1960s, few patients lived beyond the age of ten, but today those with cystic fibrosis can live to age 20 or 25 or beyond because of medical advances in managing the condition.

Down's syndrome

Down's syndrome is a congenital (present at birth) disorder characterized by moderate to severe mental retardation and a variety of physical abnormalities.

Cause

Down's syndrome is caused by an error in the fertilized egg before it divides. Normally, each cell in the human body has 46 chromosomes — the genetic "blueprints"

Normal chromosomal makeup of the human cell is 23 pairs (22 pairs plus a pair of the sex chromosomes—X or Y) as shown in this diagram. In a person with Down's syndrome, however, there is an extra number 21 chromosome (trisomy 21, as shown in the box) resulting in a total of 47 chromosomes. This extra chromosome is responsible for the collection of symptoms known as Down's syndrome.

that determine the characteristics of the person and that carry instructions for performing all body processes. The cells in someone with Down's syndrome, however, have an extra chromosome, for a total of 47. This difference, in ways yet unknown, causes all of the unusual characteristics of Down's syndrome. In 95 percent of cases, the condition is called trisomy 21 (because the extra chromosome is attached to the 21st pair of chromosomes),

and the mistake is one that apparently could happen to anyone. In 5 percent of cases, the syndrome is called a translocation, and the defect apparently is inherited.

Symptoms

Down's syndrome (also called mongolism) is marked by somewhat slanted eyes in small sockets; a small, short head, flattened in back and front; a nose flattened at the bridge; a thick tongue; short hands, feet, neck, trunk, arms, and legs; a single rather than a double crease across the top of the palm; flabby arms and legs, with poor muscle tone; a wide gap between the first and second toes; retarded physical and mental development, with an average IQ of about 50 but ranging up to 80; and various deficiencies throughout the body. A child with Down's syndrome also usually has a poorly functioning thyroid gland (which regulates metabolism, the rate at which the body uses energy) and pituitary gland (which regulates other glands including those responsible for growth, maturation, and reproduction). About one third are born with heart defects, and both the skin and mucous membranes are especially susceptible to infection. Despite these handicaps, children with Down's syndrome are known for their sweet and lovable dispositions.

Education

Slower to walk, talk, and learn, Down's syndrome children can benefit from attending special nursery schools and play groups for retarded boys and girls. Most can attend public school in classes for the mentally trainable mentally handicapped; some can handle the work in classes for the educable mentally handicapped and eventually can perform at about the third-grade level. When they become adults, they will not be able to live independently but may be able to hold a simple, routine job, perhaps in a sheltered workshop.

Prevention

Prospective parents can reduce their chances of having a Down's syndrome child by starting their families early. A 20-year-old mother has only one chance in 2,000 of producing a child with Down's syndrome, while at age 35 the chance is one in 300, at age 40 is one in 100, and at age 45 is one in 40 live births. The age of the father also has some bearing on the risk, but not as much as the mother's age. Diagnosis of Down's syndrome can be made between the twelfth and thirteenth week of pregnancy, by testing samples of amniotic fluid that surrounds the unborn baby and contains cells shed by the baby.

Hemophilia

Hemophilia is a hereditary bleeding disorder in which the blood's clotting process does not function properly. Blood normally contains several factors that enable clotting to occur. These are designated coagulation factors I through XIII. In the most common form of hemophilia, classical hemophilia or hemophilia A, factor VIII is deficient. In this case, factors I through VII function adequately, but the clotting process is interrupted by a lack of sufficient amounts of factor VIII. Hemophilia B is the other form of the common hemophilias, although it occurs significantly less often than hemophilia A. Hemophilia B is caused by a deficiency of factor IX. Hemophilia B is also known as Christmas disease.

Cause

Hemophilia is inherited as a sex-linked recessive trait. This means that the condition appears almost exclusively in males, but the trait is carried only by females. In other words, a woman can carry the disease and pass it on to her sons without being affected herself. This is because the defective gene appears in one of the chromosomes that determine sex—the X chromosome, which is the female sex chromosome. Males carry the sex chromosomes X and Y and females carry two X chromosomes. Thus a male who inherits a defective X chromosome does not have a normal X chromosome to counteract the defect. A female, however, may have a defective X chromosome but her other normal X chromosome means that she will not develop the disease but that she can pass her defective X chromosome on to her sons who will have the disease. If she passes the defective chromosome to her daughters, they, too, will be carriers but not have the disease. Similarly, a male hemophiliac will pass his defective X chromosome to his daughters who will be carriers. However, he passes on only his normal Y chromosome to his sons who therefore cannot

develop the disease. A woman can be a hemophiliac only if her mother is a carrier and her father is a hemophiliac; in this case she inherits two defective X chromosomes.

Symptoms

Although affected males are born with the disease, the onset of symptoms is variable. Milder cases may not be readily apparent. Usually the symptoms of hemophilia begin during early childhood. When a cut in the skin occurs or an injury is suffered, the bleeding may be substantial and prolonged. In severe cases, spontaneous internal bleeding may occur without any obvious cause. Blood in the urine may result from internal bleeding. Pain is also a symptom when the bleeding occurs internally, between muscles and into joints. The course of the disease may result in irreversible damage to the joints, which, in turn, results in greater pain and in limitations in movement.

Diagnosis

If a child has any of these symptoms, or if there is known hemophilia in the family history, a physician should be consulted. The physician will order laboratory tests to diagnose the disease. The most common test for hemophilia is called partial thromboplastin time (PTT), a one-stage clotting time test. Additional laboratory tests may be ordered in certain cases. In addition, today, genetic testing can detect with increasing accuracy if a woman is a carrier of hemophilia.

Treatment

Treatment of hemophilia has undergone dramatic changes over the past several years. The treatment has become more scientific and effective. Plasma, the fluid portion of blood, contains more of factor VIII and IX than whole blood. For patients with hemophilia A, the plasma of an individual donor can be quickly frozen by a special process, slowly thawed, and separated into portions rich in factor VIII. This product is called cryoprecipitate. It can be prepared later for intravenous (into the vein) administration. However, cryoprecipitate has the disadvantage of requiring hospital availability for storage and preparation. Also, since cryoprecipitate is prepared from the plasma of a single donor, the amount of factor VIII is variable.

Treatment of hemophilia A has been further advanced by a process of rapid freezing and dehydration (removal of water) of plasma, called lyophilization. Freeze-dried concentrates are prepared and packaged, yet can be readily dissolved by a single mixing procedure. (This process is similar in concept to the convenience of freeze-dried coffee.) This concentrate is particularly efficient for home use in comparison with cryoprecipitate. The concentrate quickly stops the bleeding. Nevertheless, infection may result from the donors. The recipient of concentrate is placed at increased risk for infection compared to the recipient of cryoprecipitate. Whereas the latter is prepared from a single donor, the concentrate is prepared from thousands of donors. Hepatitis, a serious infection of the liver, is an example of disease that may be transmitted from a donor. Very recently, a new condition, acquired immune deficiency syndrome (AIDS), which is thought to be carried in the blood, has developed in several hemophiliacs treated with concentrate. This syndrome increases susceptibility to serious infection. Scientists are continuing to investigate the risks and benefits of concentrate compared to cryoprecipitate for hemophilia A.

Treatment of hemophilia B involves the use of fresh or stored plasma. Concentrate is also available for hemophilia B and is known as prothrombin complex concentrate.

Huntington's chorea

Huntington's chorea is an inherited brain disease that seldom shows symptoms before early middle age. It is characterized by disorganized body movements — the word *chorea* comes from a Greek word meaning "dance" —

along with mental deterioration. It is thought that Huntington's chorea is the result of a disturbance in that part of the brain that automatically regulates voluntary movements.

Cause

The condition is transmitted in a dominant gene from a parent who has the disease. There is about a 50 percent chance of a child's inheriting the disease from an affected parent. Since the symptoms of Huntington's chorea do not appear until the victim is between 30 and 50 years of age, a person with a family history of Huntington's chorea lives through the years of adolescence and early adulthood in dread of reaching the middle years when the symptoms may begin. Even more tragic, those who are unaware of a family history of the disease but do develop the disease may have children before discovering they have Huntington's chorea. In these cases, the victims have inadvertently put their children at risk of inheriting the disorder.

Symptoms

The first symptoms of mental deterioration are usually personality changes, in which obstinacy, moodiness, lack of interest in surroundings, and inappropriate behavior may be displayed. It should be noted that all of these types of symptoms can also be due to psychological or other disorders that have nothing to do with Huntington's chorea.

These symptoms are accompanied by irregular, jerky movements that begin in the arms, the neck, and the face. They may start as a mild form of "fidgeting," and gradually develop into facial grimaces, halting speech, irregular movements of the torso, and contractions of the neck that cause the head to rotate.

In advanced cases, the stance will become wide, in an attempt to maintain balance. The gait will become prancing, as control of the legs degenerates. As the disease progresses, the victims usually become paranoid, walking ability is lost altogether, swallowing becomes difficult, and dementia (loss of intellectual functions) increases.

Treatment

No treatment has been yet found to control the symptoms or halt the disease. However, the chorea may respond somewhat to some drugs, most notably haloperidol and chlorpromazine. There is no known treatment for the mental degeneration that accompanies the physical symptoms.

Prevention

Short of genetic engineering (which may be the only hope for genetically transmitted conditions such as this), there is no known preventive for Huntington's chorea. Presently, genetic engineering is still in its infancy as a science. Even if it were possible to "engineer" the faulty gene away, this would not help those who presently have the disease. It would only prevent the transmission of the disease.

As of now, the best preventative for Huntington's chorea is advising affected patients not to have children.

Muscular dystrophy

Muscular dystrophy is the general term for a group of diseases in which the body's muscles weaken and waste away. Muscular dystrophy almost always strikes in childhood and is usually inherited. Duchenne muscular dystrophy, which is usually inherited through the mother, is probably the most common form of the disease, but all forms—including that one—are fortunately rare.

Boys under the age of three are most apt to develop Duchenne muscular dystrophy. Girls are rarely affected. The disease is progressive, that is, it becomes worse rapidly once it takes hold. In severe forms of muscular dystrophy, the child must use a wheelchair to get around by the age of eleven or twelve. Scoliosis, or curvature of the spine, may also result from the disease.

Severe cases may be fatal, often when the patient is a young adult. Pneumonia is sometimes a fatal complication for the muscular dystrophy patient because of weakening of the chest and diaphragm muscles associated with breathing.

Muscular dystrophy is sometimes confused with multiple sclerosis. The latter is a disease of the nervous system that can ultimately result in crippling. However, there is no deterioration of the nervous system in muscular dystrophy.

Symptoms

Symptoms of muscular dystrophy may vary. Muscles usually begin to weaken first in the hips, legs, and shoulders. A child of four or five who waddles from side to side, who has difficulty standing up properly, or who falls frequently should be checked by a family physician or pediatrician. Sometimes the child even has difficulty standing up straight or raising an arm high above the head.

Parents should not be overly concerned about the natural awkwardness that occasionally overtakes the older toddler. However, a child near five years of age who consistently has problems with muscular coordination should be checked.

Diagnosis

The physician may want a muscle biopsy (a small tissue sample) to confirm a diagnosis of muscular dystrophy. The biopsy may be done on an outpatient basis in a hospital or in a physician's office with a laboratory for testing the tissue sample.

Treatment

Traditionally there has been no treatment for severe cases. An exercise program designed by a physical therapist may be helpful in mild cases. In such cases, the prescribed exercises should be performed faithfully to help slow down or hinder the weakening of the muscles.

In any case, physicians advise the parents of the patient to regulate the diet so that the child does not become overweight. The patient is not as active as other children and thus cannot eat as much. Overweight taxes the child's weakening muscles and makes life more difficult.

Prevention

Because muscular dystrophy is an inherited disease, women in the family should be tested to see if they are carriers—which means they could pass on the disease to their children. Such women should receive genetic counseling regarding any pregnancy.

Phenylketonuria

Phenylketonuria (PKU) is a congenital (present at birth) disorder characterized by the presence of increased amounts of amino acids in the blood and urine. (Amino acids are the chemical building blocks of protein.) The condition is marked by the inability to convert phenylalanine, a naturally occurring amino acid essential for optimal growth in infants and for nitrogen balance in adults, into tyrosine, another amino acid. Since excess phenylalanine is eliminated from the body by converting to tyrosine, this condition permits an accumulation of phenylalanine. The result is mental retardation in infants or young children if the disorder remains undiagnosed or untreated.

Cause

Phenylketonuria is hereditary and found in most population groups, although it is very rare in Jewish and black children. Incidence in the United States is about 1 in every 16,000 live births. There is no specific disorder or condition of pregnancy connected with phenylketonuria.

Diagnosis

Early diagnosis of phenylketonuria is vital since symptoms are usually not obvious in a newborn infant. Therefore, screening tests are mandatory for babies born in most hospitals in the United States. Sometimes infants with PKU will show neurologic (nervous system) disorders, very light skin coloring, eczema (a skin disorder), and a "mousy" odor about the body; older children may be extremely hyperactive. Often the light hair and skin coloring is an early clue to the disease; the infant will have lighter skin, hair, and even eyes than other members of the family.

Treatment

Treatment of this disorder within the first few days after birth is vital if the mental retardation that is PKU's most dreaded effect is to be prevented. Treatment consists of limiting the child's phenylalanine intake so that the essential amino acid requirement is satisifed without any excess. This can be done by feeding the infant special formulas with little or no phenylalanine. Milk is a protein food, rich in phenylalanine, so it must be avoided. When the infant is started on solid foods, low-protein natural foods, such as fruits, vegetables, and certain cereals, are permitted.

If PKU is not diagnosed in the first few days of life, the later results are usually extreme hyperactivity, seizures, and mental retardation. Some physicians think that treatment and special diet must be continued throughout the child's life. Others say it can be ended when brain development is virtually complete, around five years of age.

It is important to remember that, although untreated PKU can lead to retardation and other problems, early diagnosis and treatment can enable the child to develop normally and to lead a normal life.

Sickle-cell anemia

Sickle-cell anemia is an inherited blood disorder, occurring almost exclusively in blacks, that transforms normally round red blood cells into crescent or sickle shapes. The transformation is caused by defective hemoglobin, the iron-protein substance in the red blood cells that carries oxygen, and it occurs when part or all of the body is not getting enough oxygen. Because of their hooked shapes, the blood cells tend to tangle together and pile up, temporarily clogging tiny blood vessels and slowing circulation. Tissue formerly nourished by the clogged blood vessels dies. Furthermore, the anemia (lack of red blood cells) that results from the breakdown of the cells not only weakens the body but creates more oxygen deficiency, which produces more "sickling" of the cells. The disease is chronic, marked by fatigue, breathing difficulty on exertion, swollen joints, attacks of extreme illness, complications from other diseases, and shortened life. In the past, half of all victims died by the age of 20 and few survived past 40. With new technology and forms of treatment, the outlook is much better, although sickle-cell disease remains a chronic debilitating disease.

The disease occurs in about one out of 330 blacks in the United States. About one in ten

American blacks is a carrier of the defective gene for sickle-cell anemia but has no symptoms and is not affected by the disease. However, if one carrier marries another, the chance of each child being afflicted by the disease is one in four. The chance that the child will also be a carrier is one in two. Both the carrier state and the active state of the disease can be confirmed by a blood test.

Symptoms

Symptoms of sickle-cell anemia in half the victims begin between the ages of six months and two years. Among the first signs is an unusual swelling of the fingers and toes. The bones of the hands and feet thicken, and clumping of sickle cells may affect the bone marrow, where new blood cells are produced. Youngsters are especially subject to "sickle-cell crises," marked by severe pain in the abdomen, joints, bones, and/or muscles. These may last from four days to several weeks, and commonly occur eight to ten times a year before the age of ten. They occur much less often in later years. Signs of a crisis in a sickle-cell anemia patient include pale lips, tongue, and palms; lack of energy; sleepiness with difficulty awakening; irritability; severe pain; and a temperature of 104°F or one over 100° that lasts for at least two days.

Thickening of the heart muscle; enlarged heart, liver, and spleen in children; heart murmurs; and gallstones are common. The heartbeat is usually rapid. Children with the disease are usually small for their age. Those who survive to become adults have narrow shoulders and hips, a barrel chest, curved spine, long arms and legs, and an elongated skull.

Treatment

At present there is no cure for the disease. Treatment includes giving painkillers, making the patient as comfortable as possible, and treating problems as they occur. These problems include severe anemia, which may require a blood transfusion, and frequent infections that are a result of the body's damaged immunity. Avoiding cold, fatigue, and other stress may help to reduce the number of crises.

Prevention

Screening programs are available for those who wish to know if they carry the gene for sickle-cell anemia. Those who have the gene can get genetic counseling. There is no risk of disease in the children if only one parent is a carrier, but each child would have a one in two chance of being a carrier.

Tay-Sachs disease

Tay-Sachs disease is a hereditary metabolic disorder chiefly afflicting infants of East European

Jewish descent. It is marked by an accumulation of a certain type of fatty acid in the brain. The disease, which is progressive and always fatal (often by age two or three years), is characterized by retarded development, loss of vision, paralysis, and death.

Cause

The technical cause of the disease is a deficiency of a certain enzyme (a substance in every cell, which causes changes without being altered itself), and this deficiency results in the accumulation of the fatty acids in the brain.

Diagnosis

Diagnosis of the disorder may be made before birth by amniocentesis, a procedure in which a small amount of the fluid in the sac surrounding the baby in the uterus is removed.

There is no known treatment.

CANCER

Cancer is the term used to describe a broad group of diseases which have certain common characteristics. Most cells in the body grow and reproduce in an orderly manner, as dictated by the body's genetic information. A cancer cell does not follow the same genetic direction that normal body cells do.

Cancer cells grow at an uncontrolled rate, taking over, causing the death of, or replacing normal cells as they grow inside the body. As cancer progresses, cells are often sent through the circulatory system to start growth at other parts of the body. When this occurs, it is called *metastasis*.

The term *tumor* means, literally, "a growth." A tumor may be either malignant (cancerous) or benign (noncancerous). A benign tumor commonly grows within a self-produced capsule and does not invade surrounding tissue (although it can cause trouble by pressing on the surrounding tissue), nor does it spread itself throughout the body. Malignant tissues may grow out of control and quite commonly spread.

There are over 200 types of cancer that have been identified by pathologists, the physicians who study the body's tissues. In spite of the large numbers, there are three basic categories of cancer: carcinoma (cancer of the cells, known as epithelium cells, that line organs and serve many purposes including production of mucus and protection), sarcoma (cancer of the bony, fat, and muscle tissues), and fluid cancers (leukemia is one example of a fluid cancer). Some cancers may fall into more than one category.

Warning signs

Often a patient is the first to suspect cancer. This is why it is important to learn cancer's seven warning signals:

1. Change in bowel and/or bladder habits
2. A sore that does not heal
3. Unusual bleeding or discharge
4. Thickening or lump in the breast or elsewhere
5. Indigestion or difficulty in swallowing
6. Obvious change in wart or mole
7. A nagging cough or hoarseness

Since the chances of cure are greatest for the cancer discovered at an early stage, you should learn to perform the important self-examinations. If you are a woman, you (or a mate) should learn to perform the breast self-exam-

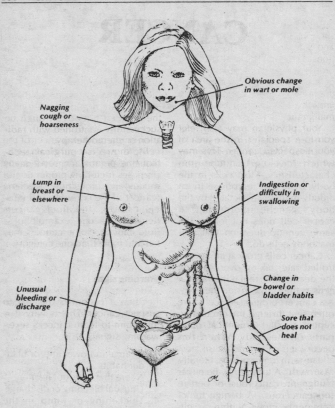

Nagging cough or hoarseness

Lump in breast or elsewhere

Unusual bleeding or discharge

Obvious change in wart or mole

Indigestion or difficulty in swallowing

Change in bowel or bladder habits

Sore that does not heal

The seven warning signals of cancer.

ination to detect suspicious lumps as early as possible. If you are a man, many physicians recommend testicle self-examination for testicular cancer.

Diagnosis

If you suspect you may have cancer, *do not delay* in seeing a physician. Following a physical examination, if the doctor suspects possible abnormal growth, he or she may order a series of tests, including X-ray examinations (for example, tomograms or CAT scans which are X rays utilizing an in-depth technique), nuclear medicine scans (liver-spleen scan, thyroid scan), ultrasound examination, cytology tests (examination of body cells such as is done in a Pap smear), and a group of laboratory evaluations. The doctor may also order a biopsy (microscopic examination of a tissue sample) to determine the cell type of the suspected growth and whether it is benign or malignant.

Your physician may also refer you to a specialist in the area of your suspected cancer. This may be an oncologist (cancer specialist), cancer surgeon, radiation therapist, hematologist (specialist in blood diseases), or a number of other specialty physicians. These physicians are specially trained to deal with diagnosis and treatment of your cancer.

Treatment

There are many ways of treating cancer. Many treatment programs (called protocols) have been developed that have been most effective in certain types of disease. Cancer therapy often includes surgery to remove the cancer, to clear obstructions of vital passageways caused by the cancer, or to cut nerve paths sending pain messages to your brain; chemotherapy (use of powerful drugs to kill cancer cells); radiation therapy (use of radioactive materials in the form of energy beams or radioactive implants to destroy cancer cells); or a number of other newly developed techniques. Often, combinations of the above therapies are used.

Surgery. Surgery is the most common method of dealing with cancers that develop into tumors. If cancer is contained in one area, surgery can sometimes completely eliminate it. New surgical techniques are continually expanding the range of tumors that can be safely removed. Furthermore, if the surgeon is able to remove only a part of the tumor, the reduced tumor can often be successfully controlled with radiation or chemotherapy.

More precise surgical techniques mean that surgery today is often less disfiguring than in the past. In addition, new developments in skin grafting make it possible to begin reconstructive work on patients — for instance, those with cancer of the head and neck —simultaneously with the cancer surgery.

Sometimes surgery is performed on a patient even though it is known that surgery will not cure the cancer. The removal of a tumor may simply make the patient more comfortable. In other cases, nerve pathways to the pain center may be cut. Certain noncancerous growths may be removed because they are a kind of growth that in some patients may develop into cancers.

Chemotherapy. Chemotherapy, the treatment of cancer with drugs, has gradually become much more significant. More than 12 kinds of cancer can now be effectively treated by chemotherapy alone. However, cancer drugs are most often used as an adjuvant, that is, as a backup to primary treatment such as surgery. Once surgery has reduced a cancer, chemotherapy can often eliminate it. Chemotherapy has proved effective against some forms of cancer that used to be almost always fatal, particularly Hodgkin's disease, acute lymphocytic leukemia (a blood disease of children), and cancer of the testes (the male sex glands).

Most cancer drugs attack any fast-reproducing cells in the body whether they are cancerous or not, producing some of the well-known side effects of chemotherapy. Destruction of normal cells that reproduce frequently, such as those in the digestive tract, the hair follicles, and the bone marrow, can lead to nausea, hair loss, and lowered red blood cell count.

Usually several drugs are administered in combination. If the cancer does not respond, or a resistance to a drug develops, another combination may be attempted.

Radiation. Radiation destroys the ability of cells to divide. Cancer cells are far more susceptible to radiation than normal cells, although not all cancers respond to radiation. Like surgery, radiation therapy is a localized treatment, directed at a particular cancer site. Radiation treatment may also involve directly implanting into a tumor a radioactive pellet that destroys from within. Radiation can be used before surgery to reduce a tumor to operable size, and frequently a patient receives radiation after surgery to destroy any cancer cells that might remain near the cancer site. In addition, some tumors can be treated by radiation alone.

Radiation can be especially useful in cancers for which surgery will impair basic bodily functions. For example, surgery for cancer of the testes may leave the patient impotent, while radiation treatment avoids this; radiation treatment of cancer of the larynx preserves the voice box; and in the case of breast cancer, radiation can prevent the disfiguring effects of surgery. However, even in these forms of cancer, surgery may often be necessary.

Radiation therapy is being continually refined. Drugs have been discovered that make cancer cells more sensitive to radiation. Different forms of radiation are being tested on resistant cancers. In addition, radiation today can be directed more precisely, and in stronger forms, with little harm to overlying tissue. However, there are still side effects including loss of appetite, nausea, and temporary hair loss. It is not certain how dangerous it is to be treated with radiation, which is itself a carcinogen; however, it is believed that a cancer in the body is far more threatening than the future effects of radiation therapy.

Immunotherapy. The goal of immunotherapy is to enable the patient's own body to produce substances that resist the growth of cancer. The basis of immunotherapy is the theory that cancer develops when, for some reason, the body fails to destroy abnormal cells. So far, immunotherapy is still in the experimental stage.

Interferon is a natural substance produced by the body to resist viruses. In the laboratory, interferon has been observed to prevent cancer cells from multiplying. Yet, so far, interferon has been very costly to produce artificially, and in tests it has not been as effective as standard treatments. It is likely that in the future strengthening the body's defenses will become an important weapon against cancer.

Heat therapy. Heat therapy, or hyperthermia, now being used experimentally, may soon become standard treatment for some kinds of cancer. Tumors have been shown to shrink when their temperature is raised. The circulation inside tumors is much more sluggish than in normal tissue—thus a tumor can usually endure far less heat. Temperatures tolerable to normal cells can be deadly to cancers. Heat therapy is largely painless. An instrument called a Magnetrode can deliver heat to inner portions of the body without harming overlying tissue. However, not all patients can be treated with hyperthermia; the location of the tumor or the weakened health of the patient may rule out heat therapy. At this point, heat therapy has been most effective when used in combination with radiation or chemotherapy.

Laetrile. Laetrile is an extract of apricot pits that some have proclaimed is a cure for cancer. This substance has been banned because it has been shown to be of no value against cancer in laboratory animals and has been shown to be poisonous.

Sometimes, in desperation, a patient or the family will seek unorthodox methods of treatment, such as laetrile. The medical community is actively researching all known methods of treating cancer and carefully evaluating those that look most promising. Many treatments are slow, and often have severe side effects. Many quack cures, however, offer — but do not deliver — rapid cure with fewer side effects. The harm done by quack practitioners is that they prevent a patient from seeking *effective* treatment until it is too late for *any* treatment to be of use. The best advice is to trust a physician to treat cancer and not waste time, money, and hope on a quack.

There are many places to get cancer treatment. Most cancers can be effectively treated at a well-equipped and staffed community hospital. There are, however, a number of large cancer centers throughout the country where specialized protocols are available. Often diagnosis and/or treatment is initiated at a special center and then continued in the community by an oncologist and/or family physician. If you need information or referrals, cancer hotlines or the American Cancer Society are valuable resources. In the event you wish a second opinion about your case, either resource, or your personal physician, should assist you in getting another evaluation.

Those at risk

Who develops cancer? This is a question that is very difficult, if not impossible, to answer. There are, however, certain risk factors that increase the possibility that you may develop cancer in your lifetime. Among these are age—as a rule, the older you are, the higher your risk of getting cancer; in some cases family history, for example, if your mother or sister had breast cancer, your risk of developing breast cancer is increased; and environmental and other factors.

The rapid increase in cancer rates during this century has been blamed, to a large part, on the environment. Polluted air and water, food additives and colorings, changes in diet from "natural" to "processed" foods all have been implicated as possible causes. Cigarette smoking has been shown to be a cause of lung and other related cancers. If you wish to reduce your risk of getting cancer, it is important to control the factors that you can control — obviously one person alone cannot clean the environment. However, you can stop smoking.

Prognostic factors

If you do develop cancer, there are a number of prognostic factors (factors that predict length of survival) that are important. Most important are the stage and the type of the disease. The earlier the stage of the disease, that is, the sooner it is diagnosed, the better the prognosis will be. The type of tumor also makes a major difference, since different tumors respond differently to treatment. Furthermore, within a specific organ there are different cell types of cancer that can occur. For example, all lung cancers are not the same type of cell. Often these types are important in determining both response to therapy and

prognosis. Your age and overall physical condition are also important in determining your ability to win the fight over cancer.

Cancer should no longer be considered the dreaded scourge that it was thought to be 20 years ago. It is not always fatal and is in many instances curable. The keys to living today should be to avoid cancer-causing materials (for example, cigarettes), to consult your physician regularly (and discuss possible increased risk factors), and to perform regularly the important self-examination procedures that your doctor suggests. Early detection is of extreme importance and you are the best source of early detection.

Types of cancer

Bladder cancer. This is the most common cancer of the urinary tract. It occurs most often between the ages of 50 and 70 and is the fourth leading cause of cancer death among men. Four times as many men as women are afflicted.

Bladder cancer has been connected with exposure to a number of carcinogens. This may be because the urinary tract comes into contact with so many foreign substances because of its excretory function. For many years it has been known that those who work with aniline dyes have a high incidence of cancer of the bladder. Bladder cancer is also associated with tar from tobacco smoke and with schistosomiasis infestation, a tropical parasite.

Blood in the urine is usually the first symptom of bladder cancer.

In addition, urination may be difficult, painful, and frequent. The appearance of blood in the urine may be intermittent, and sometimes, if this symptom disappears, a doctor is not consulted. However, anyone with blood in the urine should consult a doctor, since in early stages this disease is highly curable, and treatment is far more difficult later on. If your doctor feels the symptoms suggest bladder cancer, he or she may order a cystoscopy. Under local anesthesia a lighted tube called a cystoscope is passed into the urinary tract through the urethra (the passageway from the bladder to the outside), through which the interior of the bladder can be examined. This instrument can even take a biopsy (removal of a small piece of tissue for analysis) of a suspicious growth.

Treatment of bladder cancer depends on how far advanced the disease is. A small tumor can sometimes be completely removed by a cystoscope. More advanced cases are treated by surgery or radiation or a combination of the two.

Bone cancer. This is a rare form of cancer most common in children between the ages of five and 15. Predisposing factors to bone cancer are bone diseases, bone fractures, and exposure to radiation. Bone cancer begins with a sarcoma, the name for a tumor that develops in muscle, bone, or cartilage (the elastic tissue at the ends of bones).

Bone cancer usually develops first in the arms or legs. Pain, swelling, or brittleness of the bone may be its symptoms. Often it is far advanced by the time it is discovered. The first tool in diagnosis is the X ray, which can often tell whether the bone is cancerous and if the disease has spread. If cancer is indicated, an orthopedic surgeon should perform a biopsy. Bone cancer is usually treated by a combination of surgery, radiation, and chemotherapy.

Brain cancer. Any tumor in the brain, whether cancerous or not, is very dangerous. Because the brain occupies an enclosed space within the skull, even a small tumor that weighs only a fifth of a pound can cause crowding sufficient to bring on death. Brain cancer is most often the result of metastasis from other cancer sites, particularly the breast, lung, and skin.

Symptoms of brain cancer are of two kinds. Increased pressure in the skull can cause seizures, headaches, nausea, forgetfulness, and personality changes. However, symptoms may also arise in the part of the body controlled by the affected area in the brain. For instance, coordination, vision, or strength of limbs may be affected. In the past, brain tumors have not responded well to treatment because their presence is so difficult to detect that diagnosis occurred late in the development of the disease. Recently, however, diagnostic techniques have improved. The CAT (computerized axial tomography) scanner produces a three-dimensional image of the brain that can clearly determine the size and location of a tumor. By using a CAT scanner, doctors are also able to monitor carefully the progress of any treatment.

Surgery is the primary treatment for brain cancer when the disease has not spread throughout the body. Surgery in the brain is a delicate procedure; often a tumor deep in the brain cannot be totally removed without risking impairment of body function. However, new techniques in brain surgery—sometimes with the use of a microscope—permit treatment of tumors once considered inoperable. Radiation or chemotherapy will often follow surgery, though the sensitivity of brain tissue demands that these be administered cautiously. Steroid drugs will often be given to reduce the dangerous swelling that a tumor can produce.

Breast cancer. About one woman in 13 will develop breast cancer at some time in her life. It is the leading cause of cancer death in women, and the leading cause of all death in women between the ages of 40 and 44. The high risk group includes women over 35, women who have never had children or who have had a child for the first time after the age of 30, and women who began menstruation early or who experienced late menopause. Breast cancer also occurs more frequently in chemical workers, women with a family history of this disease, and women who have already had breast cancer.

Self-examination of the breast can often lead to early detection. All women—particularly those in the high risk category—should perform these examinations monthly at the end of the menstrual period. Approximately 90 percent of all breast tumors are first discovered by self-examination. The recommended tech-

In the shower, keep one hand overhead and examine each breast with opposite hand. Wet, soapy skin may make it easier to feel lumps.

In front of a mirror, stand with hands resting on hips. Examine breasts for swelling, dimpling, bulges, and changes in skin.

In front of mirror, examine breasts for changes with arms extended overhead. This position highlights bulges and indentations which may indicate a lump.

Lying in bed, place a pillow under one shoulder to elevate and flatten breast. Examine each breast, with the opposite hand, first with arm under head and again with arm at side.

Make rotary motions—with flat pads, not tips, of fingers — in concentric circles inward toward nipple. Feel for knots, lumps, or indentations. Be sure to include the armpit area.

Squeeze nipples gently to inspect for any discharge. Report any suspicious findings to your doctor.

nique for breast self-examination is shown in the illustration in this section.

If a lump is discovered in the breast, your doctor will probably order an X ray of the breast, known as a mammogram. The doctor may also recommend a thermogram, which can detect growths by measuring body heat. This test is based on the premise that new growths may generate more heat than the surrounding tissue. However, thermography is not as accurate as mammography and should be used only to augment a physical examination and a mammogram. The doctor may also take a biopsy (a tissue sample) of the lump to test for the presence of cancer. If cancer is indicated, surgery will probably be performed. Women with breast cancer often dread surgery because of the disfigurement that can result; however, today surgery for a breast tumor is often less extensive than in the past. At one time all breast cancer patients received a radical mastectomy, or removal of the breast, underlying chest muscles, and lymph glands in the armpit. Now it is known that in many cases the removal of the breast, or even the tumor alone, may be equally effective. In addition, there are techniques for reconstruction of the breast after surgery and rehabilitation of muscle tone in an arm that has been weakened by surgery. In some cases radiation therapy will be used after surgery to destroy any remaining cancer cells.

Cancer of the colon. About 40,000 Americans die every year of cancer of the colon and rectum. About half of all cases of cancer of the colon can be cured by surgery, and early detection can greatly improve this percentage. A simple test for blood in the stool can indicate whether further tests should be made for the presence of this cancer. Everyone over 40, or with chronic digestive problems, should have this test regularly. Chance of cure is twice as likely if the disease is discovered before symptoms occur.

Symptoms of cancer of the colon include a change in stools or in bowel movements, bleeding from the rectum, pencil thin stools, and abdominal discomfort not eased by bowel movement. If you have any of these symptoms your doctor will probably perform a rectal exam, inserting a finger into the rectum to search for unusual growths. If further examination is necessary, the doctor may introduce a sigmoidoscope (a lighted tube) into the colon through the anus, the opening at the end of the intestine. This instrument permits examination of the inside of the colon and can also take a biopsy of suspicious growths. Sometimes a noncancerous polyp is removed by a similar instrument, because such polyps may sometimes develop into cancer.

Surgery is the usual treatment for cancer of the colon. If the cancer is near to or in the rectum, the surgeon may remove all the rectum and create an artificial rectum, or colostomy, in the lower abdominal wall. A colostomy is usually covered with a bag to collect waste material.

Cancer of the cervix. The cervix is the lower part of the uterus, or womb, that extends into the vagina. Cancer of the cervix is the second most common cancer among American women. The death rate from this disease has decreased 50 percent over the last 50 years, largely as a result of early diagnosis. Early cervical cancer has no symptoms but can be detected by a Pap smear. A Pap smear is performed routinely in a doctor's office by scraping the surface of the cervix. The collected material is then tested for indications of cancer. Today two out of three cases of cervical cancer are detected by a Pap smear before they display symptoms.

Cervical cancer has a higher incidence among black women and poor women. This cancer also occurs more frequently among women who were sexually active early with many partners and among those with genital herpes.

If a Pap smear indicates the possibility of cervical cancer, a biopsy of the affected area will probably be performed. Treatment depends on how far the disease has advanced; early forms are almost always curable by surgical removal of the cervix and uterus, called a hysterectomy. If a patient still hopes to bear children, and the cancer is in an early stage, sometimes this surgery can be put off until after children have been born. However, this is possible only if the disease does not seem to be progressing, and the cancer must be monitored carefully during this phase. Eventually the uterus should be removed. More advanced forms of the disease are treated with radiation as well as surgery.

Leukemia. This is a disease of the bone marrow, the site of blood

Original cancer

Blood vessel

Cancer invading new location

The spread of cancer from its original site to other locations in the body is called metastasis. As cancer progresses, cells are often sent through the circulatory and/or lymphatic system to start growth at other parts of the body.

cell production. Blood cells called platelets control clotting; white blood cells fight infection; and red blood cells carry oxygen throughout the body. The symptoms of leukemia result from the impairment of these functions.

Leukemia is the most common form of cancer in children. In recent years the outlook has improved dramatically for children suffering from leukemia. Twenty years ago nearly all children diagnosed as having leukemia died. Today close to 50 percent are cured—and the lives of many more are prolonged.

More than half the people diagnosed as having leukemia first consult a doctor with complaints of being easily tired, a result of low red blood cell count. Other symptoms are easy bruising, bleeding from the gums, blood in the stool, fever, and frequent infections. The spleen and lymph glands are usually enlarged.

A diagnosis of leukemia should be made by a cancer specialist. The doctor will probably insert a needle into the hipbone to withdraw bone marrow cells that will be tested for the presence of cancer.

Leukemia is often treated first with intensive chemotherapy to kill all cancer cells in the body. The patient may become even sicker during treatment because of the large dosages of cancer-fighting drugs. After this initial treatment phase, radiation and additional drugs may be administered to be sure all of the disease has disappeared.

Liver cancer. Liver cancer usually results from the spread of cancer cells from another site in the body. However, cancer that originates in the liver can sometimes be traced to environmental carcinogens. It is known that anyone who has worked with vinyl chloride, a chemical used in plastics manufacture, has a higher risk of this disease. It also appears that cirrhosis of the liver, a disease in which normal liver cells are replaced by fibrous tissue, may cause an individual to be more susceptible to cancer of the liver.

Symptoms of liver cancer are difficult to identify. Often they resemble the signs of a peptic ulcer — aching or burning pain in the upper abdomen, nausea, and vomiting. A swollen or hardened liver often indicates to the doctor the need for further testing.

In the rare cases in which this cancer is diagnosed early and is confined to the liver, it can be treated surgically, but most often the prognosis is not good.

Lung cancer. Cigarette smoking is generally accepted as the major cause of lung cancer. Lung cancer is the leading cause of cancer death in men, although in recent years the incidence of lung cancer in women is growing, probably as a result of increasing numbers of women who smoke. In addition, lung cancer is also increasing among nonsmokers. This may be due to improved diagnostic techniques (many lung tumors were once diagnosed as tuberculosis), as well as to increased environmental pollution.

If you smoke, and are over 45, or have a family history of this disease, you should be on the lookout for symptoms, since the early signs can be very mild: a persistent cough or lingering respiratory discomfort. Later, coughing will increase as will chest pain and shortness of breath. The patient may also cough up blood.

A cancerous tumor in the lung is usually removed by surgery. To eliminate the entire tumor, it may be necessary to remove an entire lobe of the lung. Because lung cancers are usually not detected until they are well advanced, surgery alone may not be able to eliminate them, and radiation and chemotherapy will be used in combination with surgery.

In recent years the deadliest form of lung cancer, small-cell carcinoma, has yielded to a new drug therapy that has produced significant remission in some patients.

Lymphoma. This cancer attacks the lymphatic system, particularly the lymph nodes and the spleen. These organs manufacture lymphocytes, cells that protect the body against infection.

The first symptoms of lymphoma are usually a swollen spleen or swollen lymph glands in the neck, armpit, or groin (the juncture between the lower abdomen and the inner thigh). Fever and sweating are later symptoms. If these symptoms persist, a doctor should be consulted. If the doctor suspects cancer, he or she will probably order a biopsy (tissue sample) of the enlarged organ.

There are two major forms of lymphoma: Hodgkin's disease and non-Hodgkin's lymphoma. In recent years there have been dramatic strides in the treatment of Hodgkin's disease. In early stages, radiation alone can be very effective. Later in the development of the disease, more extensive radiation may be required, or a combination of radiation and chemotherapy. Treatment of non-Hodgkin's lymphoma is much the same as that of Hodgkin's, but far fewer patients are cured. This form of the disease is usually discovered too late for treatment.

Cancer of the ovary. This is the most dangerous form of cancer of the female reproductive organs, because it is so difficult to diagnose in its early stages. Women over 50 have a higher incidence of the disease, as do childless women and those with a family history of ovarian cancer.

Symptoms may include pelvic discomfort, constipation, abdominal swelling, and irregular menstruation. Often a diagnosis cannot be made without an exploratory operation known as a laparotomy, during which the disease can be evaluated and, in some cases, treated. In ovarian cancer usually both ovaries and the uterus are surgically removed, although sometimes it is possible to remove only one ovary. After surgery, radiation or chemotherapy may be administered.

Prostate cancer. After lung cancer, this is the most common cancer among men. Black Americans have a higher incidence of prostate cancer than any other group in the world. In general, it is more common in men over 55. Prostate cancer can develop very slowly and it often produces no symptoms until the disease is far advanced. Sometimes a routine examination turns up a lump in the prostate, which will prove to be cancerous in about 50 percent of the cases. Prostate examinations should be included in med-

ical checkups of all men over 50.

When symptoms occur, they are usually the result of an enlarged prostate, the male gland that lies at the base of the bladder. The enlargement causes difficult urination or blood in the urine. Prostate cancer often spreads to the bone, and patients may complain of bone pain before they show any other symptoms.

In the small percentage of cases in which prostate cancer is discovered before it has begun to spread, the cancer can be removed by surgery or radiation. Since surgery may cause the patient to become impotent and unable to control urine flow, radiation is the preferred treatment for small tumors. When the disease has spread, usually only its symptoms are treated as they occur. Often a patient can live a long time with this form of treatment.

Skin cancer. About 300,000 cases of skin cancer are discovered every year. Its incidence increases every year, particularly among women, perhaps because people currently are getting more exposure to sunlight. The ultraviolet rays of the sun are a major cause of skin cancer. Fair-skinned people, lacking in a protective substance in the skin called melanin, are more susceptible to the effects of these rays than are dark-skinned people. Skin cancer can also result from prolonged exposure to certain chemicals such as arsenic compounds. Burn scars and skin diseases sometimes develop into cancer.

Most skin cancers are highly treatable. Some can be removed in a doctor's office or an outpatient clinic. But since some forms of these cancers can spread throughout the body, it is important that they be treated early. The most dangerous skin cancer, the malignant melanoma, can metastasize through the lymph glands. Melanomas usually develop from moles, though only about one mole in a million ever becomes a melanoma.

Symptoms of skin cancer are a change in the surface of the skin, wounds that do not heal, and a sudden major change in a wart, mole, or birthmark. All such suspicious signs should be examined by a doctor.

Skin cancer is an unusual form of cancer in that it can be prevented easily. Fair-skinned people and anyone with a family history of skin cancer should avoid exposure to the sun. Additionally, everyone who spends time in the sun should apply a protective sunscreen to exposed portions of the body. It is important to remember that the use of certain drugs, such as barbiturates, antibiotics, and birth control pills, can increase the sensitivity of the skin. In addition, children with their more sensitive skin should be protected against the sun.

Stomach cancer. Stomach cancer has decreased 50 percent in the last 25 years. A change in diet may account for this. Stomach cancer is more common in men than women and usually occurs between the ages of 50 and 70. The high risk group includes those with a history of pernicious anemia or alcoholism, and persons with a diet rich in smoked, pickled, or salted foods.

Symptoms of stomach cancer are similar to those of peptic ulcer (heartburn and abdominal discomfort), making diagnosis more difficult. It may not be until the disease is well advanced that identifying symptoms of a bloody stool or vomit appear. To find a tumor a doctor will take a special X ray that involves swallowing barium, a substance that coats the lining of the stomach so that it will show up on a photograph. If a tumor is indicated, a flexible tube known as an endoscope may be inserted down the throat into the stomach to examine the tumor more closely and perhaps take a biopsy of it. Surgery is the most effective treatment of this disease, but only about 10 percent of victims survive more than five years after diagnosis. Surgery is most useful when the tumor has not begun to spread. Sometimes it is necessary to remove all or part of the stomach. After such surgery a patient will have to consume a low-bulk, high-protein diet.

Cancer of the uterus. This disease is most common in women over 50. Especially susceptible are women who have never borne children, and those who are obese, diabetic, or suffer from high blood pressure. Women who have taken the female hormone estrogen to control symptoms of menopause are also in the high risk group.

Vaginal bleeding after menopause is the most common symptom of uterine cancer. If a Pap smear shows no abnormalities, then minor surgery, known as dilatation and curettage, may be performed. This involves scraping the interior walls of the uterus in order to examine the tissue for the presence of cancer. If cancer is indicated, a hysterectomy (surgical removal of the uterus and the ovaries) is usually performed, although hormones may be an effective treatment against this form of cancer. Cancer of the uterus is harder to detect than that of the cervix; it is often discovered after it is too advanced.

Cancer of the vagina. Once a disease confined to women over 50, in recent years cancer of the vagina has also begun to appear in some women between the ages of 17 and 20. The mothers of most of these young women took artificial estrogens during pregnancy, particularly the drug DES (diethylstilbestrol), in order to prevent miscarriage. Any woman whose mother took artificial estrogens during pregnancy should have a Pap smear twice a year. Symptoms of vaginal cancer include vaginal pain and bleeding. The disease is usually treated by radiation.

FACTS ABOUT MEDICAL TESTS

The basis of medical care is a complete medical history and physical examination. Common health problems are primarily detected and diagnosed by means of the history and physical examination. Nevertheless, your doctor will also use a variety of diagnostic aids and tests to rule out a disease, to confirm a diagnosis, or to detect a disorder that is not apparent. Modern technology now enables medical professionals to inspect the structure of a cell, to see the inside of an organ, or to examine a detailed cross-sectional picture of an internal structure. Used properly, these tests provide vital information to aid your doctor in both the diagnosis of illness and the selection of appropriate treatment.

To help you understand what procedures are available and how they are carried out, this section is a guide to some of the more common medical tests.

Common tests

BLOOD TESTS

The complete blood count (the most common of the blood tests) and blood chemistry screening tests are usually based on blood samples drawn by venipuncture (puncture of a vein by a hypodermic needle). While some blood tests may be done from a finger prick, most tests require more blood for the sample and it will be necessary to take blood from a vein. The procedure is quick and relatively painless. The doctor who orders the tests will most often submit all the test orders together, so that multiple venipunctures are not needed.

Although some patients fear that a great volume of blood is being drawn in venipuncture, the usual laboratory tests do not ordinarily require more than 10 to

20 ml (two to four teaspoons). Remember that the total amount of blood circulating in the body of the average person is at least six quarts at any given time and is constantly being replenished. Therefore, fears about unusual blood loss from the usual testing are groundless.

Complete blood count (CBC)

A complete blood count determines the number and types of blood cells in the blood. The CBC includes:

- Hematocrit, a measure of how much of the blood is made up of red blood cells alone
- Hemoglobin test, to measure the amount of hemoglobin (the blood substance that carries oxygen to the body tissues) present in a given volume of red blood cells
- White blood cell count, to find out how many white blood cells are in the blood
- Differential count, to learn how many of each type of white blood cell are present in the blood
- Platelet count, to determine the number of platelets (the blood elements that aid in clotting the blood) that are present (usually the platelet count is expressed in terms of "adequate," "increased," or "decreased"; if a full count is needed, it must be ordered separately).

Blood chemistry panels

Besides the complete blood count, there are other blood tests that taken together constitute what is known as a blood chemistry panel. These tests, which analyze many components and chemicals in the blood, can be done from a single sample of blood within minutes using an automated blood chemistry machine.

Blood chemistries are performed routinely as screening tests for detection of certain disorders, such as diabetes or kidney disease. They are also used as particular diagnostic tests when specific diseases are suspected, such as hepatitis. Blood chemistry profiles are frequently used to determine the overall function of an organ, especially the liver (the usual profiles contain three or four indicators of liver function). These tests may not pinpoint a specific disease of the liver, but instead provide a general indication of whether or not the liver is functioning normally, leading the physician to perform more specific diagnostic tests. Many illnesses affect more than one organ; furthermore, failure in one organ may cause problems in another. It is here that blood chemistry profiles have great utility; they give information about the function of several organs (particularly the liver and kidneys) at once, using one sample.

The following list contains some of the more common blood chemistry tests with a brief description about the purpose of each:

- Blood glucose (sugar)—to measure blood glucose levels, especially in suspected or diagnosed

diabetes mellitus (in many cases, if the blood sugar is high enough on a screening panel, the diagnosis of diabetes mellitus can be made from this alone)
- Blood urea nitrogen (BUN)—to assess kidney function
- Creatinine — to assess kidney function
- Electrolytes — to check body fluid and salt balance (salts include sodium, potassium, and chloride)
- Uric acid—to aid in diagnosing gout
- Cholesterol or triglycerides—to measure fat levels in blood
- Bilirubin—to assess liver function; to evaluate jaundice; to help diagnose hemolytic anemia
- Albumin — to measure protein (albumin) in blood in order to assess general nutritional status as well as get a general idea of liver function (albumin is produced by the liver).

URINALYSIS

A routine urine analysis is a microscopic examination and a chemical analysis of the urine. Under the microscope, red or white blood cells in the urine can be seen, indicating bleeding and/or an infection somewhere along the urinary tract. Other microscopic elements such as "casts" (formations of protein with and without cellular elements that usually indicate disease in the kidney) and crystals (uric acid or calcium, for example) may also be seen. A chemical analysis can determine the presence of sugar, protein, or other substances that may indicate kidney or bladder diseases as well as other disorders unrelated to the urinary tract, such as diabetes mellitus and starvation. There is no risk to this test.

The patient is given a clean container and told to urinate directly into it. When a urine culture is indicated, a "midstream" specimen is usually requested, that is, a specimen obtained after proper cleansing of the urinary opening and after the initial spurt of urine is passed. If you are to collect the specimen at home, you should also be provided with a clean container with a cap. If not, you should use a clean glass or plastic container. A container that has held food, perfume, chemicals, or cosmetics should not be used. Such containers are difficult to empty and may still contain traces of the original contents, thus invalidating the test results.

CHEST X RAY

The most common standard X-ray examination is the chest X ray. This is an X ray usually used to check for signs of lung diseases and abnormalities. In addition, in a standard chest X ray, the heart, parts of the aorta, the ribs, the upper backbones, the shoulders, the upper arm bones, and the collar bones are seen along with the lungs. Often, diseases other than those that affect the lungs, such as osteoporosis (thin, brittle bones) and congestive heart failure (enlarged heart with the characteristic pattern of fluid in the lungs and lung vessels), may be diagnosed and followed with chest X rays.

The patient undresses from the waist up. The usual chest X ray is taken in two positions: sideways and with the patient standing with his or her front side resting against an X-ray cassette (where the film is) and with the X-ray machine at his or her back. Correct positioning and inactivity are critical in obtaining good X-ray pictures. The actual time of exposure to radiation is quite short. The test is painless but, as with any X-ray procedure (if the test is overused), it may carry a risk of long-term effects of radiation exposure. Routine X rays should be avoided by pregnant women; however, if necessary, a lead shield may be used to protect the fetus (unborn baby).

ELECTROCARDIOGRAM

An electrocardiogram (ECG) is a visual record of the heart's electrical impulses that control the rate and rhythm of beating and reflect many alterations of the heart muscle. This test, along with the history and physical examination, is used to diagnose numerous heart disorders, including previous and new myocardial infarction (heart attack), some congenital (present at birth) abnormalities of the heart, pericarditis (inflammation of the lining sac of the heart), and abnormal thickness of the muscle (such as is seen in long-term high

blood pressure), among many others. There is no risk to this test, and it is totally painless.

Electrodes (small metal disks) sensitive to the heart's impulses are taped onto the body at various points on the chest, arms, and legs. The electrode cables are connected to the electrocardiograph, a machine that produces a visual record of the impulses. A normal heart produces an ECG tracing consisting of regularly occurring wave patterns, whereas one with some other condition will produce alterations in the cadence and/or appearance of the wave patterns.

STOOL BLOOD TEST

This test is used to detect tiny quantities of occult (hidden) blood in the stool (feces or solid waste material) that are not visible to the eye and that may signal bowel disease or bleeding somewhere along the digestive tract.

The test is usually done by the patient at home and mailed to a laboratory. The patient places a small sample of stool on specially coated paper that will reveal any blood when treated with a special developer. The test may have to be done several times, since the bleeding may be intermittent, that is, it may start and stop rather than be constant. The patient will be instructed to eat a diet that is free of red meat for at least three days before taking the stool specimen (since the blood from meat, including cooked meat, may cause a false positive result on the test) and to take no aspirin-containing medications (aspirin may cause bleeding from the stomach).

This test is painless and has no risk. It is an excellent method of screening for colon cancer.

THROAT CULTURE

This common procedure is used to determine the type of microorganisms causing infection in the throat.

The test involves obtaining a sample of bacteria by rolling a cotton-tipped applicator around the swollen area. The test is painless, but may cause gagging. There is no risk.

The cell samples are placed in a culture medium (a special mixture of chemicals and nutrients designed to support growth of bacteria), so that growth of microorganisms can be detected and measured. Special procedures are used to identify the specific bacteria. This procedure usually takes from 24 to 48 hours for definitive results.

Special diagnostic tests

ALLERGY TESTS

Tests to determine the existence of various allergies are as numerous and complex as the substances (called allergens) that cause the allergic responses. One of the most common allergy tests is the skin test. This procedure can be either a scratch skin test or an intracutaneous skin test. In the scratch test, suspected allergens are applied in small amounts to individual, tiny scratches on the skin, often several at a time and in a prescribed order. In the intracutaneous skin test, small quantities of the suspected allergens are injected into or under the skin. After a short period of time — about one half hour — the doctor notes which substances have caused a reaction. In both of these tests, a swollen reddish bump at the site of the application is a positive reaction to that allergen. The skin scratches and injections can be uncomfortable while the procedures are being performed. In addition, there is a risk to the skin tests in that an extremely sensitive individual may react strongly to an applied or injected allergen.

Although skin tests are relatively safe and reliable, there is also a blood test to help diagnose allergens. The test, called radio-allergosorbent technique (RAST), measures specific (allergic-group) antibodies in the blood. Antibodies are substances formed by the immune system in response to foreign invaders, such as an allergen. The test can be used for those people who should not have skin tests: people with extremely sensitive skin, very young children, and those individuals suspected to be extremely sensitive to an injected allergen. However, the RAST may not be as sensitive as skin tests and is more expensive.

In the case of food allergies, diagnosis is often difficult. One method of identifying allergens is to have samples of suspected allergy-causing foods eaten in small quantities, at times when there is nothing in the digestive system. Symptoms, if any, are noted. Adequate time is required between food samples so that each sample can clear the system before the next food is given. Someone with a history of severe reactions should not be tested in this fashion. Skin testing can be done, but may not be accurate.

BIOPSY

A biopsy is the removal of a small sample of tissue for examination under a microscope. This procedure is done to establish a precise diagnosis of abnormalities, including cancer. The tissue may be removed by cutting, by aspirating (suctioning) with a needle, or by other methods, depending on the part of the body from which the tissue sample is removed. For example, endoscopic biopsy is removal of tissue by instruments attached to or passed through an endoscope (a device — usually a flexible lighted tube — used for direct visualization of the interior of a hollow organ) into a hollow organ, such as the colon.

The procedure varies with the type of biopsy to be performed. Some require hospitalization — especially if surgery is required to conduct a biopsy on internal organs. Other procedures, such as removal and/or biopsy of small skin growths or needle aspiration (suctioning) of a breast lump, can be done in a doctor's office or an outpatient clinic. Although many biopsies are done with some type of anesthesia, there may be some discomfort if a biopsy involves some sort of cutting or invasive (entering the body) technique. Additionally, depending on the surgical or invasive procedures involved, there is some risk, which varies with the procedure being performed. The risks of outpatient biopsies are usually minimal, but complications, such as excessive bleeding, can occur.

CONTRAST EXAMINATIONS

Contrast media, popularly known as "dyes," are materials introduced into the body that alter radiopacity (the capacity to be "seen" by X ray or fluoroscope) of one part of the body in comparison with surrounding parts. The contrast materials are opaque, that is, they are able to be seen on the X ray or fluoroscope, and are essential to visualize certain internal body areas, such as the stomach and intestines. When the contrast medium is introduced into the body, the radiologist performing the test often uses fluoroscopy (the projection of moving X rays onto a special screen) to observe the working of the internal body organs and then takes still X-ray films of the area being examined. Common contrast examinations include the upper gastrointestinal tract examination (upper GI series), lower gastrointestinal series (barium enema), intravenous pyelogram (IVP or kidney X ray), the gallbladder series, and angiogram (visualization of blood vessels).

Upper GI series

The upper GI series is a contrast medium/X-ray examination of the esophagus, stomach, and first part of the small intestine (duodenum). This X ray is used to detect ulcers, cancers, and other abnormalities. The contrast medium used is barium sulfate, and it is introduced by having the patient drink it after fasting overnight. It is necessary that the patient's stomach be empty to accommodate the barium meal and also to avoid having food particles confuse the results. The radiologist observes the filling of the stomach on the fluoroscope as the patient drinks. The time required for the exam is about 30 minutes. In some instances, such as suspected regional enteritis or an obstruction, the doctor will order what is known as "small bowel followthrough," a series of X rays following the barium throughout the small intestine. In this procedure, many films are taken at specified time intervals. This X ray may take hours. Patients can expect very light-colored stools after the test because of the presence of the barium sulfate. As with any X-ray examination, there may be a risk of effects from radiation exposure,

but modern equipment and techniques have minimized this.

Lower GI series

The lower GI series, or barium enema, is a contrast medium/X-ray examination of the large intestine (colon) that is useful in detecting tumors, polyps, and other problems in the colon. For this examination, the colon must be cleared of all fecal matter. This is usually accomplished by a liquid diet for 24 to 48 hours, accompanied by laxatives and enemas. Nothing is then allowed by mouth until the examination is completed. The time for the examination itself is usually about 30 minutes. The patient is given an enema consisting of a barium solution (that makes the colon opaque) introduced into the large intestine through a tube inserted into the anus and must retain the enema until all the films are made. When looking for polyps or when a detailed view of the lining of the colon is required, air is put into the colon to form a double contrast with the barium. This technique is referred to as an "air contrast barium enema" and is rapidly becoming more common than the plain lower GI.

At the time of the examination, the radiologist fluoroscopically observes the colon filling with the liquid suspension of barium sulfate. Before, during, and after emptying of the solution, films are made of the barium-coated colon. Afterward the patient is usually given a cleansing enema and occasionally a mild laxative to rid the colon of barium.

There is the usual risk from radiation exposure and, rarely, an obstruction of the colon by impacted (hardened) barium or a perforation of the colon because of the enema may occur.

Intravenous pyelogram (IVP)

This test is used to determine the size and functioning of as well as the presence of obstructions in the kidneys and the urinary tract. In men, an enlarged prostate gland may also be noted. The test is done by injecting contrast material—into a vein in the arm—which then is eliminated through the kidneys and urinary tract. X-ray films are made at given time intervals to observe the rate of excretion, the concentration of the contrast medium inside the kidneys, and the outlines of the ureters (tubes from kidneys to bladder) and the bladder. Since fecal matter and gas in the intestinal tract obscure the observation of urinary tract structures, the lower bowel needs to be cleared for this examination. There is the usual risk of the effects of radiation exposure. Patients with diabetes mellitus, known kidney disease, or a history of previous reactions to X-ray contrast materials may be at risk of kidney damage or serious allergic-type reactions. These patients should inform their physicians and the radiologist of these facts, since adequate precautions can be taken to minimize the chance of complication.

Gallbladder series

This series, called the oral cholecystogram is performed to test gallbladder function and to detect gallstones.

Contrast medium (a dye in tablet form) is given to the patient after the evening meal the day before the X ray. Usually nothing is given by mouth until the examination is completed. If the gallbladder does not show up (concentrate the contrast), the next day the dose of contrast is repeated and another film is taken now 48 hours after the first dose. If the gallbladder is still not visible, this indicates a diseased gallbladder (assuming that the gastrointestinal tract and liver are processing the contrast normally). In some X-ray departments, after the films of the contrast-filled gallbladder have been made, the patient is given a fatty meal to stimulate the gallbladder to empty, and then another film is made to judge this function. The time required for the examination is about one hour, excluding the time for the fatty meal. The oral cholecystogram will correctly diagnose gallbladder disease (including both poor function and/or stones) about 96 percent of the time.

For this examination, as with pyelography (kidney X ray), it is helpful to clear the intestinal tract of fecal matter and gas to allow for adequate viewing of the gallbladder. This is done with a special diet 24 hours prior to the examination and administration of enemas. Avoiding creams, butters, and other fatty foods (fats stimulate the gallbladder, which must be at rest in order to concentrate the dye well) is also required. There may be some side effects such as nausea, vomiting, or diarrhea. There is the usual risk from exposure to radiation, along with the risk (although uncommon) of allergic-type reaction to the contrast. Patients with diabetes and known kidney disease may be at risk of kidney damage and should inform their doctor so that precautions can be taken.

Cardiac catheterization

Cardiac catheterization, often referred to as the "angiogram," is required before most heart surgery and for diagnosis of some heart diseases. In this procedure the cardiologist introduces a tube (called a catheter) into the heart. This is usually done through a puncture in an artery in the groin or arm. Through this tube, an opaque contrast is injected so that moving pictures of the heart can be clearly seen. Through the catheterization, the cardiologist and the cardiovascular surgeon obtain crucial information such as the location of defects in the various walls and valves of the heart, the location and degree of narrowing of the cornary arteries (the arteries that supply the heart muscle itself with blood), and even the different pressures in the chambers, giving an idea as to the overall functional situation of the heart. Nowadays, this procedure is commonly performed, and car-

ries a very low risk potential in the hands of experienced physicians. After the procedure, there is occasional bleeding at the catheter introduction site along with some mild discomfort there. During contrast injection, many patients complain of a "hot flash" or nausea. There is the usual risk of radiation exposure in this test. Also, patients with previous history of reaction to contrast materials, diabetes, or kidney disease may be at risk from the contrast. Adequate precautions can be taken to prevent complications when the physician performing the procedure is informed of these problems prior to the test.

It is important to note that there are other (uncommon) complications that can occur with cardiac catheterization. Detailed explanations of the risks should be obtained from the doctor.

Radioactive isotopes

Radioactive isotopes, or radioisotopes, are used primarily as a diagnostic tool to detect tumors, blood clots, or malfunctioning organs in the body.

A radioisotope is a variation of a normal chemical element that contains a different number of neutrons in its unstable nucleus (which is the center of the atom, the element's smallest part). Because it is unstable, the nucleus disintegrates and gives off electrically charged energy (ionizing radiation).

Certain elements are attracted

to, or are used by, particular organs. For example, iodine, when given by mouth or injected, will travel to and is used by the thyroid gland. Radioactive iodine, when administered to a patient, will also travel to the thyroid gland, but, because of its special properties, it will show up on X rays. A machine, called a scanner, is placed near the patient and picks up the radiation emitted by the radioactive isotope as it travels to the organ being studied. The scanner converts the radiation into flashes of light and then into an image, which is put on an X-ray film or projected onto a screen.

Using this technique, a physician can determine the position, shape, and size of an organ or the presence of a tumor. By looking at the rate at which the radioisotope is absorbed and eliminated, the doctor can also see how the organ is functioning.

Radioisotopes are mainly used to study the "soft tissues" (thyroid gland, brain, liver, spleen, and kidney), which do not show well on regular X rays. The most recent advance in radioisotope diagnosis has allowed doctors to observe the heart muscle. Although the procedure is still quite costly, it holds out much promise for victims of heart attack or other abnormalities. Some conditions that can be detected by using radioisotopes are over- or under-functioning organs, tumors, blood clots, injuries, bone marrow disease, red blood cell irregularities, cirrhosis of the liver (a condition

in which the internal tissues of the liver are scarred and otherwise damaged), hepatitis (inflammation of the liver), nonabsorption of Vitamin B_{12}, and certain anemias.

Radiation poisoning poses no danger to the individual being tested. Because very small amounts of radiation can be detected and measured, only a minute amount of a radioisotope is required.

ELECTROENCEPHALOGRAM

An electroencephalogram (EEG) is a visual record of the electrical impulses discharged by the brain cells. The EEG is used to diagnose and interpret possible abnormalities in the brain.

Electrodes (small metal disks) are placed at specified points on the surface of the head (in special circumstances, disks may be inserted through the nose into the throat, which may be annoying but not painful or dangerous) and then attached to the electroencephalograph machine, which produces a visual tracing of the brain's electrical waves. When, for instance, the brain has been damaged or the patient has epilepsy, the waves produced by the electrical discharges form patterns characteristic of those disorders. Tracings are taken when the patient is awake but calm; when he or she has been asked to hyperventilate (breathe rapidly) and has been stimulated with a flashing light which may evoke changes characteristic of epileptic grand mal seizures; and when the patient is asleep. An EEG usually takes about one hour to complete. Careful pretest preparation of the patient is essential for accurate results. On the day of the test, no coffee, tea, cola drinks, or other stimulants are permitted. Alcohol, which as a depressant would affect the accuracy of the EEG, must also be avoided. The physician ordering the test must be informed of any medications the patient is taking as these can have profound effects on the EEG. After shampooing, no hair preparations should be used until after the tracing is made. Since part of the tracing may be made while you are asleep, it is helpful if no naps are taken on the day of the test.

ENDOSCOPY

Endoscopy is a method of directly viewing the inside of hollow organs by inserting an endoscope (lighted tube) into the organ. Five common endoscopic examinations are described below, in order from the most frequently to the least frequently done.

Proctosigmoidoscopy

This is an examination of the rectum and colon for detection of cancers and other ailments of the lower 12 inches of the large intestine. In addition to cancer, the examination can reveal muscle tone, swollen veins (hemorrhoids), infected areas, anal fistulas (abnormal passages in the anus), rectal polyps (growths protruding from rectal wall), abnormal narrowing of the intestine, tumors, and foreign bodies, among other problems.

The examination is frequently recommended as part of any complete checkup. It is a must for anyone with rectal bleeding and/or a change in bowel habits. The examination usually takes place on a tilting-top table with the patient in the knee-chest position or lying in a head-down position. After a manual examination (insertion of the physician's finger into the anus), the doctor inserts a lubricated anuscope to examine closely the anus (the opening from the rectum to the outside). Then the sigmoidoscope (a lighted, hollow, rigid tube also known as a proctoscope) is inserted through the anal canal into the large intestine.

Patients are advised to prepare for this examination by eating a light diet for 24 to 48 hours before the test and by emptying the lower intestinal tract with one or two enemas. If a barium X ray of the colon is to follow the sigmoidoscopic examination, a more detailed preparation involving laxatives and a number of enemas is undertaken.

There are few risks to a routine screening. Perforation of the colon is possible, but quite rare. There may be some discomfort or cramping during the examination, but there should be no actual pain.

Gastroscopy

Gastroscopy is an examination of the interior of the esophagus, stomach, and duodenum (the first part of the small intestine). The test is performed to detect and examine ulcers or tumors and to determine the cause of gastro-intestinal bleeding or any other known or suspected abnormalities. The response of an ulcer to treatment can also be followed endoscopically rather than by X ray. Often during this procedure tissue samples (biopsies) are collected or stomach contents suctioned out for examination.

In the procedure, the throat is first anesthesized by a spray and/or gargle. The patient is then given a sedative to induce relaxation. A flexible lighted tube (the gastroscope) is then passed down the throat through the esophagus into the stomach and duodenum. The patient can have no solid food for the evening meal the night before the test is done. Water may be taken in the evening, but not on the day of or within eight hours prior to the test. Smoking is prohibited on the day of the test until the examination is completed, since smoking stimulates the stomach's secretion of gastric juices. Any other stimulation, such as alcohol, caffeine, or colas, should also be avoided. There is little risk to this test (very rarely, there may be a risk of the gastroscope injuring or perforating an organ or of the patient vomiting and inhaling the contents of the stomach). The patient may experience a temporary sore throat afterward.

Colonoscopy

This procedure is similar to proctosigmoidoscopy except that the entire colon (large intestine) is examined, and the instrument is a long, flexible tube. Usually, colonoscopy is performed to detect and/or remove polyps (small growths), to do a biopsy of tumors or suspicious areas, to look for sites of occult (hidden) or obvious bleeding, and to inspect the entire colon for inflammatory bowel disease. In this test the patient is asked to stay on a liquid diet for about 48 hours before the procedure. Laxatives and enemas are also given to cleanse the colon thoroughly. During the test, mild sedatives are given to aid in relaxation. Some discomfort and cramping are common, but actual pain should not occur. The risks are mainly perforation and bleeding from the site of the biopsy or growth removal. However, both are uncommon.

Cystoscopy

Cystoscopy is the direct viewing of the interior of the urinary bladder, the urethra (the passageway from the bladder to the outside of the body), and part of the prostate gland in men. A flexible, lighted tube, called a cystoscope, is passed through the urethra into the bladder. The inside of the bladder and urethra are examined for cancer, polyps (growths), and other abnormalities. The procedure includes collecting tissue samples (biopsy), if indicated, for later examination. An overgrown prostate gland can also be "shaved down" through the cystoscope. This is referred to as a transurethral resection of the prostate and is considered a surgical procedure.

The male patient is usually given a sedative before the test and a spinal or general anesthetic during the procedure. Women frequently only need local anesthesia and often have the procedure done as outpatients. Men, however, generally enter the hospital for the procedure. There is little risk involved in the diagnostic cystoscopy, although there may be a slight chance of damage to the lining of the urethra, of perforation of the bladder, and of temporary retention of urine after the test.

Bronchoscopy

Bronchoscopy is the direct viewing of the trachea (windpipe), larynx (voice box), and bronchi (the breathing tubes through which air travels from the trachea into the lungs). This examination can be performed to pinpoint the cause of an unexplained persistent cough, wheeze, or pneumonia. It is also used to investigate an undiagnosed abnormality on a chest X ray or to diagnose a lung tumor. As with other forms of endoscopy, bronchoscopy may

also be used to take a tissue sample or remove a small obstruction, such as a foreign body.

A lighted tube, either flexible or rigid and varying in diameter, is threaded from the mouth or nose through the trachea into the bronchi. Some bronchoscopes are small enough in diameter to offer a view of even the smallest structures in the bronchial tree. A sedative and topical anesthetic are used; the anesthetic may be in a spray form for the mouth and nose and in a lubricating jelly to protect and anesthetize the tissues of the nose and throat. The patient fasts for at least eight hours prior to the test. Patients with a history of heart disease or those over age 50 are frequently monitored with an electrocardiograph. There is a minor risk of possible damage to the teeth, throat, or bronchial structures, but damage to the respiratory tract is very rare. Bleeding from biopsy sites and areas of growth removal also occurs, but uncommonly. This procedure is almost always done in a hospital setting, but admission to the hospital is often unnecessary.

LUMBAR PUNCTURE

The lumbar puncture, also called spinal tap, is a procedure used to withdraw a small amount of cerebrospinal fluid from an area (the subarachnoid space) surrounding the spinal cord. The cerebrospinal fluid is then examined microscopically and analyzed chemically to detect conditions that may exist in the brain and spinal cord (both of which comprise the central nervous system). The conditions include bleeding, infections, and other abnormalities of the brain and spinal cord. Often the appearance of the fluid, which is normally crystal clear, will provide a preliminary diagnosis of a problem; if, for example, the fluid is cloudy, an infection may be indicated.

The patient usually lies on his or her side with knees drawn up sufficiently to bow the back. After a local anesthetic is administered, the subarachnoid space (where the cerebrospinal fluid circulates) is entered with a special needle inserted through the skin and soft tissues and between two of the lower lumbar vertebrae (backbones). The pressure of the cerebrospinal fluid in the central nervous system is measured with a manometer (an instrument for measuring the pressure of liquids and gases). The fluid is then allowed to drip into a series of small, sterile test tubes.

Although patients are sometimes apprehensive about the lumbar puncture procedure, it is not usually painful. Headache after the tap is not uncommon. It is not possible, however, to predict who will develop one. It seems that maintaining a lying-flat position for an hour or so after the tap decreases the incidence of headache. Furthermore, if a headache should develop, lying flat seems to ease the pain.

There is a slight risk of nerve damage from the needle, but this is extremely rare. The site of the puncture is below the end of the spinal cord, so the cord itself cannot be injured in any way. In conditions in which pressure in the central nervous system is elevated, such as with a brain tumor or other mass, or if there is swelling of the brain because of disease or injury, a lumbar puncture may lead to a "dropping" of the brain downward. This is a serious complication, but fortunately a rare one. New procedures, such as computerized tomography (CAT scan), have minimized this problem by providing a noninvasive means of ruling out a large mass or swelling before performing a spinal tap. Also, as with any procedure that invades the body, there is a risk of infection, but the incidence of infections following lumbar punctures is quite low.

PULMONARY FUNCTION TESTS

Pulmonary function testing (PFT) is a procedure to assess the physical functioning of the lungs, especially lung capacity. The results of this group of tests often reveal the existence of various diseases of the lungs, including asthma and emphysema. Diseases that cause restriction of lung movement can also be diagnosed and differentiated from those that cause airways obstruction, such as asthma. Pulmonary function tests are also used as a baseline to monitor the course of a disease and the effects of therapy.

The routine PFT is done with a spirometer; long tubes resembling vacuum-cleaner hoses are connected to a device that measures (in graphic form) the volume of air breathed in and out against time. The patient breathes into the spirometer according to instructions given during the test. The amount of air inhaled and exhaled as well as the rate of inhalation and exhalation are measured, and sometimes specific exhaled gases are also measured. Some pulmonary function tests also require a blood sample from an artery to determine if the arterial blood (freshly oxygenated in the lungs) has adequate oxygen and a normal concentration of carbon dioxide.

The test is painless and without risk, with the possible exceptions of discomfort during and complications after an arterial puncture for the blood sample.

CARDIAC STRESS TEST

The stress test, also often called the treadmill test, is done basically to determine the reaction of the heart and circulatory system to physical exercise. Devices other than a treadmill, such as a bicycle, can also be used, depending on the situation. A stress test can be done for many reasons: to determine if the cause of chest pain is the heart; to detect the presence of coronary artery disease; and to follow the progress of a patient in cardiac rehabilitation, among others.

For this test, the patient is told to sleep well the night before the test and to eat lightly more than three hours before the test. At the lab the patient will put on exercise clothes and running shoes. The patient is questioned about recent medical history and exercise habits. An individual in good health who has not exercised for a long time may have a treadmill negative for coronary disease, but the test will indicate poor cardiovascular conditioning.

For the test, electrodes for continuous electrocardiogram are attached so that the tester (usually a cardiologist) can monitor the heart rate and the electrocardiographic response of the heart to graded exercise. A blood pressure cuff is also attached to an arm.

The patient is then started on the treadmill at a low work load. The work load (speed and incline of the treadmill) is then increased, usually at three-minute intervals until the patient either (1) attains about 90 percent of the predicted maximum heart rate for his or her age (obtained from standardized tables); (2) develops symptoms or electrocardiographic changes consistent with heart disease; or (3) cannot continue the test for any reason (for example, leg cramps or shortness of breath). The time it takes to reach the target heart rate is related to the degree of cardiovascular fitness, but not necessarily related to the presence or absence of heart disease. That is, an individual who attains his or her peak heart rate at only six minutes is less fit ("cardiovascular-wise") than someone who can exercise 12 minutes on the treadmill. Both, however, may or may not have changes or symptoms indicating heart disease. At the individual's maximum performance level, the closer he or she comes to the predicted maximum heart rate, the more meaningful the test. In other words, if the age-predicted maximum is 180 beats per minute and the patient must stop at 130 beats because of a leg cramp, fatigue, or other non-cardiovascular reason, this test is considered "submaximal." In this case, the negative ECG (meaning there is no heart disease) carries less diagnostic importance than a negative ECG at a heart rate of 180 beats.

Stress tests may cause discomfort because of fatigue, tired muscles, and so forth. The main risk is of precipitating a cardiac event, such as arrhythmia (abnormal heart rhythm) or a coronary. In centers with well-trained and well-equipped staff, and with carefully chosen patients, these risks are minimized.

TOMOGRAPHY

Tomography is a type of X-ray examination in which the shadows in front of and behind the part of the body being studied are blurred out on the X-ray picture. Successive exposures are made at different depths within the structure of the body part under study and from different angles. The effect is the same as that achieved when a microscope is adjusted back and forth and up and down while looking at a piece of tissue: it is possible to get a picture of a structure at different levels, each one pinpointed and sharply focused.

Nowadays these multiple images can be fed into a computer that has been programmed to coordinate such data, and a cross-sectional "map" of the body part under study can be constructed in picture form. The expansion of computer capabilities has led to a high degree of sophistication in tomography, resulting in what is called "Computerized Axial Tomography" (also known as the CAT scan). As the name implies, the computer produces a tomographic picture of a body part with exposures taken around the axial or longitudinal line of the body (which is a line from the head to the toes that runs exactly through the center of the body).

The most widely known use of the CAT scan has been in the detection and description of brain disorders. However, in recent years this scanning technique has been extended to other parts of the body, so, for example, cross-sectional images of organs in the abdomen, such as the liver and pancreas, can now be produced. These scans are quite sensitive and have greatly aided the effort for early detection of tumors. One of the breakthroughs that has made this possible is the development of scanners that can complete their scan in five seconds or less. The brain scan does not require such fast scanning, since the head can be easily immobilized. The abdominal area, on the other hand, is in constant movement, because of the action of the stomach, the intestines, and the diaphragm. Consequently, the scan must be made fast enough to provide a clear image in the same way that a fast shutter speed on an ordinary camera can "stop" the motion of the subject. The test is painless, but there is a risk of radiation exposure. Also, intravenous X-ray contrast solution is used to enhance the picture. Persons with kidney disease or diabetes, as well as persons with a sensitivity to the dye, may be at risk of kidney damage or serious allergic-type reactions when contrast solution is used. These individuals should tell their physician of these facts so that adequate precautions can be taken to minimize the chance of complication. This type of testing is expensive and therefore not done routinely.

Computerized Tomography is known by a variety of names, depending on the method and the sequence of scanning: Computerized Axial Tomography (CAT), Computerized Transverse Axial Tomography (CTAT), Computer-Assisted Transaxial Tomography (CATT).

ULTRASONOGRAPHY

Ultrasonography, often called ultrasound, is a method of visualizing the deep structures of the body by recording the reflection off those structures of high-frequency sound waves. The procedure is painless and uses no radiation. Ultrasound, the sound range used in diagnostic procedures, is a vibration beyond the range of human hearing. Ultrasound diagnosis is based on interactions between the sound waves and biological structures in the human body.

The instrument used in ultrasonography is called a transducer. The transducer, placed over the area to be examined, directs ultrasonic waves at the tissue. The sounds returning from the internal structure are processed by machines that produce a multidimensional, detailed visualization of the structure. Formerly, only still pictures could be obtained. Now, however, moving pictures in "real time" are routinely done, as in pregnancy, when the baby's movements and beating heart can actually be seen.

The development of sonography as an alternate way of visualizing body structures reflects not only current technological advances, but also present-day concern about the potential dangers of over-reliance on X rays. Sonography offers an alternative to X rays in the examination of soft tissues in those cases in which X rays might be ineffective or potentially harmful. Another advantage is that sonography does not require invasive procedures (for example, injections, catheterization, incisions) or the use of contrast media such as opaque dyes. There is no known risk involved in sonography, although the long-term effects of sound waves have not been determined.

Tests for women

AMNIOCENTESIS

Amniocentesis is the surgical penetration through the abdomen of the pregnant uterus and the amniotic sac surrounding the unborn baby in order to withdraw some amniotic fluid to be tested. The analysis of amniotic fluid is useful in determining the condition and health of the fetus (unborn baby), since the amniotic fluid contains cells that normally are discarded by the baby. Examination of these cells for chromosomal and chemical makeup can detect numerous genetic defects and hereditary disorders. Testing certain chemicals in the fluid itself is done to determine fetal lung maturity and to detect certain fetal abnormalities, such as spina bifida. The fetal cells will also indicate the sex of the baby. Identifying the sex of the baby before birth may be important when a sex-linked hereditary disorder (such as hemophilia, a blood-clotting disease occurring almost exclusively in males) is suspected. However, amniocentesis is never performed simply to satisfy curiosity about the sex of a baby. In fact, the test is not routine; it is performed most often in pregnant women over the age of 35 or with a family history of certain hereditary disorders. The incidence of chromosome abnormalities of the fetus increases rapidly after a woman reaches the age of 35. As each year passes, the chances of chromosome abnormalities increase.

The sample of amniotic fluid is obtained by inserting a hollow needle through the mother's abdomen into the uterus and amniotic sac and drawing out fluid with a syringe attached to the needle. The procedure should be relatively painless since a local anesthetic is used around the injection site. The test is usually done around the sixteenth to eighteenth week of pregnancy (before this time the test results are inconclusive), but final results are often not available for about three to four weeks. Therefore, the waiting period can be the most difficult part of the test. However, studies have shown that approximately 95 percent of amniocentesis results are normal.

There is some risk to this test, which is why it is not routinely used. There is a risk of miscarriage as well as a chance of striking the placenta or baby. However, much of the risk is minimized, or even eliminated, by the use of ultrasonography to reveal the position of both the fetus and placenta before the needle is inserted. In addition, as with any technique that invades the body, there is a chance of infection. A patient experiencing any pain, fever, or discharge from the puncture site or from the vagina should notify her doctor immediately.

MAMMOGRAPHY

Mammography is a simple, painless examination of the breasts by means of a special X-ray machine that is specially designed to be used for soft tissue. This procedure is especially valuable for the detection of early breast cancers before they can be manually felt by the woman or her doctor. Mammography can also differentiate between malignant (cancerous) and nonmalignant (noncancerous) lumps and can provide information about fibrocystic breast disease.

Many medical experts recommend that a baseline mammogram (of the normal breasts) be made when a woman is around the age of 40. This can later be used for comparison purposes if subsequent mammograms reveal changes in the breasts. After the first mammogram, it is recommended that the test be repeated every one to five years, depending on individual risk factors such as a family history of breast cancer. Some doctors suggest a mammogram every year for women past the age of 50, regardless of risk factors. However, a mammogram should not replace a monthly breast self-examination nor regular breast examinations by a doctor; rather, the mammogram should be done in conjunction with these manual examinations.

Other related techniques for breast examination are xerography and thermography. Xerography is a form of mammography that records the image using a photo-electric process rather than standard X-ray film. Thermography is a diagnostic technique that, unlike mammography and xerography, uses no X rays and

thus can be repeated as often as desired. Thermography records any variations in the temperature of various parts of the breast.

The basic premise of thermography is that rapidly growing cancer cells give off more heat than does normal tissue. Thermography, however, is not as accurate as mammography and should only be used to augment information obtained from a physical examination and a mammogram.

There is some question about the risk of radiation exposure in mammography, especially for those women who receive a yearly mammogram. The radiation dosage has been reduced in modern testing, and many physicians feel that because of this the benefits of early detection outweigh any risks. However, most doctors are conservative about the use of mammography, and a woman should discuss the benefits and risks of this test procedure with her doctor who knows her medical history. It is important to remember, too, that mammography should not be used on a pregnant woman; the radiation may be harmful to the baby.

PAP TEST

The Pap test (abbreviation of Papanicolaou, the scientist who developed the test) is a standard part of the gynecological examination for women. It is used to detect early cell changes that might indicate cancer or other abnormalities of the cervix, the neck of the uterus.

The Pap test involves scraping a smear of cells from the surface of the external area where the cervix opens into the vagina. The scraping is done with a small plastic spatula and the scrapings are spread to dry on a glass slide. The test is painless, and there is no risk.

The test results are categorized into five groups: Class I — no abnormal cells; Class II—atypical cells, usually caused by inflammation or infection; Class III — cells suspected to be cancerous; and Classes IV and V—cancer cells present. In some laboratories, a modification of this classification is used so that the report states that the smear is negative, doubtful, unsatisfactory, or positive.

A woman should have her first Pap test at about 18 years of age, and then every one to two years. Women over age 40 should have an annual test. Any woman with a history of cervical or uterine cancer or of abnormal Pap tests should have the test done every six months.

PELVIC EXAMINATION

The pelvic examination is a physical and visual inspection of the female reproductive tract. It is done to assess the condition of and to detect disorders in the reproductive organs, including the vagina, cervix, uterus, and ovaries. A pelvic examination can also reveal pregnancy.

The patient lies on an examination table and places her heels in metal holders resembling the stirrups on a horse's saddle. The doctor inserts into the vagina a speculum, a special instrument that expands the vagina to permit visual examination of the vagina and cervix. After removing the speculum, the doctor will also insert two fingers into the vagina while simultaneously pressing lightly on the patient's abdomen. This procedure enables the doctor to feel the uterus and ovaries and detect any abnormalities in these organs. Sometimes the doctor also inserts a finger into the rectum while pressing on the abdomen; this, too, enables the doctor to feel the uterus and ovaries.

FACTS ABOUT PRESCRIPTION DRUGS

Because of the variety of drugs now available, both over the pharmacy counter and also by prescription from our physicians, a wide range of illnesses and disorders can be controlled, relieved, or even cured. We can control hypertension, eliminate the irritating effects of allergies and hay fever, relieve cold discomfort, cure a variety of stomach and intestinal disorders, control stress and insomnia, and end bacterial and fungal infections—all by taking a medication.

The process of buying and taking a drug starts when your doctor writes out a prescription. The choice of drug is determined by many facts you have already told your doctor, including information about drugs that you have taken at various times in your life, any allergic reactions you might have suffered, any chronic conditions for which you are still taking medication, any special side effects that you have experienced with certain drugs or classes of drugs, and any chronic health problems you have. Based on this information, the doctor makes a decision as to what he or she thinks is the right drug for your particular condition. The doctor's part of the process is now complete; your part is just beginning.

As you read on, you will learn how to read a prescription correctly and how to buy, store, and use drugs.

As with other sections of the book, this section is not a substitute for informed advice from your doctor and pharmacist. You should keep these two persons informed at all times of your condition and of any reactions you are experiencing, as well as of other medication you take on a regular basis. You should also consult your doctor or pharmacist about the latest information about your medications; although every effort has been made to assure that the information here is up-to-date, new developments occur rapidly in drug research. What this section can do, however, is help you to work better with both pharmacist and doctor or other health care professionals in becoming a wise, well-informed, and aware patient who receives the maximum benefits from his or her medication and treatment.

How to read and understand your prescription

Part of the process of becoming an educated participating patient is to understand as much as possible about the medications you are taking. This process starts in the doctor's office. Make sure that you understand what medication is prescribed for you, how often and how it should be taken, and for how long. Ask specifically if you should continue the medication once the symptoms subside. Some drugs, such as antibiotics, should be taken for a certain minimum period of time, even though all the symptoms have disappeared. Other drugs should be discontinued when the symptoms subside. Make sure, too, that you understand your dosage schedule, any precautions you need to take to prevent or reduce possible side effects, and how (if at all) you should alter your normal eating or drinking habits while you are on the medication. You should also learn what side effects are to be expected that are within the "normal" range and which ones are signals that you need to consult your doctor again. Be sure that you know and understand all of these facts before you leave your doctor's office.

A more detailed step-by-step review will be helpful.

Step 1: Read your prescription. You cannot be sure that your prescription has been filled correctly unless you can read it, so your first step is to read the prescription.

John D. Jones MD
Anytown, U.S.A.

DEA # 123456789   PHONE # 123-4567

NAME _Your name_   AGE _25_
ADDRESS _Anytown, U.S.A_   DATE _12-15-85_

Rx   Darvon cpd - 65
                #24
              sig: cap ī q̄4h prn pain

REFILLS _5X_   _John D. Jones, MD_
LABEL _yes_   MD

COMMON ABBREVIATIONS AND SYMBOLS

ABBREVIATION	MEANING	DERIVATION
A₂	both ears	*auris* (Latin)
aa	of each	*ana* (Greek)
ac	before meals	*anti cibum* (Latin)
AD	right ear	*auris dextra* (Latin)
AL	left ear	*auris laeva* (Latin)
AM	morning	*ante meridiem* (Latin)
AS	left ear	*auris sinistra* (Latin)
bid	twice a day	*bis in die* (Latin)
c̄	with	*cum* (Latin)
cap	capsule	—
cc or cm³	cubic centimeter	30 cc equal one ounce
disp	dispense	—
dtd#	give this number	*dentur tales doses* (Latin)
ea	each	—
ext	for external use	—
gtts	drops	*guttae* (Latin)
gutta	drop	*gutta* (Latin)
h	hour	*hora* (Latin)
HS	bedtime	*hora somni* (Latin)
M ft	make	*misce fiat* (Latin)
mitt#	give this number	*mitte* (Latin)
ml	milliliter	30 ml equal one ounce
O	pint	*octarius* (Latin)
O₂	both eyes	*oculus* (Latin)
OD	right eye	*oculus dexter* (Latin)

There is nothing mysterious or secret about a prescription; the "indecipherable" notations are simply abbreviations of Latin and/or Greek words and phrases (actually, holdovers from a time when doctors wrote in Latin). The following chart will help you understand the abbreviations—for example, "gtts" is an abbreviation for Latin *guttae*, or "drops"; "ut dict" is from *ut dictum*, meaning "as directed"; and "bid" stands for the Latin *bis in die*, or "twice daily."

Once you have familiarized yourself with this simple table, you will be able to check your actual prescription with the label on the drug container to make sure that the two coincide. The chart lists the most commonly-used symbols and abbreviations that doctors use in writing prescriptions. Read it; then check your skills by reading the sample prescription reproduced in this book.

Step 2: Try reading a sample prescription.

The sample prescription reproduced here is for Darvon Compound-65 (appearing on the prescription as Darvon cpd-65).

ABBREVIATION	MEANING	DERIVATION
OL	left eye	*oculus laevus* (Latin)
OS	left eye	*oculus sinister* (Latin)
OU	each eye	*oculus uterque* (Latin)
pc	after meals	*post cibum* (Latin)
PM	evening	*post meridiem* (Latin)
po	by mouth	*per os* (Latin)
prn	as needed	*pro re nata* (Latin)
q̄	every	*quaqua* (Latin)
qd	once a day	*quaqua die* (Latin)
qid	four times a day	*quater in die* (Latin)
qod	every other day	—
s̄	without	*sine* (Latin)
Sig	label as follows	*signetur* (Latin)
sl	under the tongue	*sub lingua* (Latin)
SOB	shortness of breath	—
sol	solution	—
ss	half unit	*semis* (Latin)
stat	at once, first dose	*statim* (Latin)
susp	suspension	—
tab	tablet	—
tid	three times a day	*ter in die* (Latin)
top	apply topically	—
ung or ungt	ointment	*unguentum* (Latin)
UT	under the tongue	—
ut dict	as directed	*ut dictum* (Latin)
x	times	—

The prescription tells the pharmacist to give you 24 capsules (#24). It also directs you to take one capsule (cap i) every four hours (q4h) as needed (prn) for pain. In the space for refills the prescription indicates that you should receive up to five refills (5x) and that the label on the drug container states the name of the drug (LABEL-yes). It also gives your name and address, perhaps your age, the date of the prescription, and the name of the physician. Many physicians' prescription blanks will also give their office address and telephone number in case the pharmacist needs to call for clarification on anything.

Step 3: Talk with your pharmacist. Once you have read the prescription, you may feel that you understand the instructions. But you may not understand them clearly enough. Using the sample Darvon prescription as an example, the prescription states that you can take one capsule every four hours as needed. What does "as needed" mean? Surely you shouldn't take a capsule each hour even if you feel you need one. How many capsules is your maximum for the day

—four, five, six? You need to know your per day limit on this prescription.

As another example, suppose your prescription states that you should "take one tablet four times a day." Does that mean one tablet every six hours around the clock (which means getting up at night to take a tablet) or one tablet in the early morning, one at noon, one in the late afternoon or early evening, and one at bedtime? For other medications, it might mean one tablet every hour for the first four hours after arising in the morning. If you are confused about these instructions, be sure to ask the pharmacist while you are there in the pharmacy. He or she can always call the physician for clarification if necessary.

Step 4: Check with your pharmacist about how to take the drug.
For some medications, it makes a difference as to whether you take the drug before a meal, after a meal, or along with it. When you take the drug can make an important difference; often the drug's effectiveness depends upon following exactly the directions for its use. Your pharmacist can help you understand directions such as "as directed," "as needed," and "take with fluid." For example, with some drugs you may take water, while with others you should take milk or fruit juice. Some diuretics, for example, should be taken with orange, other citrus, or tomato juice to decrease potassium loss, since these foods have natural potassium. And be sure to check on the maximum number of doses per

day if your prescription simply says "as needed."

Step 5: Ask about any foods, beverages, or other drugs that you should avoid.
This is a very important step, because some drugs may interact in negative, even dangerous, ways with tobacco, alcohol, certain foods, and/or drugs you habitually take (even common nonprescription drugs like aspirin). Ask your pharmacist specifically about all these items, even if you have already discussed them with your doctor. You may have neglected to mention that you will be traveling and taking an antinausea medication, for example, or that you will be going to a dinner party where alcohol will be served, or that you take a certain medication for a chronic condition. Go over the list of items with your pharmacist just to make sure. Ask specifically about alcohol and about avoiding any foods. There are many drugs that interact dangerously with alcohol, so don't become a "drug reaction" statistic. If you are a woman and are taking oral contraceptives, be sure to mention the contraceptive you take and ask if you should continue it along with the new medication. If the pharmacist says no, check with your doctor about an alternate pill or birth control method that is safe.

Step 6: Ask about activities that you should avoid or restrict.
Some drugs now contain warnings on the label that you should not drive or operate equipment/machinery because the drug causes drowsiness and slowed

reactions. Even if your medication does not carry such a warning, ask anyway. Drowsiness is a common side effect and, in a driver, can be lethal. Also ask if you need to restrict travel or exposure to sun. Some drugs, especially in combination with other drugs, cause *photosensitivity* (sensitivity to light—that is, to sun) and you may end up with an uncomfortable rash and other side effects.

Step 7: Make sure you know how long to continue the medication.
The length of time you need to take a medication varies with your condition and also with the drug itself. In some cases, it is advisable to stop the drug as soon as your symptoms disappear in order to minimize side effects or, in some cases, to avoid building up a tolerance to the drug. In other cases, you should continue taking the drug for a specified length of time regardless of whether or not you are free from symptoms. In some special cases, such as kidney infection, the treatment is long-range and you'll need to take the medication for several weeks or months.

Step 8: Be certain you are familiar with possible side effects.
This is probably the most important step of all. Your doctor will probably have already mentioned possible side effects to you, but check again with your pharmacist. What are the most common side effects of this drug? Write down the list if you have trouble remembering. Which can you expect and which are rare? Which side effects are "just side effects" and

nothing to be concerned about and which are serious? For example, the drug Butazolidin may cause a blood disorder and one of the first symptoms of that disorder is a sore throat. Thus your pharmacist will urge you to check with your doctor if you develop a sore throat in the course of your medication. (This topic is discussed in more detail in the section on managing side effects.)

Step 9: Learn how to store your medication.
Finally, before you leave the drugstore or pharmacy, ask the pharmacist how to store the medication. This is important because many drugs can lose potency and therefore become ineffective if they are not stored correctly.

Most prescription drugs can be safely stored at room temperature, out of direct sunlight. (Even if your pills or tablets are in dark or colored bottles, keep them out of direct sunlight.)

There are some drugs that require refrigerator storage. However, "refrigerate" does not mean to store the drug in the freezer. Some medications, especially sugar-coated tablets, will crack if frozen and thawed; also some liquid medications will separate into layers and can't be remixed.

There are also some drugs that cannot be stored in the refrigerator at all—for example, a cough suppressant Tussionex, which thickens and ceases to pour when cold. Contrary to popular belief, nitroglycerin does not become more stable when refrigerated. In fact, it should not be refrigerated at all.

The bathroom medicine cabinet is not a good place to keep your medication, since the temperature and humidity changes in the bathroom can have adverse effects on the stability of many prescription drugs. Also, if there are small children in the house, a bathroom cabinet is an easily accessible place for them to reach and overdose on the drugs, which they may assume are candy or gum.

Remember to keep your medications away from children at all times. When you are finished with the prescription, flush the unused portion down the toilet or pour it in the sink. Discard capsules or tablets you no longer use. What is a small overdose to an adult can be fatal to a small child.

You will notice that prescription drugs have an expiration date on the container. This is a date established by the manufacturer to indicate a time beyond which the drug is no longer effective. In most cases the time is five years after the drug is made (not after it is purchased) and is based on the time by which 5 percent of the drug will have been lost or converted.

The expiration date on certain antibiotics, such as tetracycline, is very important, because after that date, the antibiotic becomes toxic. After the expiration date, tetracycline actually converts into another chemical that can damage the kidneys. Other antibiotics, such as penicillin, do not become toxic but completely lose their effectiveness and become worthless as medication.

DEFINITIONS OF IDEAL STORAGE TEMPERATURES

Cold	Any temperature under 46°F (8°C)
Refrigerator	Any cold place where the temperature is between 36°-46°F (2°-8°C)
Cool	Any temperature between 46°-59°F (8°-15°C)
Room temperature	Temperature usually between 59°-86°F (15°-30°C)
Excessive heat	Any temperature above 104°F (40°C)

Buying drugs: spending money, saving money

Prescription drugs can be expensive. Therefore, you might want to ask your pharmacist about substituting a generic drug for your prescription medication, particularly if your drug therapy is a long-term affair.

A "generic" drug is one that is not protected by trademark registration. The generic name of a drug is like a shortened form of its chemical name so that any manufacturer can use this generic name when the drug is marketed (for example, many manufacturers make the drug called tetracycline).

Usually a manufacturer will use both a trade name and a generic name for a drug. A trade name is registered and reserved for the manufacturer who holds that trademark. Thus, to follow our example above, only Lederle Laboratories can call their tetracycline Achromycin, and only Upjohn can use the name Panmycin for the same drug. (If you're confused about what the trade name looks like, it is usually capitalized in print and will include the register symbol ® after it.)

It is not necessarily true that trade name drugs are made by large manufacturers and generic drugs by small ones. Often a manufacturer will market large quantities of a certain drug under a trade name and then sell the base chemical to several other companies, some of which will sell the drug generically while others will sell it under their own trade name.

The major difference in trade name and generic drugs is in cost. Generic drugs are usually priced lower than trademarked equivalents because they are less widely advertised. You should be aware, however, that not all drugs are available generically. Furthermore, not every generic drug is significantly cheaper than nor

equivalent to the trademarked drug. You should seek your pharmacist's advice on these matters, since some trademarked drugs are superior to their generic equivalents, yet others are not significantly different either in quality or in price. Remember, however, that although the Food and Drug Administration reports that there is no evidence of "serious differences" between generic and trade name drugs, private research has demonstrated differences in quality between certain brands.

If you do find an acceptable, safe generic equivalent for your drug, your cost savings can be significant. One hundred capsules of Darvon Compound-65 analgesic may cost $12 to $15 while the generic equivalent can be bought for about $8. Pavabid vasodilator can cost $17 per 100 capsules, but the generic drug may be as low as $9 per 100.

In most states, it is now legal for consumers to inquire about and to request pharmacists to fill prescriptions with the cheapest generic brand. If this subsitution is not legal in your state, you might ask your doctor to prescribe drugs by their generic name so that the pharmacist will fill the prescription in this form. This is especially helpful if the medication is one that you take on a long-term or regular basis.

Your pharmacist can also help you save money by recommending the use of over-the-counter drugs (OTC drugs). These are, of course, drugs that can be purchased without a prescription and consequently can be sold anywhere. There are no legal requirements and no limitations on who can buy them.

Finally, if you are on a medication for a long period of time or if you are very sensitive to drugs and suspect that you might react badly to one, you might wish to save money by purchasing larger or smaller quantities of the medication. In the first instance, patients with chronic conditions such as heart disease, high blood pressure, or diabetes may want to purchase medication in quantity. Generally, the price per dose decreases with the amount purchased. For example, a drug that costs 6¢ per tablet when bought in amounts of 25 or 30 tablets decreases to 4 to 5¢ per tablet when bought in bottles of 100 or more. Many doctors will prescribe one to six months' supply of drugs that you take regularly.

On the other hand, if you have a history of drug reactions or allergies and are concerned about the side effects of a certain drug, you might ask the pharmacist to fill one half or one quarter of the prescription to see if the drug "agrees" with you. You may have to pay more per dose when you buy in small amounts, but you will then have a chance to test the drug on yourself. Make sure that the pharmacist realizes that you took only half the prescription (or a third, or whatever) so that you can get the rest if you want it. For many drugs, however, you must get another prescription once any part of the first has been filled.

INDEX

A

abortion
  dilatation and curettage, 400
  spontaneous (miscarriage),
    456–457
acetaminophen, 129
  fever and, 58
  in Reye's syndrome, 89
acetylcholine, in Alzheimer's
  disease, 122
Achilles tendon, 197
acidosis, 68
acne, 151–153, 418, 423
  topical drugs, 153
acquired immune deficiency
  syndrome. See AIDS
acromegaly, 385
  carpal tunnel syndrome and, 186
acrophobia, 511
ACTH, 366–367, 384
  excess in Cushing's syndrome,
   369
  in production of corticosteroids,
   369
Acyclovir, 84
Addison's disease, 367–368
additives, 9
adenocarcinoma and DES, 399
adenoids, 220
adenomas, 370
adrenal glands, 365, 366
  Addison's disease, 367–368
  adrenal hyperplasia, 377
  Cushing's syndrome, 369–371
  hirsutism, 376
adrenaline, 240
adrenocorticotropic hormone. See
  ACTH
agoraphobia, 511, 512
AIDS, 107–108
albumin, 354
  in glomerulonephritis, 354
  in nephrotic syndrome, 484
  test, 554

alcohol abuse, 22–23, 24–26
  Alcoholics Anonymous, 26
  folic acid deficiency anemia,
   257, 259
  hepatitis, 332–334
  hypoglycemia, 379–380
  impotence and, 392
  liver cirrhosis, 319
  pancreatitis, 384
  stomach cancer, 550
  thiamine deficiency in, 26
allergy, 104–107
  allergens, 105–106
  allergic purpura, 172
  allergists, 32–33
  anaphylactic shock, 105,
   108–109
  asthma attacks, 239
  contact dermatitis, 110–112
  food allergy, 112
  hay fever, 113–114
  hives, 115
  immunology and, 32–33
  immunotherapy, 106
  insect bite and sting, 118
  nasal congestion in, 63
  photodermatitis, 111
  rashes, 67
  symptoms, 105
  tests, 556
allopurinol, 190
alopecia, 155
alveoli, 236
Alzheimer's disease, 121–124
  vs. senility, 517
amblyopia, 461–462, 494
amenorrhea, 397–398
  anorexia nervosa and, 500
amino acids, 10–11
  in phenylketonuria, 533
amnesia, 124–125
  meningitis and, 138
amniocentesis, 494, 536, 569
  amniotic fluid, 447, 526

amphetamines, 141
amylase, 382
amyloid, 271
    amyloidosis and carpal tunnel
        syndrome, 186
analgesic drugs, 66
anaphylactic shock (anaphylaxis),
    105, 108–109
    vs. anaphylactoid reactions, 109
anaphylactoid purpura, 172
androgens, 366. See also
        testosterone
    in baldness, 155
    in hirsutism, 376
anemia, 257–260
    boils and, 156
    celiac disease and, 522
    hemoglobin count, 287
    sickle-cell, 534–535
anesthesiologists, 33
anesthetic drugs, 448
aneurysm, 260–262
    stroke and, 304
angina pectoris, 262–265
    vs. heart attack, 262, 282
angiogram, 262
anorexia nervosa, 62, 500–503
    hirsutism and, 376
anoscopy, 332
antacids, 48, 59, 60
anti-arrhythmic drugs, 285
antibiotics
    abnormal heart valves and, 279
    appendicitis, 316
    boils, 157
    Candida albicans and, 76
    canker sores, 159
    cystitis, 352
    dental procedures, 301
    middle ear infections, 227
    photodermatitis, 111
    photosensitivity and, 550
    prostatitis, 394
    pyelonephritis, 362
    rheumatic heart disease, 302
antibodies, 71, 102–104, 483,
        484, 522
    in gamma globulin, 111

anticholinergic drugs, 342
anticoagulants, 268, 277, 278,
        283, 297
anticonvulsant drugs, 132
antigens, 109
antihistamines, 106, 114, 115,
        136, 231
    overuse in nasal congestion, 223
antipsychotic drugs, 516
antispasmodic drugs, 345
antithyroid drugs, 378–379
antitoxins, 71
anus, 314
    anal fistula, 327
    anoscopy, 563
    gonorrhea, 82–83
    hemorrhoids, 330–332
    itching, in pinworms, 489
    proctology, 43–44
anxiety, 511
aorta, 255
    aneurysms, 260
Apgar score, 462–463
aphthous ulcers. See canker sores
aplastic anemia, 257, 259
apnea, 237–238
appendicitis, 315–316
appetite
    control, 15
    loss (anorexia nervosa), 62
arrhythmia, 284–285
    fainting and, 56
    ventricular extrasystole and, 280
artery, 260
    arteriogram (angiogram), 262
    artery diseases. See blood and
        circulatory diseases
arthritis, 179–181
    osteoporosis and, 192
    in Reiter's syndrome, 94
artificial insemination, 448–449
ascorbic acid. See Vitamin C
aseptic meningitis, 79
aspartame, 9
aspirin, 58
    arthritis and, 181
    circumcision and, 470
    fever and, 58

Reye's syndrome, role in, 78, 491
rheumatic fever and, 301
asthma, 238–241
 beta blocker drugs, danger in, 268
 cor pulmonale and, 273
 pulmonary function tests, 565–566
astigmatism, 202–203
ataxia, 125–126
atherosclerosis, 265–270
 aneurysms, 261
 angina pectoris and, 262
 cholesterol in, 12–13
 fluoride in, 14
 ischemia and, 291
 role in heart attack, 282
 stroke, 304
athlete's foot, 153–154
atopic dermatitis, 162
attention deficit disorder. *See* hyperkinesis
autism, 463–465
autoimmune diseases, 109–110, 381

B
bacilli, 73
bacitracin, 203
backache, 181–183
 in osteoporosis, 192
 slipped disk, 196
bacteremia, 278
bacteria, 72–74
bacterial infections, 69. *See also* viral infections
 bubonic plague, 74–75
 diphtheria, 80–82
 hair loss in, 155
 scarlet fever, 96
 septicemia, 96–97
 tetanus, 101
baldness, 154–156
bariatrics, 33
barium enema, 326, 344, 346
Bart's disease, 287

basal body temperature, 440
"baseball pitcher's elbow," 185
battered child syndrome, 465–467
behavior modification, 500
Bell's palsy, 126–127
 shingles and, 99
benzocaine, 228
benzophenone, 175
beta blocker drugs, 211, 268, 283, 285, 290, 379
 precautions, 240, 283
bile, 316–317
 jaundice, 338
bilirubin, 316, 317, 338, 554
biliverdin, 317
biopsy, 557
birth control, 429, 430–436
 calendar method, 432
 condom, 433
 contraceptives and vaginal irritation, 409
 contraceptive sponge, 435
 diaphragm, 432–433
 IUD, 433–434
 menopause and, 413
 mucus method, 432
 permanent, 435–436
 pills, 434–435. *See also* oral contraceptives
 post-coital, 400
 spermicides, 432
 temperature method, 431
birth defects
 amniocentesis in detecting, 569
 artificial insemination and, 449
 caffeine and, 9
 celiac disease, 521–523
 cerebral palsy, 467–469
 cleft lip/cleft palate, 471–473
 clubfoot, 473–474
 congenital hypothyroidism, 474–476
 Down's syndrome, 526–528
 patent ductus arteriosus, 486–488
 spina bifida, 493–494
 strabismus, 494–495

"black death." See bubonic plague
blackheads, 152
bladder, 347
    cancer, 542–543
    cystitis, 349–353
    cystocele, 398–399
    cystoscopy, 350
    incontinence, 356
bleeding. See hemorrhage
blepharitis, 203–204
blood, 256–257
    clots, 260, 276, 282, 294, 307
    clotting mechanism, 287
    coagulation, 294
    hemoglobin, 286–287
    lymphocytes, 292
    platelets, 294
    pressure reading, 68
    Rh factor, 302–304
    in the stools, 65, 288
    in the urine, 288
    in the vomitus, 288
    sugar levels, 379
    tests, 552–554
    transfusion, 294
blood and circulatory diseases
    anemia, 257–260
    aneurysm, 260–262
    atherosclerosis, 265–270
    coronary artery disease, 262
    coronary bypass surgery,
        268–270
    cyanosis, 274–275
    embolism, 276–278
    hemorrhage, 287–288
    ischemia, 291
    necrosis, 292
    polycythemia, 294–295
    pulmonary embolism, 295–297
    Raynaud's phenomenon and
        disease, 297–298
    restless legs syndrome, 298–299
    sickle-cell anemia, 534–535
    stroke, 304–306
    thrombocytopenia, 306–307
    thrombophlebitis, 307–309

transient ischemic attacks (TIAs),
    309–310
    varicose veins, 310–311
body's defenses, 70–71
body temperature, 68
    hypothermia, 137–138
    normal, 57
boils, 156–157
bone diseases and disorders,
    45–46. See also joint diseases;
    muscle diseases
    backache, 181–183
    bones, 177
    bunions, 183–184
    cancer, 543
    fractures, 187–189
    osteomyelitis, 485–486
    osteoporosis, 191–193
    otosclerosis, 193–194
    Paget's disease, 194–195
    slipped disk, 195–197
bone marrow, 256, 257, 292, 295
    androgens and, 366
    leukemia, 546–547
Bornholm disease, 79
botulism, 144
bowel. See also colon; intestinal
    diseases
    control, 356
    irritable bowel syndrome,
        336–337
    movement, postponing of, 331
brain and brain disorders,
    119–121
    Alzheimer's disease, 121–124
    amnesia, 124–125
    cancer, 543–544
    cerebrospinal fluid, 127
    concussion, 127–129
    electroencephalogram,
        561–562
    encephalitis, 129–130
    Huntington's chorea, 530–533
    hydrocephalus, 481–482
    hyperkinesis, 482–483
    lumbar puncture, 127, 139
    meningitis, 138–139

Tay-Sachs disease, 535–536
tomography, 567–568
tumors, 130, 135
breast(s)
cancer, 544–545
enlargement in a male, 388–390
fibrocystic disease, 405–407
mammography, 406–407
mastectomy, 410–412
mastitis, 412
breast-feeding, 448
mastitis, 412
prolactin, 384
thyroid hormone and, 475
Bright's disease. See
glomerulonephritis
Bromocriptine, 146
bronchi, 236
bronchiectasis, 241–242
bronchitis, 242–245
cor pulmonale and, 273
emphysema and, 244
nasal congestion in, 62–63
smoking and, 28
bronchodilators, 244
bronchoscopy, 564
bubonic plague, 74–75
bulimia, 501, 503
bunion, 183–184
burns and dehydration, 51
Burow's solution, 154
bursitis, 184–185
bursae, 160, 177, 184, 185
bypass surgery. See coronary
bypass surgery

C

caffeine, 10
extrasystole and, 280
migraine headache and, 133
calcitonin, 195
calcium, 20
antagonists, 265, 267
deposits, 13–14, 185
kidney stones and, 360
osteoporosis, 191–193

calluses and corns, 157–158,
159–160
calories, 7–8
cancer, 537–551
chemotherapy, 539–540
danger of immunization in, 117
heat therapy, 541
immunotherapy, 540–541
laetrile, 541
leukemia, 546–547
leukoplakia and, 167–168
oncology, 39
radiation, 540
smoking and, 27–28
surgery, 539
types of, 537, 542–551
warning signs, 537–538
Candida albicans, 75–76
in glossitis, 228
in vaginitis, 427
canker sores, 158–159
capillaries, 255
carbohydrates, 11
in diabetes mellitus, 371
carbuncles, 157
carcinoma, 537
cardiac arrest, 275
cardiac arrhythmia. See
arrhythmia
cardiac catheterization, 560. See
also angiogram
cardiac stress test, 566–567
cardiology, 33
cardiovascular diseases. See blood
and circulatory diseases; heart
diseases
cardiovascular surgery, 34
caries (tooth decay), 342
carpal tunnel syndrome, 142,
185–187
cartilage, 177
cataplexy, 141
cataracts, 204–205
retinal detachment and, 208
catatonia
catatonic symptoms, 515
electroconvulsive therapy, 516

CAT scan, 338, 370, 481, 538, 543
cavity (tooth decay), 342
celiac disease (sprue) 521–523
cerebellum, 121
cerebral hemorrhage in stroke, 304
cerebral palsy, 467–469
    ataxia in, 125
    epilepsy and, 130
cerebrospinal fluid, 127, 477, 494, 564
    in hydrocephalus, 481
cerebrovascular embolism, 304
cerebrum, 121
cervix, 395
    cancer, 546
    dilatation and curettage, 400–401
    "hostile," 439
    hysterectomy, 408–409
    Pap test, 193
cesarean section, 449–451
    genital warts and, 436
chafing vs. heat rash, 166–167
chancre, 99
change of life. See menopause
chelation therapy, 122
chemotherapy, 539–540
    side effects, 540
chest pain, 48–49
chicken pox, 76–78
    aspirin and Reye's syndrome, 78, 491
    encephalitis and, 129
    gamma globulin in, 113
    rash, 66
    shingles and, 77
    vaccine, 78
child abuse. See battered child syndrome
childbirth, 447–448. See also breast-feeding; pregnancy
    cesarean section, 449–451
    cystocele and, 398
    dysmenorrhea and, 402
    endometriosis and, 404
    episiotomy, 455

genital warts and, 436
herpes and, 450
labor, 447
oxygen starvation in, 469
oxytocin in, 384
prolapsed uterus and, 423
prostaglandins in, 385–386
vaginal fistula in, 327
childhood diseases and problems. See also infant diseases and problems
amblyopia, 461–462
aseptic meningitis, 79
aspirin in chicken pox and influenza, 58
asthma, 240
autism, 463–465
battered child syndrome, 465–467
blepharitis, 203–204
bone cancer, 543
bone fractures, 187–189
Bornholm disease, 79
bronchitis, 242–245
cavities and fluoride, 342
celiac disease, 521–523
chicken pox, 76–78
childhood schizophrenia vs. autism, 464
colds, susceptibility to, 222–224
congenital rubella syndrome, 94
coxsackie viruses, 78–80
croup, 476–477
cystic fibrosis, 223–226
diabetes, 371–374
diphtheria, 80–82
ear infections, 226–227
epidemic pleurodynia, 79
Gilles de la Tourette's syndrome, 199, 478–480
goiter, 374–376
hand, foot, and mouth disease, 79
herpangina, 79
hydrocephalus, 481–482
hyperkinesis, 482–483
immunization, 72, 116–118
interstitial keratitis, 211–212

leukemia, 546—547
measles, 89—91
meningitis, 138—139
mumps, 91—93
muscular dystrophy, 532—533
myocarditis, 80
nephrotic syndrome, 484—485
obesity in children, 14
osteomyelitis, 485—486
paralytic disease, 79
pediatricians, 41—42
pericarditis, 80
phimosis, 488
pinworms, 488—489
purpura fulminans, 172
respiratory disease, 79
Reye's syndrome, 78, 89,
    489—491
rubella, 94—96
rubella-like rash, 79—80
chlorpromazine, 531
cholecystitis, 317—318
    cholecystectomy, 318
    gallstones and, 329
cholera
    dehydration in, 51
    immunization, 117
cholesterol, 11—13
    deposits in arteries, 268
    relation to stroke, 306
    role in formation of gallstones,
        328
    test, 554
choline-acetyltransferase, 122
chorea, 301
choroid
    membrane (eye), 201, 207
    plexi, 127
chromosomes, 453, 519—521
    in color blindness, 206
chronic mountain sickness, 273
chronic obstructive pulmonary
    disease, 273
chymopapain, 197
cilia, 219, 451
cimetidine, 345
circulatory diseases. See blood
    and circulatory diseases

circumcision, 469—471
    phimosis, 488
cirrhosis, 318—320
    in hepatitis, 333
claustrophobia, 511
cleft lip/cleft palate, 471—473
climacteric. See menopause
clomiphene, 441
Clostridium tetani, 101
clotrimazole, 154
clots. See blood
clubfoot, 473—474
coagulation. See blood
cocci, 73
cochlea, 218
codeine, 233
colchicine, 190
cold. See common cold
cold sores. See fever blisters
colitis, 320—321
colon, 313—314
    cancer, 545—546
    colitis, 320—321
    colonscopy, 563
    diverticulitis, 325—326
    lower GI series, 558—559
    proctosigmoidoscopy, 562
    spastic or mucous colon,
        336—337
    ulcerative colitis, 345—346
color blindness, 205—206
colostomy, 321—323, 546
comedones, 151—152
common cold, 222—224, 460
    cough and, 50—51
    nasal congestion, 62—63
computerized tomography. See
    CAT scan
conception, 443, 451—453
    pelvic inflamatory disease and,
        421
concussion, 127—129
condom, 433
condylomata acuminata,
    436—437
cones and rods, 214
congenital hypothyroidism,
    474—476

congenital rubella syndrome, 94
congestive heart failure, 270—272
conjunctivitis, 206—207
    conjunctiva, 201
    in Reiter's syndrome, 93
constipation, 49—50
    fibroid tumors and, 408
    hemorrhoids and, 331
    rectocele and, 424
contact dermatitis, 110—112, 161
contraception. See birth control;
    oral contraceptives
contrast examinations, 557—558
COPD. See chronic obstructive
    pulmonary disease
cor pulmonale, 273—274
cornea, 201
    herpes simplex keratitis, 164
    keratitis, 211—212
    keratomalacia, 214
corns and calluses, 157—158,
    159—160
coronary artery disease, 262
    coronary artery, 262
coronary bypass surgery, 268—270
corpora cavernosa, 392
corpus callosum,
corticosteroids, 115, 195, 240,
    368—369
    hirsutism and, 377
    precautions, 240
corticotropin. See ACTH
cortisol, 369
cortisone, 163, 171, 187, 301,
    321, 368
Corynebacterium diphtheriae, 80
cough, 50—51, 460
    in croup, 476
coxsackie viruses, 78—80
creatinine, 554
crib death. See sudden infant
    death syndrome
Crohn's disease, 323—325
cromolyn, 240—241
"cross-eye." See strabismus
croup, 476—477
cryoprecipitate, 530
cryotherapy, 208

cryptorchidism. See testes,
    undescended
Cushing's syndrome, 369—371
    hirsutism and, 376—377
cyanocobalamin, B_{12}, 18
cyanosis, 274—275
cyclamates, 9
cyclothymia, 506
cystic fibrosis, 523—526
    bronchiectasis and, 241
cystitis, 349—353
cystocele, 398—399
cyst, 160—161
    birth control pills and, 407
    in breasts, 405—407
    chronic fibrocystic mastitis, 412
    cystoscopy, 350—351, 543, 563
    ovarian, 409

D
danazol, 405
D and C. See dilatation and
    curettage
Darvon, 574
deafness, 224—226. See also ear
    infections and diseases
    antituberculosis drugs, damage
        from, 254
    hearing aids, 225
    Meniere's disease, 230—231
    meningitis, 138—139
    mumps encephalitis, 129
    otosclerosis, 193—194
    Paget's disease, 194—195
decongestants, 63, 67, 223, 227
    overuse in nasal congestion, 63
    precautions, 231
defibrillation, 275—276
dehydration, 51—52
    diarrhea, 52
delirium, 503—504
    tremens, 25
delusions, 515
dental plaque, 343
dental procedures and bacterial
    infections, 301
dentistry and dentists, 34
depression, 504—507

dermatitis, 161–163
  contact dermatitis, 110–112, 161
    dermatologists, 34–35
    photodermatitis, 111
dermoid cysts, 418
DES, 399–401, 551
detached retina, 207–208
diabetes insipidus, 385
diabetes mellitus, 371–374
  Candida albicans in, 75–76
  carbohydrates in, 371
  carpal tunnel syndrome and, 186
  cataracts in, 204
  dehydration in, 51
  intravenous pyelogram and, 559
  ketosis, 382
  retinopathy, 216
  stroke and, 304
dialysis, 353–354
diaper rash, 75
diaphanography, 407
diaphragm, 335
diaphragmatic hernia, 335
diaphragm (birth control),
    432–433
diarrhea, 52–53, 460–461
  irritable bowel syndrome and,
    336
  Reiter's syndrome and, 93
  toxic shock syndrome and, 426
  ulcerative colitis and, 346
diathermy, 208
diazepam, 101
diet(s)
  balanced, 16–17
  crash and fad, 15
  vegetarian, 8
diethylstilbestrol. *See* DES
diflunisal, 402
digestive diseases, 313, 346. *See
    also* intestinal diseases
digitalis, 272, 283
dilatation and curettage, 400–401
  in miscarriage, 457
diphtheria, 80–82
  immunization, 82
discography, 197
diuretics, 231, 485

in atherosclerosis, 268
in congestive heart failure, 272
dehydration and, 51
in heart attack, 283
in hypertension, 290
diverticulitis (diverticulosis),
    325–326
dizziness and vertigo, 53–54
  Meniere's disease, 230–231
  nystagmus, 214–215
  postural hypotension, 219
DNA, 519
doctors. *See* physicians
dopamine, 146
Doppler technique, 309
"dowager's hump," 193
Down's syndrome, 526–528
drug addicts
  risk of AIDS, 107
  risk of hepatitis, 333
drugs
  generic, 578
  in pregnancy, 446
  prescriptions, 572–578
  saving money on, 578–579
DPT shots, 484
Duchenne muscular dystrophy,
    532
duodenal ulcers. *See* ulcers
duodenum, 314, 383
  gastroscopy, 563
  upper GI series, 558
dwarfism, 385
dysmenorrhea, 401–403
  fibroid tumors and, 408
dyspareunia, 403
dyspepsia. *See* indigestion
dyspnea, 245
dystrophy (muscular), 532–533

E
ear infections and diseases,
    226–227. *See also* deafness
  adenoids in relation to, 221
  mastoiditis, 229–230
  Meniere's disease, 230–231
  otosclerosis, 193–194
  stapedectomy, 194

eating, excessive. *See* bulimia
ECG. *See* electrocardiogram
echolalia, 464
echoviruses, 78—80
eclampsia. *See* toxemia of
    pregnancy
ECT. *See* electroconvulsive
    therapy
ectopic pregnancy, 453—455
    oophorectomy and, 417
eczema, 161—162
edema, 54—55
    in celiac disease, 522
    in glomerulonephritis, 355
    in kidney failure, 357
    in menstruation, 416, 422
    in nephrotic syndrome, 357
    in toxemia of pregnancy, 459
EEG. *See* electroencephalogram
egg (ovum), 395
    chromosomes and, 519
    fertilization, 453
    zygote, 443
ejaculation, 388
    retrograde, 439
Ekbom syndrome. *See* restless legs
    syndrome
electric shock. *See*
    electroconvulsive therapy
electrocardiogram
    (electrocardiograph), 267,
    286, 555
electroconvulsive therapy, 506,
    507, 516
electroencephalogram
    (electroencephalograph), 381,
    507, 561—562
electrolysis in hirsutism, 377
electrolytes, 554
embolism, 276—278
    cerebrovascular embolism, 304
    emboli, 295
embryo, 443
emotional problems. *See* mental
    problems
emphysema, 244, 245—248
    cor pulmonale and, 273
    dyspnea and, 245

pulmonary function tests,
    565—566
    smoking and, 27
encephalitis, 129—130
    amnesia and, 124
    "Parkinsonism" and, 144
    Reye's syndrome and, 489—490
    rubella and, 94
endarterectomies, 268
endocarditis, 278—279
    in septicemia, 96—97
endocrine glands, 363. *See also*
    adrenal glands; ovaries;
    pancreas; parathyroid glands;
    pituitary gland; testes; thyroid
    gland
endocrinologists, 35
endodontia, 34
endometriosis, 403—405, 439
    dysmenorrhea and, 402
    dyspareunia and, 403
    oophorectomy and, 417—418
endoscopic retrograde
    cholangiopancreatography,
    383
endoscopy, 562
enemas, 50
enteroviruses, 78
epidemic pleurodynia, 79
epidemiology, 35—36
epidermis, 150
    psoriasis, 170—172
epididymis, 387
    epididymitis, 442
epilepsy, 130—132
    incontinence and, 356
    meningitis and, 138
epinephrine, 109, 240
episiotomy, 455
    dyspareunia and, 403
erection, 390
erythrocytes, 302. *See also* red
    blood cells
erythromycin, 81, 157, 203
erythrophobia, 512
esophagus
    gastroscopy, 563
    paraesophageal hiatus hernia, 335

upper GI series, 558
estrogen, 193, 389, 395, 403, 413, 434, 439
estrogen therapy
  DES, 399—401
  hirsutism, 376—377
  osteoporosis, 193
  purpura, 173
  side effects in cancer of the uterus, 550
eustachian tube, 218
exercise
  angina pectoris and, 265
  cholesterol levels and, 13
  exercise tolerance test and, 267
  heart attack and, 283
  obesity and, 16
exfoliative dermatitis, 162
exocrine glands, 525
exodontia, 34
extrasystole, 279—281
exudative retinitis, 215
eye diseases. *See also* vision
  blepharitis, 203—204
  cataracts, 204—205
  conjunctivitis, 206—207
  glaucoma, 208—211
  herpes simplex keratitis, 164
  keratitis, 211—212
  keratomalacia, 214
  laser surgery, 208
  macular degeneration, 212
  night blindness, 214
  retina, detached, 207—208
  retinitis, 215—216
  retinopathy, 216—217
  sty, 217
  xerophthalmia, 214

F
fainting, 55—56
fallopian tubes, 395
  blocking gonorrhea, 82
  obstruction, 439
  in pelvic inflammatory disease, 421
  removal in hysterectomy, 409
  tubal pregnancy, 453—455

family doctor. *See* physicians
family therapy, 500
fatigue, 56—57
fats
  in atherosclerosis, 265—266
  gallstones and, 328
  heart attack and, 282
  ketosis, 382
  saturated, 11
fecalith, 325
feet, diseases and injuries. *See* podiatry
female reproductive system, 395—428
femoral artery occlusion, 42
fertilization, 452—453
fetus, 444, 445, 446
fever, 57—58, 460
  danger of immunization in, 117
  with joint inflammation, 299
fever blisters, 163—164
fiber,
  constipation, 50
  hemorrhoids, 332
  irritable bowel syndrome, 337
  psyllium, 326
fibrocystic disease of the breast, 405—407
  caffeine and, 407
fibroid tumors, 407—408
fistula, 324, 326—327
flooding technique, 512
flu. *See* influenza
fluoride, 13—14, 343
fluoroscopy, 557
folic acid, 320, 325
  deficiency anemia, 259
follicle-stimulating hormone (FSH), 384
fontanelles, 477
food
  additives in hyperkinesis, 483
  binges. *See* bulimia
  cancer and, 542
  digestion, 313
  groups, 9
  health food quacks, 10
food allergy, 112

fractures, 187–189
  excessive calcium in kidneys, 358
  Paget's disease, 194–195
Friedreich's ataxia, 126
frostbite, 164–166
  gangrene in frostbite, 165
FSH. *See* follicle-stimulating hormone
fungal infections
  Candida albicans, 75–76
  fungi, 73
  histoplasmosis, 85–86
  onychomycosis, 169
furuncles. *See* boils

G
gallbladder, 314
  bile, 316
  cholecystitis, 317
  gallbladder series, 559–560
  inflammation, gangrene in, 317
  jaundice, 327–328
  pancreatitis and, 383
gallstones, 327–330
gamma globulin, 112–113
  in hepatitis, 113
gastroenteritis, 330
gastroenterologists, 36
gastrointestinal series, 558–559
gastroscopy, 563
genes, 519–521
  genetic engineering, 521, 531
genital warts, 436–437
German measles. *See* rubella
giantism, 385
Gilles de la Tourette's syndrome, 199, 478–480
gingivitis, 339
  deficiency of Vitamin C, 18
GI series. *See* gastrointestinal series
glaucoma, 208–211
  cataracts and, 204
glomerulonephritis, 354–356
  glomeruli, 484
glossitis, 227–229
glucagon, 365

glucocorticoids, 369
gluten, in celiac disease, 521
goiter, 374–376
gonadotropic hormones, 384
gonorrhea, 82–83, 351, 430
  microbe, 93
  pelvic inflammatory disease and, 82
gout, 189–190
  kidney stones in, 189, 358
granulomatous colitis, 321
Graves' disease, 377–378
griseofulvin, 154, 169
group therapy, 500
growth hormone, 384, 386
gums, 338–340
gynecology/obstetrics, 38
gynecomastia, 388–390

H
hair
  baldness, 154–156
  excessive growth. *See* hirsutism
hallucinations, 504
  in schizophrenia, 516
  haloperidol, 199
  halothane, 319
hand, foot, and mouth disease, 79
hardening of the arteries. *See* atherosclerosis
hay fever, 113–114
  conjunctivitis in, 206
HDL. *See* high density lipoprotein
headaches, 132–137
hearing aids, 225
hearing loss. *See* deafness
heart, 255
  valves, 301
  ventricles, 255
heart attack (myocardial infarction), 281–284
heartbeat irregularities (arrhythmia), 284–285
heartburn, 48, 58–59
heart diseases, 48
  angina attack vs. heart attack, 262

angina pectoris, 262–265
cardiac catheterization, 560
cardiac stress test, 566–567
chest pain in, 48–49
cholesterol and, 12
congestive heart failure,
    270–272
coronary artery disease, 262
cor pulmonale, 273–274
defibrillation, 275–276
embolism, 276–278
endocarditis, 278–279
extrasystole, 279–281
hypertension, 288–290
hypotension, 290–291
pericarditis, 292–293
rheumatic fever, 299–301
rheumatic heart disease,
    301–302
sinus node, 284
heart murmurs, 285–286
heat rash, 166–167
heat therapy, 541
hematocrit, 553
hematology, 36–37
hemodialysis, 353
hemoglobin, 286–287, 553
hemolysis, 303
hemolytic anemias, 259
hemophilia, 528–530
    circumcision and, 470
    hemophiliacs, risk of AIDS, 530
Hemophilus vaginalis, 427
hemorrhage, 287–288
    brain, 129
    in ectopic pregnancy, 454
    low platelet count in, 294
    in purpura, 172–173
    in retinopathy, 216–217
    in ulcers, 344
hemorrhoids, 330–332
Henoch-Schonlein purpura, 173
heparin, 277, 297
hepatitis, 332–334
    cirrhosis and, 319
    gamma globulin in, 113
hereditary disorders
    celiac disease, 521–523

cystic fibrosis, 523–526
Down's syndrome, 526–528
hemophilia, 528–530
Huntington's chorea, 530–532
muscular dystrophy, 532–533
phenylketonuria (PKU),
    533–534
sickle-cell anemia, 534–535
Tay-Sachs disease, 535–536
hernia, 334–336
herpangina, 79
herpes, 83–85
    genital and cancer, 546
    simplex, 163
    simplex encephalitis, 130
    simplex keratitis, 164
    zoster. *See* shingles
hexachlorophene and
    photosensitivity, 169
hiatus hernia. *See* diaphragmatic
    hernia
high blood pressure. *See*
    hypertension
high density lipoprotein (HDL), 12
Hirschsprung's disease, 321–322
hirsutism, 376–377
histamine, 104
histoplasmosis, 85–86
hives, 115
HMD. *See* hyaline membrane
    disease
Hodgkin's disease, 548–549
    chemotherapy, 549
    shingles and, 98
homosexuals, risk of AIDS, 107
hookworms and iron deficiency
    anemia, 251
hormones, 363
    acne and, 151
    excessive production, 369
hot flashes, 413
human papilloma virus, 175
Huntington's chorea, 530–532
hyaline membrane disease
    (HMD), 480–481
hydrocele, 390
hydrocephalus, 481–482
    in spina bifida, 494

hydrocortisone, 346, 366
hydrophobia. See rabies
hymen
  in amenorrhea, 397
  in dyspareunia, 403
hyperactivity. See hyperkinesis
hyperemesis gravidarum,
    455–456
hyperkinesis, 482–483
hypertension, 267, 288–290
  aneurysms in, 261
  atherosclerosis, 267
  blood pressure reading, 289
  heart attack and, 282
  premature menopause and, 414
  retinal detachment in, 208
  salt and, 9
  stroke and, 304
hyperthermia. See heat therapy
hyperthyroidism, 377–379
  excessive eating and, 501
  myasthenia gravis and, 140
hyperventilation, 68, 507–508
  dyspnea, 245
hypochondria, 508–509
hypoglycemia, 379–380
hypotension, 290–291
hypothalamus, 369, 475
  appetite control, 15
  narcolepsy and, 141
  ovulation and, 420
hypothermia, 137–138
hypothyroidism, 380–382
hysterectomy, 408–409, 546
  in conjunction with
    oophorectomy, 417–418

I
ibuprofen, 181, 402
ileitis. See Crohn's disease
ileum
  Crohn's disease, 323–325
ileostomy, 336
illness, symptoms of, 47–68
immune reaction, 104
  platelets, 294

immunity, 104. See also
    autoimmune diseases;
    immunization; immunology
immunization, 72, 116–118
  children's, 116, 483–484
  foreign travel, 117–118
  precautions, 117
immunology, 32–33
immunosuppressive therapy, 173
  herpes in relation to, 84
immunotherapy, 106, 540–541
impotence, 390–392
incontinence, 356
indigestion, 59–60
  chest pain in, 48
infant diseases and problems. See
    also birth defects; childhood
    diseases and problems
  Apgar score, 462–463
  apnea, 237–238
  asthma, 238–241
  blindness and gonorrhea, 82
  cataracts and German measles,
    94
  circumcision, 469–471
  congenital pyloric stenosis, 341
  fontanelles, 477
  hearing loss, testing for, 225
  heat rash, 166–167
  Hirschsprung's disease,
    321–322
  hyaline membrane disease,
    480–481
  hydrocephalus, 481–482
  interstitial keratitis, 211–212
  jaundice, 337–338
  normal temporary
    gynecomastia, 389
  patent ductus arteriosus,
    486–488.
  phenylketonuria, 533–534
  sudden infant death syndrome
    (SIDS), 495–496
  Tay-Sachs disease, 535–536
  thrombocytopenia, 306–307
  umbilical hernia, 334
  when to call the doctor,
    460–461

infections, bacterial and viral, 69—70
infectious diseases, 69—101
  bubonic plague, 74—75
  Candida albicans, 75—76
  chicken pox, 76—78
  coxsackie viruses, 78—80
  diphtheria, 80—82
  histoplasmosis, 85—86
  mononucleosis, 86—87
  influenza, 87—89
  measles, 89—91
  mumps, 91—93
  Reiter's syndrome, 93—94
  rubella, 94—96
  scarlet fever, 96
  septicemia, 96—97
  shingles, 97—99
  syphilis, 99—101
  tetanus, 101
infectious mononucleosis, 86—87
infertility, 429—430, 437—441
  artificial insemination, 448—449
  cystic fibrosis and, 525
  female, 439
  fertilization, 441
  impotence, 390—392
  male, 438—439
  undescended testes, 496
inflammatory bowel disease, 320
influenza, 87—89
  cough in, 50—51
  immunization, 89
  nasal congestion in, 63
  Reye's syndrome and, 490
insemination, artificial, 448—449
insect bite and sting, 118
insight therapy, 512
insomnia, 60—61
insulin, 371, 372, 373, 374, 379, 382, 383
interferon
  cancer and, 540
internists, 37
intestinal diseases
  appendicitis, 315—316
  Crohn's disease, 323—325

gastroenteritis, 330
gastrointestinal series, 558
gastroscopy, 536
hemorrhoids, 330—332
hernia, 334—335
ileostomy, 336
irritable bowel syndrome, 336—337
peritonitis, 340—341
pyloric stenosis, 341—342
ulcerative colitis, 345—346
intrauterine devices (IUDs), 433—434
  in pelvic inflammatory disease, 421—422
intravenous pyelogram, 559
intrinsic factor, 258
"*in vitro*" fertilization, 441
iodine, 21, 474
  in goiter, 374
  in production of thyroid hormone, 377
iris, 201
iron, 21
  anemia and, 259
  deficiency in celiac disease, 522
  hemoglobin and, 287
  loss in menorrhagia, 414
  phlebotomy and, 295
irritable bowel syndrome, 320, 336—337
ischemia, 291
islets of Langerhans, 372
isotretinoin, 153
itching, 61—62
IUD. *See* intrauterine devices

J
jaundice, 317, 329, 332, 337—338
"jimmy legs" ("jitter legs"). *See* restless legs syndrome
joint diseases
  arthritis, 179—181
  bunions, 183—184
  bursitis, 184—185
  carpal tunnel syndrome, 185—187

lupus erythematosus, 190–191
slipped disk, 195–197

K
Kaposi's sarcoma, 107
keratitis, 211–212
keratomalacia, 214
ketoacidosis. See ketosis
ketones, 373, 382
ketosis, 382
kidneys, 347
  antacids and, 60
  dehydration and, 51
  dialysis, 353–354
  glomerulonephritis, 354–356
  intravenous pyelogram, 559
  kidney disease from obstruction
    in arteries, 265
  kidney failure, 356–358
  kidney stones, 358–360
  nephrology, 37–38
  nephrotic syndrome, 484–485
  proteinuria, 360–361
  pyelonephritis, 361–362
Koplik's spots, 90
Korsakoff's syndrome, 124

L
labor. See childbirth
lactose
  diarrhea and, 52
  irritable bowel syndrome and,
    337
laetrile, 541
laparascopy, 404, 441
laparotomy, 549
laryngitis, 229
laryngopharynx, 219
larynx, 219, 220
  bronchoscopy, 564
  croup, 476–477
laser
  detached retina, 208
  glaucoma, 211
  macular degeneration, 212
  therapy in herpes, 84
laxatives, 332
  appendicitis, 315

irritable bowel syndrome,
    337
  overuse, 50
"lazy eye." See amblyopia
lens (eye), 201
  cataracts, 204–205
leukemia, 546–547
  chemotherapy in, 540
  danger of immunization, 117
  prostaglandins and, 386
  shingles and, 98
leukoplakia, 167–168
leukorrhea, 409–410
leukotomy, 480
levodopa, 146
lice (in blepharitis), 203
lidocaine, 228
lifestyle changes for better health,
    290
ligaments, 177
  transverse carpal ligament, 186
lipase, 382
lipids, in the bloodstream, 267
lithium carbonate, 506, 509
liver, 315
  bile, 316
  cancer, 547–548
  cirrhosis, 318–320
  dehydration and, 51
  gallstones and, 329
  hepatitis, 332–334
  jaundice, 317, 329, 332
  Reye's syndrome and, 490
lockjaw (tetanus), 101
lumbar disk, 148
lumbar puncture, 127, 139,
    564–565
lumpectomy, 410
lung diseases, 44. See also
    respiratory diseases
  bubonic plague, 74–75
  cancer, 548
  cystic fibrosis, 523–526
  emphysema, 245–248
  pleurisy, 248–250
  pneumonia, 250–252
  psittacosis, 252–253
  pulmonary embolism, 295–297

pulmonary function tests, 565–566
pulmonary medicine, 44
tuberculosis, 253–254
lupus erythematosus, 190–191
hair loss and, 156
luteinizing hormone, 384
lymph
glands and fever blisters, 164
Hodgkin's disease and shingles, 98
lymph nodes, 71–72, 102
lymphoma, 548–549
lymphocytes, 292. See also white blood cells
lyophilization, 530

M

macular degeneration, 212
magnetrode, 541
malaria, immunization, 118
male reproductive system, 387–394
hydrocele, 390
impotence, 390–392
male sex hormones. See androgens; testosterone
malnutrition
amenorrhea and, 397
anorexia nervosa and, 500
celiac disease and, 522
Crohn's disease and, 324
cystic fibrosis and, 525
mammary glands. See breast(s)
mammography, 406–407, 545, 569–570
mania, 509
manic depressive condition, 506, 509
marijuana, 23, 26–27
masculinization, 376
mastectomy, 410–412, 545
mastitis, 412
mastoid infection, 229–230
measles, 89–91
encephalitis and, 90
gamma globulin, administration of, 113

immunization, 72, 91, 484
rash, 79–80
meclofenamate sodium, 402
medical specialties, 31–46
medical tests, 552–571
mefenamic acid, 402
melanoma, 550
prostaglandins and, 386
sunburn and, 174
memory, loss of
Alzheimer's disease, 121–124
amnesia, 124–125
Meniere's disease, 230–231
meningitis, 138–139
complication of sinusitis, 232
encephalitis and, 129
meningoencephalitis, 92
menopause, 412–414
DES therapy, 399
osteoporosis and, 191
premature in oophorectomy, 418
purpura and, 172
menorrhagia, 414–415
menstruation, 395, 415–417
amenorrhea, 397–398
dilatation and curettage, 400–401
dysmenorrhea, 401–403
endometriosis, 403–405
iron deficiency anemia and, 259
menorrhagia, 414–415
menstrual cramps and IUD, 434
menstrual cycle, 416
ovulation and, 415, 420
premenstrual tension, 416, 422–423
mental problems
anorexia nervosa, 500–503
autism, 463–465
bulimia, 503
delirium, 503–504
depression, 504–507
electroconvulsive therapy, 507
hyperventilation, 507–508
hypochondria, 508–509
mania, 509
Munchausen's syndrome, 513–514

paranoia, 509–510
phobia, 510–512
professional help, 499
psychosomatic illness, 512–514
schizophrenia, 514–517
senility, 517–518
warning signs, 498–499
metatarsus varus, 474
methotrexate, 319
methylxanthine, 407
metronidazole, 428
miconazole, 154
microorganisms, 69
migraine headache, 133–135
miliaria. See heat rash
milium, 161
milk, role in kidney stones, 358.
    See also lactose
milk glands and ducts, 412
mineralcorticoids, 366, 368
minerals, 19–22
    deficiency symptoms, 16–17
minimal brain dysfunction. See
    hyperkinesis
miscarriage, 456–457
    DES and, 457
    dilatation and curettage in, 400
moles, 168
mongolism. See Down's syndrome
moniliasis, 75
mononucleosis, 86–87
    hepatitis and, 333
monophobia, 511
morning-after pill, 399
morning sickness, 443, 455
mountain sickness, chronic, 273
mucous colitis. See irritable bowel
    syndrome
mucous glands, 161
    in cystic fibrosis, 523
mucous membranes, 71
    cysts, 161
    leukoplakia, 167
multiple sclerosis, 139–140
    gamma globulin as a diagnostic
        tool, 113
    vs. muscular dystrophy, 532

mumps, 91–93
    encephalitis and, 129
    immunization, 93, 484
Munchausen's syndrome,
    513–514
muscle diseases
    backache, 181–183
    muscles, 177–178
    tendonitis, 197–198
    tic, 198–199
    trichinosis, 199–200
muscular dystrophy, 532–533
mutation, 521
myasthenia gravis, 140–141
myelin sheath, 139
myelogram, 197
myocardial infarction. See heart
    attack
myocarditis, 80
    in trichinosis, 200
myomectomy, 408
myopia, 212–214
    retinal detachment and, 208
myxedema in carpal tunnel
    syndrome, 186

N

nail abnormalities
    carpal tunnel syndrome,
        185–187
    onychogryphosis, 168–169
    onychomycosis, 169
    psoriasis, 170–172
Naproxen sodium, 402
narcolepsy, 141
nasal congestion, 62–63
nasopharynx, 219
nausea and vomiting, 63–65
    in pregnancy, 443
    in pyloric stenosis, 341
nearsightedness. See myopia
necrosis, 292
neostigmine, 141
nephrology, 37–38
nephrotic syndrome, 484–485

nervous system disorders,
    119–149. *See also* brain and
    brain disorders
  ataxia, 125–126
  Bell's palsy, 126–127
  carpal tunnel syndrome,
    142, 185–187
  epilepsy, 131–132
  headaches, 132–137
  lumbar puncture, 564–565
  multiple sclerosis, 139–140
  myasthenia gravis, 140–141
  narcolepsy, 141
  neuralgia, 142–143
  neurology, 38
  neurotransmitters, 143
  paralysis, 143–144
  Parkinson's disease, 144–146
  rabies, 146–148
  sciatica, 148–149
  shingles, 97–99, 142–143
"nervous tic," 198
neuralgia, 142–143
neurodermatitis, 162
neurology, 38
neurons, 119
neurotransmitters, 143
  in hyperkinesis, 482
NGU. *See* nongonococcal
    urethritis
nicotinic acid. *See* niacin
night blindness, 214
nitrates, 265
nitroglycerin, 265
nocturia. *See* urination
nongonococcal urethritis, 83, 442
nosebleeds, 231
nose disorders. *See also* ear
    infections and diseases; throat
    infections and diseases
  bleeding, 231
  sinusitis, 231–233
nuclear medicine, 44–45, 538
nummular dermatitis, 162
nutrition, 7–10, 444
nyctalopia. *See* night blindness
nystagmus, 214–215

O
obesity, 14–16
  apnea and, 238
  backache and, 181
  bariatrics, 33
obstetrics/gynecology, 38
occlusion, 42
occult blood, 65
  stool blood test, 555–556
occupational medicine, 38–39
oncology, 39, 539
onychogryphosis, 168–169
onychomycosis, 169
oophorectomy, 417–418
ophthalmology, 40
oral cholecystogram, 559
oral contraceptives, 405, 407,
    434–435
  amenorrhea and, 398
  contraindications, 435
  depression as a side effect, 504
  endometriosis, 405
  fibrocystic disease, 407
  heart attack and, 282
  hirsutism, 377
  hypertension and, 169
  photosensitivity and, 169
  thrombophlebitis and, 307
orchitis, 92
oropharynx, 219
orthodontia, 34
orthopedics, 40
  and sports medicine, 45–46
osteitis deformans. *See* Paget's
    disease
osteoarthritis, 179
osteomyelitis, 485–486
  as a complication of sinusitis,
    232
  necrosis in, 292
osteoporosis, 191–193, 418
  bone fractures in, 189
  fluoride and, 13
  menopause and, 191, 414
otitis media, 224
otorhinolaryngology, 40–41
otosclerosis, 193–194

ovarian cysts, 418—419
ovaries, 365, 395
  cancer, 549
  cysts, 418—419
  DES and, 399
  ectopic pregnancy, 453—455
  oophorectomy, 417—418
  polycystic and hirsutism, 376
  removal and osteoporosis, 191
ovulation, 419—421
  birth control and, 431
  endometriosis and, 405
oxygen
  in sickle-cell anemia, 534
oxyhemoglobin, 286
oxyphenisatin, 319
oxytocin, 384
oxyurids, 488

P

pacemakers, 285
Paget's disease, 194—195
  osteoporosis and, 192
pain, 65—66
pancreas, 314
  cystic fibrosis, 523—526
  hypoglycemia, 379—380
  pancreatitis, 365, 382—384
panic attacks. See phobia
Pap smear (Pap test), 414,
    570—571
  estrogen therapy and, 193
para-aminobenzoic acid, adverse
    reactions, 174
paralysis, 143—144
paralytic disease (coxsackie
    viruses), 79
paranoia, 509—510
paraplegia, 144
parathyroid glands, 365
  calcium absorption and, 359
Parkinson's disease, 144—146
paronychia, 75
parotid glands, 91
partial thromboplastin time (PTT),
    529
patent ductus arteriosus, 486—488

pathology, 41, 537
pediatrics, 41—42
pelvic inflammatory disease,
    421—422, 439
  gonorrhea and, 82
  nongonococcal urethritis and,
    83
  pelvic examination, 571
  as a reaction to IUD, 434
penicillin, 81, 96, 101, 157, 227,
    251, 302
  gonorrhea, 83
  nongonoccocal urethritis, 83
  syphilis, 100
penis, 387
  circumcision, 469—471
  gonorrhea, 82
  penile implants, 391—392
  phimosis, 488
peptic ulcers. See ulcers
perceptual disorders, 515
pericarditis, 80, 292—293
  pericardial sac, 270
periodontal disease, 338—340
  fluoride and, 13
  periodontia, 34
peripheral neuropathy, 142
peripheral vascular diseases, 42
peritoneal dialysis, 353
  in hypothermia, 137
peritonitis, 340—341
  in relation to diverticulitis, 325
pernicious anemia, 259
  stomach cancer and, 550
pertussis. See whooping cough
pessary, 399
phagocytes, 74. See also white
    blood cells
phenylalanine, 534
phenylketonuria (PKU), 533—534
phimosis, 488
phlebotomy, 295
phobia, 510—512
photosensitivity, 169—170
  PABA, adverse reaction, 174—175
  photodermatitis, 111
physical medicine and
    rehabilitation, 42—43

physicians
  choosing a family doctor, 29–31
  choosing a dentist, 34
  choosing a specialist, 31–46
phytanic acid, 125
  in retinitis pigmentosa, 215
phytols, 215
PID. See pelvic inflammatory
  disease
"pigeon toe," 474
piles. See hemorrhoids
pill. See oral contraceptives
pimples, 161. See also acne; boils
pinkeye. See conjunctivitis
pinworms, 488–489
pituitary gland, 363, 367, 376,
  384–385, 434
  ACTH, 366
  growth hormone and, 384
  ovulation and, 420
  thyroid hormone and, 377
PKU. See phenylketonuria
placenta, 447
placenta previa, 457–459
plaque. See dental plaque
plasma, 256
  in hemophilia, 530
platelets, 294, 547, 553
  thrombocytopenia, 306
pleurisy, 48, 248–250
  pleura, 236
pneumonia, 250–252
  bronchiectasis and, 241–242
  cough and, 50
  measles and, 90
  muscular dystrophy and, 532
podiatry, 43
poison ivy, 105
poison oak, 105
polio, immunization, 484
polioviruses, 78
polycythemia, 294–295, 287
polymorphonuclear leukocytes,
  292
polyuria, 349
prednisone, 126, 200, 306
preeclampsia. See toxemia of
  pregnancy

pregnancy, 443–448. See also
  breast-feeding; childbirth
  alcohol and, 446
  amniocentesis, 569
  anemia in, 257
  carpal tunnel syndrome and, 186
  cleft lip/cleft palate,
    development of, 471–472
  common cold preparations,
    precautions, 223
  conception, 451–453
  danger of immunization, 117
  DES and, 399
  diabetes and, 374
  drugs in, 446
  ectopic (tubal) pregnancy,
    453–455
  endometriosis, 404
  fibroid tumors and, 408
  genital warts, 436
  heartburn in, 59
  hemorrhoids, 331
  herpes, 446
  hyperemesis gravidarum,
    455–456
  miscarriage, 456–457
  moniliasis in, 75
  placenta previa, 457–459
  Rh factor, 303
  rubella, 94, 95, 446
  sexually transmitted diseases
    and, 430
  syphilis, 99
  thrombocytopenia in, 307
  toxemia of, 459
  urination in, 349
  vaginal bleeding during, 456
  varicose veins, 310
  vomiting, excessive, 455–456
premenstrual tension, 422–423
prenatal care, 444–446
prescriptions, understanding of,
  573–578
preventive medicine, 43
prickly heat. See heat rash
primary pneumonic plague, 75
proctology, 43–44
proctoscopy, 321

proctosigmoidoscopy, 562, 563
prodrome, 84
progesterone, 395, 414
prolactin, 384
prolapse, 423
propranolol, 378
prostaglandins, 385–386
prostate, 387
  cancer, 549
  cystoscopy, 563–564
  gonorrhea and, 82
  pyelogram, intravenous, 559
  urination and, 348
prostatitis, 392–394
proteins
  amino acids, 10–11
  gamma globulin, 113
  low-protein diet in gout, 190
  low-protein diet in kidney
    failure, 358
  phenylketonuria, 533–534
  poor absorption in celiac
    disease, 521
proteinuria, 360–361
protocols (in cancer), 539
protozoa, 73
pseudocyst, 383
psittacosis, 252–253
psoriasis, 170–172
psychiatry
  psychiatrists, 44, 499
  psychiatrists vs. psychologists, 44
psychoanalysis, 500
psychophysiological illness. See
    psychosomatic illness
psychosomatic illness, 512–514
psychotherapy, 500
  in schizophrenia, 516
psyllium, 326
PTT. See partial thromboplastin
    time
pulmonary angiography, 297
pulmonary artery, 273
pulmonary diseases. See lung
    diseases
pulmonary edema, 271
pulmonary embolism, 42,
    295–297

thrombophlebitis and, 307
pulmonary function tests,
    565–566
pulmonary medicine, 44
pulmonary surfactant, 480
pulse rate, 68
pupil, 201
purpura, 172–173
PUVA therapy, 171
pyelogram, 559
pyelonephritis, 351, 361–362
pyloric stenosis, 341–342
pyloromyotomy, 342
pyorrhea, 338–340
pyrantel pamoate, 489
pyridostigmine, 141
pyridoxine, 18

R
rabies, 146–148
  immunization, 147
radial keratotomy, 214
radiation, 540
  and cataracts, 204
  side effects, 540
  therapists, 44–45
radioactive iodine, 561
radioactive isotopes, 560–561
radioallergosorbent technique,
    556
radiology, 44–45
radionuclide scanning, 317
radiotherapy, 44–45
ranitidine, 345
rash, 66–67
RAST test. See radioallergosorbent
    technique
Raynaud's phenomenon and
    disease, 297–298
reactive hyperemia, 298
reactive hypoglycemia, 379
recommended daily allowances,
    19
recommended dietary allowances
    (RDA), 19
rectocele, 423–425
rectum, 314
  anal fistula, 327

cancer and Crohn's disease, 324
hemorrhoids, 330–332
ileostomy, 336
proctology, 43–44
proctosigmoidoscopy, 562
prolapse, 423
rectocele, 423–425
ulcerative proctitis, 321
red blood cells, 256. *See also*
    erythrocytes
    anemia, 257–260
    leukemia, 546–547
    sickle-cell anemia, 534–535
Refsum's syndrome, 125
regional enteritis. *See* Crohn's
    disease; colitis
regional sympathectomy, 298
rehabilitation and physical
    medicine, 42
Reiter's syndrome, 93–94
relaxation training, 500
relaxin, 443
reproductive system. *See* female
    reproductive system; male
    reproductive system
reserpine, 298
respiratory diseases. *See also* lung
    diseases
    apnea, 237–238
    asthma, 238–241
    bronchiectasis, 241–242
    bronchitis, 242–245
    coxsackie viruses, 79
    dyspnea, 245
respiratory rate, 68
restless legs syndrome, 298–299
retina, 201
    cataracts in detached, 208
    detached, 207–208
retinitis, 215–216
retinopathy, 216–217
Reye's syndrome, 489–491
    aspirin and, 78, 79
rheumatic fever, 299–301
rheumatic heart disease, 301–302
rheumatoid arthritis, 179
    carpal tunnel syndrome and, 186
rheumatology, 45

Rh factor, 302–304
rhinoviruses, 222–224
rhodopsin, 214
ringworm
    athlete's foot, 153
    in hair loss, 156
rods and cones, 214
rubber band ligation, 332
rubella, 94–96
    encephalitis and, 94, 129
    immunization, 95–96, 484
    rash, 95
    rubella-like rash, 79–80
rubeola. *See* measles

S

saccharin, 9
saliva, 314
salpingectomy, 417
salpingitis. *See* pelvic
    inflammatory disease
salt, 20
sarcoma, 537
scarlet fever, 96
schistosomiasis infestation, 542
schizophrenia, 514–517
    paranoid vs. paranoia, 510
sciatica, 148–149
sclera, 201
    scleroderma and Raynaud's
        phenomenon, 297
scoliosis, 491–493
    Friedreich's ataxia and, 126
    muscular dystrophy and, 532
scrotum, 390, 452
    hydrocele, 390
    varicose veins in, and infertility, 439
seborrheic dermatitis, 162
    blepharitis and, 203
sebum, 150
sedatives
    in heart attack, 283
    insomnia and, 61
    precautions in emphysema, 248
seizures
    autistic children, 464
    encephalitis, 129
    epileptic, 130

semen, 347, 388
senility, 517–518
septicemia, 96–97, 486
sex
  cells, 519–521
  impotence, 390–392
  therapists, 392
sexual abuse. See battered child
  syndrome
sexual intercourse, 388
  dyspareunia and, 403
  erection, 390
  frequent, and sperm count, 439
  genital warts and, 437
  hysterectomy and, 409
  urethritis, 351
sexually transmitted diseases, 430,
  436, 446
shingles, 97–99, 142–143
  chicken pox and, 97
  rash, 66–67
  vaccine, 72
shock treatments. See
  electroconvulsive therapy
SIDS. See sudden infant death
  syndrome
sickle-cell anemia, 534–535
sigmoidoscopy, 321, 346, 546
sinuses, 219
  headache and, 136
  sinusitis, 231–233
skin, 150–176
  acne, 151–153
  athlete's foot, 153–154
  baldness, 154–156
  blackheads, 152
  boils, 156–157
  calluses, 157–158
  cancer, 549–550
  canker sores, 158–159
  corns, 159–160
  cysts, 160–161
  dermatitis, 161–163
  fever blisters, 163–164
  frostbite, 164–166
  heat rash, 166–167
  leukoplakia, 167–168
  mole, 168

onychogryphosis, 168–169
onychomycosis, 169
photosensitivity, 169–170
psoriasis, 170–172
purpura, 172–173
sty, 217
sunburn, 173–175
warts, 175–176
whiteheads, 152
slipped disk, 195–197
smallpox, immunization, 117
smoking, 23–24, 27–28
  angina pectoris and, 263
  atherosclerosis and, 12
  cancer and, 27
  cholesterol and, 12-13
  chronic bronchitis and, 243
  cor pulmonale and, 273
  extrasystole and, 280
  fibrocystic disease and, 407
  heart attack and, 282
  obesity and, 15
  smoker's patches (tongue), 167
  stroke and, 304
sodium chloride. See salt
somatotropin. See growth
  hormone
sore throat, 67–68, 460
  rheumatic fever and, 299
spastic colon. See irritable bowel
  syndrome
specialists, 31–46
sperm, 387, 395, 443
  artificial insemination, 448–449
  chromosomes and, 519–520
  count, 439
  fertilization, 453
  "hostile" cervix and, 439
  ovulation and, 419–420
  undescended testes, 496
spermicides, 432
spina bifida, 493–494
spinal column in osteoporosis,
  193
spinal cord, 127
  cerebrospinal fluid, 127, 477,
    494, 564
  lumbar puncture, 564–565

spina bifida, 493
spinal tap. *See* lumbar puncture
sports medicine, 45—46
sprue. *See* celiac disease
"squint eye." *See* strabismus
stapedectomy, 194
Staphylococcus aureus, 203
starvation. *See* anorexia nervosa
stasis dermatitis, 162—163
Stein-Leventhal syndrome, 418
sterility, 429
    gonorrhea and, 82
    vs. infertility, 441
sterilization, 435—436
steroid, 111, 368, 544
stoma, 321, 336
stomach, 460
    cancer, 550
    diaphragmatic hernia, 335—336
    gastroenteritis, 330
    gastrointestinal series, 558
    gastroscopy, 563
    ulcers, 343—345
stool blood test, 546, 555—556
strabismus, 494—495
strep throat. *See* sore throat
streptococcus bacteria, 234
streptomycin, 75
stress test, 267
stridor, 476
stroke, 304—306
    aneurysms in, 260
    TIAs as a precursor of, 309
sty, 217
sucralfate, 345
sudden infant death syndrome,
    495—496
    nongonococcal urethritis and, 442
sugar, refined, 11
    dental plaque and, 343
suicide, 506, 515
sulfa drugs (sulfonamides), 427
sulfasalazine, 346
sunburn, 173—175. *See also*
    photosensitivity
surgery, 46
swearing, compulsive. *See* Gilles
    de la Tourette's syndrome

sweat glands, 395
sweeteners, synthetic, 9
syphilis, 99—101
    aneurysms in, 260
    glossitis and, 227
    interstitial keratitis and, 211
    leukoplakia as a symptom, 167
    locomotor ataxia in, 125

T
talipes equinovarus, 473
tampons, 409
    toxic shock syndrome and, 425
Tay-Sachs disease, 535—536
teeth, 342—343
    fluoride and, 13—14
tendonitis, 197—198
tendons, 177
testes, 365, 387
    cancer and DES, 399
    hydrocele in, 390
    mumps and, 93
    undescended, 496—497
testosterone, 193, 391, 441. *See
    also* androgens
    impotence and, 391
    osteoporosis and, 193
tests, diagnostic, 552—571
test-tube fertilization, 441
tetanus, 101
    immunization, 101
tetracycline, 75, 153, 252, 442
thalamus, 121
theophylline, 240
thermography, 545
thiabendazole, 200
thirst, in diabetes, 373
throat infections and diseases
    adenoids, 220—222
    gonorrhea of the throat, 82
    laryngitis, 229
    sore throat, 67—68
    throat culture, 556
    tonsillitis, 234—235
thrombi, 42
thrombocytes. *See* platelets
thrombocytopenia, 306—307
thrombocytopenic purpura, 173

thrombophlebitis, 307—309
thrush, 75
thymus gland, 292
  myasthenia gravis and, 141
thyroid gland, 363—365
  congenital hypothyroidism, 380
  goiter, 374—376
  hyperthyroidism, 377—379
  hypothyroidism, 380—382
thyroid hormone, 377
thyroid stimulating hormone
    (THS), 384
thyrotropic hormone. See thyroid
    stimulating hormone
TIAs. See transcient ischemic
    attacks
tic, 198—199
  Gilles de la Tourette's syndrome,
    199, 478
tic douloureux, 142
tinea pedis. See athlete's foot
tolnaftate, 154
tomography, 567—568
tongue
  burning, 257
  glossitis, 227—229
tonsillitis, 234—235
  tonsils, 220
tooth decay, 342—343
Tourette's syndrome, 199,
    478—480
toxemia of pregnancy, 459
toxic multinodular goiter, 378
toxic shock syndrome, 425—426
toxins, 102
toxoplasmosis, 446
trachea, 236
tranquilizers
  insomnia and, 61
transient ischemic attacks (TIAs),
    309—310
translocation, 527
transverse carpal ligament, 186
treadmill test. See cardiac stress
    test
tretinoin, 153
trichinosis, 199—200
trichomonad, 410

Trichomonas vaginalis, 427
trigeminal neuralgia, 142
"triple vessel disease," 270
trisomy, 527
TSS. See toxic shock syndrome
tuberculosis, 253—254
  test for children, 484
tumor, 537
typhoid, immunization, 117
"typist's shoulder," 185

U

ulcerative colitis, 345—346
ulcerative proctitis, 321
ulcers, 343—345
ultrasonography (ultrasound),
    538, 568
umbilical
  cord prolapse, 423
  hernia, 334
undescended testes, 496—497
urethra, 347, 387
  cystoscopy, 350—351
  urethritis, 351, 352
uric acid, 360
  deposits, 189
  test, 554
uricosurics, 190
urinary system diseases. See
    bladder; kidneys; urethra
urination
  excessive in diabetes, 373
  fibroid tumors and, 408
  increased frequency, 347
  painful, 347
  prostatitis, 392
  urethritis, 351, 352
urine
  blood in, 542
  changes in, 347
  urinalysis, 393, 554
  volume in kidney failure, 357
urology, 46
urticaria. See hives
uterus, 395
  cancer, 550—551
  dilatation and curettage, 400—401
  endometriosis, 403—405

fibroid tumors, 407—408
hysterectomy, 408—409
prolapsed, 423

V

vaccination. See immunization
vagina, 395
cancer, 551
cystocele, 398—399
in gonorrhea, 82
vaginal bleeding during
pregnancy, 458, 459
vaginal fistula, 327
vaginal infections, 409—410
vaginal lubricants, 403
vaginal medications, 410
vaginitis, 76, 352, 426—428
varicella zoster, 97
varicose veins, 310—311
vas deferens, 387
vasectomy, 435
vascular diseases. See blood and
circulatory diseases
vasodilators, 291
vasopressin, 384
veins, 255
venereal diseases. See sexually
transmitted diseases
venipuncture, 552
venous thrombosis, 42
ventricular fibrillation, 275
verapamil, 265
vertigo, dizziness and, 53—54
Meniere's disease, 230—231
nystagmus, 214—215
TIAs, 309—310
viral infections, 69—70. See also
bacterial infections
chicken pox, 76—78
coxsackie viruses, 78—80
hepatitis, 332—334
influenza, 87—89
measles, 89—91
mononucleosis, 86—87
mumps, 91—93
Reiter's syndrome, 93—94
Reye's syndrome and, 490
rubella, 94—96

shingles, 97—99
virilization, 376
viruses, 69
coxsackie, 78—80
Epstein-Barr, 86
types of, 78—80
vision
amblyopia, 461—462
astigmatism, 202—203
cataract, 204—205
color blindness, 205—206
detached retina, 207—208
glaucoma, 208—211
keratitis, 211—212
macular degeneration, 212
myopia, 212—214
night blindness, 214
nystagmus, 214—215
retinitis, 215—216
retinopathy, 216—217
rhodopsin, 214
strabismus, 494—495
visual purple, 214
vital signs, 68
vitamins, 16—19
deficiency symptoms, 16—17
vitiligo, 367
vitreous humor, 201
vomiting, 63—65, 460
dehydration and, 51
excessive, in pregnancy,
455—456
induced, in bulimia, 501
pancreatitis, 383
pyloric stenosis, 341
toxic shock syndrome, 426

W

warfarin, 277, 297
warts, 175—176
genital, 436—437
weight loss
in anorexia nervosa, 501
appetite control, 15
crash and fad diets, 15
white blood cells, 553. See also
lymphocytes; phagocytes
whiteheads, 152

whooping cough (pertussis)
  bronchiectasis and, 241–242
  immunization, 116
"widow's hump," 193
wrist disorders
  carpal tunnel syndrome,
    185–187

X
xerography, 570
xerophthalmia, 214
X ray, 554–555

Y
yeast infections, 75
  vaginal, 426–428
yellow fever, immunization, 117
Yersinia pestis, 74

Z
zygote, 443